BIOPSY INTERPRETATION SERIES

BIOPSY INTERPRETATION OF THE BLADDER

Fourth Edition

Jonathan I. Epstein, MD
Professor of Pathology, Urology and Oncology
The Reinhard Professor of Urological Pathology
Director of Surgical Pathology
The Johns Hopkins Medical Institutions
Baltimore, Maryland

Victor E. Reuter, MD
Attending Pathologist and Member
Memorial Sloan Kettering Cancer Center
Professor of Pathology and Laboratory Medicine
Weill Medical College of Cornell University
New York, New York

Mahul B. Amin, MD
Professor and Chairman Emeritus
Department of Pathology and Laboratory Medicine
Cedars-Sinai Medical Center
Professor of Pathology and Laboratory Medicine
UCLA David Geffen School of Medicine
Visiting Professor
Department of Urology
USC Keck School of Medicine
Los Angeles, California
Visiting Professor
Department of Pathology & Immunology
Baylor College of Medicine
Houston, Texas

Wolters Kluwer

Philadelphia • Baltimore • New York • London
Buenos Aires • Hong Kong • Sydney • Tokyo

Acquisitions Editor: Nicole Dernoski
Development Editor: Ariel S. Winter
Editorial Coordinator: Remington Fernando
Editorial Assistant: Kristen Kardoley
Marketing Manager: Kirsten Watrud
Production Project Manager: Catherine Ott
Manager, Graphic Arts & Design: Stephen Druding
Manufacturing Coordinator: Lisa Bowling
Prepress Vendor: Straive

9 8 7 6 5 4 3 2 1

Printed in Mexico

Cataloging-in-Publication Data available on request from the Publisher
ISBN-13: 978-1-9751-9920-3

shop.lww.com

QUADM0623

CONTRIBUTORS

Syed Z. Ali, MD, FRCPath, FIAC
Director of Cytopathology
Professor of Pathology
Department of Pathology
The Johns Hopkins University School of Medicine
Baltimore, Maryland

Mahul B. Amin, MD
Professor and Chairman Emeritus
Department of Pathology and Laboratory Medicine
Cedars-Sinai Medical Center
Professor of Pathology and Laboratory Medicine
UCLA David Geffen School of Medicine
Visiting Professor
Department of Urology
USC Keck School of Medicine
Los Angeles, California
Visiting Professor
Department of Pathology & Immunology
Baylor College of Medicine
Houston, Texas

Jonathan I. Epstein, MD
Professor of Pathology, Urology and Oncology
The Reinhard Professor of Urological Pathology
Director of Surgical Pathology
The Johns Hopkins Medical Institutions
Baltimore, Maryland

Victor E. Reuter, MD
Attending Pathologist and Member
Memorial Sloan Kettering Cancer Center
Professor of Pathology and Laboratory Medicine
Weill Medical College of Cornell University
New York, New York

Christopher J. VandenBussche, MD, PhD
Associate Professor of Pathology
Department of Pathology
The Johns Hopkins University School of Medicine
Baltimore, Maryland

PREFACE

In the modern era of a multidisciplinary approach to personalized medicine, we strive to live up to our responsibility to contribute to the management of patients with urothelial diseases. This requires constant reevaluation of established principles and classification schemes, adoption of novel concepts, definition of new pathologic entities, and incorporation of markers and molecular data that help in the classification, treatment, and outcome prediction of urothelial tumors. The fourth edition of *Biopsy Interpretation of the Bladder* is a significant and timely revision from the prior edition. It incorporates new concepts and classification schemes included in the 2022 fifth edition of the World Health Organization Classification of urothelial tumors, as they apply to biopsy/transurethral resection specimens. Every chapter has been revised to some degree. Newly proposed terminology, in keeping with the new WHO nomenclature and dealing with flat and papillary thickened lesions without cytologic atypia, is outlined. The chapter dealing with flat lesions has been updated to include new concepts on precursor lesions. Best practice recommendations are discussed on how to use immunohistochemistry in the classification of bladder tumors. The morphologic spectrum of glandular lesions is expanded, including tumors with müllerianlike features as well as urachal tumors with mucinous and cystic features. The section on both schistosomiasis- and non–schistosomiasis associated squamous cell carcinoma has been updated. The morphologic spectrum, immunophenotype, and clinical relevance of divergent differentiation (morphologic subtypes) are discussed in greater detail, as are subtypes of urothelial carcinoma. The chapter on prognostic and predictive factors has been entirely updated and now includes a section on molecular markers. A new chapter has been added on Biopsy of the Renal Pelvis and Ureter with many new figures, as biopsies from these sites have unique diagnostic difficulties. We hope the fourth edition will continue to be a useful reference in your daily practice.

Jonathan I. Epstein, MD
Victor E. Reuter, MD
Mahul B. Amin, MD

CONTENTS

1

NORMAL BLADDER ANATOMY AND VARIANTS OF NORMAL HISTOLOGY

Understanding the normal anatomy of the bladder is of paramount importance since its landmarks are used to stage, establish clinical risk, and select therapy in cases of bladder cancer. One must also be aware that local injury, instrumentation, and prior therapy can influence the appearance of the bladder wall as well as the overlying urothelium significantly.

The epithelium of the urinary bladder and urethra is entirely derived from endoderm of the urogenital sinus, while the lamina propria, muscularis propria, and adventitia develop from the surrounding splanchnic mesenchyme. Despite their different histogenesis, the entire urinary excretory passages are lined by the urothelium, previously known as transitional epithelium. During early embryologic development, the caudal portions of the mesonephric ducts contribute to the formation of the mucosa of the bladder trigone but are eventually replaced by endoderm.[1]

The urinary bladder is formed by four layers: (1) urothelium, (2) lamina propria, (3) muscularis propria, and (4) adventitia or serosa (eFigs. 1.1-1.5). Depending on the location, these layers may be surrounded by perivesical fat.[2,3] The thickness of the urothelium varies, as does the shape of the epithelial cells, depending on the degree to which the bladder is distended. In the empty bladder, the epithelium can be up to seven cells thick. The deepest (basal) cells have a cuboidal or columnar shape, above which are the intermediate cells that are composed of several layers of irregularly polyhedral to columnar cells (Fig. 1.1). The most superficial or luminal layer consists of large, sometimes binucleated, cells with abundant eosinophilic cytoplasm and a rounded free surface. They are descriptively called umbrella or superficial cells.[2] In the distended bladder, the epithelial lining can be as few as two cells thick, with a basal layer of cuboidal cells and a superficial layer of elongated and flattened umbrella cells (see Chapter 2 for histology of normal urothelium).

A thin basement membrane separates the urothelium from the underlying lamina propria. The latter is formed of abundant connective tissue containing a rich vascular network, lymphatic channels, sensory nerve endings, and a few elastic fibers. We prefer the term lamina propria over submucosa in the bladder since a muscularis mucosae, if present, is

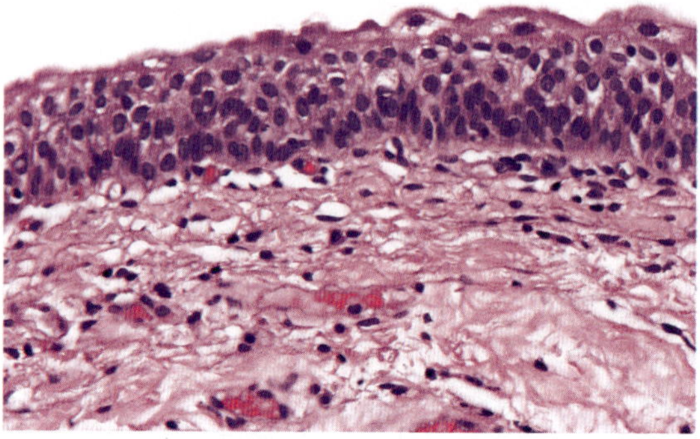

FIGURE 1.1 Normal urothelium.

usually discontinuous. The term submucosa is used for the layer of tissue between the muscularis mucosae and muscularis propria. Occasionally, in some areas of the bladder, a muscularis mucosae layer may be absent, and hence, technically in these areas, the tissue below the mucosa is the submucosa; however, the term lamina propria rather than submucosa is traditionally used in the bladder. In the ureter, pelvicalyceal mucosa, and urethra where there is no muscularis mucosae, the term subepithelial connective tissue is more appropriate. This nomenclature is also used in the AJCC staging systems for the respective sites (bladder, ureter, and pelvis), which is based on the paradigm of depth of invasion in tumors. In the bladder, the lamina propria varies in thickness in the empty vs the distended bladder but is generally thinner in the areas of the trigone and bladder neck. It is unlikely to encounter muscularis mucosae at these sites since muscularis propria extends closer to the urothelial surface. It is important to note that wisps or small fascicles of smooth muscle may be found within the superficial lamina propria, either isolated or forming a complete or incomplete muscularis mucosae[3-6] (Figs. 1.2 and 1.3, eFigs. 1.5-1.9).

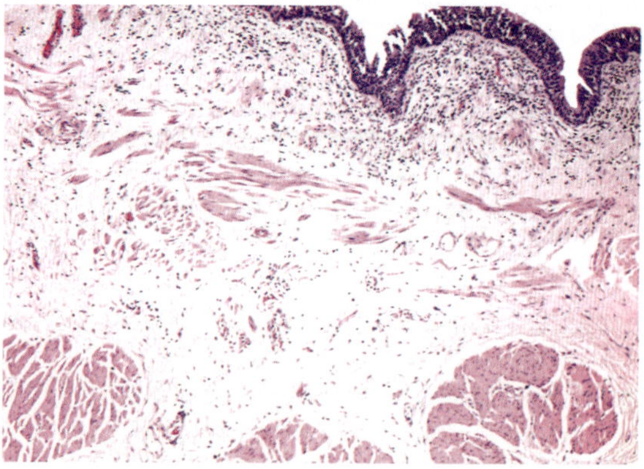

FIGURE 1.2 Normal histology with urothelium, lamina propria with muscularis.

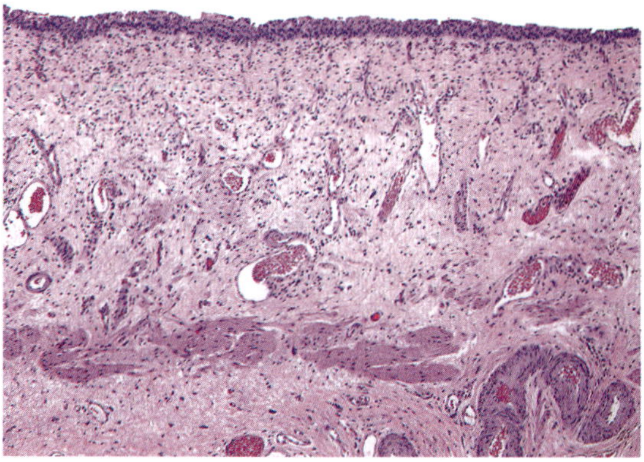

FIGURE 1.3 Normal histology with urothelium, lamina propria with muscularis mucosae, and muscularis propria.

This muscularis mucosae, if present, is frequently seen in association with medium-sized vessels, which are also prominently seen within the lamina propria (Fig. 1.4). It must not be confused with the smooth muscle bundles of the muscularis propria since this might result in errors of tumor staging and treatment. Occasionally, the muscularis mucosae may take on a hyperplastic appearance.[5,6] The most common setting is when the muscle fascicles are thick rather than wispy, even though they retain haphazard outlines. On rare occasions, the muscularis mucosae may present as muscularis propria–like muscle bundles but characterized by a superficial location and scattered distribution. On small or superficial biopsies, these may be impossible to distinguish from true muscularis propria. It may also be impossible to make this determination at the site of prior biopsy where the

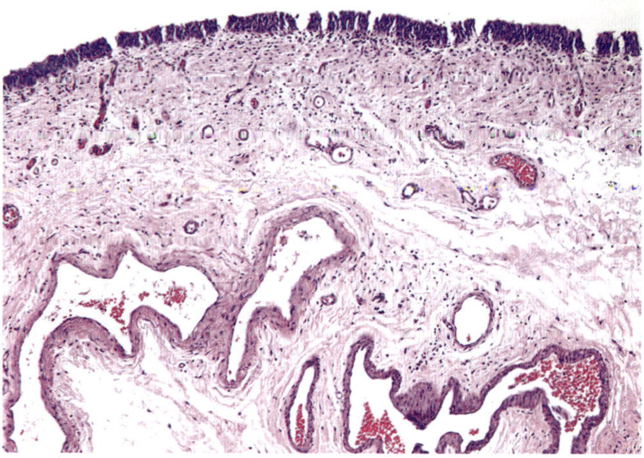

FIGURE 1.4 Normal histology with urothelium, lamina propria, and numerous prominent blood vessels at the level of the muscularis mucosae.

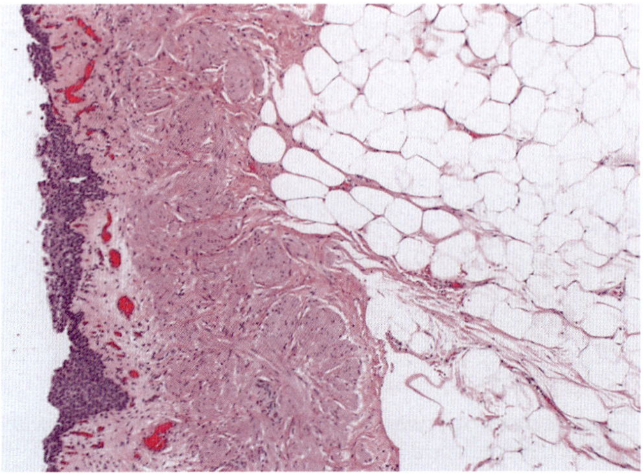

FIGURE 1.5 **Hyperplastic muscularis mucosae associated with a bladder diverticulum.**

normal anatomy is disrupted. The muscularis mucosae may also become hyperplastic in association with bladder diverticula where it can take on a thick, bandlike appearance without the formation of muscle bundles (Fig. 1.5). Some studies suggest that smoothelin is differentially expressed in the muscularis mucosae as compared to the muscularis propria, with the latter positive while the former is either negative or only weakly and focally immunoreactive (Fig. 1.6).[7,8] However, the utility of this antibody in routine practice remains controversial.[9,10] In bladder diverticula, where the muscularis propria may become hyperplastic, negative or weak, staining for smoothelin may help in differentiate it from muscularis propria.[11] We and others have noticed that there may be differential expression of vimentin

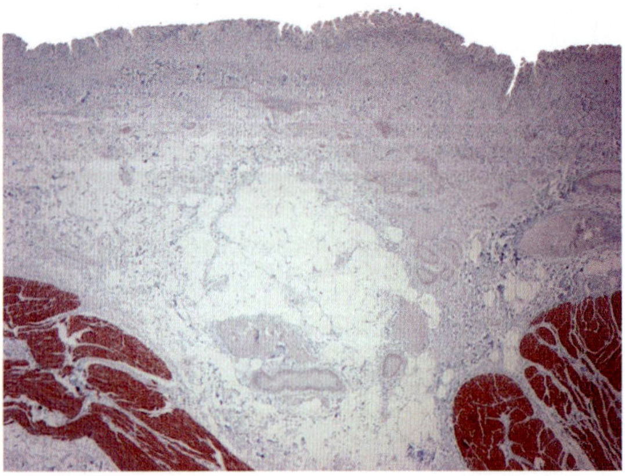

FIGURE 1.6 **Smoothelin with strong labeling of muscularis propria.** Muscularis mucosae only shows weak positivity.

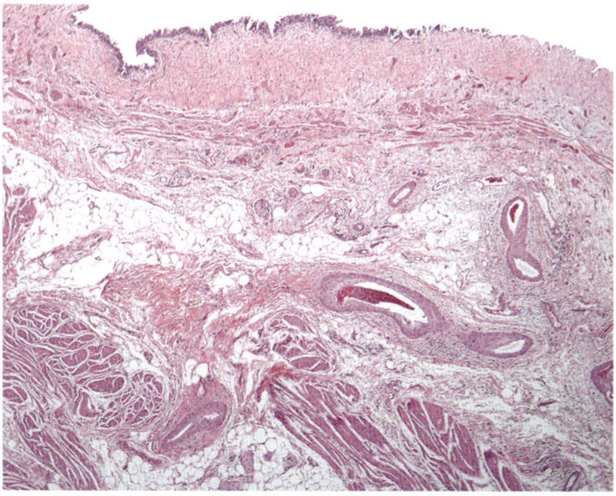

FIGURE 1.7 Normal histology with adipose tissue in deep lamina propria.

with muscularis mucosae exhibiting strong staining, whereas muscularis propria tends to be either negative or weak. It is also important to note that one may encounter fat within the lamina propria as well as in the muscularis propria[12] (Figs. 1.7 and 1.8, eFigs. 1.10-1.12). Fat may be found in bladders that have never been instrumented or in areas of prior transurethral resection and may rarely be present in the lamina propria (usually scant or focal when present). It is more common in the muscularis propria; typically, more abundant in the deeper muscularis propria. Whether its presence is due to a normal anatomic variant, a function of the patient's body habitus, or a metaplastic phenomenon is not known. It is important that the presence of invasive tumor at the level of smooth muscle fibers or fat in a transurethral resection specimen does not necessarily warrant a diagnosis of muscularis propria invasion or extravesical extension, respectively. Within the lamina propria, one may also encounter paraganglia, commonly in intimate association with small-caliber vessels or nerve twigs

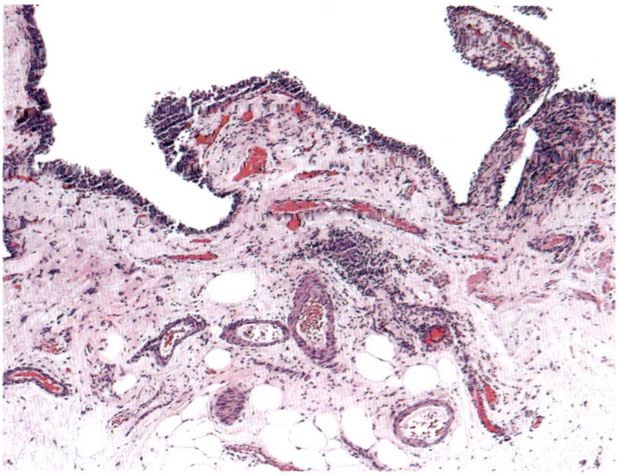

FIGURE 1.8 Normal histology with adipose tissue in deep lamina propria.

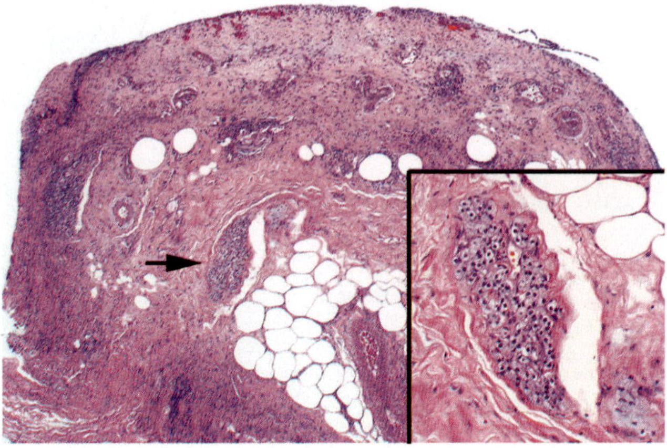

FIGURE 1.9 Paraganglia in lamina propria (higher magnification of paraganglia (*arrow*) [*inset*]).

(Figs. 1.9 and 1.10). These usually present as small aggregates of cells with basophilic granular cytoplasm and small- to medium-sized round nuclei. In a small biopsy, these aggregates may be difficult to differentiate for a bona fide or even invasive carcinoma. As expected, paraganglia will be strongly and diffusely immunoreactive for chromogranin but negative for cytokeratins. Dispersed paraganglia may also be encountered within the muscularis propria and perivesical fat. Rarely, one may encounter urachal remnants in biopsies of the dome or anterior wall of the bladder. These present as one of several epithelial-lined structures in which the epithelial cells have the morphologic appearance of urothelium or glandular (usually enteric) epithelium. These cells are lined by an imperceptible basement

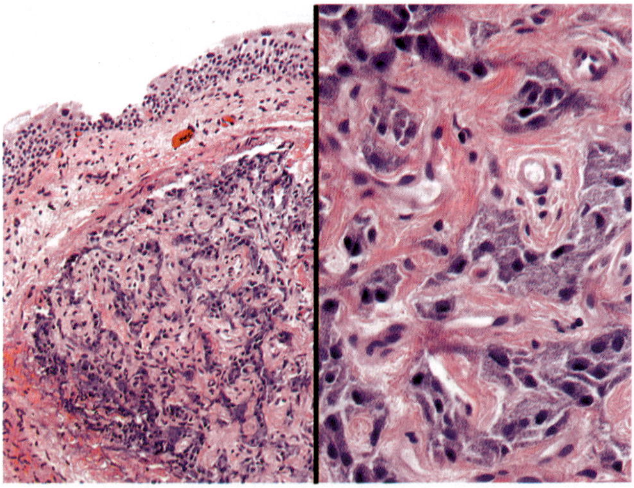

FIGURE 1.10 Paraganglia in lamina propria (higher magnification of paraganglia [*inset*]).

membrane and a variably thin layer of fibromuscular tissue. Rarer yet, one may encounter müllerian or mesonephric rests within the bladder wall. The morphology and clinical repercussions of these lesions are discussed in Chapter 8.

The vascular plexus of the lamina propria, although most classically associated with the muscularis mucosae, may vary somewhat in location from case to case and section to section. Similar to the muscularis mucosae, it may be seen in a superficial, mid, or deep location.

The muscularis propria, also known as detrusor muscle, has loosely anastomosing, ill-defined internal and external longitudinal layers and a more prominent middle circular layer of muscle (Fig. 1.11). For staging purposes, the muscularis propria is divided into the superficial and deep layers (pT2a vs pT2b); substaging of bladder cancer is not performed in biopsies of transurethral resection specimens. The bundles of muscle of the muscularis propria are generally much larger than those of the muscularis mucosae, a feature that is useful as an anatomic landmark. In the bladder neck of the male, the fascicles of the muscularis propria are continuous with the fibromuscular tissue of the prostate (Fig. 1.12).[2] In the trigone and bladder neck area, the muscularis propria is distinct in that the muscles appear as stacked medium-sized muscle bundles/fascicles as they extend to an almost suburothelial location; in these sites, a well-defined distinct overlying muscularis mucosae is not present (Fig. 1.13). In the area of the bladder neck not only may the muscularis propria be anatomically approach the surface urothelium but the smooth muscle may not form distinct bundles. As previously mentioned, fat may be present between the muscle bundles of the muscularis propria.[12] The boundary between the muscularis propria and the perivesical fat is typically ill defined, occasionally compounding staging difficulties in cystectomy specimens.

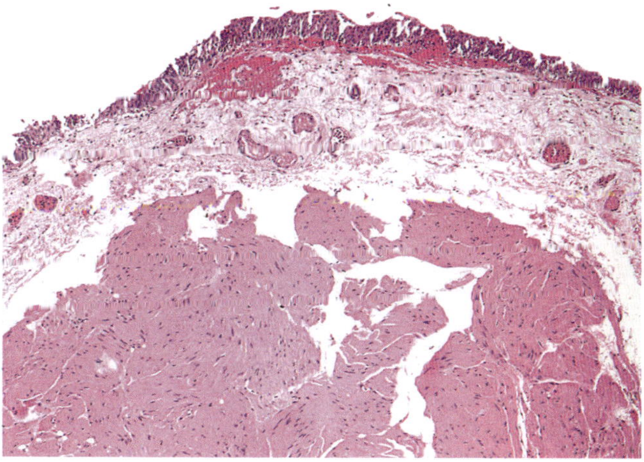

FIGURE 1.11 Muscularis propria (detrusor muscle) extending close to mucosal surface.

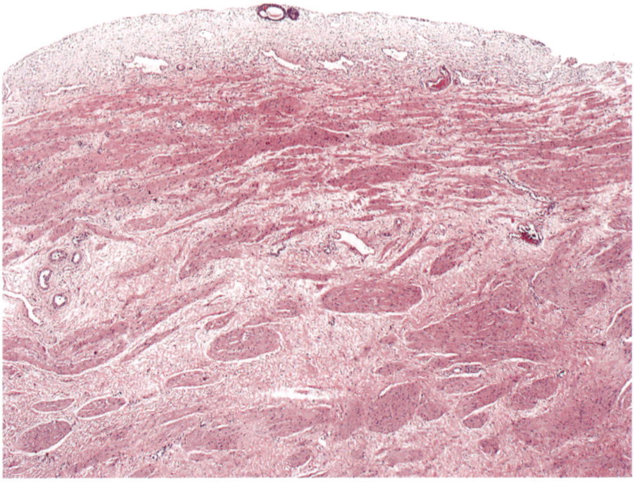

FIGURE 1.12 Bladder neck with fascicles of muscularis propria extending close to urothelial surface.

The outermost layer of the viscus is an adventitia of connective tissue; only the superior surface is covered by serosa of the pelvic peritoneum. Since most of the organ is not covered by a serosa, the outmost layer of muscularis propria has irregular contours (Fig. 1.14). Together with the fact that fat is commonly present within the muscularis propria, establishing extravesical extension by tumor in a resection specimen can be difficult.[13] Occasionally, lymph nodes, usually small, are found in the perivesical fat.

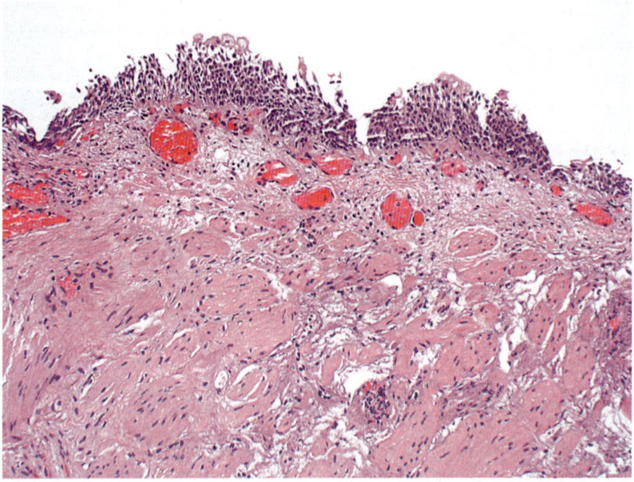

FIGURE 1.13 Bladder neck with gradual diminution of muscularis propria bundles as they extend to the surface.

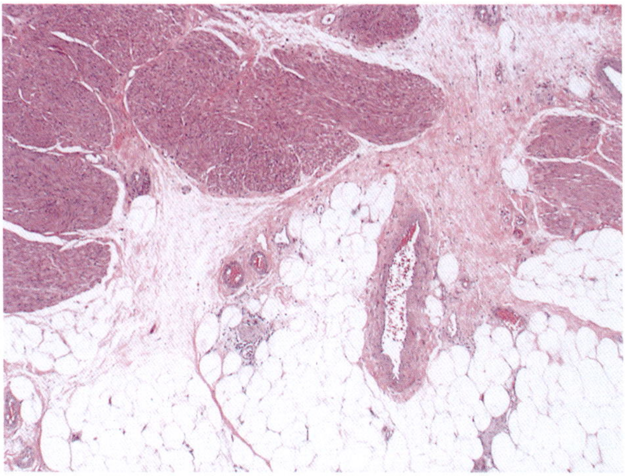

FIGURE 1.14 Irregular interface between the deep muscularis propria of the bladder and the perivesical fat.

The intramural ureter is a difficult area to evaluate on cystoscopic resections and biopsies. Well-circumscribed nests of tumor seen within the wall of the bladder in the area of the trigone may very well represent noninvasive ureteral disease or at least this possibility must be considered (Fig. 1.15).

The adult empty bladder has the shape of a four-sided inverted pyramid and is enveloped by the vesical fascia.[14] The superior surface faces superiorly and is covered by the pelvic parietal peritoneum. The posterior surface, also known as the base of the bladder, faces posteriorly and inferiorly. It is separated from the rectum by the uterine cervix and the

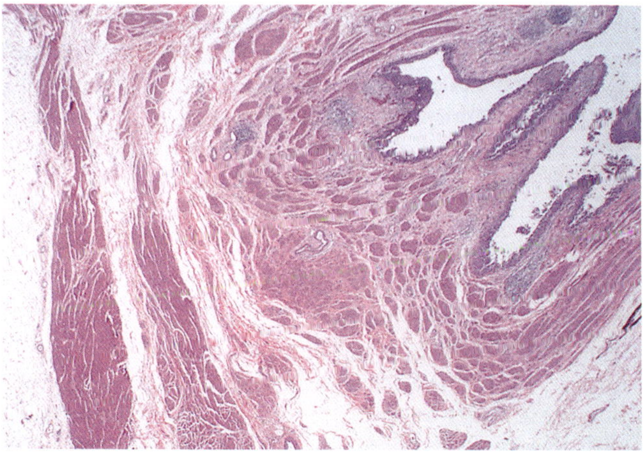

FIGURE 1.15 **Intramural ureter.** Ureter contains a lamina propria of variable thickness and longitudinal fibers of muscularis propria, which intermingles with the muscularis propria of the bladder.

proximal portions of the vagina in females and by the seminal vesicles and the ampulla of the vasa deferentia in males. These posterior anatomic relationships are very important clinically. Since most bladder neoplasms arise in the posterior wall adjacent to the ureteral orifices, invasive tumor may extend into adjacent soft tissue and organs. The intimate relationships to the previously mentioned organs explain why hysterectomy and partial vaginectomy are commonly performed at the time of radical cystectomy in women. Conversely, we know that seminal vesicle involvement is associated with a poor prognosis in bladder carcinoma in males, a reflection of high pathologic stage.

The bladder bed (structures on which the bladder neck rests) is formed posteriorly by the rectum in males and vagina in females. Anteriorly and laterally, it is formed by the internal obturator and levator ani muscles as well as the pubic bones. These structures may be involved in advanced tumors occupying the anterior, lateral, or bladder neck regions and render the patient inoperable.

The most anterosuperior aspect of the bladder is known as the apex or dome and is located at the point of contact of the superior surfaces and the two inferolateral surfaces. The apex marks the point of insertion of the median umbilical ligament and consequently is the area where urachal carcinomas occur.

VARIANTS OF NORMAL HISTOLOGY

A very important feature of the urothelium is its ability to transform its morphologic appearance, most likely as a reaction to a local stimulus (usually some sort of injury). The end result is that the urothelium may take on a host of benign morphologic features that are so common that they are considered variants of normal histology. One such example is the squamous mucosa routinely encountered in the trigone in women. The urothelial cells take on a distinct squamous appearance but lack keratinization. Often, the cytoplasm will contain ample amounts of clearing, hence the name glycogenated squamous metaplasia, which is said to vary in relation to the menstrual cycle, similar to what is seen in the uterine cervix (see Chapters 2 and 9).

Brunn (von Brunn) Nests

The most common reactive proliferative change within the urothelium is the formation of Brunn nests, which represent invaginations of the surface urothelium into the underlying lamina propria[15-18] (Figs. 1.16 and 1.17, eFigs. 1.10 and 1.11). Basal and intermediate cells are readily identifiable. In some cases, these solid nests of benign-appearing urothelium may lose continuity with the surface, becoming isolated within the superficial lamina propria. Such proliferations may mimic the nested variant of urothelial carcinoma, particularly if the nests lie relatively deep in the lamina propria or have elongation and branching complexity. In contrast to nested variant

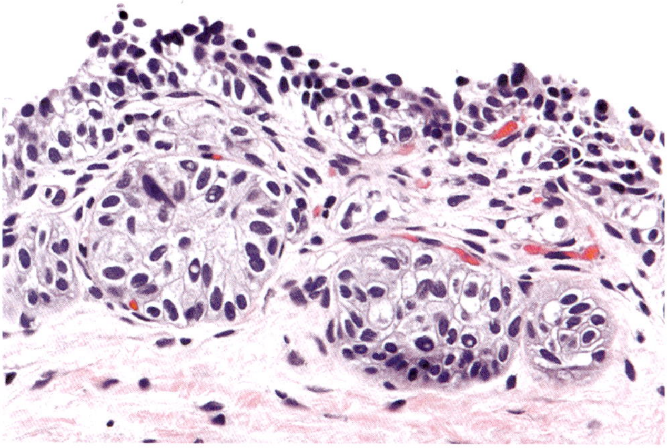

FIGURE 1.16 von Brunn nests with slightly enlarged nuclei relative to surface urothelium.

of urothelial carcinoma, examples of florid Brunn nests in the bladder generally show larger nests with more regular shapes and regular spacing.[19] Nests that are irregular in size and shape and are stacked up on each other should alert the pathologist to consider the possibility of a nested variant of carcinoma.[20,21] Cystic formation is more pronounced in florid Brunn nests and involves a higher proportion of nests. Occasionally, there may be prominent clear cell change. In Brunn nests, apical glandular differentiation and eosinophilic secretions are also more common, and atypia is absent, although nuclei may be minimally enlarged compared to surface urothelial cells (Fig. 1.16), and the lesions have a flat noninfiltrative base. Cases of florid Brunn nests in the ureter show small nests similar to nested

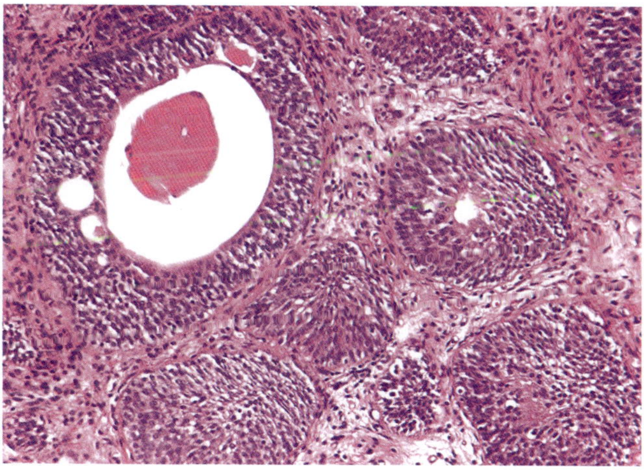

FIGURE 1.17 von Brunn nests and cystitis cystica.

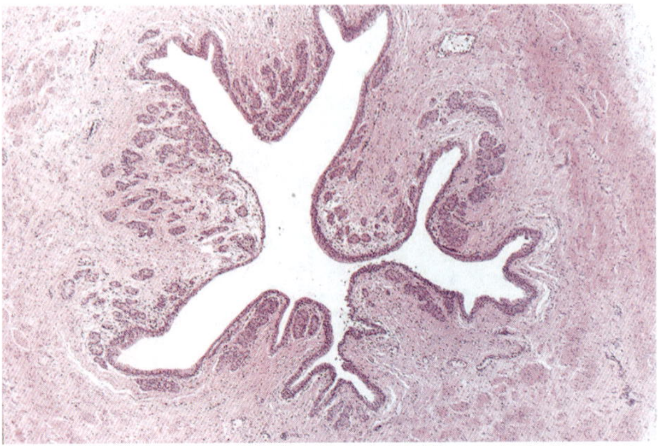

FIGURE 1.18 Ureter with florid proliferation of von Brunn nests.

variant of urothelial carcinoma. Distinguishing features of florid Brunn nests include a noninfiltrative base, a lobular or linear array of the nests, and a lack of cytologic atypia (Figs. 1.18-1.20). Wide variation in staining for MIB-1, p53, p27, and cytokeratin 20 is seen in both florid Brunn nests and nested variant of urothelial carcinoma, such that except for a few cases, a specific cutoff value cannot be determined for diagnostic purposes.[19]

Cystitis Cystica/Cystitis Glandularis

The term cystitis cystica has been coined to describe when the nests become cystically dilated, acquiring a luminal space (Figs. 1.21-1.25, eFigs. 1.12-1.15). In this setting, the umbrella cell layer may take on a cuboidal or columnar appearance. In some cases, the epithelial lining undergoes

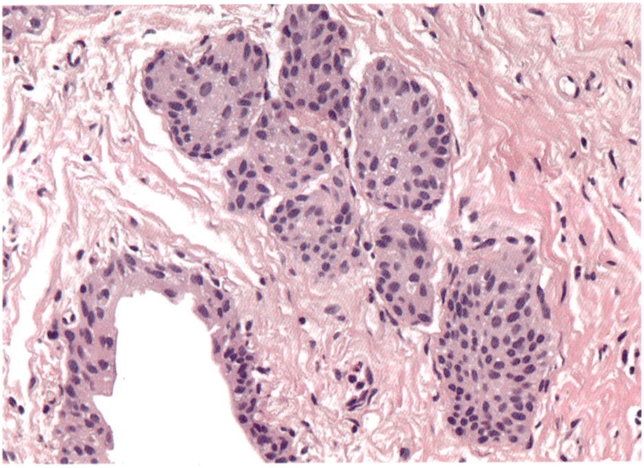

FIGURE 1.19 Ureter with florid proliferation of von Brunn nests (high magnification of Fig. 1.15).

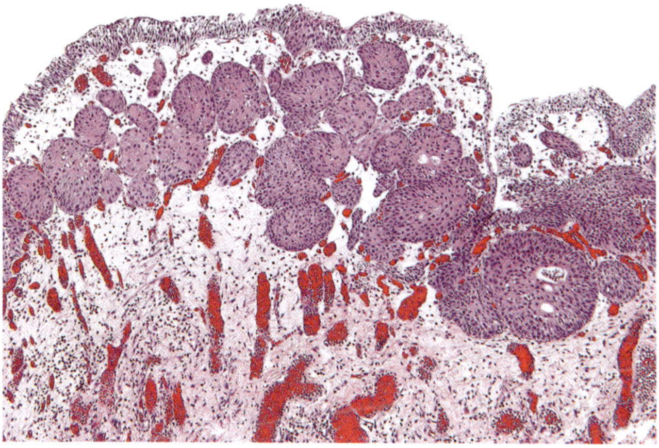

FIGURE 1.20 Proliferation of Brunn nests in the bladder with uniform-sized nests in the superficial lamina propria and a noninfiltrative base.

glandular metaplasia, giving rise to what is called cystitis glandularis. The cells become cuboidal or columnar and mucin secreting. If the epithelium acquires intestinal-type goblet cells, this variant is called cystitis glandularis with intestinal metaplasia (see Chapter 8). Rarely, intestinal metaplasia may be associated with extravasated mucin.[22] Some cases of Brunn nests/cystitis cystica/cystitis glandularis may mimic invasive urothelial carcinoma (eFigs. 1.16-1.36). The absence of frank cytologic atypia/dysplasia is important if one is to make a benign diagnosis. The presence of enteric form of dysplasia may be a marker for the presence of adenocarcinoma.[23]

Brunn nests, cystitis cystica, and cystitis glandularis represent a continuum of proliferative or reactive changes seen along the entire urothelial tract, and it is common to see all three in the same specimen. Most inves-

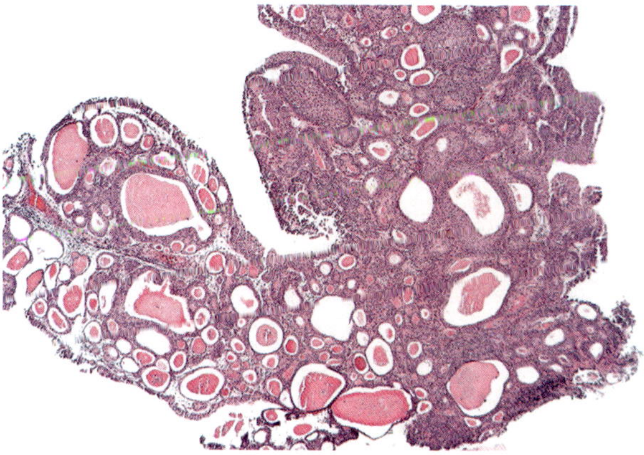

FIGURE 1.21 Florid cystitis cystica et glandularis.

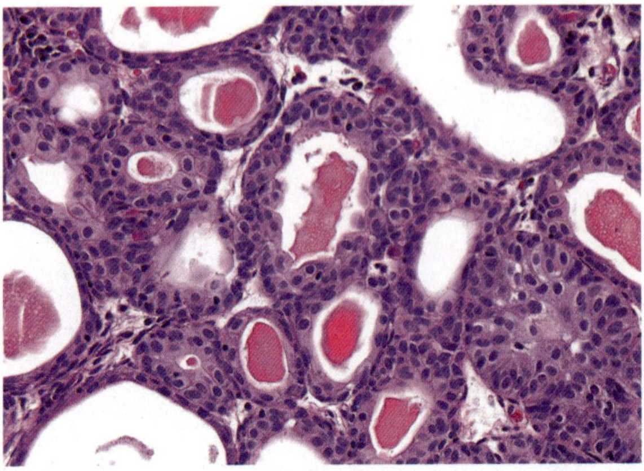

FIGURE 1.22 Florid cystitis cystica et glandularis (high magnification of Fig. 1.20).

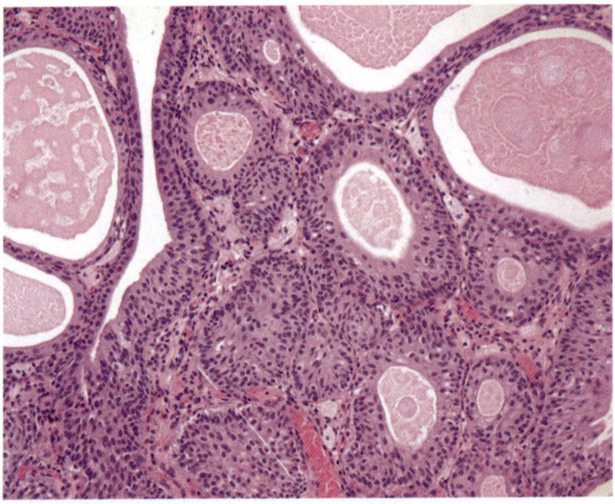

FIGURE 1.23 Florid cystitis cystica et glandularis with cystic dilatation.

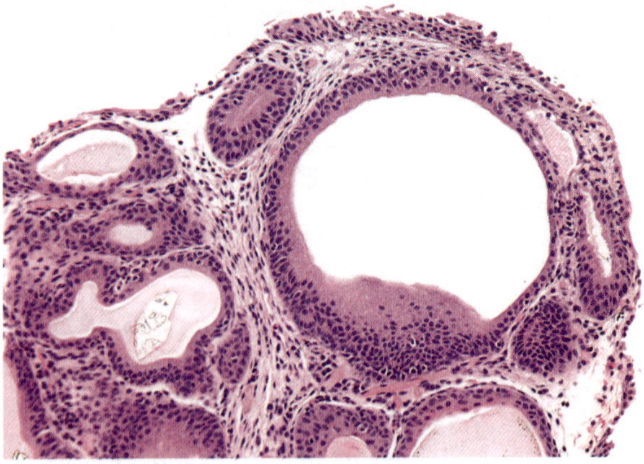

FIGURE 1.24 Florid cystitis cystica et glandularis with cystic dilatation.

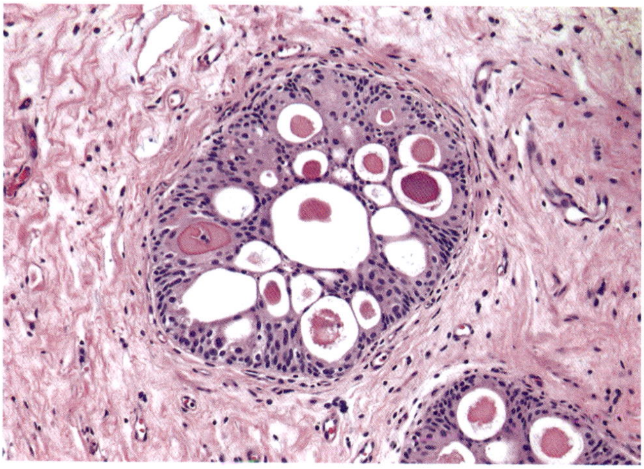

FIGURE 1.25 Cystitis cystica et glandularis.

tigators believe that they occur as a result of local inflammatory insult.[13,14] Nevertheless, these proliferative changes are seen in the urothelium of patients with no evidence of local inflammation so that it is possible that they also represent either normal histologic variants or the residual effects of prior inflammatory processes.[15,16]

Much has been written about the association of Brunn nests, cystitis cystica and especially cystitis glandularis, and urothelial carcinoma.[13-17,21-23] The high incidence of these proliferative changes in normal bladder would argue that they are not likely premalignant changes and that there is no cause-effect relationship between their presence and the appearance of bladder cancer. It is true that one or all of these changes are commonly present in biopsy specimens containing bladder cancer, but the coexistence may be coincidental or the cancer itself may be producing the local inflammatory insult that causes them and not vice versa. The fact that exceptional cases may occur in which carcinoma clearly arises within the epithelium of these reactive lesions does not alter this argument.[24,25]

REFFRENCES

1. Moore KL, Persaud TVN. *The Developing Human: Clinically Oriented Embryology*. Saunders; 2003.
2. Fawcett DW, Bloom W. *A Textbook of Histology*. Saunders; 1986.
3. Reuter V. Urinary bladder and ureter. In: Sternberg SS, ed. *Histology for Pathologists*. Raven Press; 1997:835-847.
4. Ro JY, Ayala AG, el-Naggar A. Muscularis mucosa of urinary bladder. Importance for staging and treatment. *Am J Surg Pathol*. 1987;11:668-673.
5. Paner GP, Ro JY, Wojcik EM, et al. Further characterization of the muscle layers and lamina propria of the urinary bladder by systematic histologic mapping: implications for pathologic staging of invasive urothelial carcinoma. *Am J Surg Pathol*. 2007;31: 1420-1429.

6. Vakar-Lopez F, Shen SS, Zhang S, et al. Muscularis mucosae of the urinary bladder revisited with emphasis on its hyperplastic patterns: a study of a large series of cystectomy specimens. *Ann Diagn Pathol.* 2007;11:395-401.
7. Paner GP, Shen SS, Lapetino S, et al. Diagnostic utility of antibody to smoothelin in the distinction of muscularis propria from muscularis mucosae of the urinary bladder: a potential ancillary tool in the pathologic staging of invasive urothelial carcinoma. *Am J Surg Pathol.* 2009;33:91-98.
8. Lindh C, Nilsson R, Lindstrom ML, et al. Detection of smoothelin expression in the urinary bladder is strongly dependent on pretreatment conditions: a critical analysis with possible consequences for cancer staging. *Virchows Arch.* 2011;458(6):665-670.
9. Miyamoto H, Sharma RB, Illei PB, et al. Pitfalls in the use of smoothelin to identify muscularis propria invasion by urothelial carcinoma. *Am J Surg Pathol.* 2010;34:418-422.
10. Amin MB, Trpkov K, Lopez-Beltran A, et al. Best practices recommendations in the application of immunohistochemistry in the bladder lesions: report from the International Society of Urologic Pathology consensus conference. *Am J Surg Pathol.* 2014;38(8):e20-e34.
11. Hansel DE, Paner GP, Nese N, et al. Limited smoothelin expression within the muscularis mucosae: validation in bladder diverticula. *Hum Pathol.* 2011;42(11):1770-1776.
12. Philip AT, Amin MB, Tamboli P, et al. Intravesical adipose tissue: a quantitative study of its presence and location with implications for therapy and prognosis. *Am J Surg Pathol.* 2000;24:1286-1290.
13. Ananthanarayanan V, Pan Y, Tretiakova M, et al. Influence of histologic criteria and confounding factors in staging equivocal cases for microscopic perivesical tissue invasion (pt3a): an interobserver study among genitourinary pathologists. *Am J Surg Pathol.* 2014;38:167-175.
14. Moore KL, Dalley AF, Agur AMR. *Clinically Oriented Anatomy*. 6th ed. Lippincott Williams & Wilkins; 2010.
15. Morse HD. The etiology and pathology of pyelitis cystica, ureteritis cystica and cystitis cystica. *Am J Pathol.* 1928;4:33-50.
16. Mostofi FK. Potentialities of bladder epithelium. *J Urol.* 1954;71:705-714.
17. Goldstein AM, Fauer RB, Chinn M, et al. New concepts on formation of Brunn's nests and cysts in urinary tract mucosa. *Urology.* 1978;11:513-517.
18. Wiener DP, Koss LG, Sablay B, et al. The prevalence and significance of Brunn's nests, cystitis cystica and squamous metaplasia in normal bladders. *J Urol.* 1979;122:317-321.
19. Volmar KE, Chan TY, De Marzo AM, et al. Florid von Brunn nests mimicking urothelial carcinoma: a morphologic and immunohistochemical comparison to the nested variant of urothelial carcinoma. *Am J Surg Pathol.* 2003;27:1243-1252.
20. Drew PA, Furman J, Civantos F, et al. The nested variant of transitional cell carcinoma: an aggressive neoplasm with innocuous histology. *Mod Pathol.* 1996;9:989-994.
21. Cox R, Epstein JI. Large nested variant of urothelial carcinoma: 23 cases mimicking von Brunn nests and inverted growth pattern of noninvasive papillary urothelial carcinoma. *Am J Surg Pathol.* 2011;35:1337-1342.
22. Young RH, Bostwick DG. Florid cystitis glandularis of intestinal type with mucin extravasation: a mimic of adenocarcinoma. *Am J Surg Pathol.* 1996;20:1462-1468.
23. Gordetsky J, Epstein JI. Intestinal metaplasia of the bladder with dysplasia: a risk factor for carcinoma? *Histopathology.* 2015;67(3):325-330.
24. Edwards PD, Hurm RA, Jaeschke WH. Conversion of cystitis glandularis to adenocarcinoma. *J Urol.* 1972;108:568-570.
25. Lin JI, Yong HS, Tseng CH, et al. Diffuse cystitis glandularis. Associated with adenocarcinomatous change. *Urology.* 1980;15:411-415.

2

FLAT UROTHELIAL LESIONS

There are four main reasons a surgical pathologist is asked to evaluate flat (cystoscopically apparent or unapparent) lesions. The first two indications involve multiple random biopsies by cold cup biopsy technique (1) in patients previously diagnosed with noninvasive or lamina propria–invasive papillary tumors who are on surveillance for bladder cancer and (2) in patients who are diagnosed with papillary bladder carcinoma for the first time. The aim of the biopsies is to detect flat intraurothelial disease, which suggests urothelial instability, multifocality, and proclivity for disease progression. The third indication is in patients with hematuria, dysuria, and increased frequency of micturition, who have positive urine cytology, positive FISH UroVysion, or are at high risk of development of bladder cancer. The aim is to detect urothelial carcinoma *in situ* (CIS), which may or may not be cystoscopically apparent. The fourth indication is in patients without a high risk of bladder cancer but who present with urinary symptoms similar to those listed but who do not respond to routine medical treatments, for example, patients being evaluated for symptomology related to interstitial cystitis. In this setting, biopsies are performed to evaluate other causes for the symptoms. Significant flat urothelial disease may be inapparent by cystoscopy, and this has promulgated the concept of performing random bladder biopsies in patients with cancer, resulting in most of the flat lesions seen clinically.[1] Recently, techniques to enhance recognition of CIS lesions (blue light and narrow-band imaging), cystoscopy may be helpful in identifying lesions not visible using white light cystoscopy.[2]

APPROACH TO THE EVALUATION AND DIAGNOSIS OF FLAT LESIONS

The widely used and recommended classification is the World Health Organization (WHO)/International Society of Urological Pathology (ISUP) classification of flat intraurothelial lesions, which is outlined in Table 2.1.[3-5] The system first proposed as the WHO/ISUP (1998) system, with minor modifications, has subsequently been largely adopted during revisions of the WHO Blue Books (2004, 2016, and 2022). The approach to the diagnosis of lesions within this classification requires attention to several organizational and cytologic features within the urothelium, the

TABLE 2.1 The Classification of Flat Intraurothelial Lesions
Normal
Hyperplasia
Flat lesions with atypia
Reactive (inflammatory type)
Dysplasia (low-grade intraurothelial lesion)
Carcinoma *in situ* (high-grade intraurothelial lesion)

constellation of the presence or absence of which helps make the correct diagnosis [6-8] (Table 2.2).

On low-power examination, one should pay attention to several features including the thickness of the urothelium, overall polarity, presence or absence of cytoplasmic eosinophilia, and neovascularity at the base of the urothelium. Observation regarding the thickness of the urothelium may provide useful clues. It is normally three to seven layers in thickness, depending on the state of distention. Denudation may be seen in reactive conditions (trauma or infection) or CIS. Hyperplastic urothelium may be encountered in the entire spectrum of flat intraepithelial lesions (reactive atypia, dysplasia, and CIS), and its presence merits evaluation of cytologic features, on the basis of which the diagnosis is ultimately made. Other features assessed at low power include polarity, nuclear crowding, and cytoplasmic clearing. In the normal urothelium, the cells are arranged perpendicularly to the basement membrane with orderly organization of the basal cells, intermediate cells, and superficial umbrella cells. Loss of

TABLE 2.2 Histologic Parameters Useful in the Evaluation of Flat Lesions With Atypia
Thickness of urothelium
Polarity
Cytoplasmic clearing
Nuclear size
Nuclear crowding
Nuclear borders including notches
Nuclear chromatin distribution
Nucleoli
Mitoses including atypical forms
Accompanying inflammation
Neovascularity and inflammation at the base of the lesion

normal polarity and presence of nuclear crowding are often indicative of intraurothelial neoplasia. Loss of cytoplasmic clearing (increased eosinophilia) is also a sign of dysplasia or CIS. Nucleomegaly is objectively determined by comparison if clearly normal urothelium is present in the biopsy. If normal urothelium is not present, stromal lymphocytes may also be used for size comparison. The larger nuclei in CIS are often five times the size of a normal lymphocyte, whereas the nuclear size of normal urothelium and dysplastic urothelium is only approximately twice the size of lymphocytes, aiding in their distinction from CIS.[9] The presence of dysplasia is confirmed by unequivocal nuclear atypia (nuclear border and nuclear chromatin abnormalities) but does not meet the threshold for CIS. The presence of nuclear pleomorphism, frequent mitoses (including atypical mitotic figures or surface mitoses), and prominent nucleoli (single or multiple) throughout much of the urothelium favor a diagnosis of urothelial CIS over that of urothelial dysplasia or reactive changes. Nucleolar pleomorphism (multiple nucleoli of varying sizes and shapes) may be seen in CIS and is a helpful feature when present. Neovascularization in a bladder biopsy without a history of previous treatment suggests the presence of a host response to an intraurothelial neoplastic process and is more commonly seen in CIS. Ultimately, the diagnosis of flat lesions is based on a constellation of features, which have to be viewed in the aggregate, as none of the above features on their own unequivocally point to a certain diagnostic category. For example, denudation, mitotic activity, or prominent nucleoli may be seen in reactive conditions and CIS, and pleomorphism may be seen in CIS and posttreatment regenerative atypia.

HISTOLOGIC FEATURES OF FLAT INTRAUROTHELIAL LESION CATEGORIES

Normal

The normal urothelium, as mentioned previously, is composed of three cell types: basal, intermediate, and superficial cells arranged in three to seven cell layers, with the thickness varying depending on the state of distention (Fig. 2.1, eFigs. 2.1-2.7). The nuclei of basal cells are small and hyperchromatic, and the cells usually form a single layer. The intermediate cells constitute the bulk of the urothelium, the cells are oriented perpendicular to the basement membrane, and the nuclei are usually oval to round in tissue sections. Nuclear grooves are frequently identified. The cytoplasm is clear to amphophilic. The superficial or umbrella cells are arranged parallel to the basement membrane and are large, with one cell typically spanning or covering several intermediate cells (like an umbrella). The nucleus is small, and cytoplasm is voluminous and clear or eosinophilic. Mild degrees of architectural variation (apparent loss of polarity) but without cytologic atypia are considered acceptable to be designated as normal (Figs. 2.2 and 2.3). This is often due to tangential or thick sectioning.

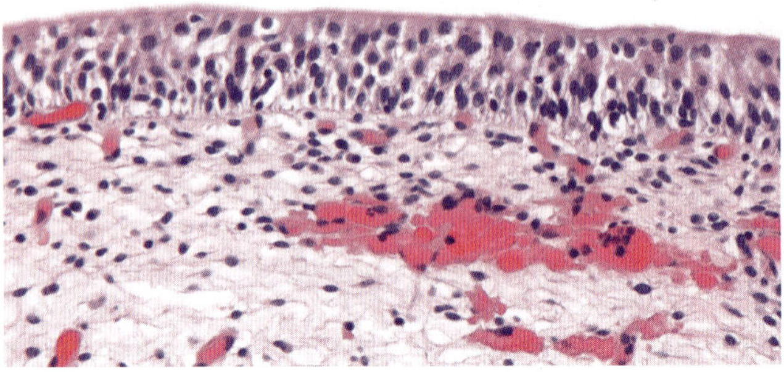

FIGURE 2.1 Normal urothelium.

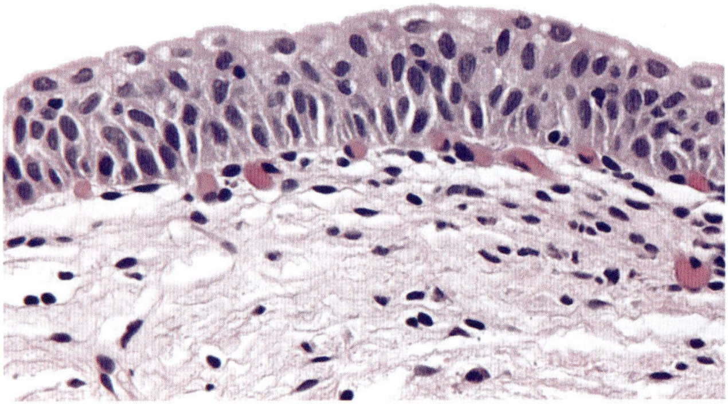

FIGURE 2.2 Although there is slight disorganization and minimal variation in nuclear size and shape, this urothelium is within the range of "normal" urothelium.

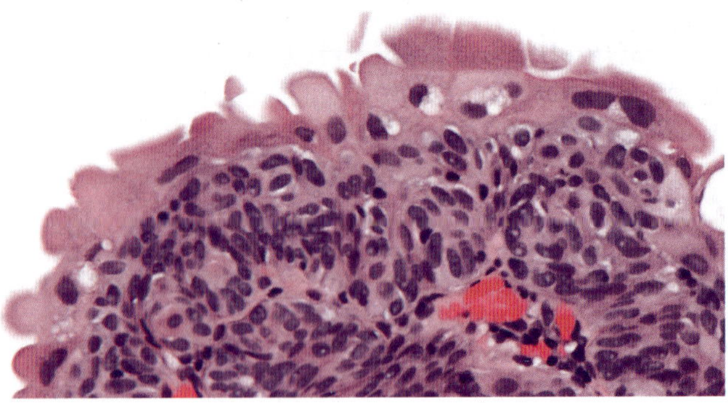

FIGURE 2.3 Tangentially sectioned cytologically appearing normal urothelium with umbrella cells showing slight atypia.

Squamous Metaplasia

Nonkeratinizing squamous epithelium metaplasia, particularly in the area of the trigone, is a common finding in premenopausal women and is responsive to estrogen production (eFigs. 2.8-2.12). This type of squamous mucosa is characterized by abundant intracytoplasmic glycogen and lack of keratinization, making it histologically similar to vaginal or cervical squamous epithelium (Fig. 2.4) (see Chapter 9 for additional images).[10] It is likely that trigonal squamous mucosa in women represents a normal histologic variant unassociated to local injury. Under other pathologic conditions, the metaplastic squamous epithelium, that is, nonkeratinizing squamous mucosa in males and/or in nontrigonal locations or mucosa with keratinization in either sexes, may exhibit parakeratosis and even a granular layer[11] (Fig. 2.5, eFig. 2.13). This metaplastic epithelium is not preneoplastic *per se* but under some circumstances may lead to squamous carcinoma (see Chapter 9), particularly where multifocal and extensive.

Flat Urothelial Hyperplasia

The term flat hyperplasia has undergone nomenclatural changes recently. In the original WHO/ISUP 1998 and the third edition of the WHO (2002), lesions with thickened mucosa without cytologic atypia in flat lesions were referred to as flat hyperplasia. The term urothelial proliferation of uncertain malignant potential (UPUMP) was used to encompass flat and papillary lesions in the fourth (2016) edition of the WHO.[7] In 2021, the Genitourinary Pathology Society (GUPS) white paper recommended separating flat from papillary hyperplasia, with the former to be designated as atypical urothelial hyperplasia-flat.[12] The recent fifth edition of the WHO does not have any equivalent terminology for flat lesions.[8] In our clinical

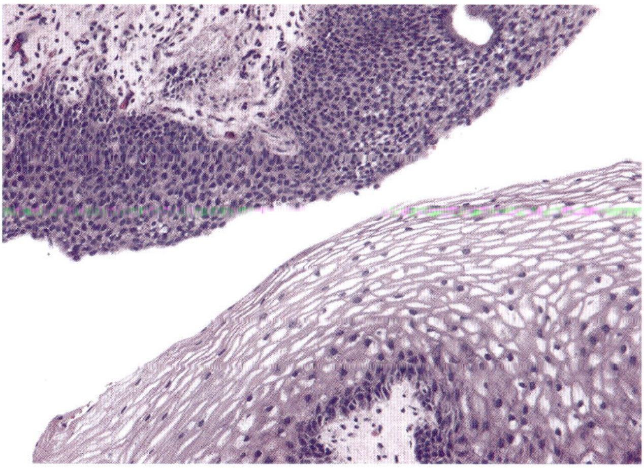

FIGURE 2.4 Normal trigone in a woman with glycogenated squamous metaplasia (*bottom*) compared to normal urothelium (*top*).

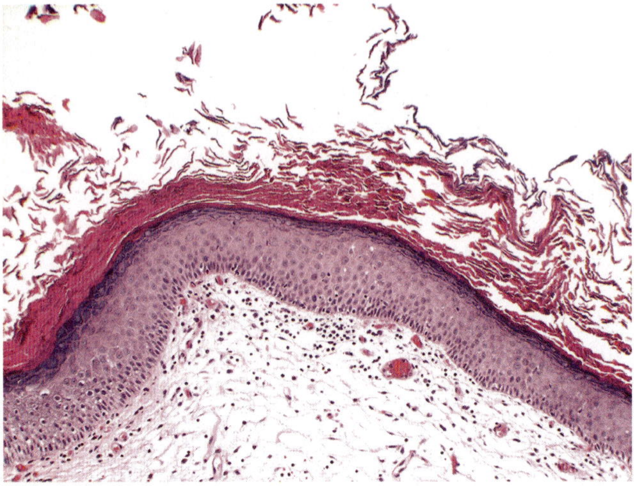

FIGURE 2.5 Keratinizing squamous metaplasia.

practice, and therefore for the purposes of this book, we still recognize flat hyperplasia using the traditional simplistic criteria–markedly thickened urothelium, often with increased cellular density and lacking atypia.

Hyperplasia may present as a discernable bladder mucosal bump that may draw the attention of the examining urologist on cystoscopy with concern for a small papillary tumor. This is likely not an uncommon scenario, since thickening in hyperplasia is often pronounced; obvious enough to be sampled on cystoscopy. Furthermore, hyperplasia are frequently detected as "false-positive" lesion in photodynamic diagnosis.[2] Studies on hyperplasia reported as UPUMP that included *de novo* lesions (38%) and those with flat architecture (69% of *de novo*) showed that most *de novo* hyperplasias had associated symptoms including 61% of patients presenting with hematuria.[13] Reporting hyperplasia thus provides a pathologic diagnosis, corresponding to and explaining a cystoscopic abnormality and possible clinical symptoms.

While evaluating the histology, one notes that the urothelium is markedly thickened and, importantly, lacks cytologic atypia (Fig. 2.6, eFigs. 2.14-2.16). Rather than requiring a specific number of cell layers, marked thickening and/or increased cell density within the urothelium (increased cells per unit area) is needed to diagnose flat hyperplasia. Tangentially sectioned and/or distorted urothelium may mimic hyperplasia. However, the effect of tangential sectioning is typically focal and not seen in other fragments. Further, the increase in cell layers is not that striking and the increase in cellularity is not that dense; both features may recede on deeper levels. Hyperplasia may be seen in a *de novo* setting or it may be seen in the flat mucosa adjacent to low-grade papillary urothelial lesions. Identification of hyperplasia in a repeat TUR as a pure lesion (without residual papillary tumor) should prompt a comment that the hyperplasia

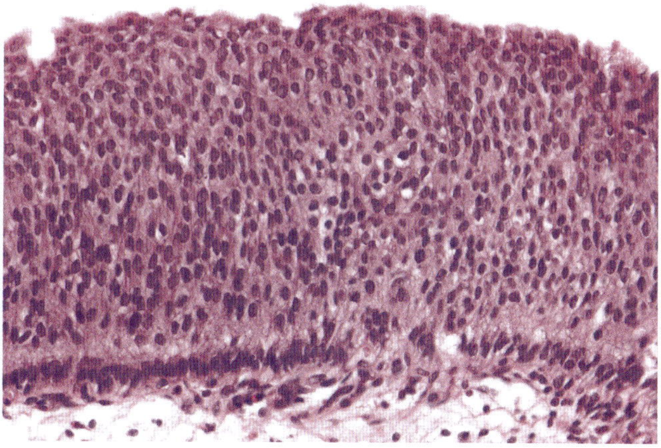

FIGURE 2.6 Flat urothelial hyperplasia.

may represent lateral extension of the prior papillary tumor. Diagnosis of the uncommon *de novo* flat hyperplasia should also prompt a comment for reasonable clinical follow-up. In evaluation of such lesions, we emphasize for the pathologist, the utmost importance of accessing patient diagnostic and clinical history, requisite correlation with cystoscopic reports describing the lesion sampled, and judicious use of recuts and deeper level sections to document or exclude more worrisome findings (cytologic atypia or true papillary cores) deeper in tissue blocks.

Deletion of chromosome 9 is present in 37%-70% of hyperplasia [14-16]; other chromosomal losses, gains, and amplification have also been detected in hyperplasia.[15-17] *FGFR3* mutation, common in low-grade papillary tumors, is detected in 23% of hyperplasia, including those with no prior or concomitant urothelial neoplasm (*de novo* hyperplasia).[16] Polysomy of at least one chromosome is detected in 17% of hyperplasia cases,[18] and a recent whole organ mapping of bladders with cancer detected *TERT* mutations in 33% of hyperplasia.[19] Presence of these alterations suggests that at least a significant subset of hyperplasia is preneoplastic or neoplasia associated. From an outcome perspective, 5% of patients with flat hyperplasia (UMPUMP–flat in study) progressed to neoplasia.[13,20]

Reactive Urothelial Changes

As "reactive urothelial atypia" may in some instances lead to confusion with dysplasia or cause concern for patients, some of the current authors have substituted the term "reactive urothelial changes." Nucleomegaly is the most prominent finding in reactive urothelial changes, but the cells often have a single prominent nucleolus and evenly distributed vesicular chromatin (Fig. 2.7, eFigs. 2.17-2.28). The nuclear borders are smooth. The nuclei are frequently round, and nuclear pleomorphism is lacking.[21]

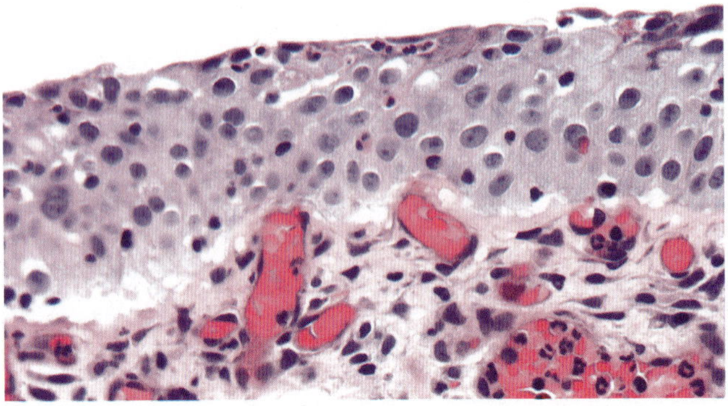

FIGURE 2.7 Reactive urothelium with scattered neutrophils within the urothelium.

Architecturally, the cells maintain their polarity perpendicular to the basement membrane, although a minimal loss of polarity may be evident. The mitotic rate may be increased with mitoses present predominantly in the basal and intermediate urothelium, but atypical forms are not seen. Intraurothelial acute or chronic inflammation is commonly identified (Figs. 2.8-2.10). It is important to recognize that even intraepithelial lymphocytes, by themselves, can result in reactive changes. The cytoplasm may become more basophilic or eosinophilic with loss of cytoplasmic clearing. Clinical history of stones, infection, or frequent instrumentation may be present.[22] Reactive urothelium may be denuded with only a single residual layer of basal cells remaining; the residual cells are not hyperchromatic, not enlarged, and do not possess nuclear membrane irregularity. The umbrella cells frequently undergo reactive change alone and exhibit multinucleation

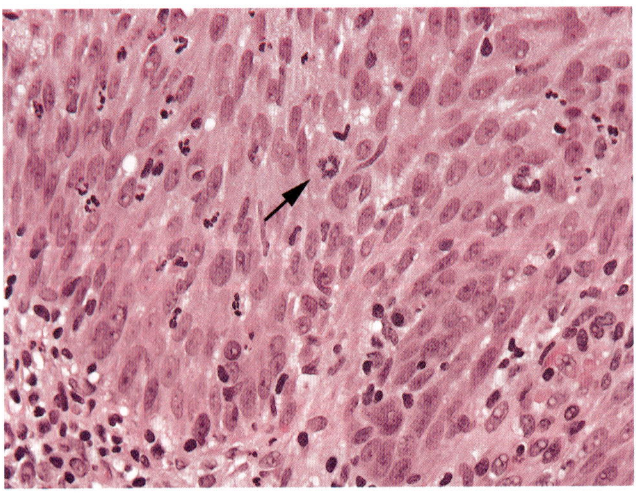

FIGURE 2.8 Reactive urothelium with scattered lymphocytes and neutrophils within the urothelium showing mitotic figure (*arrow*).

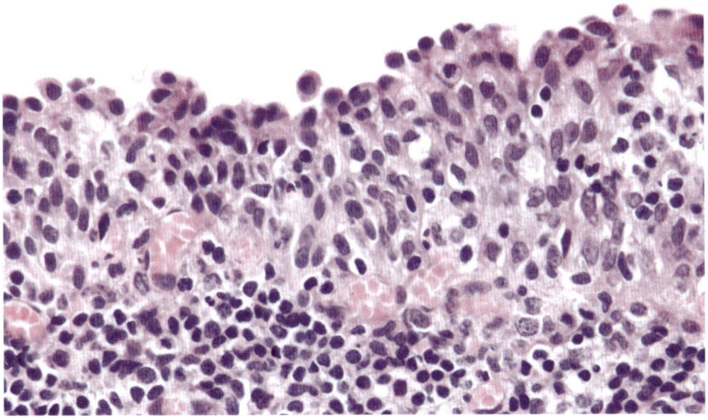

FIGURE 2.9 Reactive urothelium with lymphocytes within the urothelium.

or nucleomegaly, often with cytoplasmic vacuolation. Although reactive conditions share the presence of enlarged nuclei, prominent nucleoli, and frequent mitoses with CIS, in reactive conditions, nuclei are uniform in size and shape with vesicular nuclei as opposed to the often hyperchromatic nuclei of CIS. Furthermore, most cases of CIS are not associated with intraepithelial inflammation. Treatment-related reactive and regenerative atypia can have only the aforementioned histologic features or may have additional features based on specific etiology–see "Problems and Pitfalls in the Diagnosis of Flat Lesions With Atypia" section.

Urothelial Atypia of Unknown Significance

This term was originally proposed as a descriptive category in cases with inflammation in which the severity of atypia appears to be out of proportion to the extent of inflammation such that dysplasia or CIS could not be confidently excluded (Figs. 2.11 and 2.12, eFigs. 2.29). The message conveyed to the urologist by use of this diagnostic terminology was that the

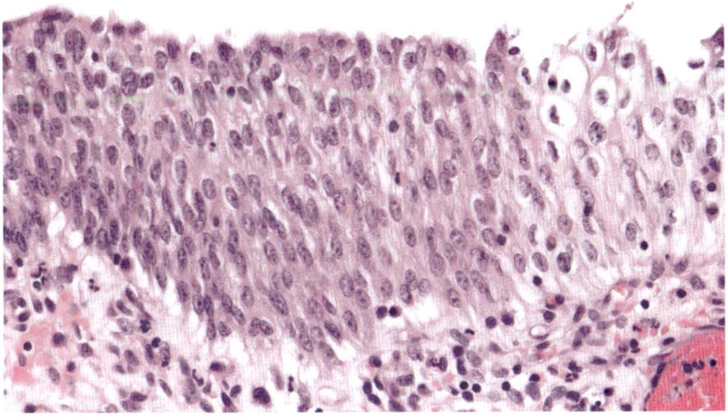

FIGURE 2.10 Reactive urothelium with lymphocytes within the urothelium.

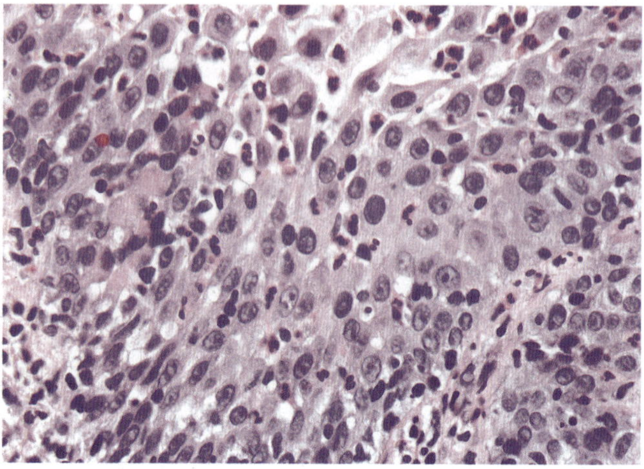

FIGURE 2.11 Atypia of unknown significance with scattered hyperchromatic nuclei yet prominent inflammation.

patient should be followed up after inflammation subsides. This was not a disease or diagnostic entity but merely a descriptive term that may be designated in a biopsy in which the flat lesion with atypia cannot be diagnosed with certainty into reactive, dysplastic, or CIS categories. Since this term is often used loosely and potentially as a "wastebasket" term by pathologists for lesions with minimal atypia that may well fall into the spectrum of "normal," we dissuade the use of this term and suggest that pathologists acknowledge the level of diagnostic difficulty in cases where it is not possible to reliably exclude reactive from neoplastic atypia, than use this term. Studies have shown that cases diagnosed as reactive atypia and atypia of unknown significance have similar clinical features and are not associated

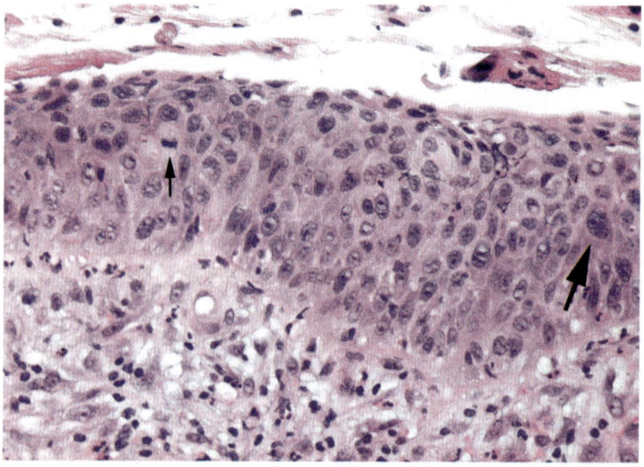

FIGURE 2.12 Atypia of unknown significance with variably sized and shaped nuclei (*large arrow*) showing a mitotic figure (*small arrow*) associated with prominent inflammation, difficult to distinguish between reactive and neoplastic atypia.

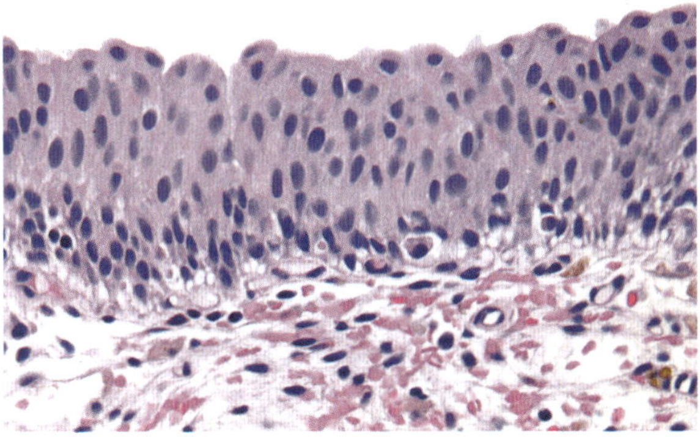

FIGURE 2.13 Urothelial dysplasia with scattered, enlarged nuclei.

with progression to bladder cancer[23,24] further supporting our position. Recently, specialized genitourinary pathologists were able to reclassify a subset of atypia of unknown significant into CIS after re-review and with the aid of ancillary CK20, CD44, and p53 panel of immunostains.[25] See section on CIS (below) for the potential role of immunohistochemistry; we strongly suggest employing and interpreting immunohistochemical findings strictly in the context of morphology and the clinical scenario.

Urothelial Dysplasia

Distinct appreciable nuclear abnormalities in the urothelium that occur in the absence of inflammation or that appear disproportionate to the amount of inflammation (if present), but that are not severe (ie, falling below the threshold of CIS), may be designated as urothelial dysplasia/ low-grade intraurothelial neoplasia (Figs. 2.13-2.16, eFigs. 2.20-2.39). It

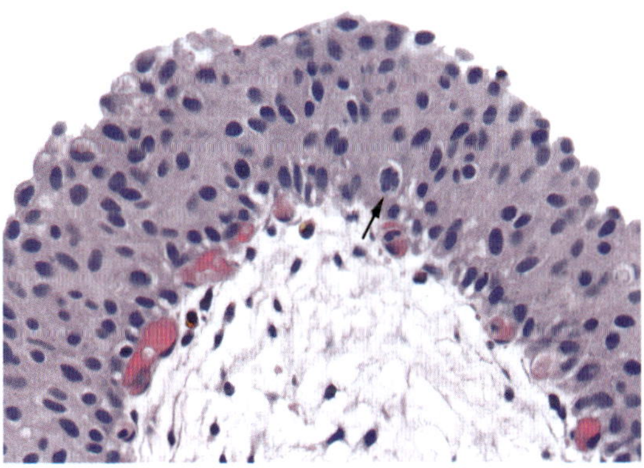

FIGURE 2.14 Urothelial dysplasia with loss of polarity, scattered small yet hyperchromatic nuclei, and a mitotic figure (*arrow*).

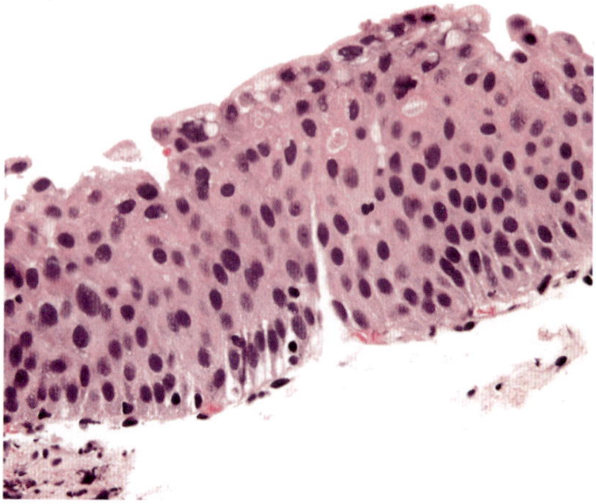

FIGURE 2.15 **Urothelial dysplasia with scattered hyperchromatic nuclei.** Although there is considerable nuclear atypia, the collective features fall short of the diagnosis of CIS.

has been proposed that bladder intraepithelial lesions, like intraepithelial lesions of the cervix, be graded on the basis of level of involvement of atypical cells (ie, mild dysplasia for lesions showing atypia confined to the lower one-third, moderate dysplasia for atypia up to the middle third, and so on).[26] However, observations in animal models and in clinical specimens indicate the importance of cytologic features (degree of cytological atypia) rather than histologic pattern (extent of atypia from the basal layer).[27]

In dysplasia, the thickness of the urothelium is usually normal (three to seven layers) but may be decreased or increased (Fig. 2.17). Flat lesions with a benign cytology and minimal disorder should be considered within the spectrum of "normal".[28] Dysplastic lesions show loss of polarity (normal

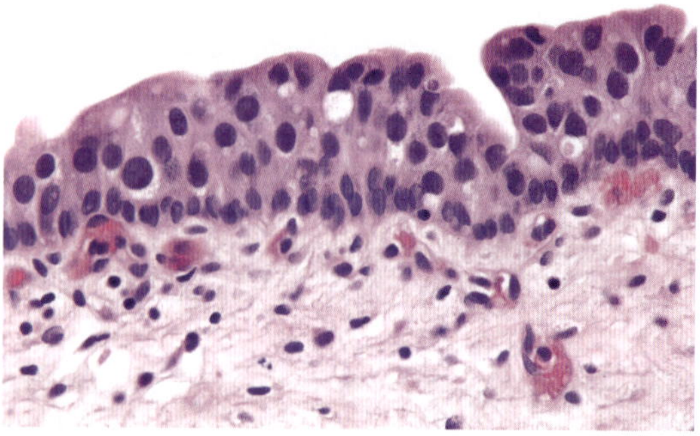

FIGURE 2.16 **Urothelial dysplasia with scattered, enlarged nuclei.** Although there is considerable nuclear atypia, the collective features fall short of the diagnosis of CIS.

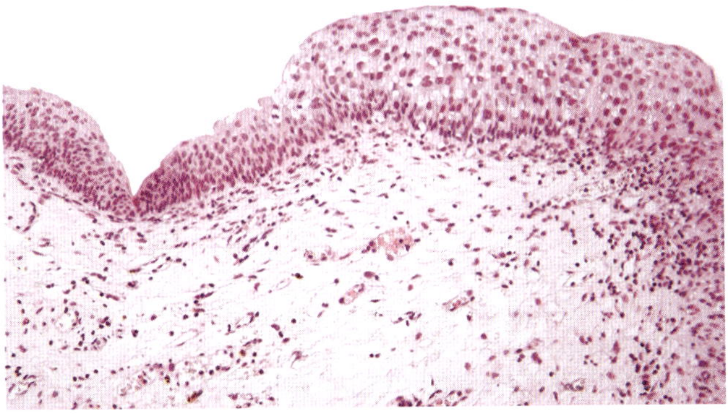

FIGURE 2.17 **Hyperplastic urothelium with dysplasia.** These findings may be a precursor lesion to noninvasive low-grade papillary urothelial carcinoma and in some cases may be seen next to noninvasive low-grade papillary urothelial carcinoma.

cells are columnar to oval with nuclei perpendicular to the basement membrane) evidenced by crowding of nuclei. The cells are more rounded to polygonal cells with nuclei parallel to the long axis. Nuclear atypia is evident but is not severe enough to merit a diagnosis of CIS. Often, increased cytoplasmic eosinophilia, nucleomegaly, irregularity of nuclear contours with notching of cell borders, and altered chromatin distribution are seen. Nucleoli are usually not conspicuous or are only randomly present in the mucosa but are not typically present throughout. Only a minimal degree of pleomorphism is allowable in dysplasia, and the mitotic activity is variable, although usually not in the higher layers. The lamina propria is usually unaltered, but it may contain increased inflammation or neovascularity. Denudation with atypical cells clinging to the submucosa is not a common feature of dysplasia. Comparison with more normal-appearing urothelium, if present in the same biopsy specimen or in another simultaneously obtained biopsy specimen from the same patient, may help in assessing features such as nucleomegaly, loss of clearing, and loss of polarity. In some patients on surveillance for low-grade papillary urothelial carcinoma, due to increased frequency of cystoscopy, early lesions may be found, which histologically show thickened urothelium with dysplasia. Early papillary formation or neovascularity at the base, similar to papillary hyperplasia, may be present. Recently, the 2021 GUPS white paper suggested using the term "early low-grade PUC" for such challenging scenarios presented by lesions demonstrating overall flat dysplasia with foci of early papillary formation.[12] This preferred term is less ambiguous than "dysplasia with early papillary features," an alternative term. Both early low-grade papillary urothelial carcinoma and dysplasia with early papillary features are descriptive designations and it must be acknowledged that it is not yet entirely clear if such lesions truly can evolve into a well-developed papillary carcinoma. Similar abnormalities in the urothelium may be seen in the mucosa immediately adjacent to a low-grade papillary urothelial carcinoma (shoulder effect). Another way to conceptualize the difference between dysplasia and CIS is that the cytological findings seen in dysplasia are analogous to those seen in noninvasive low-grade papillary urothelial carcinoma, whereas CIS is analogous in its histology to noninvasive high-grade papillary urothelial carcinoma. Immunostaining is not recommended in the distinction between dysplasia and CIS (for potentially useful immunoprofile, see section on CIS below) as the distinction is based purely on morphologic grounds with the former denoting distinct nuclear atypia falling short of the threshold to be designated as CIS.

A diagnosis of primary dysplasia (ie, no prior history or concomitant urothelial neoplasia) should be made with great caution.[29,30] Dysplasia is usually a histologic diagnosis seen most commonly in patients with bladder neoplasia, in whom the incidence is 22%-86%. The incidence approaches 100% in patients with invasive carcinoma. Little is known about *de novo* dysplasia because there is a lack of screening in the general population. Furthermore, *de novo* dysplasia is usually cystoscopically and clinically silent, although it may appear as a slightly raised and mildly erythematous patch. The patients are predominantly middle-aged men presenting occasionally with irritative bladder symptoms with or without hematuria. The few studies published on *de novo* dysplasia indicate that 5%-19% of patients progress to have urothelial neoplasia.[20,31-33] The finding of dysplasia in patients with bladder cancer suggests that it is a marker for progression (increased recurrences or future invasion).[23,34,35] Whole-bladder genomic characterization has shown the presence of mutations in dysplasia that overlap in cancer, with both showing significantly different mutational landscapes and with lesser copy number change.[36] Significant allelic losses on multiple chromosomes,[37] deletions in chromosome 9 and p53,[38] and *TERT* promoter mutation have also been shown in dysplasia in keeping with its preneoplastic potential.[19] However, the definition of dysplasia used in all these studies has been variable, so their true clinical meaning remains in doubt. In general, the diagnosis of dysplasia suffers from poor interobserver reproducibility, even among expert genitourinary pathologists.

Urothelial Carcinoma *In Situ*

Unequivocal severe cytologic atypia (ie, changes thought to represent clear-cut neoplasia at the light microscopic level) is necessary for the diagnosis of CIS (Fig. 2.18, eFigs. 2.40-2.85). The urothelium may be denuded, reflecting the discohesive nature of the cells; it may be diminished in thickness, be of normal thickness, or even be hyperplastic. Denudation, however, may be produced artifactually by the biopsy procedure, especially if

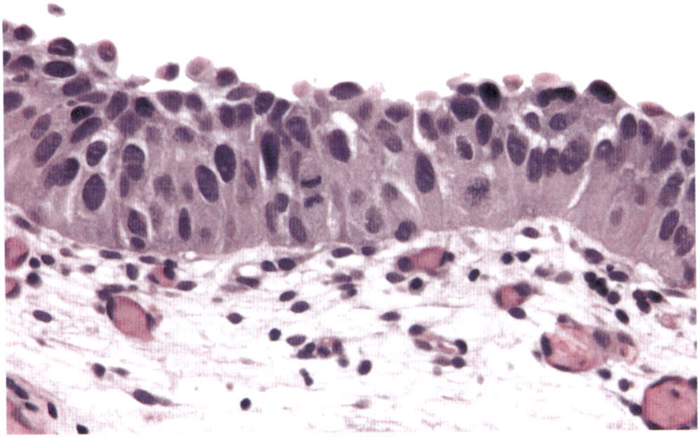

FIGURE 2.18 Carcinoma *in situ*.

the biopsy is performed with a hot wire loop.[39] Disordered urothelium at low power is commonly seen. There may be alteration or complete loss of polarity, marked crowding, pleomorphism, and frequent mitoses. Atypical mitoses and mitoses toward the surface may be present and useful in distinction from both dysplasia and reactive conditions. The lamina propria is frequently hypervascular and inflamed (presumably due to neovascularization as a host reaction), reflecting the erythematous appearance witnessed on cystoscopy. The nuclear anaplasia is generally obvious, although a spectrum of severity may exist. Involvement may be preceded by concurrent or metachronous with CIS of the upper tract or prostatic urethra. Multifocality is common in CIS, and multiple patterns have been described to embrace the wide cytologic and histologic range of manifestations[40,41] (Fig. 2.19; Table 2.3).

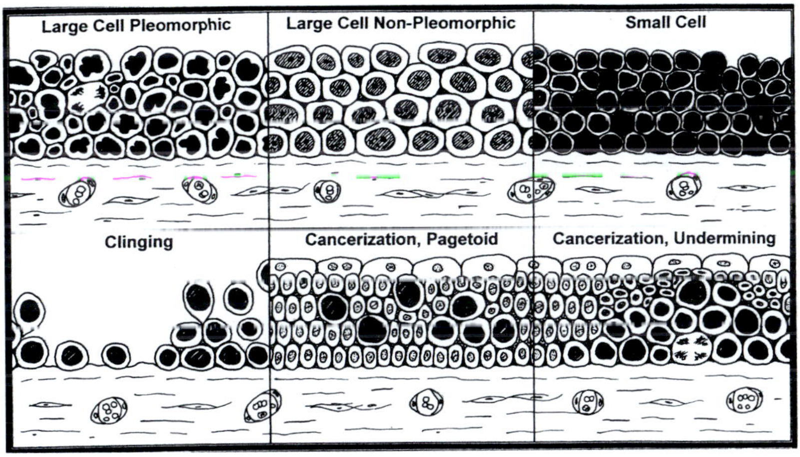

FIGURE 2.19 Schematic representations of CIS.

TABLE 2.3 Histologic Patterns of Urothelial Carcinoma *In Situ*[a]

Large cell, pleomorphic
Large cell, nonpleomorphic
Small cell
Clinging
Micropapillary
CIS with glandular differentiation
Plasmacytoid
CIS with early papillary formations
Cancerization of normal urothelium
Pagetoid
Undermining/overriding

[a]It is important for pathologists to be aware of the different histologic patterns of CIS; however, they need not be subclassified in the pathology report because individual patterns do not carry any known clinical significance.

The pattern of CIS that is most easily recognized is large cell CIS with pleomorphism (Figs. 2.20-2.22). The neoplastic cells show considerable loss of polarity and nucleomegaly with marked variation in nuclear shape and size but retain abundant eosinophilic cytoplasm. The neoplastic cells in other examples of CIS may be monomorphic (large cell CIS without pleomorphism) (Figs. 2.23 and 2.24). These lesions may mimic reactive urothelial atypia because of the uniformity of the cells with conspicuous eosinophilic cytoplasm; however, they have markedly enlarged nuclei with high-grade cytologic features diagnostic of CIS. These lesions may have enlarged nuclei with consistent prominent nucleoli or may lack nucleoli but show unequivocal irregular nuclear chromatin distribution and irregular cell borders. Nucleolar pleomorphism may be present in cases with

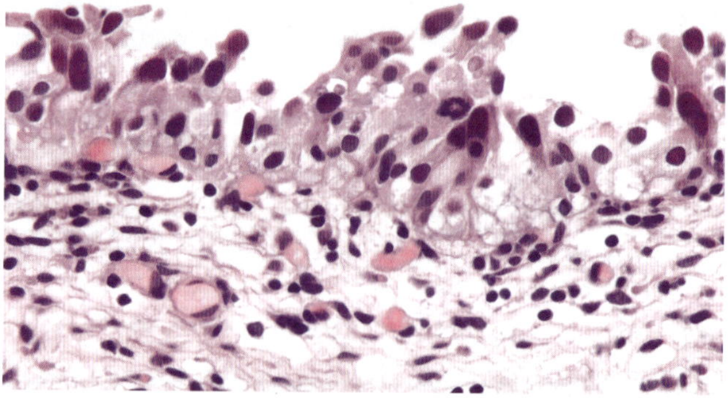

FIGURE 2.20 Carcinoma *in situ*.

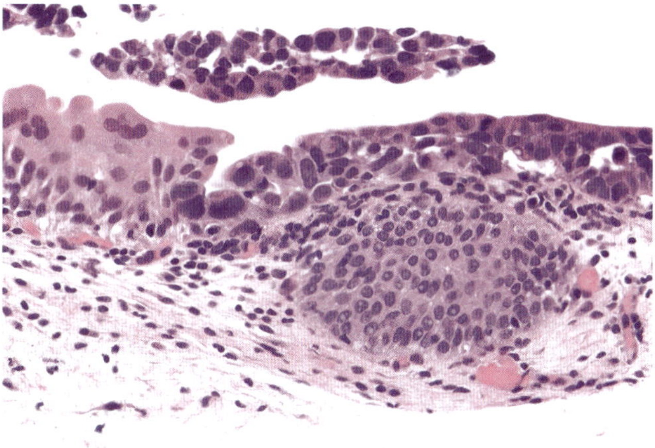

FIGURE 2.21 **Carcinoma *in situ*.** Compare to uninvolved von Brunn nest with bland cytology.

multiple nucleoli; this is a feature helpful in the distinction from reactive conditions in which nucleoli are typically single and variably prominent. "Small cell" CIS has nuclear features identical to large cell CIS without pleomorphism, but it has scant cytoplasm (Fig. 2.25). There is neither precursor relationship to small cell carcinoma of the bladder nor any neuroendocrine connotation; this is merely a descriptive designation. Although the cells appear smaller because of the absence of significant cytoplasm,

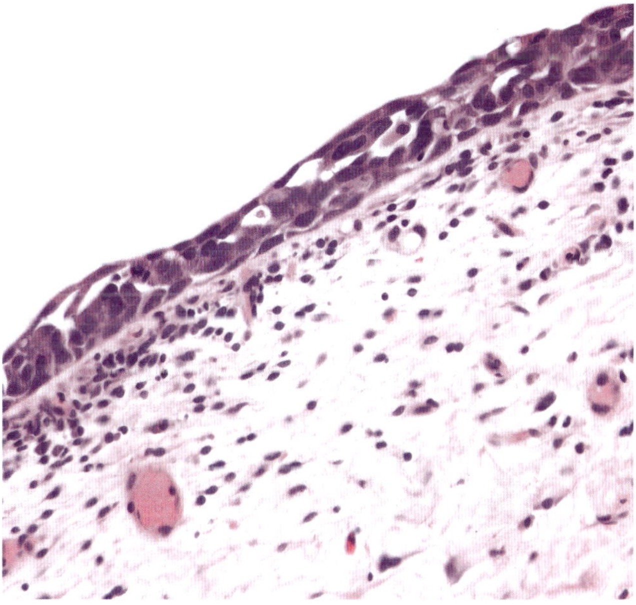

FIGURE 2.22 **CIS with thinned mucosa and preserved umbrella cell layer.**

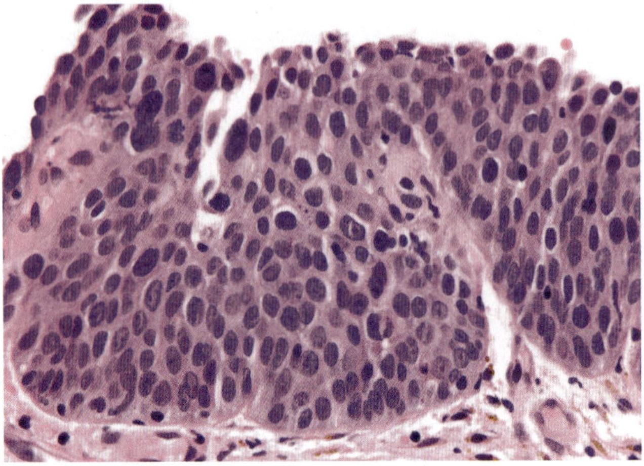

FIGURE 2.23 CIS with prominent nucleoli.

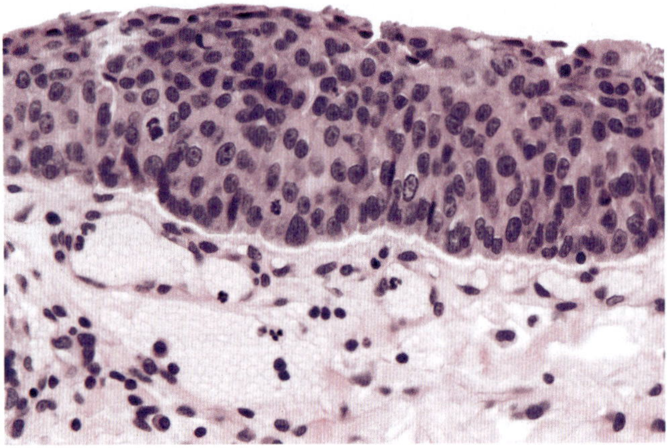

FIGURE 2.24 CIS with prominent nucleoli.

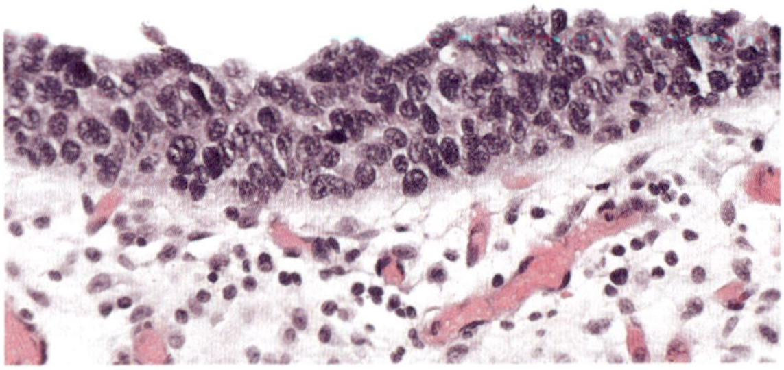

FIGURE 2.25 Small cell urothelial CIS.

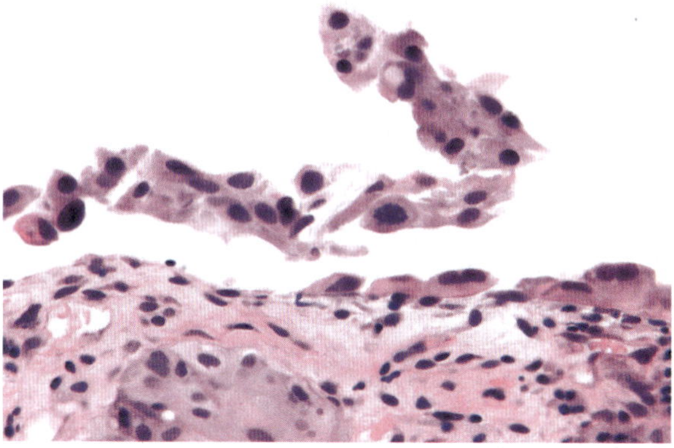

FIGURE 2.26 Discohesive cells of CIS.

the nuclei are still markedly enlarged with significant nuclear chromatin abnormalities. CIS nuclei irrespective of the descriptive pattern are four to six times larger than those in lymphocytes.[9] "Plasmacytoid CIS" is characterized by a triad of morphologic findings that include abnormal architecture of atypical cells within the urothelium, enlarged nuclei with eccentric nuclear localization, and dense globular eosinophilic cytoplasm.[42] Urothelial CIS may show glandular differentiation (distinct from adenocarcinoma *in situ* or glandular dysplasia) and is recognized due to the primarily urothelial nature of the CIS within which glandular architecture is present (see Chapter 8).[43] CIS cells also tend to be discohesive, wherein they can be seen lifting off the basement membrane (Fig. 2.26). Clinging CIS is characterized by a partially denuded urothelium with a patchy, usually single, layer of residual urothelial cells meeting the morphologic criteria for CIS (Figs. 2.27 and 2.28). The lamina propria may be hypervascular

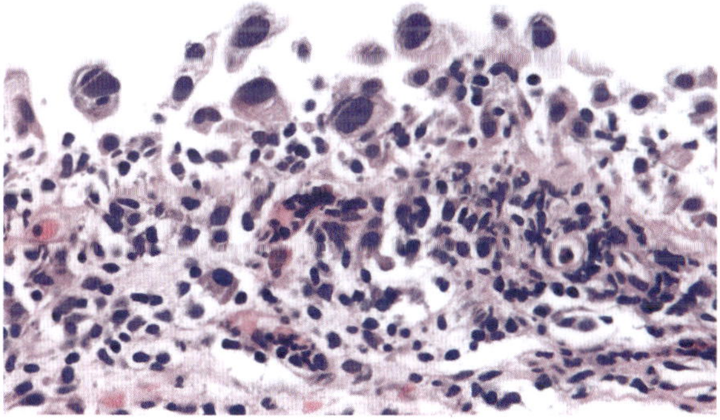

FIGURE 2.27 Clinging CIS.

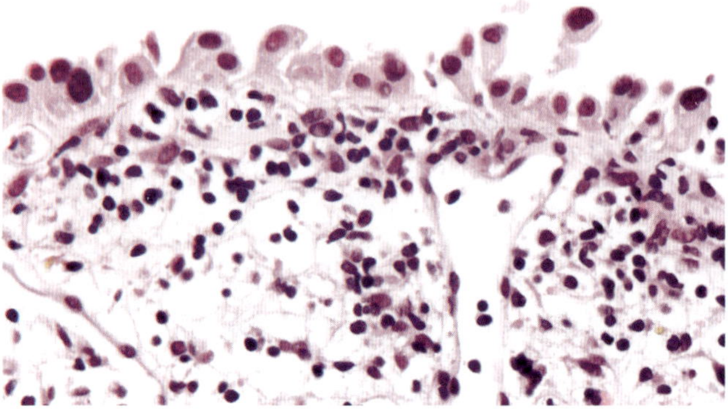

FIGURE 2.28 Clinging CIS.

and inflamed, which is a clue that the overlying epithelium, if absent, was abnormal. Judicious use of recuts may help identify clinging CIS cells. Correlation with cytology is always helpful, particularly in clinging patterns, as the cells are frequently shed in urine. The cytological findings of CIS are indistinguishable from those of other lesions in "The Paris System (TPS)" category of high-grade urothelial carcinoma (see chapter 15 on Urinary Tract Cytopathology).

CIS may also show cancerization of normal urothelium in two patterns: (1) pagetoid spread with the presence of clusters or isolated single cells with features of CIS within normal urothelium and (2) undermining or overriding of the normal urothelium by adjacent CIS (Figs. 2.29 and 2.30). Rare cases of CIS may also show glandlike differentiation or

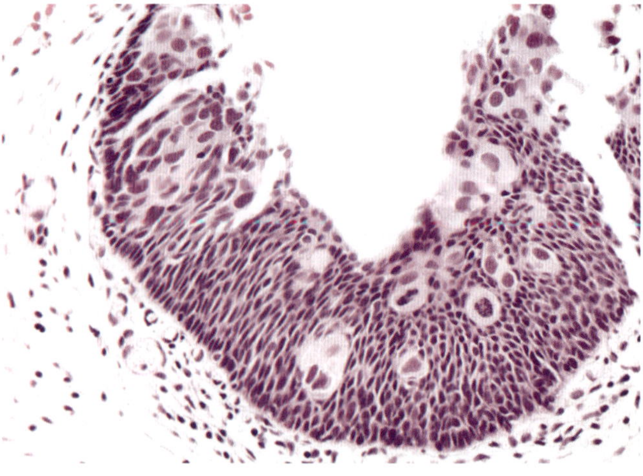

FIGURE 2.29 Pagetoid CIS.

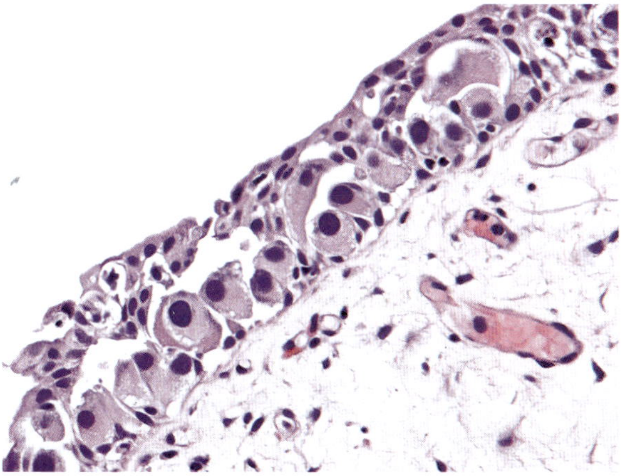

FIGURE 2.30 Pagetoid CIS.

pagetoid spread into squamous metaplasia of the urothelium (Figs. 2.31 and 2.32). The pagetoid pattern of spread is commonly seen in cases with diffuse, multifocal CIS of the bladder and may sometimes be the only pattern seen along the upper and lower urinary tract in these patients, either synchronously or at the time of recurrence. In routine diagnostic practice, we report all CIS cases as simply "urothelial carcinoma *in situ*" and do not include a descriptor of any of the descriptive patterns of CIS in the diagnosis. The terms *large cell nonpleomorphic* and *clinging* merely help pathologists recognize the important lesion of CIS, especially because there is a wide range in its morphologic presentation. On rare occasions, CIS may have a micropapillary architecture, that is, a flat surface but with filigree pattern of micropapillae (pseudopapillae without vascular cores) lined by markedly atypical cells.[6,44] It is important for the pathologist that if the

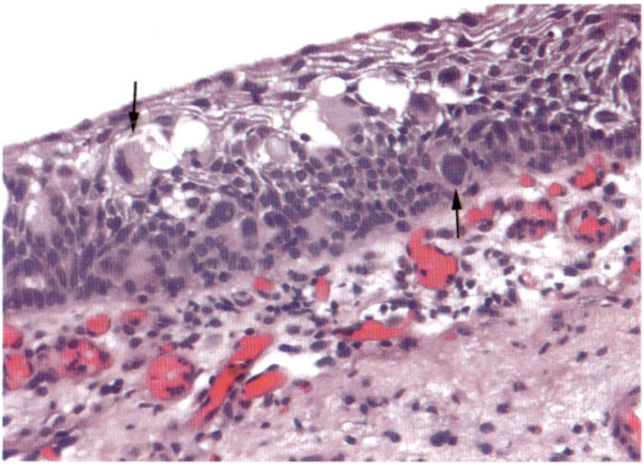

FIGURE 2.31 Pagetoid spread of CIS (*arrows*) within squamous metaplasia.

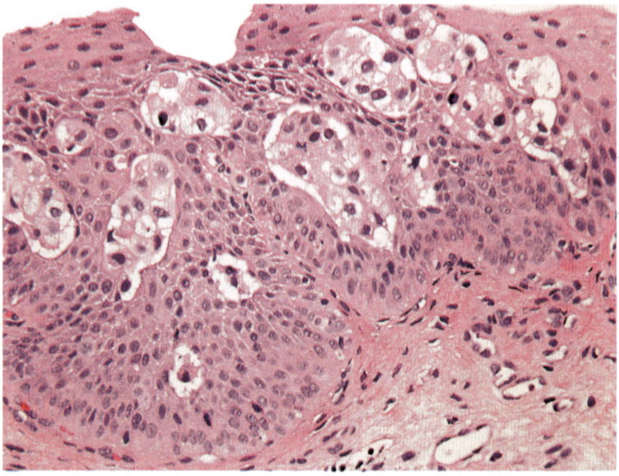

FIGURE 2.32 **Pagetoid spread of CIS within squamous metaplasia.**

term micropapillary CIS is used, that they clarify whether it is associated or not associated with invasive micropapillary carcinoma.

Patients with noninvasive high-grade papillary cancer undergo routine surveillance by protocol and during cystoscopy may have high-grade intraepithelial changes in the mucosa without true papillary formations (also see section below on "Truncated Papillae of Treated or Early Papillary Carcinoma" in Problems and Pitfalls in the Diagnosis of Flat Lesions With Atypia). Absence of true papillary formation may preclude the outright diagnosis of noninvasive high-grade papillary carcinoma, and presence in a predominantly flat or early papillary lesion may raise the question of CIS. The term CIS with early papillary formation may be used in such cases.

The prognostic implications of the different patterns of CIS are not known, and the use of descriptors of CIS, such as clinging or pagetoid, in the surgical pathology report could potentially lead to confusion on the part of the treating urologist. One study has shown that the different subtypes of CIS do not have prognostic significance, although the number of cases studied were small.[45] CIS must also be distinguished from *in situ* squamous cell carcinoma (see Chapter 9).

Distinction of CIS from reactive conditions can be difficult, although in most instances, it is straightforward based on nuclear characteristics. A panel of immunohistochemical antibodies consisting of cytokeratin 20 (CK20), p53, and CD44 (standard isoform) may have utility in the distinction of CIS from reactive atypia and has been the one most studied in the literature.[21,46-49] Although, in experienced hands, immunohistochemistry may be useful, it is a consensus opinion that morphology remains the gold standard in diagnosing CIS.[50] A panel consisting of these three antibodies is important because not all cases of CIS consistently exhibit the characteristic immunostaining specified in the subsequent discussion. Normal urothelium shows reactivity for CK20 only in the superficial umbrella cell

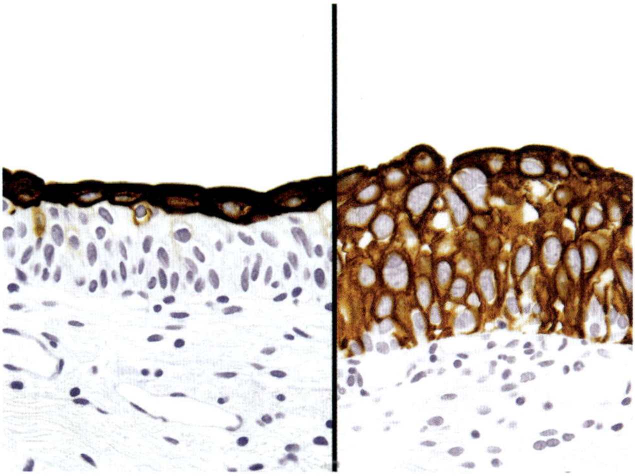

FIGURE 2.33 CK20 labeling only on the umbrella cells in normal urothelium (*left*) contrasted with full-thickness staining in CIS (*right*).

layer, whereas CD44 staining is limited to the basal and parabasal urothelial cells (Figs. 2.33 and 2.34). Nuclear staining for p53 is absent to focal in normal urothelium. Urothelium with reactive atypia shows increased reactivity for CD44 in all layers of the urothelium, particularly in cases with marked atypia. In reactive urothelium, CK20 and p53 reactivity patterns are usually identical to those seen in normal urothelium. In contrast, CIS frequently shows diffuse, strong cytoplasmic reactivity for CK20 and diffuse nuclear reactivity for p53 throughout the full thickness of the urothelium (Figs. 2.33 and 2.35). CD44 reactivity is often absent in CIS. These findings are based on immunohistochemical correlation in morphologically unequivocal cases of CIS and reactive atypia, performed retrospectively. This panel is potentially useful as an adjunct to morphology in several diagnostic situations: (1) in cases in which the pathologist strongly favors the diagnosis of CIS but has reservations making a definitive diag-

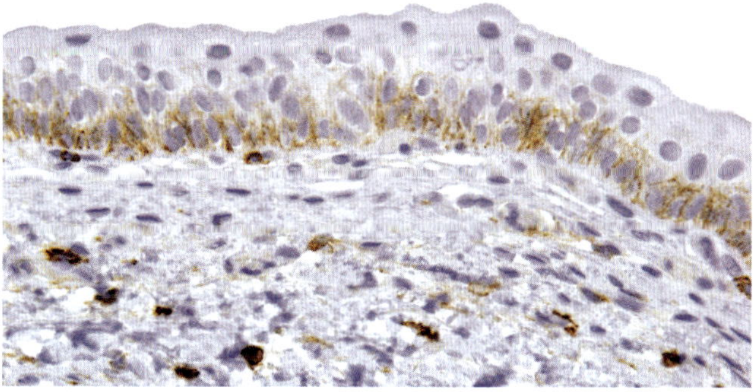

FIGURE 2.34 CD44 labeling of basal cell layer only in normal urothelium.

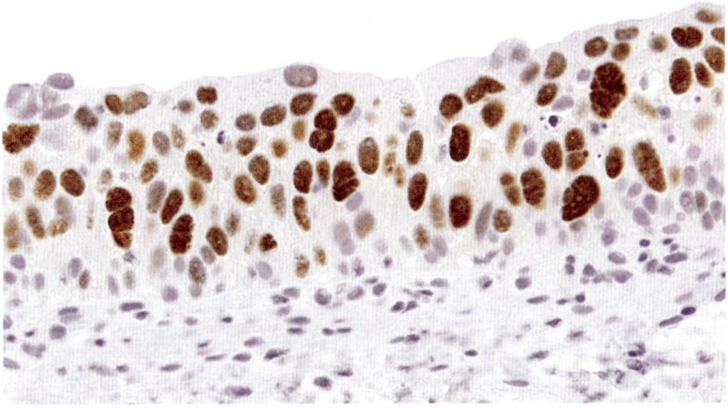

FIGURE 2.35 **Diffuse p53 nuclear labeling in CIS.**

nosis, (2) in the diagnosis of CIS at initial presentation with no known history of a papillary lesion (*de novo* or primary CIS), and (3) in confirming unusual morphologic presentations of CIS such as the cancerization of normal urothelium. This panel is not applicable, in our opinion, in the distinction of dysplasia from CIS as this distinction is one based on threshold at H&E examination. A recent study has examined the utility of this panel in the distinction of radiation-induced atypia from CIS and has found utility, though it is important to interpret the panel strictly in the context of morphology.[48] Other markers such as Ki-67, p16, E-cadherin (for cases with plasmacytoid morphology), Her2/neu, racemase, and UroVysion FISH have been used in this distinction, but their utility in routine practice remains in question.[18,29,51-54] Use of immunohistochemistry in the conformation of CIS must be made in the context of morphology alone as the described immunostaining patterns for CIS may not be seen even in classic cases and we have noted significant overlap between CIS and reactive conditions in our clinical practice or in consultation material. Ki-67, for example, can be briskly positive in both conditions, and morphologically normal urothelium may show prominent CK20 positivity.

The clinical course and biologic potential of CIS is better understood chiefly because it is more often symptomatic and may be detected by cystoscopy, rendering it recognizable by experienced urologists in a primary or *de novo* form. Most patients present with frequency, dysuria, nocturia, and suprapubic fullness; hematuria is typically microscopic.[4,55,56] Approximately 3% of CIS present as primary disease (*de novo* CIS), most CIS that is clinically encountered occurs secondarily and in approximately half to two-thirds of cases of high-grade papillary and invasive urothelial carcinoma. The bladder at cystoscopy appears erythematous or granular, although no abnormality may be present. The biologic potential of CIS is somewhat unpredictable, although the current dogma states that it is a precursor to invasive carcinoma. Almost all CIS lesions recur, and the aggregate evidence in the literature suggests that invasive carcinoma will develop in up to one-half of the patients within 5 years.[23] Guidelines for treatment and follow-up are well established, including for refractory cases. In patients undergoing cystectomy for refractory CIS, ~15%-25% of patients will have microinvasive disease (invasion <2 mm). Patients with CIS are also predisposed to upper tract disease as well as involvement of the prostatic urethra,[57] and the presence of CIS in a cystectomy is significantly predictive of a higher rate of upstaging at radical cystectomy.[58]

The evolution from CIS to invasion may be highly variable with some cases having rapid progression and others a more protracted time course. From a clinical perspective, extent of disease (focal, multifocal, or extensive), involvement of prostatic urethra, and response to therapy are the principal determinants of clinical outcome. Patients with primary (*de novo*) CIS are more likely to have no evidence of disease (62% vs 45%) and are less likely to progress (28% vs 59%) or die of disease (7% vs 45%) when compared with patients with CIS occurring in patients with papillary bladder neoplasia.[59] Whether this fact is due to the presence of papillary disease, multifocality, or extent of disease remains unknown. Cheng et al.[60] reported disease progression in 35% of CIS cases, of which 20% died of urothelial carcinoma. Davis et al.[61] estimated 55% 10-year progression-free survival for patients with CIS treated with BCG.

Contemporary sequencing has shown several recurrent mutations in CIS: TERT promoter mutation (50%), mutation in cell cycle genes (TP53, MDM2, CCND1, CDKN1A, CDKN2A, CCNE1, and FBXW7) in >70% of cases, mutations in chromatin-modifying factors (ARID1A, KDM6A, CREBBP, and EP300) in 60%-70% of cases, mutations in DNA damage response genes (BRCA2, ATM, BRCA1, and ERCC2) in 60% of cases, and mutations in PI3K/MAPK genes (ERBB2 [HER2], FGFR1, PIK3CA, EGFR, RAF1, and NF1) in ~30%-40% of cases.[62]

PROBLEMS AND PITFALLS IN THE DIAGNOSIS OF FLAT LESIONS WITH ATYPIA

Innate Vagaries of Normal Urothelium and Histologic Sectioning

The thickness of the normal urothelium varies with the state of distention of the bladder. If the sections are thick, the urothelium may appear hyperchromatic, and this artifact, compounded with tangential sectioning, may result in changes thought to represent dysplasia. The urothelium of the renal pelvis, urethra, and bladder neck is usually composed of cells with slightly larger nuclei and diminished cytoplasmic clearing and, hence, may be misinterpreted as dysplasia. Occasionally, typical umbrella cells can be displaced so that they are not on the surface, mimicking CIS (Fig. 2.36). Cells within von Brunn nests also have slightly enlarged nuclei mimicking dysplasia (Fig. 1.15).

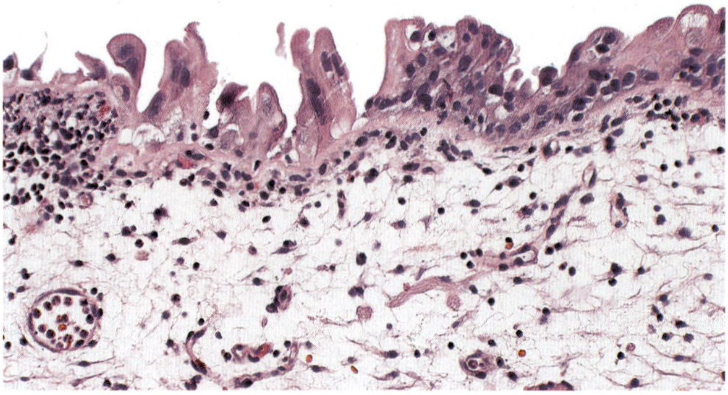

FIGURE 2.36 **Displaced umbrella cells mimicking CIS.**

Inflammatory Atypia

Inflammatory atypia and nonpleomorphic forms of CIS share in common the presence of enlarged nuclei with prominent nucleoli. Attention to other nuclear characteristics of neoplasia is necessary to diagnose CIS in such settings. The presence of acute or significant chronic inflammation, particularly in an intraurothelial location, warrants caution in the interpretation of dysplasia or CIS, although inflammatory atypia may coexist with dysplasia or CIS (Figs. 2.37 and 2.38). The presence of nuclear chromatin irregularities, atypical mitoses, multiple nucleoli with nucleolar pleomorphism argue against a reactive condition.

Therapy-Associated Atypia

While the changes inflicted by therapy, at an overarching level argue for a reactive condition, different therapies may have varying impact on

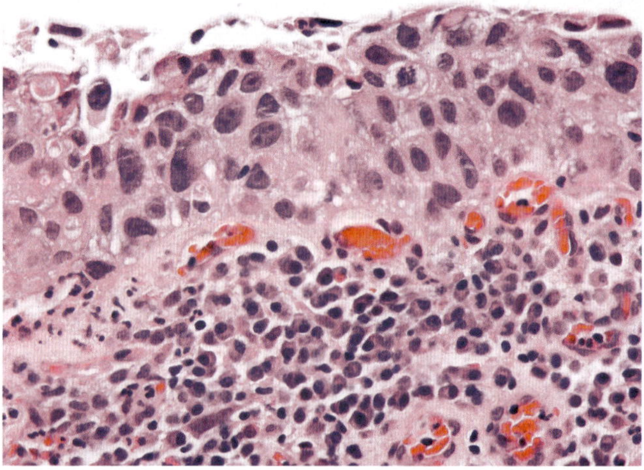

FIGURE 2.37 **CIS with intense lamina propria inflammation.** Nuclei vary in size and shape compared to nuclei with reactive changes.

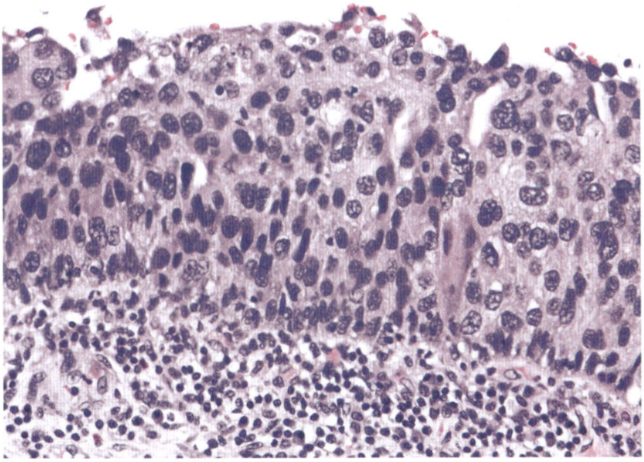

FIGURE 2.38 **CIS with intense lamina propria inflammation.** Nuclei are more hyperchromatic compared to nuclei with reactive changes.

the bladder, which depending on severity of changes significantly mimic intraepithelial neoplasia. Table 2.4 provides a summary of these therapy-associated changes.[12,63-65] The regenerative and reactive changes imparted by therapy to some extent vary upon the type of therapy.[48,65] Intravesical BCG therapy is the most common therapy for CIS, and pathologic alterations include denudation and ulceration of the urothelium, non-caseating granulomas, lamina propria edema and inflammation, and regenerative atypia (enlarged uniform nuclei with even chromatin distribution and prominent nucleoli). The urothelium may be entirely normal. Thiotepa and mitomycin C induce atypical changes primarily on the surface umbrella cells (large cells with multinucleation, smudged nuclear chromatin, and cytoplasmic vacuolation) (Fig. 2.39). In some patients, a range of findings from reactive/regenerative urothelium, normal urothelium, and CIS may be present concurrently in biopsies. Systemic cyclophosphamide therapy may result in large multinucleated urothelial cells with smudged to vacuolated nuclear chromatin, identical to changes seen with radiation. Other changes include hemorrhagic cystitis, encrusted cystitis, and reactivation of polyomavirus infection. Bladder cancer following cyclophosphamide treatment has been reported. Radiation can induce full thickness atypia closely mimicking CIS; however, there are often multinucleated cells with bizarre nuclei not typical of intraurothelial neoplasia (see Chapter 10). The cytoplasm in radiation atypia is often prominent and may show degenerative changes with vacuolization. Other associated changes may be identified in the bladder wall, including atypical fibroblasts and radiation vasculopathy. Pseudocarcinomatous epithelial proliferation, mimicking invasive carcinoma, may be seen (see Chapter 10). Effects of some other treatment modalities are summarized in Table 2.4.

TABLE 2.4 Summary of Treatment-Related Changes in Bladder Cancer	
Type of Therapy	**Histopathologic Features**
Intravesical immunotherapy (BCG, interferon-α)	BCG-induced granulomatous inflammation Extensive denudation and ulceration with reactive atypia Interferon-α: lamina propria edema with mild perivascular inflammation
Intravesical mitomycin C chemotherapy	Denudation and ulceration with surface umbrella cells atypia (low nuclear to cytoplasmic ratio). Abnormalities are more subtle or lesser in basal and intermediate cell layers
Cyclophosphamide therapy (systemic)	Necrosis of urothelium; large, bizarre nuclei with coarse chromatin and small- to medium-sized nucleoli; frequent multinucleation
Neoadjuvant chemotherapy	Minor atypia of nonneoplastic urothelium; persistence of native disease–urothelial CIS or non–muscle-invasive disease. Invasive tumor necrosis (variable to complete) and xanthoma cells
Radiation therapy	Mucosal ulceration, denudation, and reactive atypia with raised nuclear to cytoplasmic ratio; multinucleation. Reactive atypical stromal cells and vascular thrombosis in lamina propria. Pseudocarcinomatous hyperplasia. Squamoid change and bladder wall fibrosis (late stage)
Surgery-related pathologic features	Nonspecific granulomatous reaction; postsurgical necrobiotic granuloma; postoperative spindle cell nodule and suture granuloma
Ketamine use	Urothelial denudation and ulceration with prominent granulation tissue. Severe reactive atypia mimicking CIS
Gene therapy	Marked cytoplasmic vacuolization of tumor cells in early phases. B cells and macrophage inflammatory infiltrate. Nonneoplastic tissues usually unaffected and demarcated. Apoptosis-mediated tumor necrosis
Photodynamic and laser therapy	Spindling artifact of urothelial cells. Minimal but variable changes with edema in lamina propria to coagulative to hemorrhagic necrosis. Dystrophic calcifications

Modified and adapted from Amin MB, Comperat E, Epstein JI, et al. The genitourinary pathology society update on classification and grading of flat and papillary urothelial neoplasia with new reporting recommendations and approach to lesions with mixed and early patterns of neoplasia. *Adv Anat Pathol*. 2021;28(4):179-195; Lopez-Beltran A, Montironi R, Raspollini MR, et al. Iatrogenic pathology of the urinary bladder. *Semin Diagn Pathol*. 2018;35(4):218-227; Lopez-Beltran A, Paner GP, Montironi R, et al. Iatrogenic changes in the urinary tract. *Histopathology*. 2017;70(1):10-25; Lopez-Beltran A, Luque RJ, Mazzucchelli R, et al. Changes produced in the urothelium by traditional and newer therapeutic procedures for bladder cancer. *J Clin Pathol*. 2002;55(9):641-647.

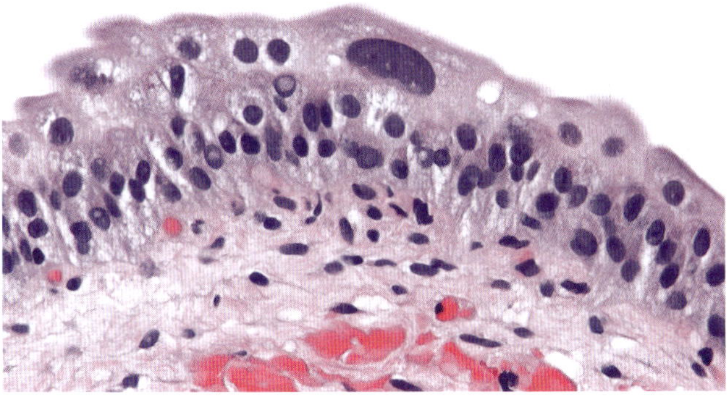

FIGURE 2.39 Mitomycin-induced atypia of umbrella cells.

Extensive Denudation

Trauma due to instrumentation, prior therapy, and CIS are the main conditions associated with denudation. The presence of a few atypical single cells clinging to the surface is sometimes the only sign of CIS ("denuding cystitis"); deeper sections through the block may reveal diagnostic cells. In the absence of atypical cells, the finding of extensive denudation, particularly that associated with neovascularity and chronic inflammation in the lamina propria, must be included in the report, and correlation with urine cytology findings may be suggested (Fig. 2.40). In cases of true denuding cystitis resulting from CIS, urine or bladder wash cytology may contain a large number of neoplastic cells.[66]

Truncated Papillae of Treated or Early Papillary Carcinoma

Mitomycin C and thiotepa therapy destroys the tips of the papillae of papillary urothelial carcinoma because they act as surface abrasives (Fig. 2.41).

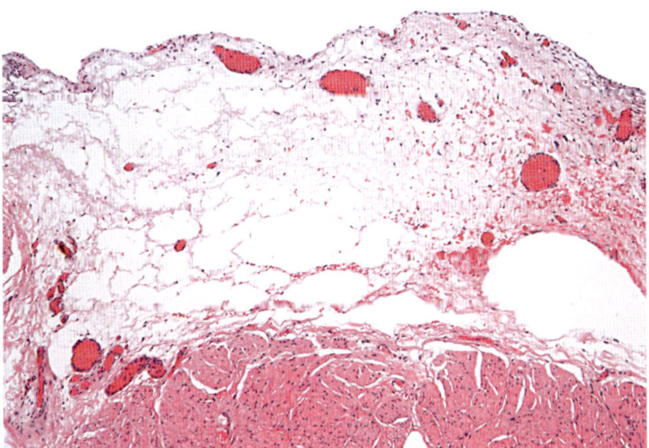

FIGURE 2.40 Bladder with urothelial denudation.

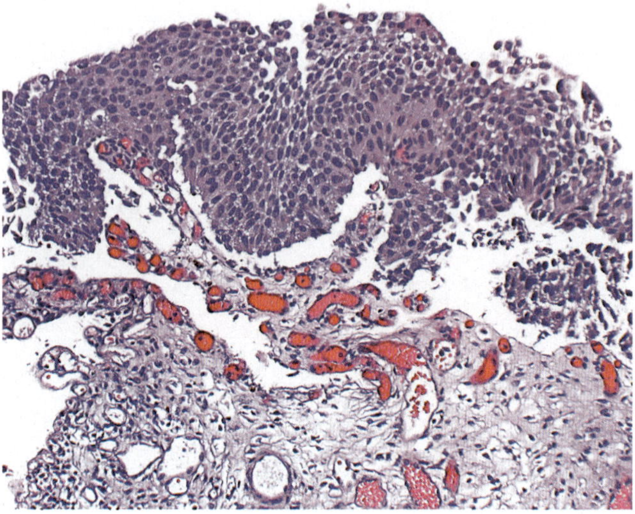

FIGURE 2.41 Truncated papillae in papillary urothelial carcinoma following intravesical chemotherapy.

When these truncated papillae are seen in areas associated with denudation and inflammation, they may be mistaken for CIS or dysplastic changes instead of residual papillary urothelial carcinoma.[67] An unusual form of CIS that could mimic truncated papillae of treated papillary carcinoma is CIS with micropapillary features (Fig. 2.42). One may also see urothelium having the cytology of dysplasia or CIS with tenting of the urothelium (ie, architecture seen in papillary urothelial hyperplasia). These cases are often seen in patients who are undergoing surveillance cystoscopy where

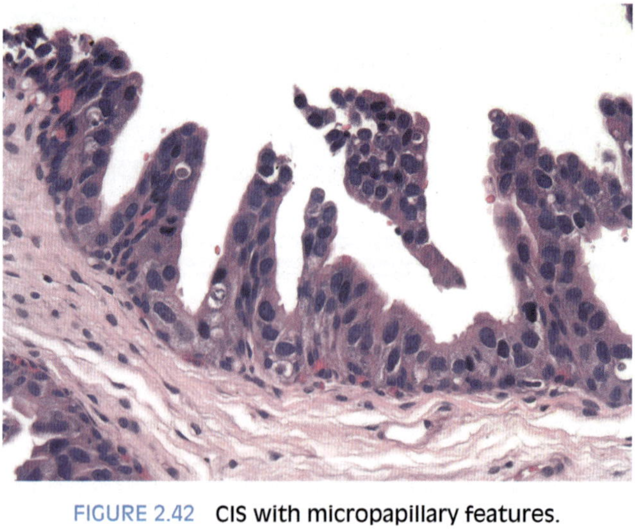

FIGURE 2.42 CIS with micropapillary features.

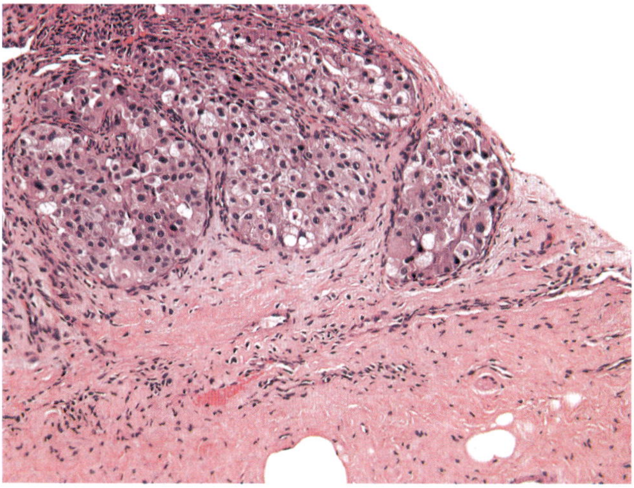

FIGURE 2.43 CIS within von Brunn nests.

the earliest papillary urothelial neoplasms are biopsied. In the absence of a clinical history of treatment, terminology such as "dysplasia with early papillary formation" or "CIS with early papillary formation" may be used (see Chapter 3). Correlation with clinical history of previous grade and stage of bladder cancer and cystoscopy is necessary.

Carcinoma *In Situ* Involving von Brunn Nests: Overdiagnosis of Invasion

CIS can involve von Brunn nests, resulting in the presence of nests of neoplastic cells within the superficial lamina propria (Figs. 2.43-2.45). In general, von Brunn nests have a round contour and lack retraction artifact or

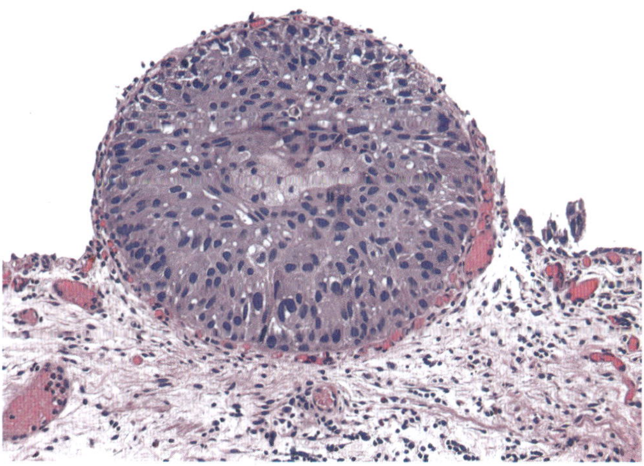

FIGURE 2.44 CIS within von Brunn nests.

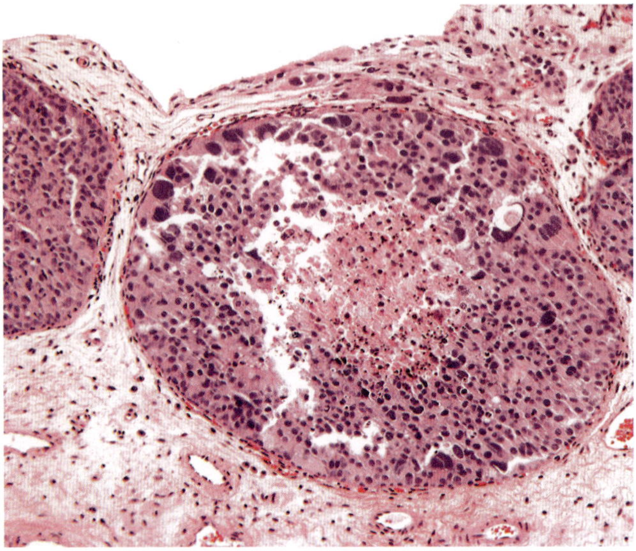

FIGURE 2.45 CIS with central necrosis involving von Brunn nests.

surrounding stromal changes. In the presence of inflammation, however, the basement membrane may be obscured and distorted, simulating invasion.

Carcinoma *In Situ* With Microinvasion: Underdiagnosis of Invasion

A histologically subtle, but potentially ominous, clinical situation arises when CIS is associated with microinvasion (see Chapter 5). The urologist is most often unsuspecting of invasive disease on the basis of cystoscopic evaluation, and the pathologist may fail to recognize single cell invasion or small clusters of invasion that may be camouflaged by background inflammation. Desmoplasia or retraction artifact is useful in recognizing invasion, but a stromal response may be absent.[21,68] Although infrequent, it is imperative that one pays attention to the lamina propria just below the CIS or denuded urothelium to look for early (microinvasion) as it could be a clinically significant finding.

Polyomavirus Infection

Infection of immunocompromised patients with the human polyomavirus, usually a nonpathogenic virus, results in large homogeneous inclusions in enlarged nuclei of urothelial cells or "decoy cells" (see Chapter 10). The findings are more frequently seen in urine cytology but may rarely be found on biopsy; in both specimens, malignancy (CIS) is mimicked.[69,70] Morphology is usually diagnostic, although immunohistochemical stains for the polyoma virus using the large T antigen of SV40 as a surrogate may be useful.

REFERENCES

1. Karl A, Tritschler S, Stanislaus P, et al. Positive urine cytology but negative white-light cystoscopy: an indication for fluorescence cystoscopy? *BJU Int.* 2009;103(4):484-487.
2. Veeratterapillay R, Gravestock P, Nambiar A, et al. Time to turn on the blue lights: a systematic review and meta-analysis of photodynamic diagnosis for bladder cancer. *Eur Urol Open Sci.* 2021;31:17-27.
3. Eble JN, Epstein JI, Sesterhenn IA. *Pathology & Genetics of Tumors of the Urinary System and Male Genital Organs.* IARC. 2004.
4. Nese N, Gupta R, Bui MHT, Amin MB. Carcinoma in situ of the urinary bladder: review of clinicopathologic characteristics with an emphasis on aspects related to molecular diagnostic techniques and prognosis. *J Natl Compr Cancer Netw.* 2009;7(1):48-57.
5. Tavora F, Epstein JI. Bladder cancer, pathological classification and staging. *BJU Int.* 2008;102(9 Pt B):1216-1220.
6. Amin MB, McKenney JK. An approach to the diagnosis of flat intraepithelial lesions of the urinary bladder using the World Health Organization/International Society of Urological Pathology consensus classification system. *Adv Anat Pathol.* 2002;9(4):222-232.
7. *WHO Classification of Tumours of the Urinary System and Male Genital Organs.* 4th ed. WHO Press; 2016.
8. Raspolini MR, Amin MB, Hartmann A, Moch H, Srigley JR. Tumours of the urinary tract: introduction. In: Comperat EM, Netto GJ, Tsuzki T, eds. *WHO classification of tumours. Urinary and Male Genital Tumours.* 5th ed. International Agency for Research on Cancer; 2022:2-3. Chapter 3, Section 5.0.0.1.
9. Milord RA, Lecksell K, Epstein JI. An objective morphologic parameter to aid in the diagnosis of flat urothelial carcinoma in situ. *Hum Pathol.* 2001;32(9):997-1002.
10. Guo CC, Fine SW, Epstein JI. Noninvasive squamous lesions in the urinary bladder: a clinicopathologic analysis of 29 cases. *Am J Surg Pathol.* 2006;30(7):883-891.
11. Tannenbaum M. Inflammatory proliferative lesion of urinary bladder: squamous metaplasia. *Urology.* 1976;7(4):428-429.
12. Amin MB, Comperat E, Epstein JI, et al. The genitourinary pathology society update on classification and grading of flat and papillary urothelial neoplasia with new reporting recommendations and approach to lesions with mixed and early patterns of neoplasia. *Adv Anat Pathol.* 2021;28(4):179-195.
13. Lowenthal BM, Sahoo D, Amin MB, Hansel DE. Urothelial proliferation of unknown malignant potential involving the bladder: histopathologic features and risk of progression in de novo cases and cases with prior neoplasia. *Arch Pathol Lab Med.* 2020;144(7):853-862.
14. Hartmann A, Moser K, Kriegmair M, et al. Frequent genetic alterations in simple urothelial hyperplasias of the bladder in patients with papillary urothelial carcinoma. *Am J Pathol.* 1999;154(3):721-727.
15. Obermann EC, Junker K, Stoehr R, et al. Frequent genetic alterations in flat urothelial hyperplasias and concomitant papillary bladder cancer as detected by CGH, LOH, and FISH analyses. *J Pathol.* 2003;199(1):50-57.
16. van Oers JMM, Adam C, Denzinger S, et al. Chromosome 9 deletions are more frequent than FGFR3 mutations in flat urothelial hyperplasias of the bladder. *Int J Cancer.* 2006;119(5):1212-1215.
17. Mazzucchelli R, Barbisan F, Stramazzotti D, et al. Chromosomal abnormalities in macroscopically normal urothelium in patients with bladder pT1 and pT2a urothelial carcinoma: a fluorescence in situ hybridization study and correlation with histologic features. *Anal Quant Cytol Histol.* 2005;27(3):143-151.
18. Schwarz S, Rechenmacher M, Filbeck T, et al. Value of multicolour fluorescence in situ hybridisation (UroVysion) in the differential diagnosis of flat urothelial lesions. *J Clin Pathol.* 2008;61(3):272-277.

19. Weyerer V, Eckstein M, Strissel PL, et al. TERT promoter mutation analysis of whole-organ mapping bladder cancers. *Genes.* 2021;12(2):230.
20. Paner GP, Smith SC, Hartmann A, et al. Flat intraurothelial lesions of the urinary bladder–do hyperplasia, dysplasia, and atypia of unknown significance need to exist as diagnostic entities? and how to handle in routine clinical practice. *Mod Pathol.* 2022;35(10):1296-1305.
21. McKenney JK, Desai S, Cohen C, Amin MB. Discriminatory immunohistochemical staining of urothelial carcinoma in situ and non-neoplastic urothelium: an analysis of cytokeratin 20, p53, and CD44 antigens. *Am J Surg Pathol.* 2001;25(8):1074-1078.
22. Amin MB, Young RH. Intraepithelial lesions of the urinary bladder with a discussion of the histogenesis of urothelial neoplasia. *Semin Diagn Pathol.* 1997;14(2):84-97.
23. Cheng L, Cheville JC, Neumann RM, Bostwick DG. Flat intraepithelial lesions of the urinary bladder. *Cancer.* 2000;88(3):625-631.
24. Ziemba JB, Golan R, Skokan A, et al. The clinical presentation and outcome of urothelial atypia on biopsy of the bladder. *Urol Oncol.* 2014;32(5):645-647.
25. Lawless ME, Tretiakova MS, True LD, Vakar-Lopez F. Flat urothelial lesions with atypia: interobserver concordance and added value of immunohistochemical profiling. *Appl Immunohistochem Mol Morphol.* 2018;26(3):180-185.
26. Ayala AG, Ro JY. Premalignant lesions of urothelium and transitional cell tumors. In: Young RH, ed. *Contemporary Issues in Surgical Pathology: Pathology of the Urinary Bladder.* Churchill Livingstone; 1989:65-101.
27. Murphy WM, Soloway MS. Developing carcinoma (dysplasia) of the urinary bladder. In: Sommers SC, Rosen PP, eds. *Pathology Annual.* Vol. 17. Appleton-Century-Crofts; 1982:197-217.
28. Epstein JI, Amin MB, Reuter VR, Mostofi FK. The World Health Organization/International Society of Urological Pathology consensus classification of urothelial (transitional cell) neoplasms of the urinary bladder. Bladder Consensus Conference Committee. *Am J Surg Pathol.* 1998;22(12):1435-1448.
29. Amin MB, McKenney JK, Paner GP, et al. ICUD-EAU International consultation on bladder cancer 2012: pathology. *Eur Urol.* 2013;63(1):16-35.
30. Amin MB, Smith SC, Reuter VE, et al. Update for the practicing pathologist: The International Consultation On Urologic Disease-European association of urology consultation on bladder cancer. *Mod Pathol Off J U S Can Acad Pathol Inc.* 2015;28(5):612-630.
31. Althausen AF, Prout GR, Daly JJ. Non-invasive papillary carcinoma of the bladder associated with carcinoma in situ. *J Urol.* 1976;116(5):575-580.
32. Murphy WM, Miller AW. In: Javadpour NE, ed. *Bladder Cancer.* Lippincott Williams & Wilkins; 1984:100-122.
33. Smith G, Elton RA, Beynon LL, et al. Prognostic significance of biopsy results of normal-looking mucosa in cases of superficial bladder cancer. *Br J Urol.* 1983;55(6):665-669.
34. Cheng L, Cheville JC, Neumann RM, Bostwick DG. Natural history of urothelial dysplasia of the bladder. *Am J Surg Pathol.* 1999;23(4):443-447.
35. Mostofi FK, Sesterhenn IA. Pathology of epithelial tumors & carcinoma in situ of bladder. *Prog Clin Biol Res.* 1984;162A:55-74.
36. Majewski T, Yao H, Bondaruk J, et al. Whole-organ genomic characterization of mucosal field effects initiating bladder carcinogenesis. *Cell Rep.* 2019;26(8):2241-2256.e4.
37. Czerniak B, Li L, Chaturvedi V, et al. Genetic modeling of human urinary bladder carcinogenesis. *Genes Chromosomes Cancer.* 2000;27(4):392-402.
38. Hartmann A, Schlake G, Zaak D, et al. Occurrence of chromosome 9 and p53 alterations in multifocal dysplasia and carcinoma in situ of human urinary bladder. *Cancer Res.* 2002;62(3):809-818.
39. Levi AW, Potter SR, Schoenberg MP, Epstein JI. Clinical significance of denuded urothelium in bladder biopsy. *J Urol.* 2001;166(2):457-460.

40. Amin MB, Murphy WM, Reuter VE. Controversies in the pathology of transitional cell carcinoma of the urinary bladder. Part I, Chapter 1. In: Rosen PP, Fechner RE, eds. *Reviews of Pathology*. Vol. 1. ASCP Press; 1996:1-39.
41. McKenney JK, Gomez JA, Desai S, et al. Morphologic expressions of urothelial carcinoma in situ: a detailed evaluation of its histologic patterns with emphasis on carcinoma in situ with microinvasion. *Am J Surg Pathol.* 2001;25(3):356-362.
42. Sangoi AR, Falzarano SM, Nicolas M, McKenney JK. Carcinoma in situ with plasmacytoid features: a clinicopathologic study of 23 cases. *Am J Surg Pathol.* 2019;43(12):1638-1643.
43. Yang Z, Epstein JI. Urothelial carcinoma in situ of the bladder with glandular differentiation: report of 92 cases. *Am J Surg Pathol.* 2018;42(7):971-976.
44. Amin A, Epstein JI. Noninvasive micropapillary urothelial carcinoma: a clinicopathologic study of 18 cases. *Hum Pathol.* 2012;43(12):2124-2128.
45. Compérat E, Jacquet SF, Varinot J, et al. Different subtypes of carcinoma in situ of the bladder do not have a different prognosis. *Virchows Arch Int J Pathol.* 2013;462(3):343-348.
46. Harnden P, Eardley I, Joyce AD, Southgate J. Cytokeratin 20 as an objective marker of urothelial dysplasia. *Br J Urol.* 1996;78(6):870-875.
47. Sarkis AS, Dalbagni G, Cordon-Cardo C, et al. Association of P53 nuclear overexpression and tumor progression in carcinoma in situ of the bladder. *J Urol.* 1994;152(2 Pt 1):388-392.
48. Oliva E, Pinheiro NF, Heney NM, et al. Immunohistochemistry as an adjunct in the differential diagnosis of radiation-induced atypia versus urothelial carcinoma in situ of the bladder: a study of 45 cases. *Hum Pathol.* 2013;44(5):860-866.
49. Neal DJ, Amin MB, Smith SC. CK20 versus AMACR and p53 immunostains in evaluation of urothelial carcinoma in situ and reactive atypia. *Diagn Pathol.* 2020;15(1):61.
50. Amin MB, Trpkov K, Lopez-Beltran A, et al. Best practices recommendations in the application of immunohistochemistry in the bladder lesions: report from the International Society of Urologic Pathology consensus conference. *Am J Surg Pathol.* 2014;38:e20-e34.
51. Yin H, He Q, Li T, Leong ASY. Cytokeratin 20 and Ki-67 to distinguish carcinoma in situ from flat non-neoplastic urothelium. *Appl Immunohistochem Mol Morphol.* 2006;14(3):260-265.
52. Yin M, Bastacky S, Parwani AV, et al. p16ink4 immunoreactivity is a reliable marker for urothelial carcinoma in situ. *Hum Pathol.* 2008;39(4):527-535.
53. Aron M, Luthringer DJ, McKenney JK, et al. Utility of a triple antibody cocktail intraurothelial neoplasm-3 (IUN-3-CK20/CD44s/p53) and α-methylacyl-CoA racemase (AMACR) in the distinction of urothelial carcinoma in situ (CIS) and reactive urothelial atypia. *Am J Surg Pathol.* 2013;37(12):1815-1823.
54. Gunia S, Koch S, Hakenberg OW, et al. Different HER2 protein expression profiles aid in the histologic differential diagnosis between urothelial carcinoma in situ (CIS) and non-CIS conditions (dysplasia and reactive atypia) of the urinary bladder mucosa. *Am J Clin Pathol.* 2011;136(6):881-888.
55. Lamm DL. Carcinoma in situ. *Urol Clin North Am.* 1992;19(3):499-508.
56. Murphy WM, Soloway MS. Urothelial dysplasia. *J Urol.* 1982;127(5):849-854.
57. Youssef RF, Shariat SF, Lotan Y, et al. Prognostic effect of urinary bladder carcinoma in situ on clinical outcome of subsequent upper tract urothelial carcinoma. *Urology.* 2011;77(4):861-866.
58. Yafi FA, Aprikian AG, Chin JL, et al. Impact of concomitant carcinoma in situ on upstaging and outcome following radical cystectomy for bladder cancer. *World J Urol.* 2014;32(5):1295-1301.
59. Orozco RE, Martin AA, Murphy WM. Carcinoma in situ of the urinary bladder. Clues to host involvement in human carcinogenesis. *Cancer.* 1994;74(1):115-122.

60. Cheng L, Cheville JC, Neumann RM, et al. Survival of patients with carcinoma in situ of the urinary bladder. *Cancer.* 1999;85(11):2469-2474.
61. Davis JW, Sheth SI, Doviak MJ, et al. Superficial bladder carcinoma treated with bacillus Calmette-Guerin: progression-free and disease specific survival with minimum 10-year followup. *J Urol.* 2002;167:494-500.
62. Garczyk S, Ortiz-Brüchle N, Schneider U, et al. Next-generation sequencing reveals potential predictive biomarkers and targets of therapy for urothelial carcinoma in situ of the urinary bladder. *Am J Pathol.* 2020;190(2):323-332.
63. Lopez-Beltran A, Montironi R, Raspollini MR, et al. Iatrogenic pathology of the urinary bladder. *Semin Diagn Pathol.* 2018;35(4):218-227.
64. Lopez-Beltran A, Paner GP, Montironi R, et al. Iatrogenic changes in the urinary tract. *Histopathology.* 2017;70(1):10-25.
65. Lopez-Beltran A, Luque RJ, Mazzucchelli R, et al. Changes produced in the urothelium by traditional and newer therapeutic procedures for bladder cancer. *J Clin Pathol.* 2002;55(9):641-647.
66. Parwani AV, Levi AW, Epstein JI, Ali SZ. Urinary bladder biopsy with denuded mucosa: denuding cystitis-cytopathologic correlates. *Diagn Cytopathol.* 2004;30(5):297-300.
67. Murphy WM, Soloway MS, Finebaum PJ. Pathological changes associated with topical chemotherapy for superficial bladder cancer. *J Urol.* 1981;126(4):461-464.
68. Amin MB, Gómez JA, Young RH. Urothelial transitional cell carcinoma with endophytic growth patterns: a discussion of patterns of invasion and problems associated with assessment of invasion in 18 cases. *Am J Surg Pathol.* 1997;21(9):1057-1068.
69. Koss LG. *Diagnostic Cytology and Its Histopathologic Basis*. 4th ed. JB Lippincott; 1992.
70. Weinreb DB. BK virus and carcinoma of the prostate, kidney and bladder. *Br J Cancer.* 2006;94:1948 author reply 1949-1950.

3

PAPILLARY UROTHELIAL NEOPLASMS AND THEIR PRECURSORS

PAPILLARY UROTHELIAL HYPERPLASIA

Papillary urothelial hyperplasia is the term used by one of the current authors in 1996 and further studied in 2010 to describe a well-defined entity considered to be a precursor to low-grade papillary urothelial neoplasms.[1-3] Prior to these works, *papillary urothelial hyperplasia* was used, in addition, less restrictively to describe polypoid cystitis and urothelial papillomas. In the 2004 WHO (third edition) Classification of Tumours under the category of *Urothelial hyperplasia*, the only mention of this entity was that "Within the spectrum of hyperplasia a papillary architecture may be present; most of these patients have concomitant papillary tumors."[4] In the 2016 WHO (fourth edition) blue book, the term "*urothelial proliferation of uncertain malignant potential (UPUMP)*" was introduced and defined as a "marked thickening of the urothelium with no or minimal cytological atypia and no true papillary fronds."[5] Both a flat lesion and one with mucosal folds were included in this category. Arguments against the term *papillary urothelial hyperplasia* were that the lesion lacked true papillary fronds so that *papillary* and *hyperplasia* were mutually exclusive. The term *UPUMP* never caught on, and in 2021, the Genitourinary Pathology Society recommended the term "atypical proliferative lesion, papillary" for papillary urothelial hyperplasia.[6] In the latest 2022 WHO (fifth edition) blue book, the entity is not listed as an entity and not illustrated.[7] The only mention of it is within the introduction to the Urinary Tract section where it refers to *papillary urothelial hyperplasia/UPUMP* as follows: "In this fifth-edition WHO classification, such lesions are no longer recognized as a unique entity; rather, they are considered early low-grade noninvasive papillary carcinoma or an extension of such tumors." As will be discussed below, the authors of this book recognized that in some instances, the WHO viewpoint has merit, yet in other situations, it does a disservice to patients by labeling them as having carcinoma for a lesion that morphologically and biologically does not warrant such a diagnosis. The pros and

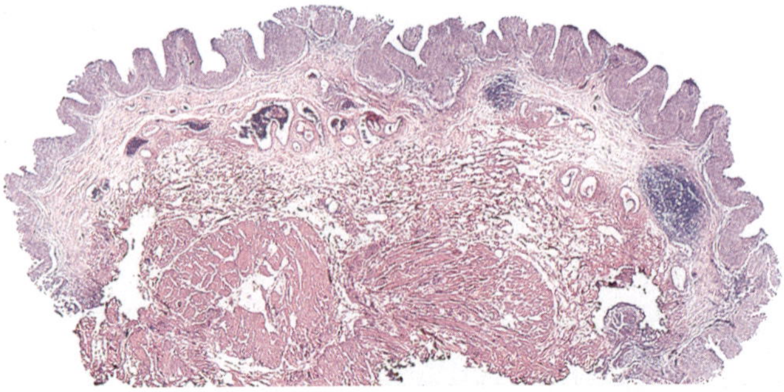

FIGURE 3.1 **Papillary urothelial hyperplasia.**

cons for different terminology and recommendations for using the term in clinical practice have been recently reviewed.[8] Within this book, *papillary urothelial hyperplasia* will be used.

Papillary urothelial hyperplasia may be a precursor lesion to low-grade papillary urothelial neoplasms.[1-3] Typically, they are discovered on routine follow-up cystoscopy for papillary urothelial neoplasms and less frequently in the workup for microhematuria or urinary obstructive symptoms. In most cases at cystoscopy, a focal elevated or roughened lesion is identified that is variably described as "bleblike," "papillary," "raised," "sessile," or "frondular."

Histologically, papillary urothelial hyperplasia consists of undulating urothelium arranged into mucosal narrow papillary folds of varying heights (Figs. 3.1-3.4, eFigs. 3.1-3.7). Both the urothelium within papillary hyperplasia and the adjacent flat mucosa are often thicker than normal. In addition to the diagnostic mucosal folds, in some cases, there are also tent-shaped, somewhat broader folds that lack the edema and inflammation typical of polypoid cystitis. The cytological findings in typical papillary urothelial hyperplasia are similar to that in normal urothelium. Some cases show increased vascularity in the stroma at the base of the papillary

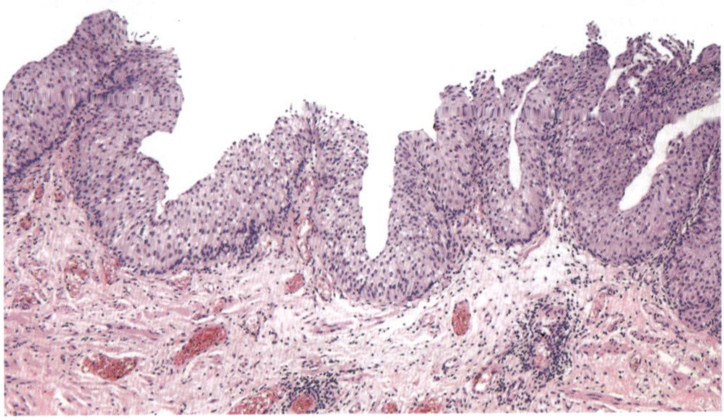

FIGURE 3.2 **Papillary urothelial hyperplasia.**

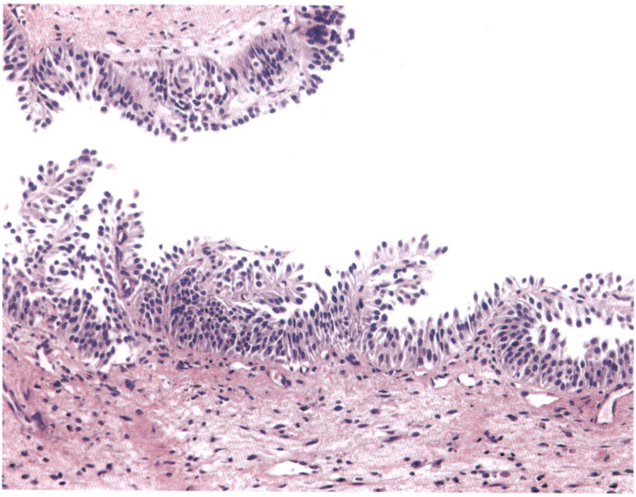

FIGURE 3.3 **Papillary urothelial hyperplasia.**

folds. An occasional case may also demonstrate early slight branching beginning at the top of one of the folds of the papillary hyperplasia. Papillary urothelial hyperplasia is distinguished from papillary urothelial neoplasms by lack of true fibrovascular cores within the hyperplastic mucosa, lack of complex arborization, and hence the absence of the appearance of "detached" papillary fronds (Figs. 3.5 and 3.6). It is distinguished from papillary urothelial proliferation of low malignant potential (PUNLMP) (lacking true fibrovascular cores) and low-grade papillary urothelial carcinoma (lacking cytological atypia and true papillary structures).

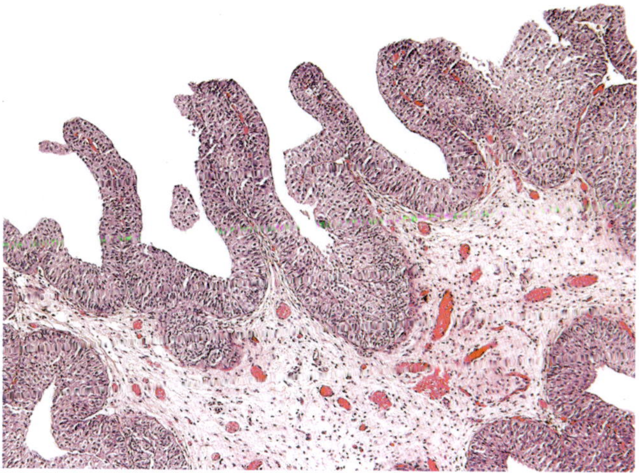

FIGURE 3.4 **Papillary urothelial hyperplasia with tall folds.** Some would regard as early papilloma.

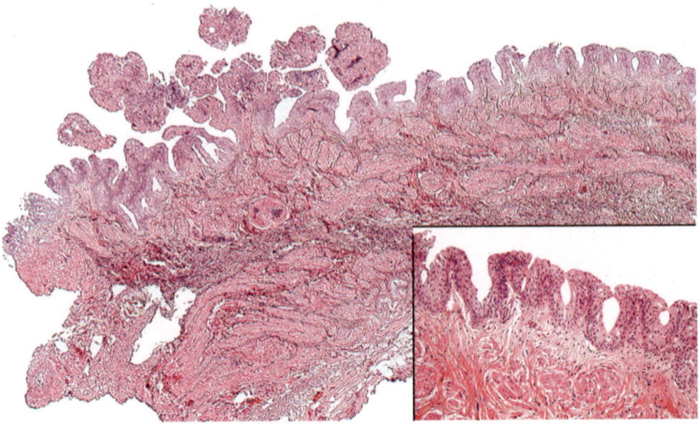

FIGURE 3.5 Papillary urothelial hyperplasia (*right* and *inset*) adjacent to urothelial papilloma (*left*).

In the study by Readal and Epstein, 11/30 (37%) patients with prior urothelial neoplasia subsequently developed bladder tumors compared to 4/23 (17%) patients with *de novo* lesions.[2] In the other sizeable study on papillary urothelial hyperplasia, Lowenthal et al. found that 3/7 (43%) with *de novo* lesions and 10/18 (56%) with a history of prior urothelial neoplasms subsequently developed urothelial tumors.[3] Even though *de novo* papillary hyperplasia will not inevitably progress to urothelial neoplasia, it is reasonable to suggest that patients should be followed up more closely than individuals in the general population, although the surveillance interview may be altered. However, given that most patients with papillary urothelial hyperplasia occurring *de novo* do not subsequently

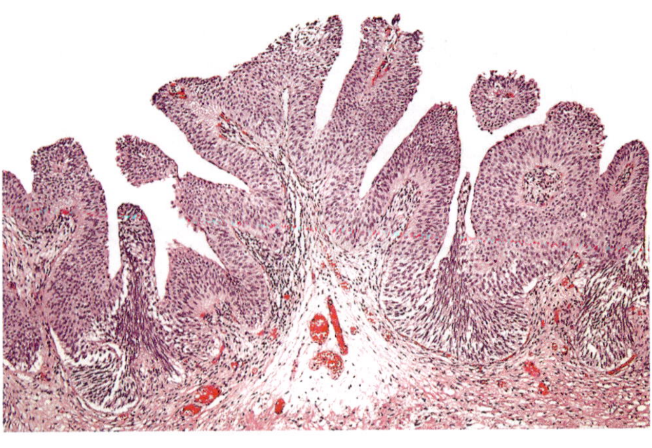

FIGURE 3.6 Papillary urothelial hyperplasia starting to develop branched fronds and "detached-appearing" papillary fronds diagnostic of early urothelial papilloma.

develop urothelial carcinoma and morphologically papillary urothelial hyperplasia lacks any cytological atypia, we disagree with the 2022 WHO blue book recommendation that patients with *de novo* papillary urothelial hyperplasia should be labeled as having noninvasive low-grade papillary urothelial carcinoma. We agree with the WHO 2022 that if papillary urothelial hyperplasia is diagnosed in someone with a history of urothelial neoplasia, it most likely indicates early recurrence of their low-grade papillary urothelial neoplasm; in some cases, it may represent a shoulder lesion at the edge of a PUNLMP. Molecular data also demonstrate that at least a proportion of papillary urothelial hyperplasia represents precancerous lesions of the bladder that subsequently progress to papillary bladder cancer.[9]

Less commonly, the overlying urothelium in a lesion with the architectural pattern of papillary hyperplasia reveals varying degrees of cytological atypia ranging from dysplasia to CIS[10] (eFigs. 3.8 and 3.9). These lesions should not be designated as papillary urothelial hyperplasia with atypia but rather as early noninvasive low-grade or high-grade papillary urothelial carcinoma, depending on the severity of the cytological atypia (see subsequent sections "Low-Grade Papillary Urothelial Carcinoma" and "High-Grade Papillary Urothelial Carcinoma").

PAPILLARY UROTHELIAL NEOPLASMS

Background

The World Health Organization (WHO)/International Society of Urological Pathologists (ISUP) classification of noninvasive papillary urothelial lesions is outlined in Table 3.1, taking into account architectural and cytologic features within the urothelium.[11]

The classification and grading of papillary urothelial neoplasms has been a long-standing source of controversy.[12] There are numerous grading systems, most of which have poor interobserver reproducibility, with most cases falling into an intermediate category.[13-20] The most commonly used grading systems for bladder tumors have been those proposed by the WHO. In 1973, the WHO system proposed that tumors be categorized into benign urothelial papillomas and three grades of carcinoma (grades 1, 2, and 3).[1] A major limitation of the WHO (1973) grading system was the lack of precise definition of the various grades and lack of specific histologic criteria. The following statement is the sole description of the difference between WHO grades 1, 2, and 3 as written in the original WHO (1973) system: "Grade 1 tumors have the least degree of anaplasia compatible with the diagnosis of malignancy. Grade 3 applies to tumors with the most severe degrees of cellular anaplasia, and grade 2 lies in between." In December 1998, members of WHO and ISUP published the WHO/ISUP consensus classification of urothelial (transitional cell) neoplasms of the urinary bladder.[9] This new classification system arose out of the

TABLE 3.1 Histologic Features of Papillary Urothelial Lesions

	Papilloma	Papillary Neoplasm of Low Malignant Potential	Low-Grade Papillary Carcinoma	High-Grade Papillary Carcinoma
Architecture of papillae	Delicate	Delicate; occasionally fused	Fused; branching; delicate	Fused; branching; delicate
Organization of cells	Identical to normal	Polarity identical to normal; any thickness; cohesive	Predominantly ordered, yet minimal crowding and minimal loss of polarity; any thickness; cohesive	Predominantly disordered with frequent loss of polarity; any thickness; often discohesive
Cytology nuclear size	Identical to normal	May be uniformly enlarged	Enlarged with variation in size	Enlarged with variation in size
Nuclear shape	Identical to normal	Elongated; round-oval; uniform	Round-oval; slight variation in shape and contour	Moderate-marked pleomorphism
Nuclear chromatin	Fine	Fine	Mild variation within and between cells	Moderate-marked variation within and between cells with hyperchromasia
Nucleoli	Absent	Absent to inconspicuous	Usually inconspicuous[a]	Multiple prominent nucleoli may be present
Mitoses	Absent	Rare; basal	Occasional, at any level	Usually frequent, at any level; may be atypical
Umbrella cells	Uniformly present	Present	Usually present	May be present

[a]If present, small and regular and not accompanied by other features of high-grade carcinoma.

need to develop a more detailed classification system for bladder neoplasia and because many of the tumors classified as "transitional cell carcinoma, grade 1" had no potential for malignant behavior once completely excised. Subsequent WHO books in 2004, 2016, and 2022 have adopted the WHO/ISUP system.[4-6] This system has been adopted by the College of American Pathologists checklists/synoptic reporting for bladder cancer and by the eighth edition of the AJCC staging system.

WHO/ISUP System

The WHO/ISUP system is a modified version of the scheme proposed by Malmström and colleagues.[18] One of the major contributions of the WHO/ISUP system is a detailed histologic description of the various grades, using specific cytologic and architectural criteria. These criteria are based on the architectural features relating to the histology of the papillae and the overall organization of the cells. Cytologic features encompassed in the WHO/ISUP system include nuclear size, nuclear shape, chromatin content, nucleoli, mitoses, and umbrella cells. Papillary tumors may show heterogeneity of grade. Tumors are graded based on the highest grade exhibited, although it remains to be defined what percentage is minimally needed to place tumors in a higher category when the highest grade is focal (see section "Mixed Low- and High-Grade Papillary Carcinoma"). The terminology used in the WHO/ISUP system for carcinomas is consistent with that used in urine cytology. Criteria and terminology for papillary urothelial neoplasms with an inverted growth pattern are described in Chapter 4.

Soon after the publication of the WHO/ISUP consensus classification in 1998, Holmang et al. published a suite of papers applying it to a set of well-annotated bladder tumors[21,22] and demonstrated that PUNLMP had a lower rate of recurrence than low-grade or high-grade papillary carcinoma while none progressed to invasive disease, although some increased in grade. Representative data on the prognosis of the WHO 2004 grading system come from Pan et al. who studied 1515 patients who underwent TURB for non–muscle-invasive bladder cancer (NMIBC) (Fig. 3.7). The recurrence rates for papillary urothelial neoplasms of low malignant potential (PUNLMPs), low-grade, and high-grade carcinomas were 18%, 35%, and 34%, respectively.[23] Tumor stage progression occurred in 2%, 6%, and 29% of patients with PUNLMP, low-grade, and high-grade papillary carcinoma, respectively. None of the patients with PUNLMP presented with an associated invasive component or died of the disease. Of patients with an initial diagnosis of low-grade and high-grade papillary carcinoma, 2% and 22%, respectively, eventually died of these cancers. PUNLMPs had a significantly lower recurrence rate than the low- and high-grade cancers, and the differences between all three tumor grades were significant in terms of stage progression and death due to cancer. In a subsequent study from this group, they developed nomograms to predict progression-free and cancer-specific survival factoring grade, stage, and intravesical therapy.[24] Similar

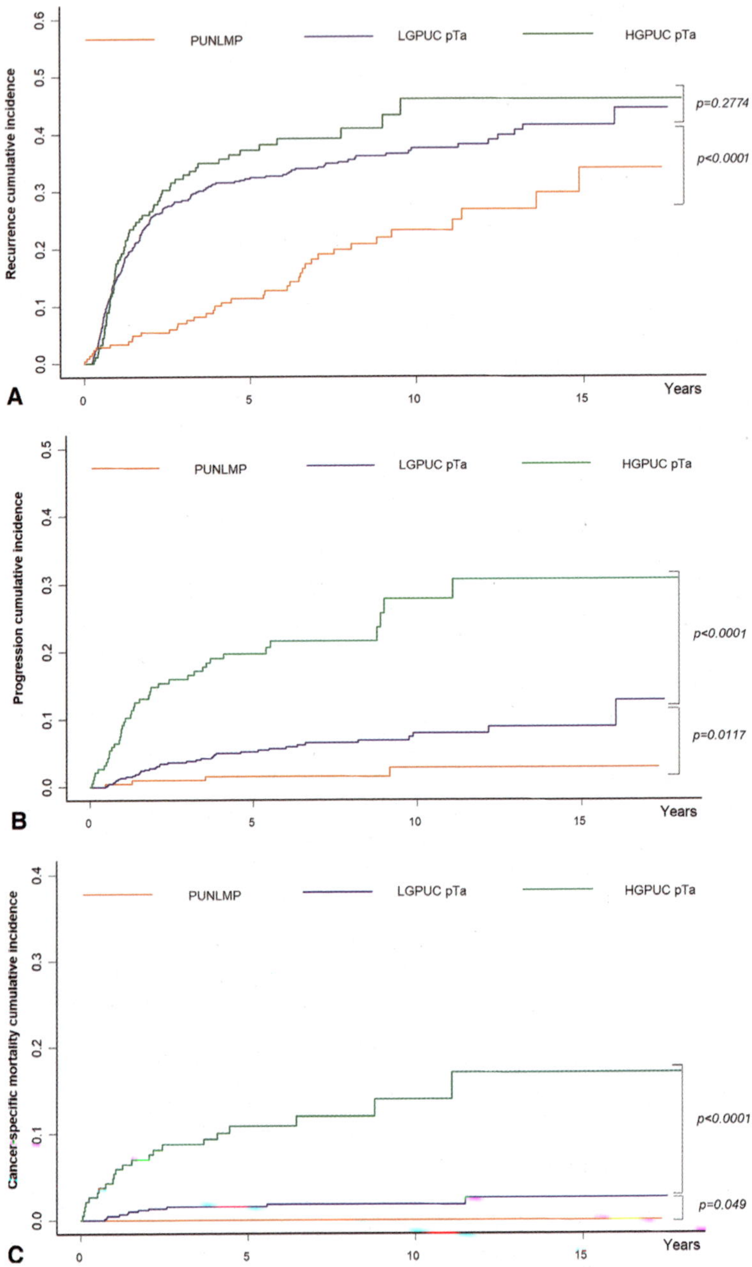

FIGURE 3.7 Cumulative incidence plots of recurrence **(A)**, progression **(B)**, and cancer-specific mortality **(C)** for patients with non-muscle-invasive bladder tumors of different grades. HPUC indicates noninvasive high-grade papillary urothelial carcinoma; LPUC, noninvasive low-grade papillary urothelial carcinoma; PUNLMP, papillary urothelial neoplasm of low malignant potential. (From Pan CC, Chang YH, Chen KK, et al. Prognostic significance of the 2004 WHO/ISUP classification for prediction of recurrence, progression, and cancer-specific mortality of non-muscle-invasive urothelial tumors of the urinary bladder: a clinicopathologic study of 1,515 cases. *Am J Clin Pathol.* 2010;133(5):788–795. Reproduced by permission of American Society for Clinical Pathology.)

findings showing differences between PUNLMP, low-grade, and high-grade noninvasive papillary urothelial carcinoma in recurrence, progression, and death have been published by other authors.[25-29]

Relation of WHO (1973) to WHO/ISUP

A major misconception in the application of the WHO/ISUP classification is that there is a one-to-one translation between it and the WHO (1973) classification system (Fig. 3.8). Only at the extremes of grades in the WHO (1973) classification does this one-to-one correlation hold true. Lesions called papilloma in the WHO (1973) classification system are also called papilloma in the WHO/ISUP system. At the other end of the grading extreme, lesions called WHO (1973) grade 3 are by definition high-grade carcinoma in the WHO/ISUP system. However, for WHO (1973) grades 1 and 2, there is no direct translation to WHO/ISUP classification system. Rather, lesions must be analyzed using the criteria of the WHO/ISUP classification system without regard to how they were diagnosed in WHO (1973) system. Lesions formerly called WHO (1973) grade 1, which upon review show no cytologic atypia and merely thickened urothelium with, at most, nuclear enlargement and minimal disorder in orientation, would be called papillary urothelial neoplasms of low malignant potential (PUNLMP). However, other WHO (1973) grade 1 lesions with definite yet slight cytologic atypia would be diagnosed in the WHO/ISUP system as low-grade urothelial carcinomas.

Within the WHO (1973) system, grade 2 is a very broad category. It includes lesions that are relatively bland, which in some places would be diagnosed as WHO (1973) grades 1-2; these lesions in the WHO/ISUP

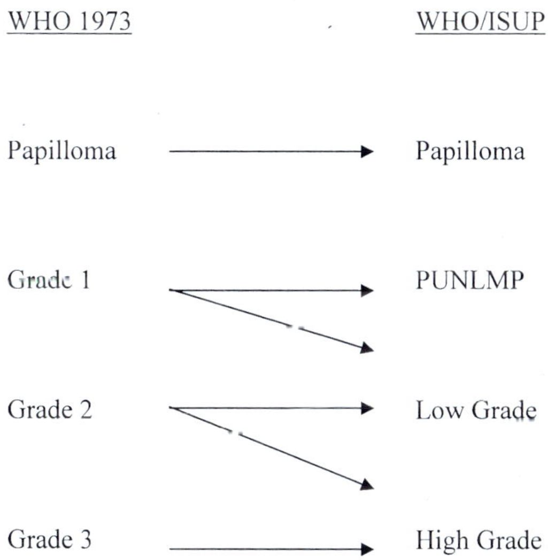

FIGURE 3.8 Relationship of WHO (1973) to WHO (2003)/ISUP classification of papillary urothelial tumors.

system would be called low-grade papillary urothelial carcinoma. In other cases, WHO (1973) grade 2 lesions border on higher-grade lesions and, in many institutions, were called WHO (1973) grades 2-3; these lesions in the WHO (2004)/ISUP classification system would be called high-grade carcinoma. In the old WHO (1973) system, a large percentage of patients with noninvasive papillary urothelial carcinomas were called grade 2, an ambiguous group that the urologists did not know how to treat. In the WHO/ISUP grading system, these grade 2 tumors can be segregated roughly equally into low- and high-grade cancers with correspondingly low and high risks of progression.[30-32] When WHO (1973) grade 2 tumors are reclassified as high-grade tumors, they show molecular aberrations usually associated with cancers of higher grade and poor outcome, further supporting that the WHO (1973) grade 2 tumors form a heterogeneous group that can be subdivided into low- and high-grade cancer.[33]

There have been several studies comparing WHO (1973) and the WHO/ISUP system. Most have demonstrated a superiority of WHO/ISUP in predicting recurrence and progression or interobserver reproducibility.[30,34-39] However, the WHO (1973) three-grade system is still in use in Europe and is incorporated with the WHO/ISUP system in prognostic factor risk groups for NMIBC.[40] Whether routine ancillary studies such as immunohistochemical or molecular markers will aid us in better stratifying these tumors into distinct risk groups remains to be proven but the strength of the data and associated cost of performing the assays should be taken into consideration. In addition, it is unlikely that this approach can be adapted globally due to cost and availability.

A significant number of publications document poor interobserver reproducibility with both the WHO (1973) and the WHO/ISUP system.[11,41-47] In a summary of 20 articles that included 3593 patients, the reproducibility and the intraobserver reproducibility of both the 1973 and the WHO/ISUP systems were poor to moderate.[44]

Papilloma

Using the WHO (1973) system, some experts applied very restrictive criteria for the diagnosis of urothelial papilloma, in part based on the number of cell layers, and regarded all other papillary neoplasms as carcinomas. Others applied a broader definition of "urothelial papilloma" so as not to label all patients with papillary lesions with minimal cytologic and architectural atypia as having carcinoma; many if not all of these latter cases would now fall into the PUNLMP category.

The WHO/ISUP system has very restrictive histologic features for the diagnosis of papilloma, requiring papillary fronds to be lined by normal-appearing urothelium[9] (Figs. 3.9-3.14, eFigs. 3.10-3.45). Most papillomas present as single lesions that are relatively small. However, multifocal tumors and larger lesions may be only occasionally seen.

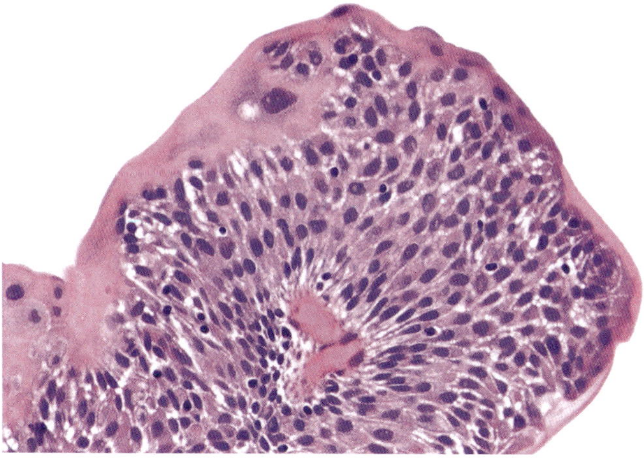

FIGURE 3.9 **Urothelial papilloma with atypical umbrella cells.**

Most papillomas have a simple nonbranching or minimally branching arrangement, slender fibrovascular stalks, and a predominantly exophytic pattern. In some papillomas, more complex anastomosing papillae, marked stromal edema within the papillae, and endophytic areas can be identified (Figs. 3.15 and 3.16). When strict criteria are applied to render this diagnosis, molecular studies have shown that it harbors KRAS/HRAS mutations rather than TERT promoter, PIK3CA, and FGFR3 mutations commonly seen in papillary urothelial carcinoma.[46]

Within the limits of normal urothelial thickness, there is some variability. Uncommon cases may be composed of only one to two cell layers of urothelium. There is no need to count the maximum number of

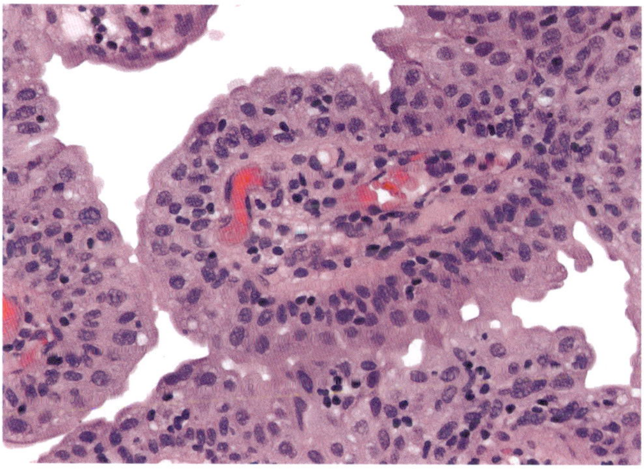

FIGURE 3.10 **Urothelial papilloma.** There is a consistent umbrella cell layer in which the cells appear slightly enlarged: this feature does not argue against a diagnosis of papilloma.

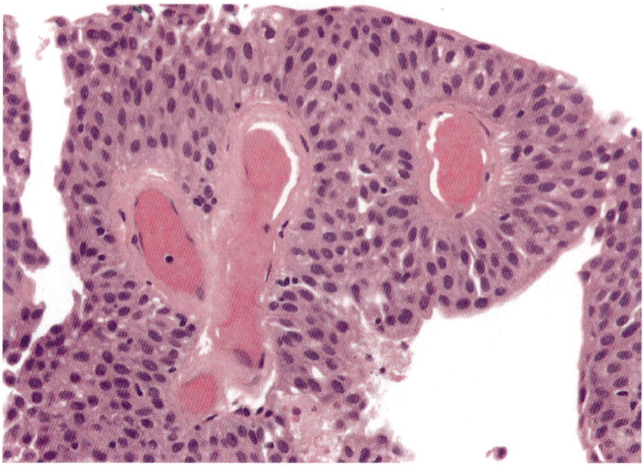

FIGURE 3.11 Urothelial papilloma.

cell layers, as long as it is not obviously thicker than the normal urothelial lining. In most cases, the urothelium is tightly cohesive, although in some cases, there may be the appearance of discohesion. Umbrella cells vary in their morphology from being inconspicuous, to being cuboidal with slightly enlarged nuclei and paler cytoplasm, to having a hobnail appearance with abundant eosinophilic cytoplasm. Occasional cases of urothelial papilloma have an umbrella cell layer with prominent vacuolization. Single, enlarged umbrella cells may also drape themselves over several underlying urothelial cells, where the umbrella cell nuclei may demonstrate degenerative atypia. Urothelial atypia, other than that which can be seen in umbrella cells, excludes the diagnosis of papilloma. Mitotic figures are absent.

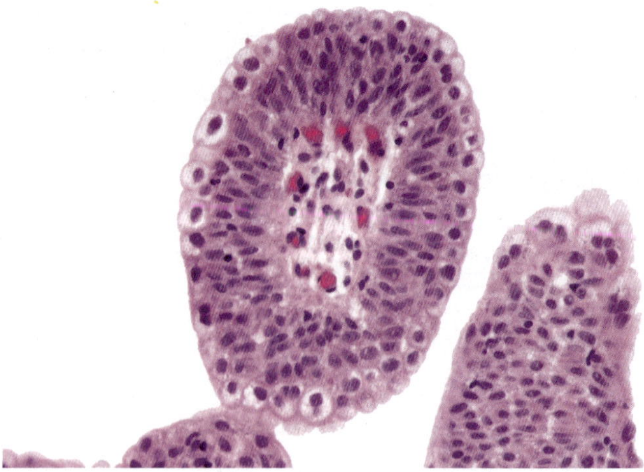

FIGURE 3.12 Urothelial papilloma with cuboidal umbrella cells with clear cytoplasm.

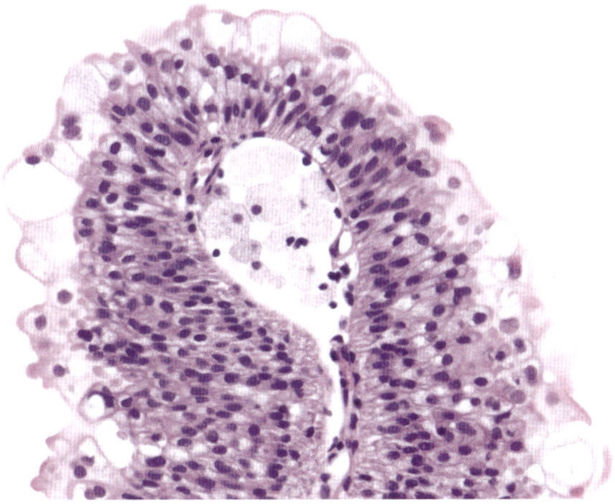

FIGURE 3.13 **Urothelial papilloma with vacuolated umbrella cells.** Note foam cells in a papillary core.

Papillomas are rare and more commonly, but not exclusively, occur in younger patients. Papillomas may occur in association with a prior or concurrent history of other urothelial tumors. However, if a papilloma is the first manifestation of urothelial neoplasia, only about 7% to 8% recur, typically within 5 years of the initial diagnosis.[32,48-52] Lesions typically recur as papilloma and less commonly as papillary urothelial neoplasm of low malignant potential (PUNLMP) or noninvasive low-grade papillary urothelial carcinoma. Of the four largest series on papillomas totaling 153 patients, only 1 patient experienced stage progression; invasive urothelial carcinoma was found extending out of the bladder 4 years after the

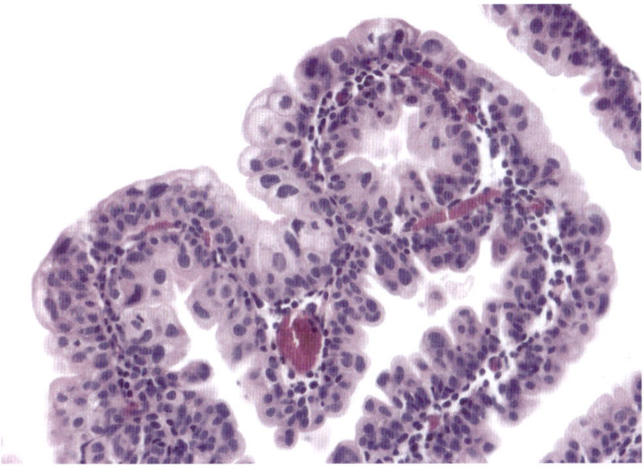

FIGURE 3.14 **Urothelial papilloma with prominent umbrella cells showing hobnail morphology.**

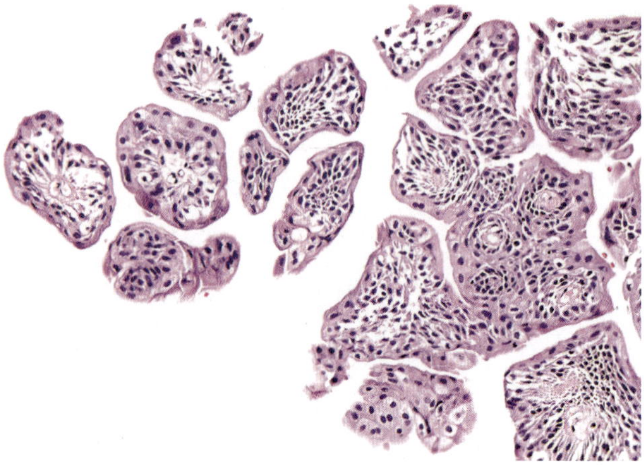

FIGURE 3.15 Urothelial papilloma.

diagnosis of papilloma.[49-52] A caveat to this exceptional case is that the patient was immunosuppressed following renal transplantation.

Papillary Urothelial Neoplasm of Low Malignant Potential

The category of PUNLMP was included to describe lesions that do not have cytologic features of malignancy, yet have thickened urothelium or have more cells per unit area (greater cellularity of urothelium) compared to papilloma (Figs. 3.17-3.22, eFigs. 3.46-3.76). Having a category of PUNLMP avoids labeling a patient as having cancer, which has psychosocial and financial (eg, insurance) implications, although since it is not labeled

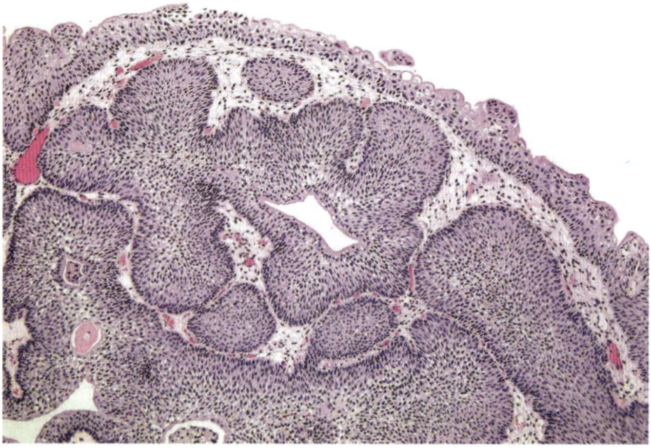

FIGURE 3.16 Areas of the tumor seen in Figure 3.15 showed inverted papilloma consistent with mixed exophytic and inverted urothelial papilloma.

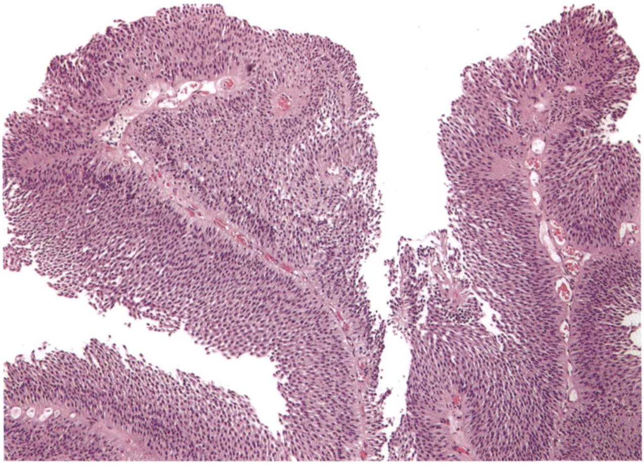

FIGURE 3.17 Papillary urothelial neoplasm of low malignant potential.

as an unequivocal benign lesion (eg, papilloma), its diagnosis implies that the patient should be adequately followed.

PUNLMPs at low power differ from papillomas by having thicker urothelium. Otherwise, there are no architectural abnormalities, because the lesion has no loss of polarity (ie, no loss of order). Cytologically, PUNLMPs have a monotonous appearance, with each cell being virtually identical to each other. At high magnification, slight variability in the nuclear contour may be evident. At most, nuclei are slightly enlarged and more crowded relative to those in normal urothelial nuclei. Nuclear grooves, a feature of normal urothelium, may be seen in these tumors and in papillomas but are not a common feature in higher-grade lesions. Nucleoli are

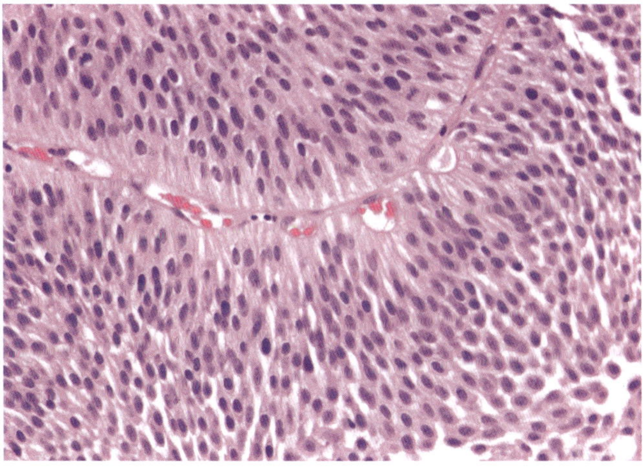

FIGURE 3.18 Higher magnification of papillary urothelial neoplasm of low malignant potential seen in Figure 3.17.

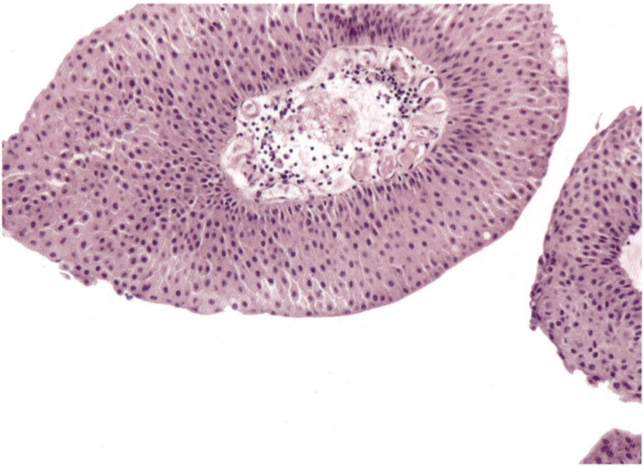

FIGURE 3.19 Papillary urothelial neoplasm of low malignant potential.

either absent or inconspicuous. The chromatin is uniformly even without the scattered hyperchromatic nuclei seen in low-grade papillary carcinoma. Mitoses are exceedingly rare and usually limited to the basal layer. Areas of the tumor that lack tangential sectioning, show proper orientation, and are evenly cut are optimal areas for evaluation of cytoarchitectural features and to prevent artifactual overgrading due to crowding or hyperchromasia.

Low-Grade Papillary Urothelial Carcinoma

To simplify the WHO (1973) system and avoid an intermediate cancer grade group (WHO 1973 grade 2), which is often the default diagnosis for

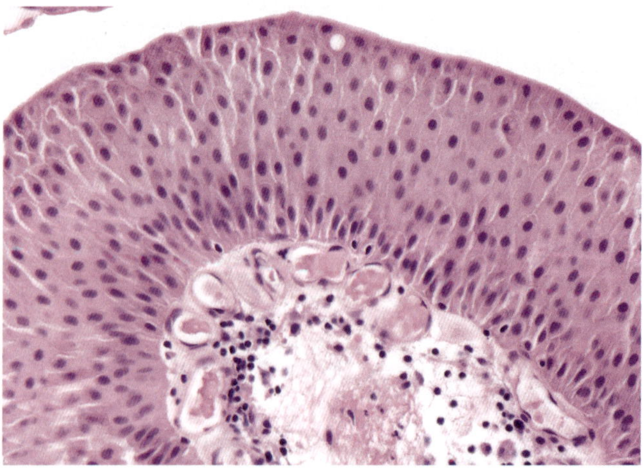

FIGURE 3.20 Higher magnification of papillary urothelial neoplasm of low malignant potential seen in Figure 3.19.

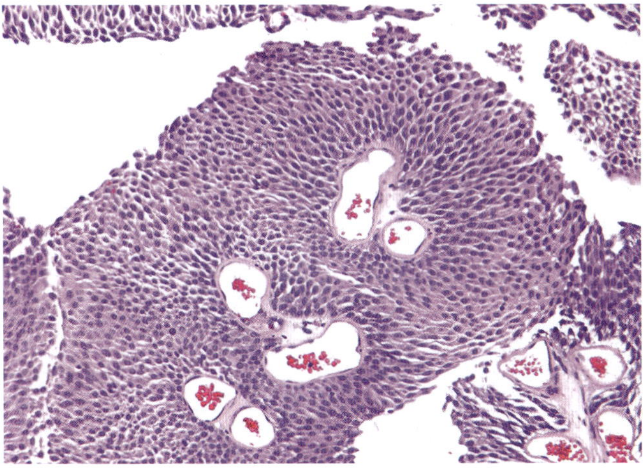

FIGURE 3.21 Papillary urothelial neoplasm of low malignant potential.

many pathologists, the WHO/ISUP system classifies papillary urothelial carcinoma into only two grades. Additional reasons for having a two-tier grading system are described above under "Relation of WHO (1973) to WHO/ISUP." Low-grade papillary urothelial carcinoma exhibits an overall orderly appearance but has minimal variability in architecture and cytologic features, which are easily recognizable at scanning magnification (Figs. 3.23-3.29, eFigs. 3.77-3.110). When analyzing for the presence of order vs disorder in all papillary tumors, it is preferable to assess only those fibrovascular cores that have been cut perpendicular to the long axis of the papillary frond, because tangential sections near the base of the frond may be misleading. It is common to see fusion of adjacent papillae, a feature that may lead to overgrading because of its appearance of disorder.

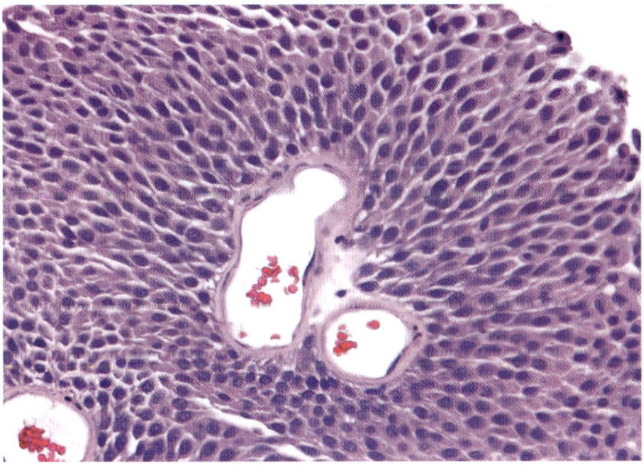

FIGURE 3.22 Higher magnification of papillary urothelial neoplasm of low malignant potential seen in Figure 3.21.

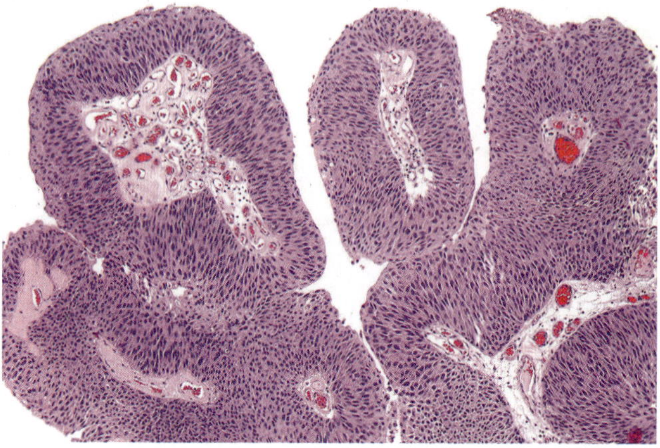

FIGURE 3.23 **Noninvasive low-grade papillary urothelial carcinoma.**

Variability in polarity, nuclear size, shape, outlines, and chromatin texture are minimal but comprise the hallmarks of the cytologic atypia seen in low-grade papillary urothelial carcinoma. Mitotic figures are infrequent. Although mitoses may be seen at any level of the urothelium, they are usually limited to the lower (inner) half. Among these features, the finding of scattered hyperchromatic nuclei, minimal nuclear membrane irregularities seen at 100× magnification, and scattered "typical" mitotic figures best distinguishes this lesion from PUNLMP. Occasionally, one sees similar cytologic features in thickened urothelium adjacent to a papillary neoplasm (Fig. 3.31, eFigs. 3.111-3.114). Degenerative atypia with low ki67 proliferation rate should not be graded as high grade (Fig. 30).[52] This

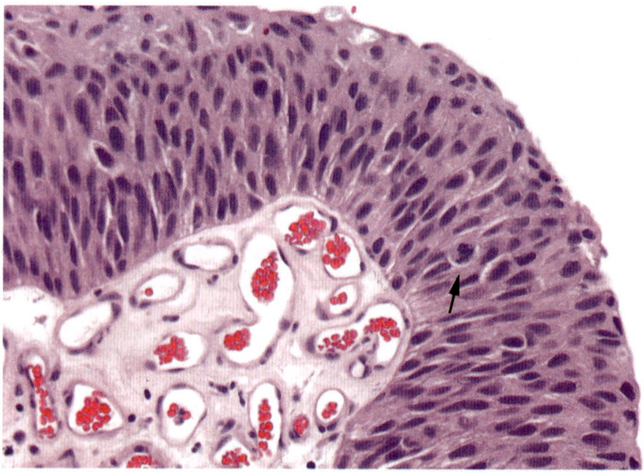

FIGURE 3.24 **Higher magnification of noninvasive low-grade papillary urothelial carcinoma seen in Figure 3.23.** Note mitotic figure (***arrow***) midway up the urothelium.

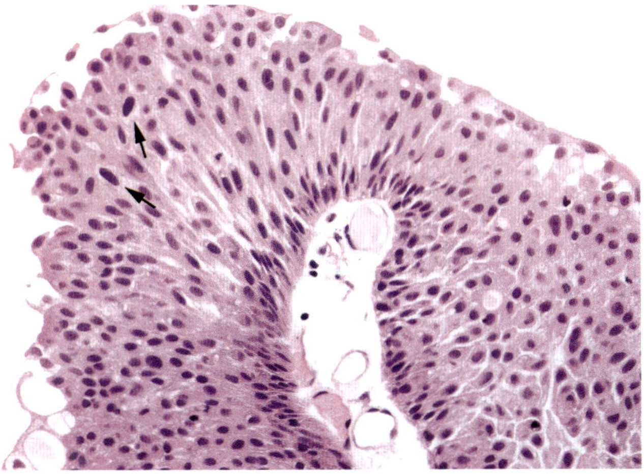

FIGURE 3.25 **Noninvasive low-grade papillary urothelial carcinoma.** Note scattered hyperchromatic nuclei (***arrows***) and irregularity of size and shape of nuclei.

thickened flat urothelium may have the identical features of cytologic and architectural disorder seen in the adjacent papillary lesion and thus represent the "shoulder" (lateral extension) of the neoplasm. One can also see rudimentary papillary projections with mild cytological atypia that represent early noninvasive low-grade papillary urothelial carcinomas, often found during cystoscopic surveillance of men with prior history of papillary carcinoma (Figs. 3.32 and 3.33). In these subtle cases, it is helpful to correlate with the presence of a papillary lesion seen on cystoscopy. Umbrella cell atypia should be discounted when graded.

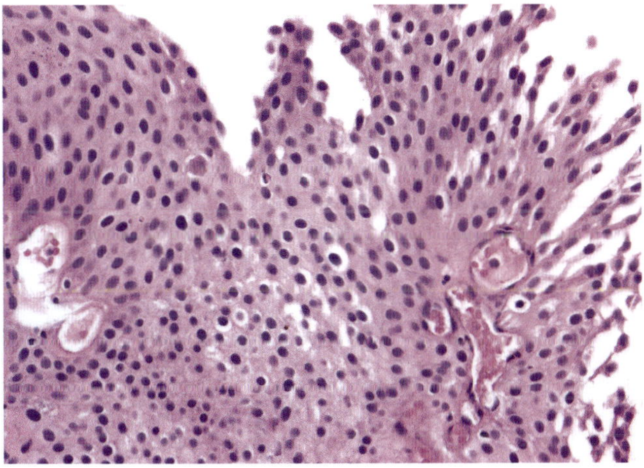

FIGURE 3.26 **Noninvasive low-grade papillary urothelial carcinoma.** Cells in this are uniformly enlarged, yet have scattered hyperchromatic nuclei.

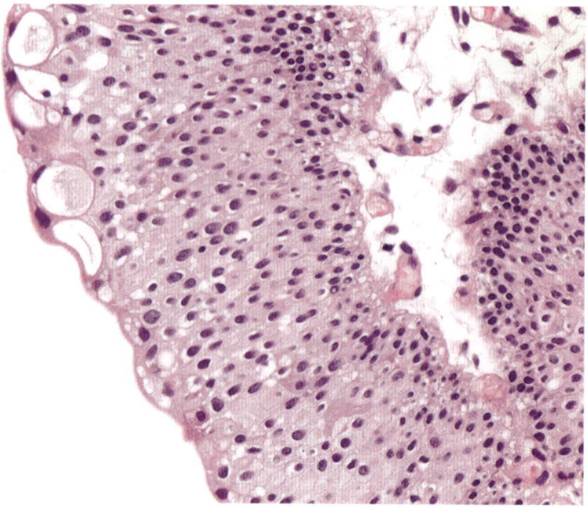

FIGURE 3.27 Noninvasive low-grade papillary urothelial carcinoma.

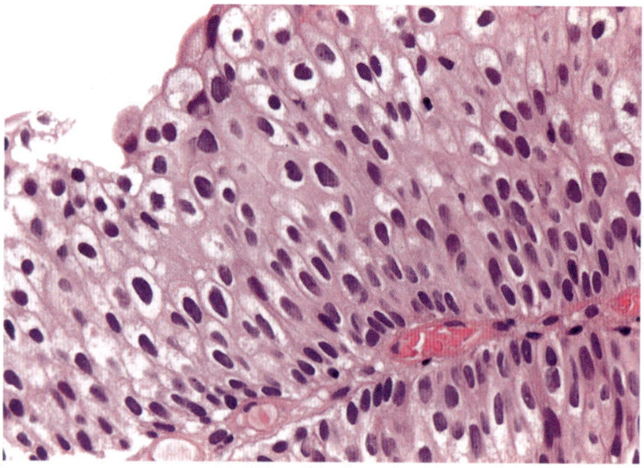

FIGURE 3.28 Noninvasive low-grade papillary urothelial carcinoma (high magnification).

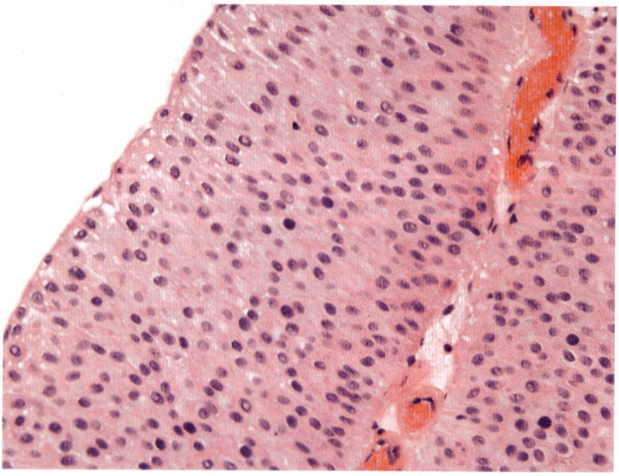

FIGURE 3.29 Noninvasive low-grade papillary urothelial carcinoma.

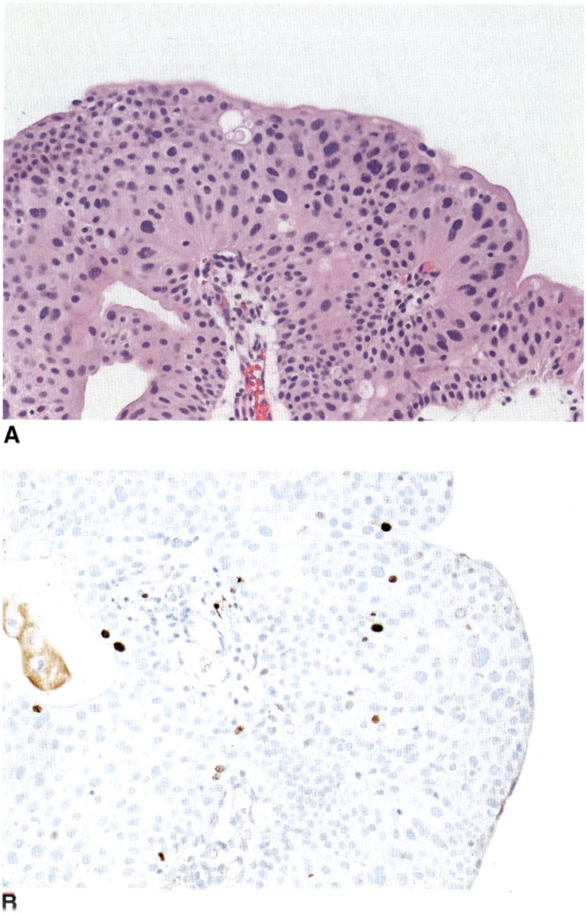

FIGURE 3.30 **A:** Low grade papillary urothelial carcinoma with degenerative atypia. **B:** Ki67 proliferation rate is low and large degenerative-appearing nuclei lack ki67 immunoreactivity.

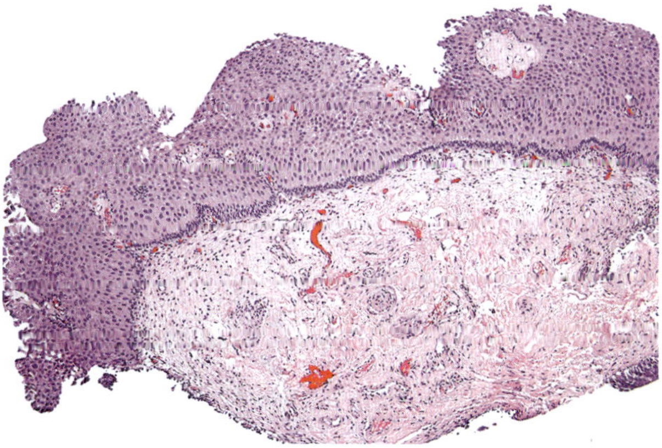

FIGURE 3.31 **Thickened urothelium adjacent to low-grade papillary urothelial carcinoma having similar cytology.** The association of numerous blood vessels within the hyperplastic urothelium suggests a subtle papillary lesion.

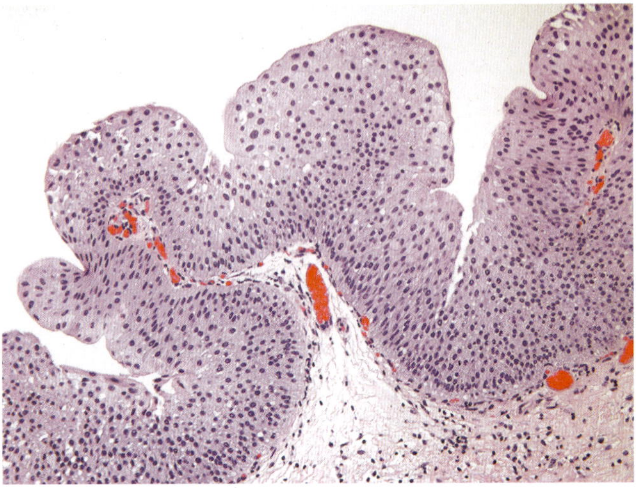

FIGURE 3.32 **Early noninvasive papillary urothelial carcinoma with thickened dysplastic urothelium, early papillary formation, and congested capillaries at the base.**

High-Grade Papillary Urothelial Carcinoma

High-grade papillary urothelial carcinomas are characterized by a disorderly appearance resulting from marked architectural and cytologic abnormalities, for the most part recognizable at low magnification (Figs. 3.34-3.43, eFigs. 3.115-3.169). Architecturally, the cells are irregularly oriented and disorganized. Cellular pleomorphism ranges from moderate to marked. The nuclear borders may be irregular, often with clefts or notches. The nuclear chromatin tends to be clumped, and nucleoli may be prominent

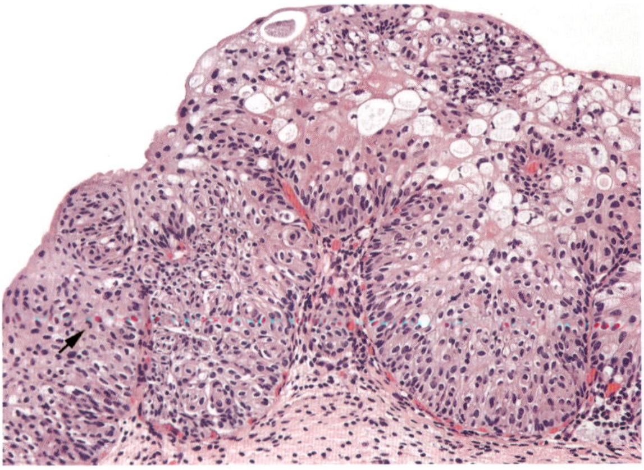

FIGURE 3.33 **Early noninvasive low-grade papillary urothelial carcinoma with minimal atypia, a mitotic figure (*arrow*), and thin fibrovascular cores, which are beginning to branch.** The lesion has whirling of the urothelium (eddies) that are more common in low-grade papillary tumors.

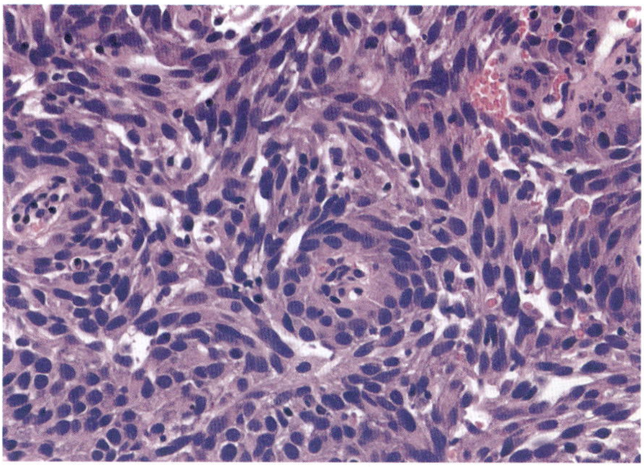

FIGURE 3.34 Noninvasive high-grade papillary urothelial carcinoma.

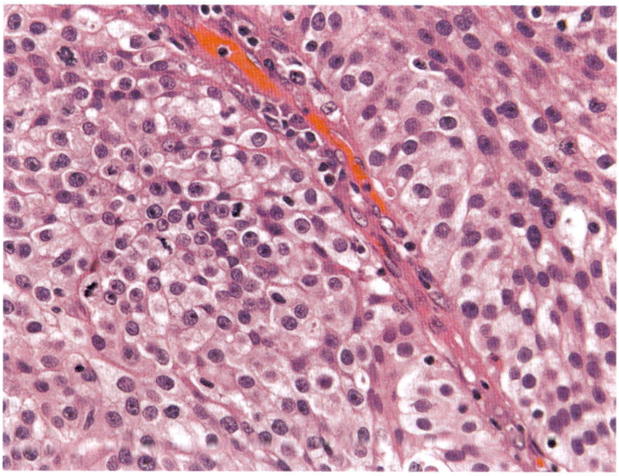

FIGURE 3.35 Noninvasive high-grade papillary urothelial carcinoma.

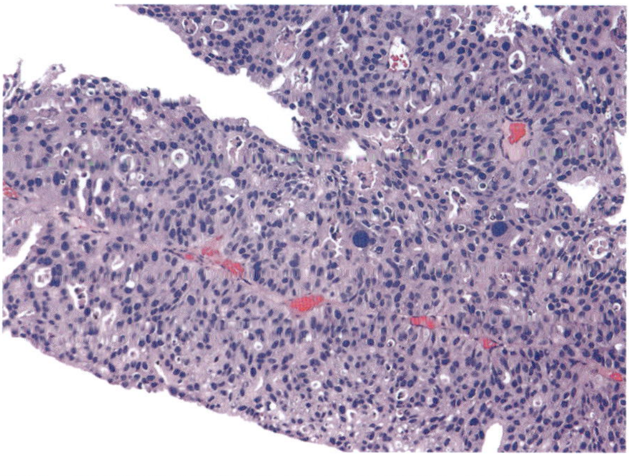

FIGURE 3.36 Noninvasive high-grade papillary urothelial carcinoma.

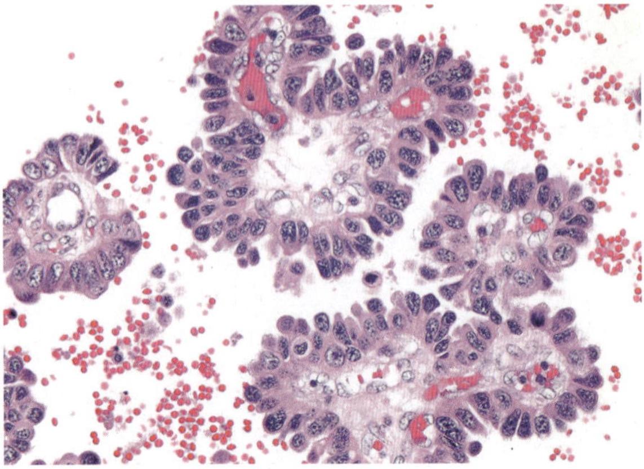

FIGURE 3.37 Noninvasive high-grade papillary urothelial carcinoma.

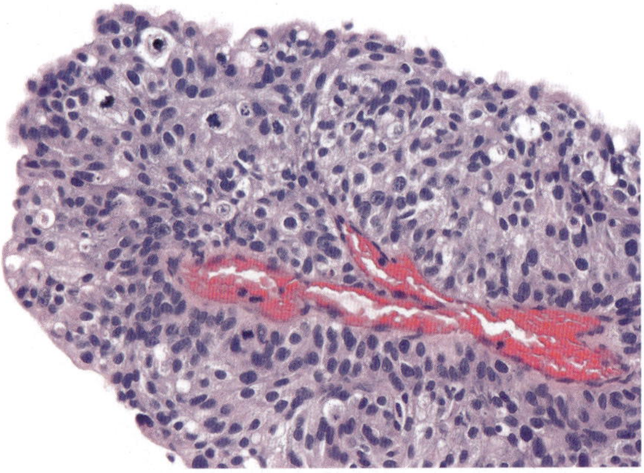

FIGURE 3.38 Noninvasive high-grade papillary urothelial carcinoma.

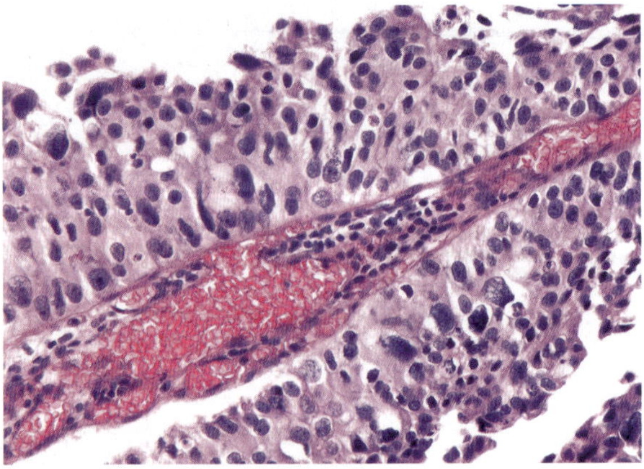

FIGURE 3.39 Noninvasive high-grade papillary urothelial carcinoma.

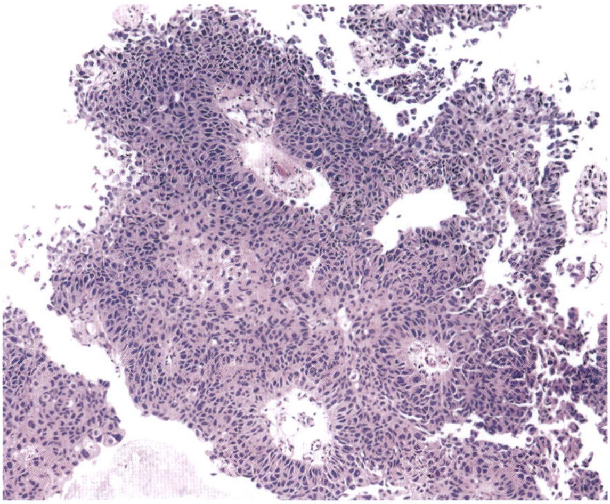

FIGURE 3.40 Noninvasive high-grade papillary urothelial carcinoma.

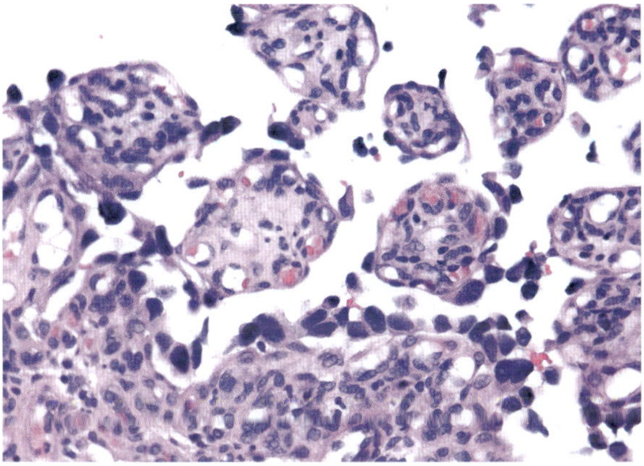

FIGURE 3.41 Noninvasive high-grade papillary urothelial carcinoma.

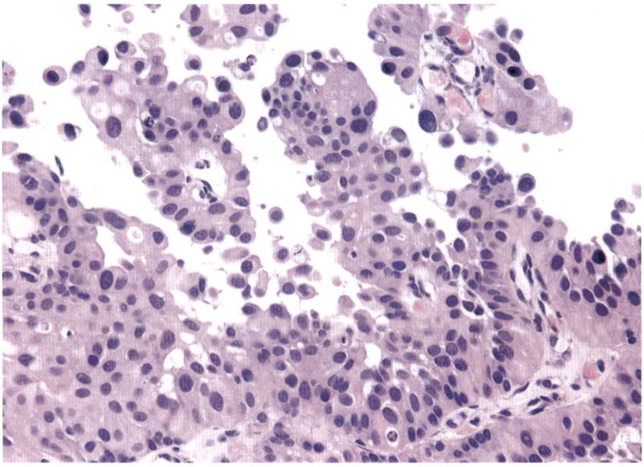

FIGURE 3.42 Noninvasive high-grade papillary urothelial carcinoma.

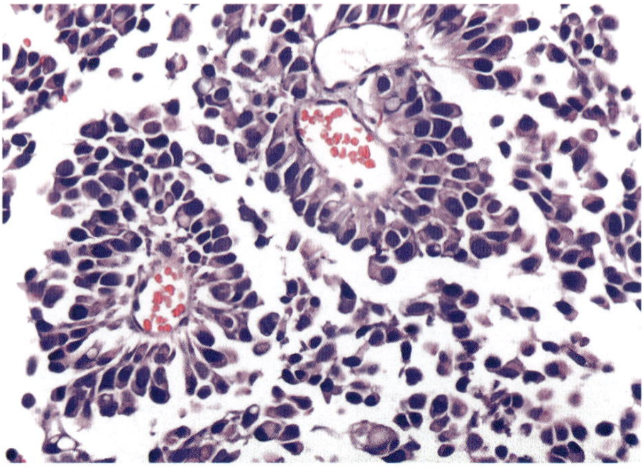

FIGURE 3.43 Noninvasive high-grade papillary urothelial carcinoma.

and irregular; occasionally, multiple nucleoli and nucleolar pleomorphism may be present. Mitotic figures, including atypical forms, may be frequently seen at all levels of the urothelium. Rarely, one can have papillary urothelial carcinoma with squamous differentiation (Fig. 3.44). As with CIS, high-grade papillary urothelial carcinomas are more likely than lower-grade papillary neoplasms to have discohesive cells and some denudation (Fig. 3.45). The majority of papillary urothelial lesions associated with prominent urothelial denudation are high grade, often occurring with either prominent cautery artifact or in anatomically confined areas (ie, ureter, renal pelvis, urethra), suggesting both iatrogenic and mechanical contributing

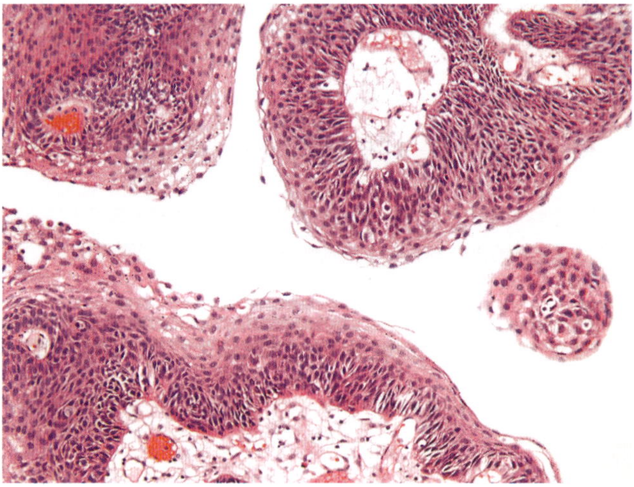

FIGURE 3.44 Noninvasive high-grade papillary urothelial carcinoma with squamous features (elsewhere lesion had features of high-grade papillary urothelial carcinoma).

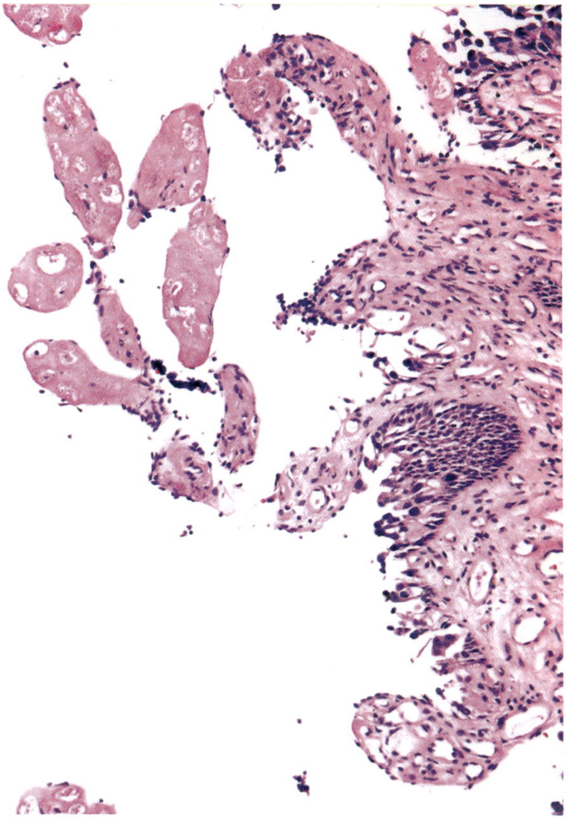

FIGURE 3.45 Noninvasive high-grade papillary urothelial carcinoma with prominent denudation.

factors, respectively.[53] Prominent urothelial denudation in papillary lesions should prompt careful examination of these specimens for rare clinging high-grade carcinoma cells, although in a minority of cases, the underlying lesion will be low grade. Invasion (and microinvasion) into superficial lamina propria should be diligently ruled out in high-grade lesions.

Analogous to early noninvasive low-grade papillary urothelial carcinomas discussed above, the same situation can occur with high-grade papillary carcinoma. In this setting, it can be difficult and somewhat arbitrary whether to diagnoses *early noninvasive high-grade papillary urothelial carcinoma* or *carcinoma in situ (CIS) with early papillary formation* (Fig. 3.46). This distinction can have clinical significance given that the presence of CIS can affect therapy (see section "Treatment of Papillary Urothelial Neoplasms"). In the absence of data, the current authors recommend diagnosing *early noninvasive high-grade papillary urothelial carcinoma* when there is a cystoscopic correlate of a papillary or even subtle elevated appearing lesion. In contrast, *carcinoma in situ (CIS) with early papillary formation* is diagnosed when cystoscopy shows a flat mucosa (ie, erythematous lesion).

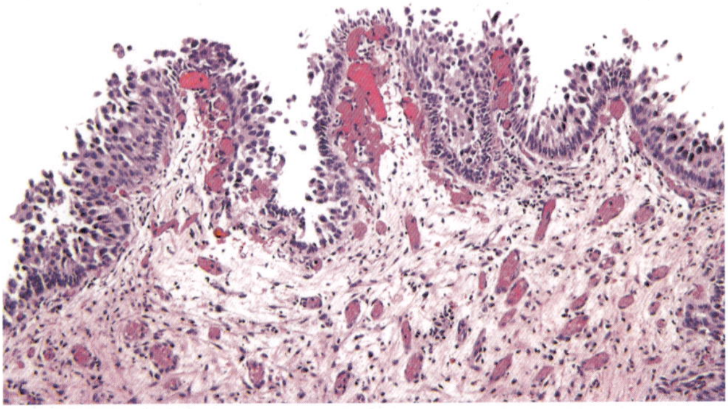

FIGURE 3.46 CIS with early papillary formation vs early noninvasive high-grade papillary urothelial carcinoma.

Mixed Low- and High-Grade Papillary Carcinoma

Most papillary carcinomas have the same grade throughout. However, a single papillary urothelial neoplasm may contain a spectrum of cytologic and architectural abnormalities (Figs. 3.47-3.49). When the high-grade component is >10%, there is consensus to grade the tumor as high grade. However, there is a lack of consensus on grading cases with mixed grades when the percentage of high-grade component is limited to <5% or <10% of the tumor, the latter occurring in ~5% of papillary urothelial carcinomas. Some experts diagnose a tumor as high grade regardless of how limited the high-grade component, whereas others make an exception when the high-grade component is very limited and

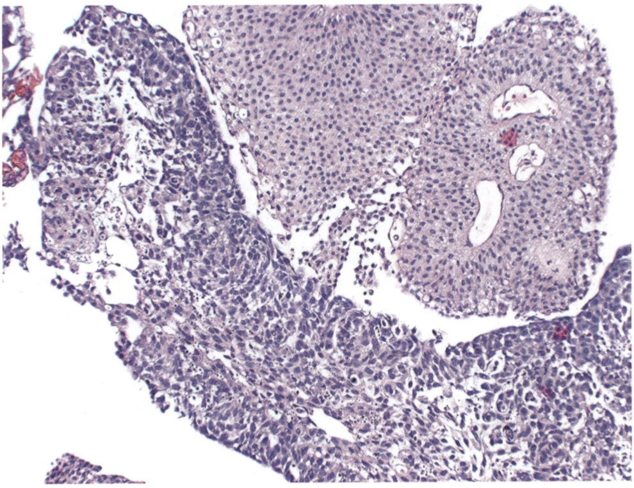

FIGURE 3.47 Noninvasive high-grade papillary urothelial carcinoma areas showing low-grade cytology.

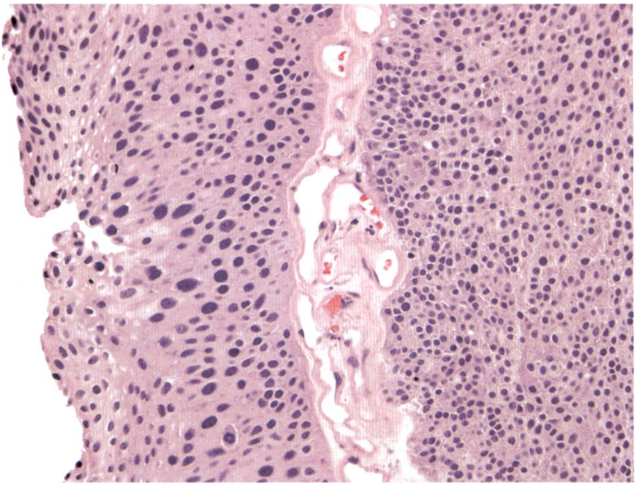

FIGURE 3.48 Noninvasive papillary urothelial carcinoma with both low- and high-grade cytologies.

grade these tumors as low grade, noting the minor high-grade component. The two largest reports on these cases have shown consistent findings. In a study of 31 mixed grade carcinomas with <5% high-grade component, stage progression and death of disease rates are comparable to that of low-grade urothelial carcinoma.[54] In the second study of 32 cases of mixed grade papillary carcinoma with <10% high-grade component, stage progression and disease-specific survival was comparable in the mixed grade carcinomas and the low-grade papillary

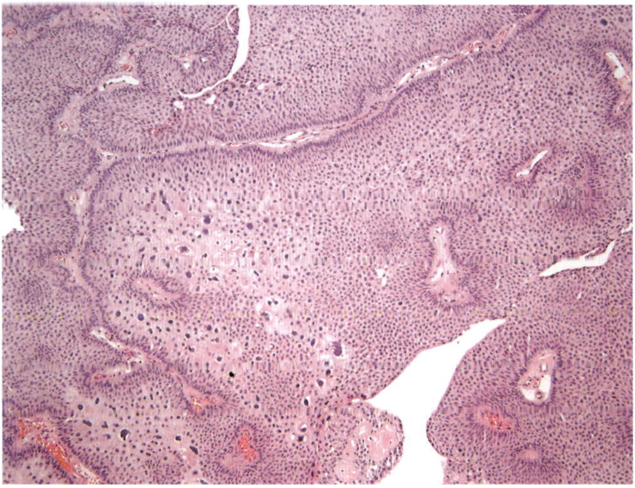

FIGURE 3.49 Predominantly noninvasive low-grade papillary urothelial carcinoma with focal high-grade cytology.

carcinomas.[55] The 2022 WHO recommends using 5% as a cutoff and reporting these cases as "noninvasive low-grade papillary urothelial carcinoma with <5% high-grade component."[7] Tumor with >5% high-grade features are diagnosed as "noninvasive high-grade papillary urothelial carcinoma." In order to account for different grades within a given tumor, a combined grading system has been proposed adding the primary (most common) and secondary (second most common) grade of bladder cancer, regardless of extent, analogous to the Gleason grading for prostate cancer.[56,57] Although a combined grading system for papillary urothelial carcinoma appears to improve prediction of prognosis, further studies are needed before this system can be recommended for routine clinical practice. Given the inherent problems of interobserver reproducibility, we doubt this approach will become standard of practice.

Borderline Lesions Between Low and High Grade

In a minority of papillary tumors, it can be challenging to decide whether a noninvasive papillary urothelial carcinoma is low or high grade. In such cases, one approach is to recognize this uncertainty whereby urologists can consider other information to determine whether the patient's tumor is more likely to require therapy for a high-grade tumor. This information would include historical data (grade of prior urothelial neoplasia, frequency of recurrence, lack of response to prior intravesical therapy), as well as salient clinical (size, focality/multifocality, cystoscopic appearance) and pathologic (concurrent CIS, urine cytology results) observations. It is especially critical to not arbitrarily diagnosis high-grade papillary urothelial carcinoma in a histologically borderline lesion arising in the renal pelvis, where this diagnosis may lead to nephroureterectomy or neoadjuvant systemic therapy.

Comment on Muscularis Propria in Noninvasive Papillary Urothelial Tumors

Whereas there is a consensus on the need to comment on the presence of muscularis propria in the setting of invasive urothelial carcinoma, there is no such information on the need to include this information in the pathology report when only a noninvasive papillary urothelial neoplasm is present. It is not recommended that a repeat TUR be performed if there was no muscularis propria in the initial resection of low-grade papillary tumors (papilloma, PUNLMP, low-grade papillary carcinoma), such that for these tumors, it is not necessary to note the presence or absence of muscularis propria.[58] In the setting of a noninvasive high-grade papillary urothelial carcinoma, such information may be useful as there could be invasion elsewhere if the lesion has not been totally resected. It could also be useful information in cases where there is residual papillary carcinoma at the site of a prior TUR for invasive disease.

PUNLMP vs Low-Grade Carcinoma

Probably, the most controversial aspect of the WHO/ISUP grading system is the category of PUNLMP. One of the earliest articles analyzing PUNLMPs was submitted before the WHO/ISUP classification system was even published and before there were detailed illustrations or descriptions on how to classify tumors using the new system.[59] In the article, lesions that were formerly called WHO (1973) grade 1 were designated as PUNLMP. According to the article, tumors classified as PUNLMP had a significant risk of recurrence, progression, and death from bladder cancer. However, if these lesions were analyzed using the WHO/ISUP criteria for PUNLMP, a subset of these tumors would have been classified as low-grade urothelial carcinomas.

A few studies have demonstrated a low level of agreement in the histological distinction between PUNLMP and low-grade carcinoma or have failed to show a difference in prognosis between the two entities.[34,45,47,61-63] However, a much larger number of studies have demonstrated that PUNLMP has a more favorable outcome compared to papillary low-grade urothelial carcinoma. These studies have shown that PUNLMPs have a lower risk of recurrence than low-grade urothelial carcinoma.[21-24,32,37,63-67] In addition, whereas a small percentage of noninvasive low-grade papillary urothelial carcinomas progress either to invasive carcinoma or to high-grade noninvasive papillary carcinoma, the majority of studies have reported that PUNLMPs do not progress either in stage or grade.[37,63-66]

Because PUNLMPs have a risk of recurrence, all patients with this diagnosis will be followed in the same manner as those diagnosed with low-grade urothelial carcinoma. One could argue that if the treatment is the same and if there are difficulties in differentiating PUNLMP from low-grade urothelial carcinoma, why make the distinction. Taking this argument one step further, some experts have argued that papillary neoplasms should be dichotomized into low-grade papillary neoplasms vs high-grade papillary cancer, since papillomas, PUNLMPs, and low-grade cancers share the same treatment and have problems with reproducibility. However, as discussed above, most studies have demonstrated prognostic differences between papilloma, PUNLMP, and low-grade carcinoma. Papillomas uncommonly recur and do not progress and are distinct at the molecular level. PUNLMPs recur at a frequency intermediate between papillomas and low-grade papillary carcinomas and rarely progress. Low-grade papillary urothelial carcinomas recur more frequently and have a low but increased risk of progression compared to PUNLMPs. "Papilloma" and "PUNLMP" are useful diagnostic categories in that they provide noncancerous diagnoses for a group of patients with indolent disease. PUNLMP is especially useful as a diagnosis for the younger patient with a newly diagnosed noninvasive papillary tumor that would not fulfill the criteria of papilloma because of its thicker urothelium.[67-69] In a study of patients aged 20 years or younger with papillary urothelial neoplasia, almost one-half of the patients were diagnosed as having a PUNLMP, thereby avoiding a cancer diagnosis.[67] Similarly, in a study of patients under 30 years of age with urothelial tumors, 40% had a diagnosis of PUNLMP.[68] Additionally, some investigators have proposed that patients with PUNLMP may be submitted to fewer follow-up cystoscopies if the number of lesions are few and no recurrences are seen during the initial surveillance period.[63]

Papillary Carcinomas: Two Grades or Three?

Another controversial area in the WHO/ISUP classification system is that carcinomas are dichotomized as low or high grade, recognizing that high-grade cancer has a spectrum of atypia with some cases showing marked anaplasia and that cases with marked anaplasia have a worse prognosis than other high-grade cancers.[22,30]

The major argument against subdividing high-grade cancers is that high-grade noninvasive papillary cancers with marked anaplasia comprise only a small percentage of noninvasive papillary cancers. In Holmang's study of the 363 noninvasive papillary carcinomas, only 13 (3.6%) were classified as WHO (1973) grade 3, compared with 28% of the cases classified as high-grade carcinoma by the WHO/ISUP system.[22] These data are similar to ours in which only 4.5% of noninvasive papillary tumors were WHO (1973) grade 3 compared with 21.6% classified as WHO/ISUP high grade.[32] There are so few WHO (1973) grade 3 noninvasive papillary carcinomas because most cases of WHO (1973) grade 3 are aggressive tumors in which there is already coexisting invasive cancer. Because patients with high-grade noninvasive papillary carcinoma are not treated with definitive therapy (eg, cystectomy), the goal should not be to restrict the high-risk group to a small population but to expand it to be more inclusive of all patients at significant risk of progression so that they can be monitored closely and treated earlier in the course of the disease.

Use of Artificial Intelligence (AI) and Immunohistochemistry for Grading Papillary Tumors

In analyzing tumors using the WHO/ISUP classification system for p53 expression and proliferation as measured by Ki-67, a progressive increase in p53 expression and proliferation measured by Ki-67 has been documented in cases of PUNLMP, low-grade carcinoma, and high-grade carcinoma, respectively.[70-72] However, there is sufficient overlap such that its use in clinical practice is premature and not recommended for routine use.

CK20 labels the umbrella cells only in normal urothelium and shows increasing thickness of staining in dysplasia to full-thickness staining and CIS.[73] In papillary lesions, a normal pattern of CK20 labeling is seen in 87% of papillomas, 59%-100% of PUNLMPs, 21%-45% of low-grade papillary urothelial carcinomas, and 0%-18% of high-grade papillary urothelial carcinomas.[64,66] In another study, diffuse staining of CK20 was seen in 0%, 25%, and 80% of PUNLMPs, low-grade papillary urothelial carcinomas, and high-grade papillary urothelial carcinomas, respectively.[72] A conflicting study showed no difference in CK20 staining between the three types of papillary tumors.[70] Although the above immunohistochemical markers in general correlate with grade, there is sufficient overlap that they are not that useful in a given case for classification of a papillary urothelial tumor. There have also been some data suggesting that the immunohistochemical pattern of CK20 and high molecular weight cytokeratin can be used to predict recurrence, although these stains are not routinely used in clinical practice.[60] Loss of CD44 immunoreactivity is also associated with increasing tumor grade.[66] Proliferation rates as shown by MIB-1 have also been correlated with progression and recurrence but again are not routinely used in current practice.[76] There have been a few studies using AI for grading papillary bladder tumor, but to date, these are not in use clinically.[74-79]

Papillary Neoplasms in Young Patients

There have been several studies examining bladder cancer in young patients. In a study based primarily on consult material on patients <20 years of age, there were 2 urothelial papillomas, 10 PUNLMPs, 8 low-grade, and 3 high-grade papillary urothelial cancers, all without invasion.[68] Mean patient age was 13.2 years (range 4-20), 19 patients were male, and 19 patients presented with gross hematuria. All lesions were solitary. Only one patient had a history of smoking, and one other had parents who smoked. Three patients (13%) had recurrences classified as either urothelial papilloma ($n = 1$) or PUNLMP ($n = 2$). All patients were alive with no evidence of disease after a mean follow-up of 4.5 years. In a similar sized study of 18 patients diagnosed at <18 years old with a mean age of 11 (range 3-17), there were 8 papillomas, 8 PUNLMPs, 1 low-grade, and 1 high-grade papillary urothelial carcinoma. After a median follow-up of 5 years, no patient experienced recurrence or progression.[78] Genetic alterations frequently seen in older adults were extremely rare in these young patients.[79] Comperat et al. studied a large cohort of patients with bladder tumors <40 years with 40% of those <30 years of age diagnosed with PUNLMP.[69] Overall patients had a favorable prognosis, but it was correlated with grade, stage, and multifocality. In summary, urothelial neoplasms in younger individuals more commonly occur in males and are predominantly low grade with a favorable clinical outcome.

TREATMENT OF PAPILLARY UROTHELIAL NEOPLASMS

Papillomas are typically treated by TUR alone without adjuvant therapy.[58] Patients are followed with routine cystoscopy in the same fashion as papillary carcinoma (see below) because there is a risk of recurrence, albeit low. There is no consensus as to how long patients should be followed, although the risk of recurrence is very low and most recurrences occur within 5 years after diagnosis.

The National Comprehensive Cancer Network (NCCN) guidelines have adopted the American Urology Association (AUA)/Society of Urological Oncology (SUO) guidelines.[80] Low-risk NMIBC includes PUNLMPs and noninvasive low-grade urothelial carcinoma that are solitary Ta and <3 cm. For these tumors, risk of recurrence or progression is low following TURBT and no further treatment is necessary, although a single instillation of intravesical chemotherapy immediately post-TURBT can be helpful in reducing the risk of recurrence.

Intermediate-risk NMIBC includes low-grade noninvasive papillary urothelial carcinomas that have any of the following characteristics: size >3 cm, multifocal, or recurrence within 1 year. In addition, high-grade noninvasive papillary urothelial carcinomas that are solitary and <3 cm are also considered intermediate risk. Although a complete TURBT alone can eradicate intermediate-risk NMIBC, there is a relatively high risk for recurrence. Therefore, after TURBT and immediate intravesical chemotherapy, a 6-week induction course of intravesical therapy is recommended, although surveillance is an option.

High-risk NMIBC includes noninvasive high-grade papillary urothelial carcinoma that has any of the following characteristics: concurrent CIS, size >3 cm, or multifocal. For patients who have not received BCG (BCG-naive), these tumors are typically treated with BCG, potentially for longer duration than intermediate-risk disease. However, for some patients, BCG is not an option due to adverse side effects, BCG shortages, or a tumor that is BCG unresponsive. For these patients, cystectomy is preferred, although intravesical chemotherapy or pembrolizumab are also options.

The European Association of Urology (EAU) has developed similar guidelines for NMIBC.[81] The EAU uses a weighted scoring factoring in number of tumors, tumor diameter, prior recurrence rate, concurrent CIS, and grade (based on the WHO 1973 system) resulting in four tiers with a low, intermediate, high, and very high risk of recurrence and progression.

Repeat TURBT may also be considered for select patients with noninvasive papillary urothelial tumors (Ta) on initial TURBT, particularly if the tumor is large and/or there was no muscle present in the initial TURBT specimen. In one study, restaging TURBT detected residual disease in 27% of patients with Ta disease, even when muscle was present in the original TURBT.[82]

MIMICKERS OF PAPILLARY UROTHELIAL NEOPLASMS

The most common mimicker of a papillary urothelial neoplasm is polypoid cystitis, which is covered in Chapter 10. Another often difficult differential diagnosis is between a papillary urothelial neoplasm with a prominent inverted growth pattern vs an inverted urothelial papilloma (Chapter 4). Finally, nephrogenic adenoma and clear cell adenocarcinoma may have

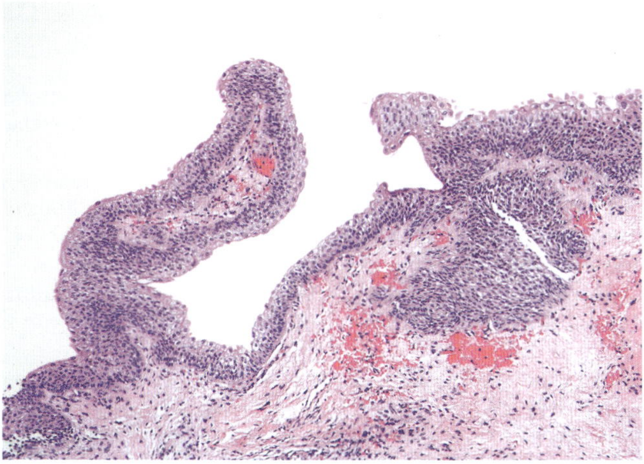

FIGURE 3.50 **Artifactual papillary fold lined by urothelium of normal thickness and cytology.** Note similarity to surround flat normal urothelium. No lesion was seen at cystoscopy.

a surface papillary component with slender fibrovascular core mimicking papillary urothelial neoplasia (Chapter 8). The key difference is that in these two entities, the lining is columnar or glandular rather than urothelial in appearance. One can also occasionally have tangential sections of normal urothelium mimicking a papillary urothelial tumor. Papillary urothelial hyperplasia is distinguished from PUNLMP by lack of true fibrovascular cores. One should be cautious diagnosing a papillary urothelial tumor on one or two fronds with no cytological atypia, particularly is associated with inflammation or reactive stromal changes in the lamina propria. Correlation with findings at cystoscopy is helpful, and if no papillary lesion is noted, then the isolated papillary-appearing structure should be considered artifactual (Fig. 3.50). Occasionally, prostatic adenocarcinoma when it involves the bladder or urethra may have a villoglandular appearance and may mimic a high-grade papillary urothelial carcinoma[83] (see Chapter 13). Immunostains and underlying invasive adenocarcinoma usually resolve the differential diagnosis. Fibroepithelial polyp and prostatic polyps in the bladder may rarely clinically be mistaken for papillary urothelial neoplasia.

REFERENCES

1. Taylor DC, Bhagavan BS, Larsen MP, et al. Papillary urothelial hyperplasia. A precursor to papillary neoplasms. *Am J Surg Pathol.* 1996;20:1481-1488.
2. Readal N, Epstein JI. Papillary urothelial hyperplasia: relationship to urothelial neoplasms. *Pathology.* 2010;42:360-363.
3. Lowenthal BM, Sahoo D, Amin MB, Hansel DE. Urothelial proliferation of unknown malignant potential involving the bladder: histopathologic features and risk of progression in de novo cases and cases with prior neoplasia. *Arch Pathol Lab Med.* 2020;144(7):853-862.

4. Eble JN, Sauter G, Epstein JI, Sesterhenn I, eds. *WHO Classification of Tumours. WHO Classification of Tumours of the Urinary System and Male Genital Organs*. Vol. 7. 3rd ed. IARC Press; 2004.
5. Moch H, Humphrey PA, Ulbright TM. In: Reuter VE, ed. *WHO Classification of Tumours. WHO Classification of Tumours of the Urinary System and Male Genital Organs*. Vol. 8. 4th ed. IARC Press; 2016.
6. Paner GP, Smith SC, Hartmann A, et al. Flat intraurothelial lesions of the urinary bladder–do hyperplasia, dysplasia, and atypia of unknown significance need to exist as diagnostic entities? And how to handle in routine clinical practice. *Mod Pathol.* 2022;35(10):1296-1305.
7. WHO Classification of Tumours Editorial Board. *WHO Classification of Tumours. WHO Classification of Tumours of the Urinary and Male Genital Organs*. Vol. 8. 5th ed. IARC Press; 2022.
8. Amin MB, Comperat E, Epstein JI, et al. The Genitourinary Pathology Society update on classification and grading of flat and papillary urothelial neoplasia with new reporting recommendations and approach to lesions with mixed and early patterns of neoplasia. *Adv Anat Pathol.* 2021;28(4):179-195.
9. Chow NH, Cairns P, Eisenberger CF, et al. Papillary urothelial hyperplasia is a clonal precursor to papillary transitional cell bladder cancer. *Int J Cancer.* 2000;89:514-518.
10. Swierczynski SL, Epstein JI. Prognostic significance of atypical papillary urothelial hyperplasia. *Hum Pathol.* 2002;33:512-517.
11. Epstein JI, Amin MB, Reuter VR, et al. The World Health Organization/International Society of Urological Pathology consensus classification of urothelial (transitional cell) neoplasms of the urinary bladder. Bladder Consensus Conference Committee. *Am J Surg Pathol.* 1998;22:1435-1448.
12. Eble JN, Young RH. Benign and low-grade papillary lesions of the urinary bladder: a review of the papilloma-papillary carcinoma controversy, and a report of five typical papillomas. *Semin Diagn Pathol.* 1989;6:351-371.
13. Broders AC. Epithelioma of the genito-urinary organs. *Ann Surg.* 1922;75:574-604.
14. Bergkvist A, Ljungqvist A, Moberger G. Classification of bladder tumours based on the cellular pattern. Preliminary report of a clinical-pathological study of 300 cases with a minimum follow-up of eight years. *Acta Chir Scand.* 1965;130:371-378.
15. Mostofi FK, Sobin LH, Torloni H. *Histological Typing of Urinary Bladder Tumours*. Vol. 19. World Health Organization; 1973.
16. Ooms EC, Anderson WA, Alons CL, et al. Analysis of the performance of pathologists in the grading of bladder tumors. *Hum Pathol.* 1983;14:140-143.
17. Jordan AM, Weingarten J, Murphy WM. Transitional cell neoplasms of the urinary bladder. Can biologic potential be predicted from histologic grading? *Cancer.* 1987;60:2766-2774.
18. Malmström PU, Busch C, Norlen BJ. Recurrence, progression and survival in bladder cancer. A retrospective analysis of 232 patients with greater than or equal to 5-year follow-up. *Scand J Urol Nephrol.* 1987;21:185-195.
19. Abel PD, Henderson D, Bennett MK, et al. Differing interpretations by pathologists of the pT category and grade of transitional cell cancer of the bladder. *Br J Urol.* 1988;62:339-342.
20. Carbin BE, Ekman P, Gustafson H, et al. Grading of human urothelial carcinoma based on nuclear atypia and mitotic frequency. II. Prognostic importance. *J Urol.* 1991;145:972-975; discussion 975-976.
21. Holmäng S, Hedelin H, Anderström C, et al. Recurrence and progression in low grade papillary urothelial tumors. *J Urol.* 1999;162(3 Pt 1):702-707. doi:10.1097/00005392-199909010-00019
22. Holmäng S, Andius P, Hedelin H, et al. Stage progression in Ta papillary urothelial tumors: relationship to grade, immunohistochemical expression of tumor markers, mitotic frequency and DNA ploidy. *J Urol.* 2001;165(4):1124-1128. discussion 1128-1130.

23. Pan CC, Chang YH, Chen KK, et al. Prognostic significance of the 2004 WHO/ISUP classification for prediction of recurrence, progression, and cancer-specific mortality of non-muscle-invasive urothelial tumors of the urinary bladder: a clinicopathologic study of 1,515 cases. *Am J Clin Pathol.* 2010;133:788-795.
24. Pan CC, Chang YH, Chen KK, et al. Constructing prognostic model incorporating the 2004 WHO/ISUP classification for patients with non-muscle-invasive urothelial tumours of the urinary bladder. *J Clin Pathol.* 2010;63:910-915.
25. Chaux A, Karram S, Miller JS, et al. High-grade papillary urothelial carcinoma of the urinary tract: a clinicopathologic analysis of a post-World Health Organization/International Society of Urological Pathology classification cohort from a single academic center. *Hum Pathol.* 2012;43:115-120.
26. Lee TK, Chaux A, Karram S, et al. Papillary urothelial neoplasm of low malignant potential of the urinary bladder: clinicopathologic and outcome analysis from a single academic center. *Hum Pathol.* 2011;42:1799-1803.
27. Maxwell JP, Wang C, Wiebe N, et al. Long-term outcome of primary papillary urothelial neoplasm of low malignant potential (PUNLMP) including PUNLMP with inverted growth. *Diagn Pathol.* 2015;10:3. doi:10.1186/s13000-015-0234-z
28. Miyamoto H, Brimo F, Schultz L, et al. Low-grade papillary urothelial carcinoma of the urinary bladder: a clinicopathologic analysis of a post-World Health Organization/International Society of Urological Pathology classification cohort from a single academic center. *Arch Pathol Lab Med.* 2010;134:1160-1163.
29. Miyamoto H, Miller JS, Fajardo DA, et al. Non-invasive papillary urothelial neoplasms: the 2004 WHO/ISUP classification system. *Pathol Int.* 2010;60:1-8.
30. Bircan S, Candir O, Serel TA. Comparison of WHO 1973, WHO/ISUP 1998, WHO 1999 grade and combined scoring systems in evaluation of bladder carcinoma. *Urol Int.* 2004;73:201-208.
31. Genega EM, Kapali M, Torres-Quinones M, et al. Impact of the 1998 World Health Organization/International Society of Urological Pathology classification system for urothelial neoplasms of the kidney. *Mod Pathol.* 2005;18:11-18.
32. Samaratunga H, Makarov DV, Epstein JI. Comparison of WHO/ISUP and WHO classification of noninvasive papillary urothelial neoplasms for risk of progression. *Urology.* 2002;60:315-319.
33. Brunner A, Schonhuber G, Waldner M, et al. Chromosomal aberrations in urothelial carcinoma of the bladder and the World Health Organization 2004 grading system. *Anal Quant Cytol Histol.* 2008;30:297-305.
34. Burger M, Denzinger S, Wieland WF, et al. Does the current World Health Organization classification predict the outcome better in patients with noninvasive bladder cancer of early or regular onset? *BJU Int.* 2008;102:194-197.
35. Gonul II, Poyraz A, Unsal C, et al. Comparison of 1998 WHO/ISUP and 1973 WHO classifications for interobserver variability in grading of papillary urothelial neoplasms of the bladder. Pathological evaluation of 258 cases. *Urol Int.* 2007;78:338-344.
36. Cao D, Vollmer RT, Luly J, et al. Comparison of 2004 and 1973 World Health Organization grading systems and their relationship to pathologic staging for predicting long-term prognosis in patients with urothelial carcinoma. *Urology.* 2010;76:593-599.
37. Mamoon N, Iqbal MA, Jamal S, et al. Urothelial neoplasia of the urinary bladder—comparison of interobserver variability for WHO Classification 1972 with WHO/ISUP Consensus Classification 1998. *J Ayub Med Coll Abbottabad.* 2006;18:4-8.
38. May M, Brookman-Amissah S, Roigas J, et al. Prognostic accuracy of individual uropathologists in noninvasive urinary bladder carcinoma: a multicentre study comparing the 1973 and 2004 World Health Organization classifications. *Eur Urol.* 2010;57:850-858.
39. Pich A, Chiusa L, Formiconi A, et al. Biologic differences between noninvasive papillary urothelial neoplasms of low malignant potential and low-grade (grade 1) papillary carcinomas of the bladder. *Am J Surg Pathol.* 2001;25:1528-1533.

40. Sylvester RJ, Rodríguez O, Hernández V, et al. European Association of Urology (EAU) prognostic factor risk groups for non-muscle-invasive bladder cancer (NMIBC) incorporating the WHO 2004/2016 and WHO 1973 classification systems for grade: an update from the EAU NMIBC Guidelines Panel. *Eur Urol.* 2021;79(4):480-488.
41. Compérat EM, Burger M, Gontero P, et al. Grading of urothelial carcinoma and the new "World Health Organization Classification of Tumours of the Urinary System and Male Genital Organs 2016". *Eur Urol Focus.* 2019;5(3):457-466.
42. Bosschieter J, Hentschel A, Savci-Heijink CD, et al. Reproducibility and prognostic performance of the 1973 and 2004 World Health Organization classifications for grade in non-muscle-invasive bladder cancer: A Multicenter study in 328 bladder tumors. *Clin Genitourin Cancer.* 2018;16(5):e985-e992.
43. Rieken M, Shariat SF, Kluth L, et al. Comparison of the EORTC tables and the EAU categories for risk stratification of patients with nonmuscle-invasive bladder cancer. *Urol Oncol.* 2018;36(1):8.e17-8.e24.
44. Varma M, Delahunt B, van der Kwast T. Grading noninvasive bladder cancer: World Health Organization 1973 or 2004 may be the wrong question. *Eur Urol.* 2019;76(4): 413-415.
45. Soukup V, Čapoun O, Cohen D, et al. Prognostic performance and reproducibility of the 1973 and 2004/2016 World Health Organization grading classification systems in non-muscle-invasive bladder cancer: a European Association of Urology non-muscle invasive bladder cancer guidelines panel systematic review. *Eur Urol.* 2017;72(5):801-813.
46. Isharwal S, Hu W, Sarungbam J, et al. Genomic landscape of inverted urothelial papilloma and urothelial papilloma of the bladder. *J Pathol.* 2019;248(3):260-265. doi:10.1002/path.5261
47. Yorukoglu K, Tuna B, Dikicioglu E, et al. Reproducibility of the 1998 World Health Organization/International Society of Urologic Pathology classification of papillary urothelial neoplasms of the urinary bladder. *Virchows Arch.* 2003;443:734-740.
48. Oosterhuis JW, Schapers RF, Janssen-Heijnen ML, et al. Histological grading of papillary urothelial carcinoma of the bladder: prognostic value of the 1998 WHO/ISUP classification system and comparison with conventional grading systems. *J Clin Pathol.* 2002;55:900-905.
49. Cheng L, Darson M, Cheville JC, et al. Urothelial papilloma of the bladder. Clinical and biologic implications. *Cancer.* 1999;86:2098-2101.
50. Magi-Galluzzi C, Epstein JI. Urothelial papilloma of the bladder: a review of 34 de novo cases. *Am J Surg Pathol.* 2004;28:1615-1620.
51. McKenney JK, Amin MB, Young RH. Urothelial (transitional cell) papilloma of the urinary bladder: a clinicopathologic study of 26 cases. *Mod Pathol.* 2003;16:623-629.
52. Matoso A, Parimi V, Epstein JI. Noninvasive low-grade papillary urothelial carcinoma with degenerative nuclear atypia: a grading pitfall. *Hum Pathol.* 2021;113:1-8.
53. Owens CL, Epstein JI. Significance of denuded urothelium in papillary urothelial lesions. *Am J Surg Pathol.* 2007;31:298-303.
54. Reis LO, Taheri D, Guner G, et al. Significance of a minor high grade component in a low grade non-invasive papillary urothelial carcinoma of bladder. *Hum Pathol.* 2016;47(1):20-25.
55. Gofrit ON, Pizov G, Shapiro A, et al. Mixed high and low grade bladder tumors–are they clinically high or low grade? *J Urol.* 2014;191:1693-1696.
56. Billis A, Carvalho RB, Mattos AC, et al. Tumor grade heterogeneity in urothelial bladder carcinoma–proposal of a system using combined numbers. *Scand J Urol Nephrol.* 2001;35:275-279.
57. Cheng L, Neumann RM, Nehra A, et al. Cancer heterogeneity and its biologic implications in the grading of urothelial carcinoma. *Cancer.* 2000;88:1663-1670.

58. Babjuk M, Burger M, Zigeuner R, et al. EAU guidelines on non-muscle-invasive urothelial carcinoma of the bladder: update 2013. *Eur Urol.* 2013;64:639-653.
59. Cheng L, Neumann RM, Bostwick DG. Papillary urothelial neoplasms of low malignant potential. Clinical and biologic implications. *Cancer.* 1999;86:2102-2108.
60. Ramos D, Navarro S, Villamón R, et al. Cytokeratin expression patterns in low-grade papillary urothelial neoplasms of the urinary bladder. *Cancer.* 2003;97(8):1876-1883.
61. Murphy WM, Takezawa K, Maruniak NA. Interobserver discrepancy using the 1998 World Health Organization/International Society of Urologic Pathology classification of urothelial neoplasms: practical choices for patient care. *J Urol.* 2002;168:968-972.
62. Tuna B, Yorukoglu K, Duzcan E, et al. Histologic grading of urothelial papillary neoplasms: impact of combined grading (two-numbered grading system) on reproducibility. *Virchows Arch.* 2011;458:659-664.
63. Herr HW, Donat SM, Reuter VE. Management of low grade papillary bladder tumors. *J Urol.* 2007;178(4 Pt 1):1201-1205.
64. Alsheikh A, Mohamedali Z, Jones E, et al. Comparison of the WHO/ISUP classification and cytokeratin 20 expression in predicting the behavior of low-grade papillary urothelial tumors. World/Health Organization/International Society of Urologic Pathology. *Mod Pathol.* 2001;14:267-272.
65. Campbell PA, Conrad RJ, Campbell CM, et al. Papillary urothelial neoplasm of low malignant potential: reliability of diagnosis and outcome. *BJU Int.* 2004;93:1228-1231.
66. Desai S, Lim SD, Jimenez RE, et al. Relationship of cytokeratin 20 and CD44 protein expression with WHO/ISUP grade in pTa and pT1 papillary urothelial neoplasia. *Mod Pathol.* 2000;13:1315-1323.
67. Fujii Y, Kawakami S, Koga F, et al. Long-term outcome of bladder papillary urothelial neoplasms of low malignant potential. *BJU Int.* 2003;92:559-562.
68. Fine SW, Humphrey PA, Dehner LP, et al. Urothelial neoplasms in patients 20 years or younger: a clinicopathological analysis using the world health organization 2004 bladder consensus classification. *J Urol.* 2005;174:1976-1980.
69. Comperat E, Larre S, Roupret M, et al. Clinicopathological characteristics of urothelial bladder cancer in patients less than 40 years old. *Virchows Arch.* 2015;466:589-594.
70. Cina SJ, Lancaster-Weiss KJ, Lecksell K, et al. Correlation of Ki-67 and p53 with the new World Health Organization/International Society of Urological Pathology Classification System for Urothelial Neoplasia. *Arch Pathol Lab Med.* 2001;125:646-651.
71. Shim JW, Cho KS, Choi YD, et al. Diagnostic algorithm for papillary urothelial tumors in the urinary bladder. *Virchows Arch.* 2008;452:353-362.
72. Yin H, Leong AS. Histologic grading of noninvasive papillary urothelial tumors: validation of the 1998 WHO/ISUP system by immunophenotyping and follow up. *Am J Clin Pathol.* 2004;121:679-687.
73. Edgecombe A, Nguyen BN, Djordjevic B, et al. Utility of cytokeratin 5/6, cytokeratin 20, and p16 in the diagnosis of reactive urothelial atypia and noninvasive component of urothelial neoplasia. *Appl Immunohistochem Mol Morphol.* 2012;20:264-271.
74. Barbisan F, Mazzucchelli R, Santinelli A, et al. Immunohistochemical evaluation of global DNA methylation and histone acetylation in papillary urothelial neoplasm of low malignant potential. *Int J Immunopathol Pharmacol.* 2008;21(3):615-623.
75. Jansen I, Lucas M, Bosschieter J, et al. Automated detection and grading of non-muscle-invasive urothelial cell carcinoma of the bladder. *Am J Pathol.* 2020;190(7):1483-1490.
76. Choi HK, Jarkrans T, Bengtsson E, et al. Image analysis based grading of bladder carcinoma. Comparison of object, texture and graph based methods and their reproducibility. *Anal Cell Pathol.* 1997;15(1):1-18.
77. Spyridonos P, Cavouras D, Ravazoula P, et al. Neural network-based segmentation and classification system for automated grading of histologic sections of bladder carcinoma. *Anal Quant Cytol Histol.* 2002;24(6):317-324.

78. Berrettini A, Castagnetti M, Salerno A, et al. Bladder urothelial neoplasms in pediatric age: experience at three tertiary centers. *J Pediatr Urol.* 2015;11:26.e1-26.e5.
79. Wild PJ, Giedl J, Stoehr R, et al. Genomic aberrations are rare in urothelial neoplasms of patients 19 years or younger. *J Pathol.* 2007;211:18-25.
80. Flaig TW, Spiess PE, Abern M, et al. NCCN Guidelines® Insights: Bladder Cancer, Version 2.2022. *J Natl Compr Canc Netw.* 2022;20(8):866-878.
81. Babjuk M, Burger M, Compérat EM, et al. European Association of Urology guidelines on non-muscle-invasive bladder cancer (TaT1 and carcinoma in situ)–2019 update. *Eur Urol.* 2019;76(5):639-657.
82. Grimm MO, Steinhoff C, Simon X, et al. Effect of routine repeat transurethral resection for superficial bladder cancer: a long-term observational study. *J Urol.* 2003;170 (2 Pt 1):433-437.
83. Gordetsky J, Epstein JI. Pseudopapillary features in prostatic adenocarcinoma mimicking urothelial carcinoma: a diagnostic pitfall. *Am J Surg Pathol.* 2014;38(7):941-945.

4

UROTHELIAL NEOPLASMS WITH INVERTED GROWTH PATTERNS

INVERTED UROTHELIAL PAPILLOMA

This is a benign tumor, most commonly occurring in the bladder neck and trigone of the bladder and less commonly in the renal pelvis, ureter, and urethra, constitutes <1% of urothelial neoplasms. Cystoscopically, they appear as solitary, raised, pedunculated, or, rarely, polypoid lesions with a smooth surface.[1] Lesions occur in a wide age range of patients (10-94 years), with a peak frequency in the sixth and seventh decades; there is a striking male predilection,[2,3] as is the case with most urothelial neoplasms. Tumor size varies from small (<1-50 mm, mean 12.8 mm). Most lesions are solitary (<5% are multifocal) and present with hematuria.[4]

Histologically, two variations have been described: trabecular and glandular. The trabecular type is the classic lesion that most pathologists think of when considering inverted papilloma, histologically showing cords and trabeculae of cells arising from a smooth surface and invaginating into the lamina propria. The trabeculae are no more than 5-10 layers in thickness representing inversion of papillary urothelium of normal thickness (Figs. 4.1-4.3, eFigs. 4.1-4.22). Due to their inverted nature, the periphery is composed of darker cells that are often palisaded (the basal cells), and the central portions show maturing cells occasionally with superficial umbrella cells lining central luminal spaces filled with colloid material (Figs. 4.4-4.6). It is not uncommon to see focal nonkeratinizing squamous and occasionally true glandular differentiation (so-called glandular type) within the center of the urothelial cords (Figs. 4.7 and 4.8). In the latter setting, mimicry with florid cystitis cystica is considerable, and we rely on the overall organization and architecture of the lesion to designate a lesion as inverted neoplasia. The surrounding stroma is fibrotic and nonreactive without inflammation.

Cytologic atypia, by definition, is minimal to absent, although occasionally degenerative atypia may be present, albeit focally (Fig. 4.9, eFigs. 4.23 and 4.24). Exceptional cases may have the classic features of benign inverted urothelial papilloma, yet have focal nondegenerative atypia. One of the authors has studied inverted papillomas with very focal atypia

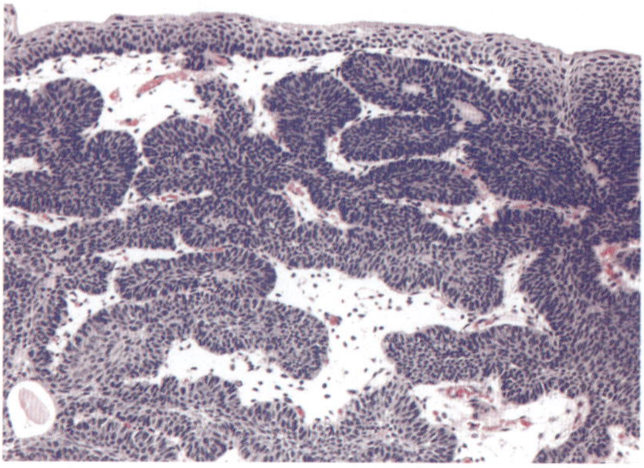

FIGURE 4.1 **Inverted urothelial papilloma with focal downgrowth from overlying benign urothelium (*upper right*).**

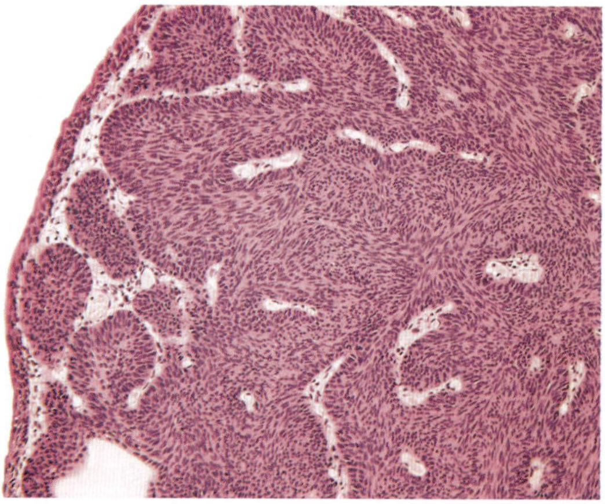

FIGURE 4.2 **Inverted urothelial papilloma with undermining overlying benign urothelium.** There is prominent spindling in this case with peripheral palisading.

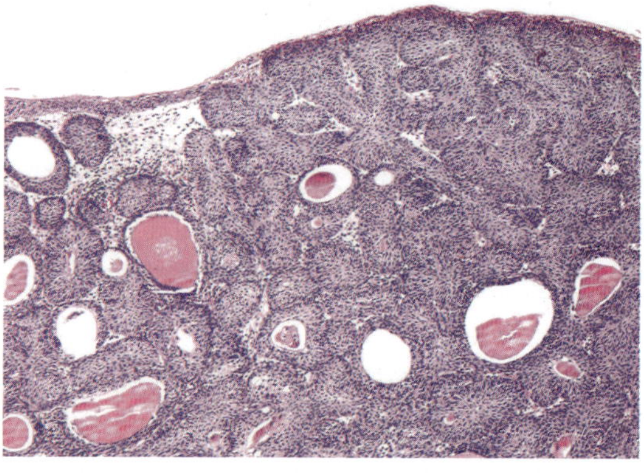

FIGURE 4.3 **Inverted urothelial papilloma with undermining overlying benign urothelium.** Note colloid cysts.

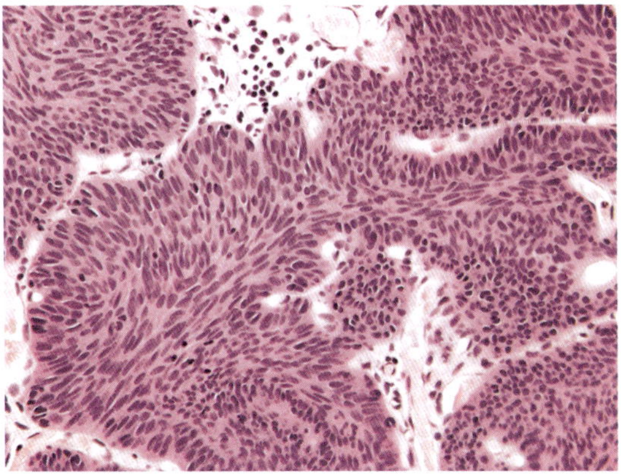

FIGURE 4.4 **Inverted urothelial papilloma with cords of epithelium showing peripheral palisading and central streaming of urothelium parallel to the cords.** High power of Figure 4.2.

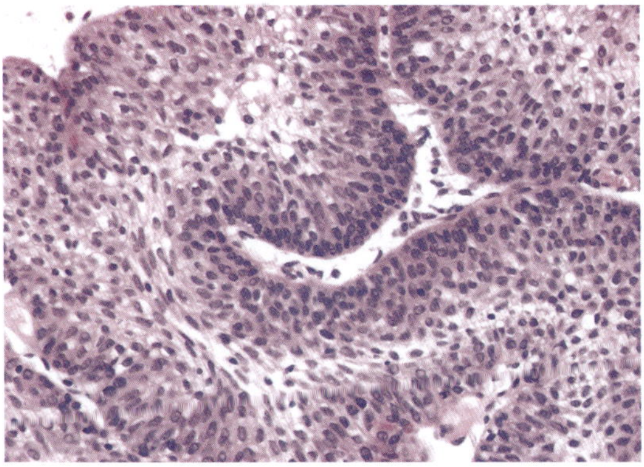

FIGURE 4.5 **Inverted urothelial papilloma with peripheral palisading and central streaming of urothelium.**

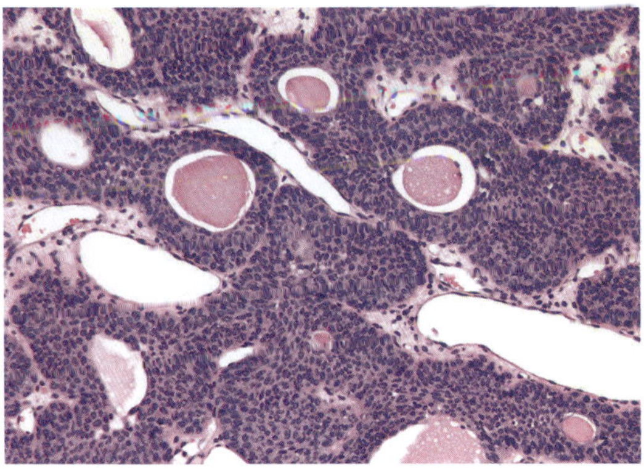

FIGURE 4.6 **Inverted urothelial papilloma with numerous colloid cysts.**

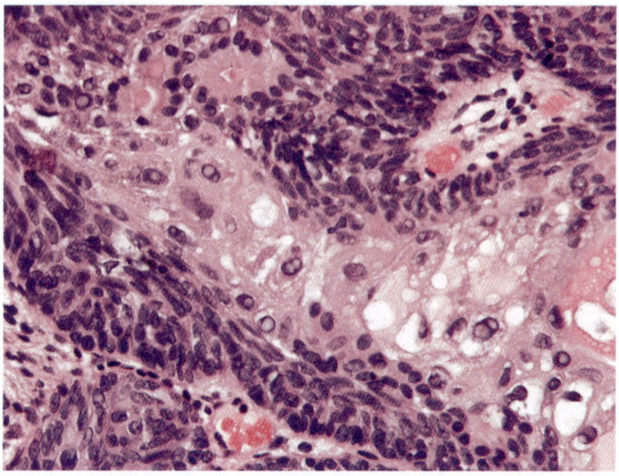

FIGURE 4.7 Nonkeratinizing squamous differentiation in inverted urothelial papilloma.

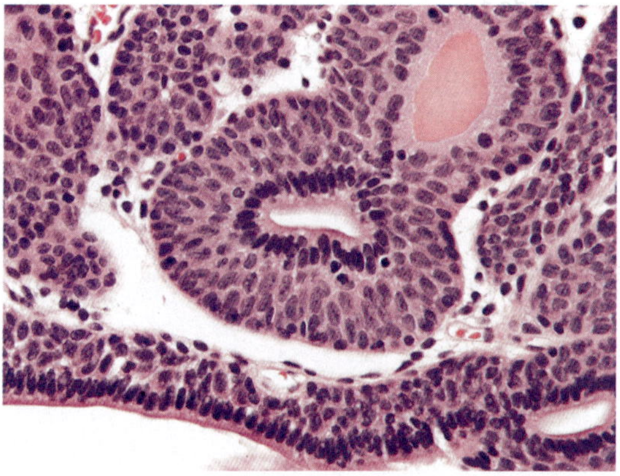

FIGURE 4.8 Glandular differentiation in inverted urothelial papilloma.

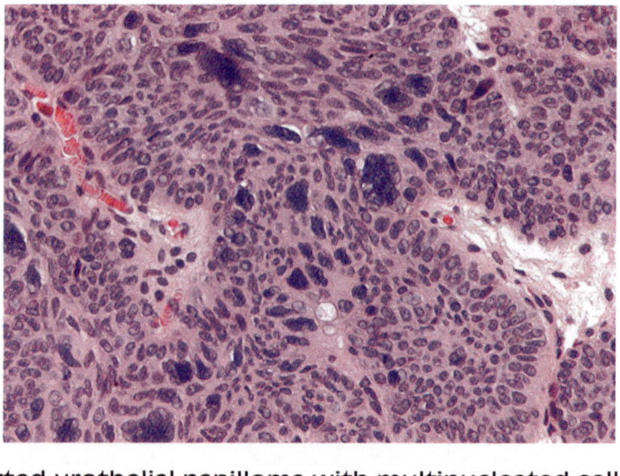

FIGURE 4.9 Inverted urothelial papilloma with multinucleated cells with degenerative atypia.

subdivided into the following groups: (1) areas containing prominent nucleoli; (2) foci with atypical squamous features; and (3) foci with areas of dysplasia, approaching the level of carcinoma *in situ* (Fig. 4.10, eFigs. 4.25-4.32). These lesions are controversial, as some experts consider that any neoplastic (nondegenerative) atypia should lead to the diagnosis of urothelial carcinoma with inverted features. Others consider that if the lesion is otherwise architecturally and cytologically classic for inverted papilloma with the exception of focal cytological atypia, it is justified to diagnose these lesions as inverted papilloma with a comment on the atypia. In the only study to investigate this phenomenon, albeit with only a few cases and limited follow-up, the clinical course was benign.[5] Regardless of the nomenclature used, any atypical features in an inverted urothelial papilloma warrant periodic cystoscopic follow-up.

Mitotic figures are rare and are only seen at the periphery of the trabeculae. The trabeculae are orderly, of relatively uniform width, with considerable ramifications and interanastomosis. The urothelium in the center of the trabeculae tends to stream parallel to the cords. Occasionally, there may be marked von Brunn nest proliferation in the adjacent mucosa. Paneth cell–like neuroendocrine differentiation is exceptionally rare.[6] Other unusual variants include those with xanthomatous or vacuolated cytoplasm (Figs. 4.11 and 4.12).[6] A cribriform adenoid cystic–like appearance may be rarely present.[7]

Inverted urothelial papillomas may have focal polypoid exophytic areas, yet lack true papillae (Figs. 4.13 and 4.14, eFig. 4.19). Within these broader projections are solid nests and cords of urothelium, cytologically characteristic of inverted urothelial papilloma, differing from a central fibrovascular core lined by urothelium seen in urothelial carcinoma and exophytic urothelial papilloma. Exceptionally, classic inverted papillomas may have one or two small apparently true fronds; in these cases, a diagnosis of inverted papilloma is still acceptable as the fronds may

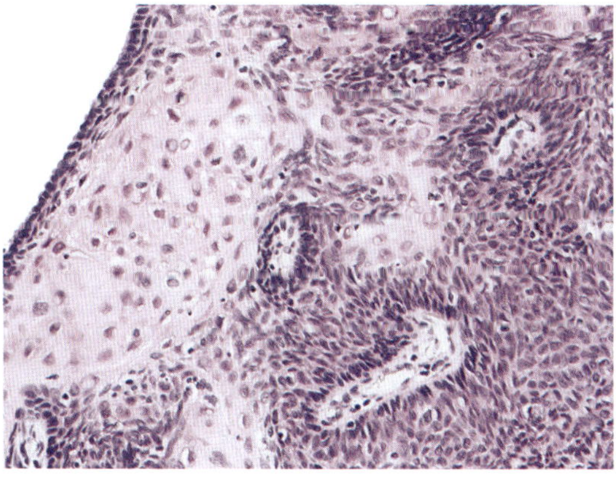

FIGURE 4.10 Inverted urothelial papilloma with focal atypical squamous epithelium.

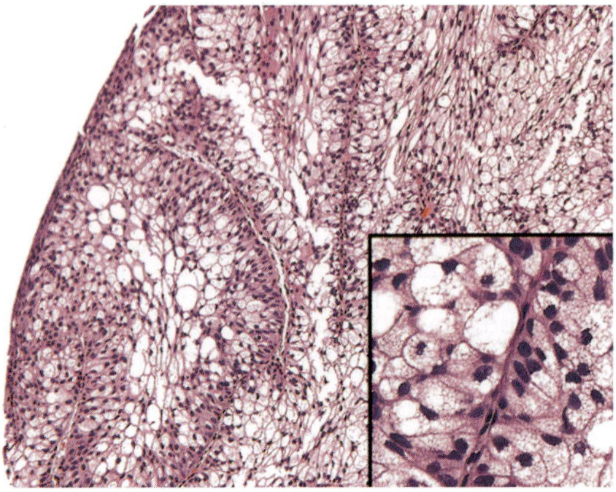

FIGURE 4.11 Inverted urothelial papilloma with xanthomatous cytoplasm (inset higher magnification).

represent a tangential section off of a polypoid growth (Fig. 4.15). In rare cases, there may be the classic findings of benign inverted urothelial papilloma with areas typical of exophytic urothelial papilloma. These cases are referred to as mixed inverted and exophytic urothelial papilloma. There are only anecdotal data on the behavior of these hybrid lesions, most behaving indolently although it is recommended that they be followed as if they had an exophytic papilloma with repeat periodic cystoscopic examinations.[8]

Inverted urothelial papilloma is a benign neoplasm, which if completely resected does not need routine cystoscopic follow-up, in contrast to what is performed for urothelial carcinoma and exophytic urothelial papilloma. The recurrence rate is 1%-2%.[9] Older studies suggested that inverted urothelial papilloma, especially in the upper urinary tract, was associated with an increased likelihood of prior, concurrent, or subsequent urothelial carcinoma.[10,11] However, multiple more recent studies

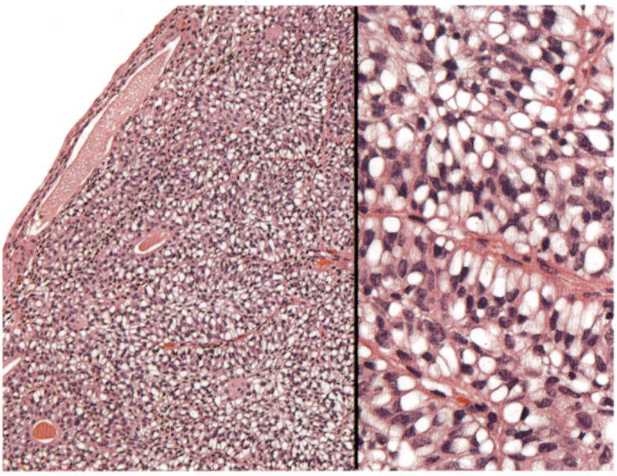

FIGURE 4.12 Inverted urothelial papilloma with prominent cytoplasmic vacuoles.

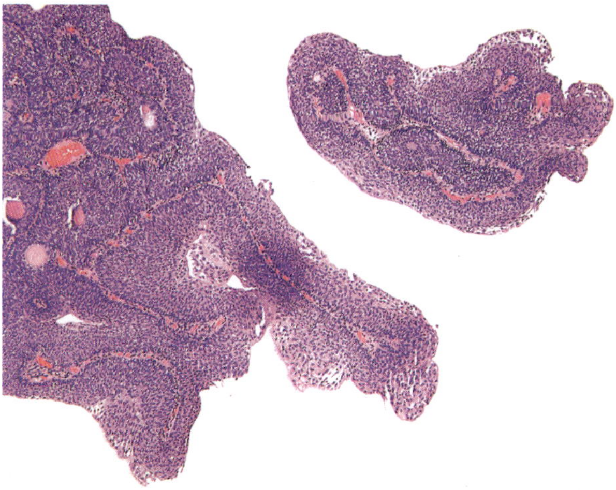

A

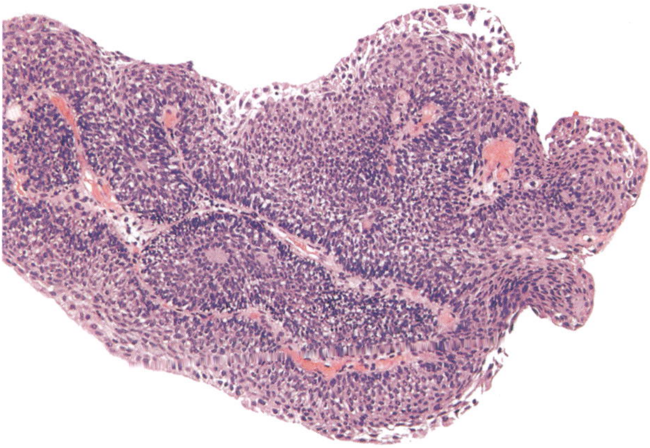

B

FIGURE 4.13 Classic inverted urothelial papilloma (A). Polypoid projection of inverted urothelial papilloma with surface and underlying nests of cells showing peripheral palisading and central streaming. High power (B).

have not shown an increased risk of urothelial carcinoma.[9,12] A review of the literature of over 348 cases has shown that 1.7% of inverted papillomas of the bladder had previous urothelial carcinoma, 1.4% had synchronous urothelial carcinoma, and 1.1% had subsequent urothelial carcinoma; time to recurrence was <45 months, average ~28 months.[4] Bladder urothelial papillomas are typically not associated with urothelial carcinoma of the upper tract such that surveillance of the upper tract in patients with inverted papilloma of the lower tract is not always deemed necessary.[4] Several studies have explored molecular changes in inverted lesions (studied by immunohistochemistry, fluorescence, *in situ* hybridization, microsatellite and loss of heterozygosity analysis, and

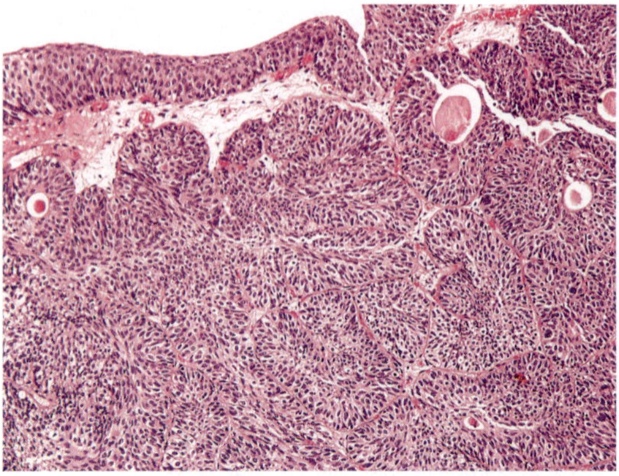

A

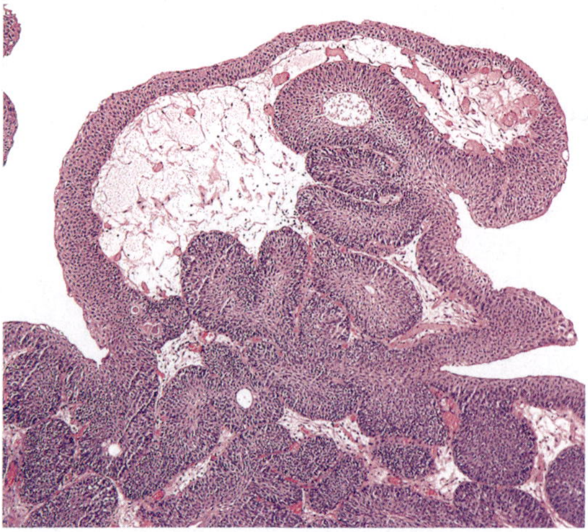

B

FIGURE 4.14 Inverted urothelial papilloma **(A)**. Focally, the lesion had a polypoid architecture filled with nests typical of inverted papilloma **(B)**.

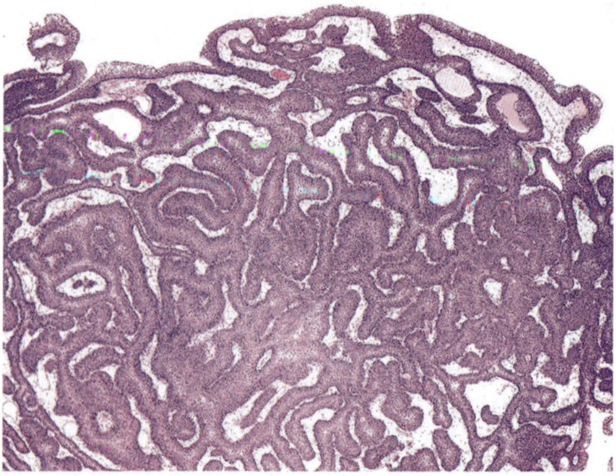

FIGURE 4.15 Classic inverted urothelial papilloma with solitary papillary frond (*left upper*).

mutational analyses), but none of these studies to date have applications to routine diagnostic surgical pathology, although they support the benign nature of these lesions.[5,9,13-15] HRAS and fibroblast growth factor receptor 3 (FGFR3) mutations have been detected in a small subset of cases.[5,16,17]

UROTHELIAL NEOPLASMS WITH INVERTED GROWTH PATTERNS (EXCLUDING INVERTED PAPILLOMAS)

Urothelial neoplasms exhibit two patterns of endophytic or inverted growth: (1) broad-front verrucous carcinoma–like growth and (2) inverted papilloma–like growth.[18] The two patterns may coexist, and either pattern may or may not be associated with frank stromal invasion. In broad-front growth, like verrucous carcinoma, broad bulbous tongues of neoplastic urothelium extend deep into the lamina propria and sometimes may reach up to the muscularis propria. In our opinion, despite the deep penetration, invasion is not present if the basement membrane is smooth, and the likelihood of metastasis is minimal. If, however, there is irregularity of the basement membrane of the bulbous endophytic tongues of broad-front growth, and if there is retraction artifact, desmoplasia, or other features suggestive of destructive invasion, the tumor must be designated as invasive.[18]

The nomenclature for inverted lesions with inverted papilloma–like architecture has been promulgated by the International Consultation on Urologic Disease/European Association of Urology consultation on bladder cancer (outlined in Table 4.1) with an aim to foster consistent terminology and foster study of cases to better understand their true biologic potential. The classification used for exophytic tumors is extrapolated for inverted lesions, and overall, there is an analogy in nomenclature and approach for flat lesions.[19-21] While inverted lesions except inverted papillomas are not separately dealt with in the WHO 2022 fifth edition, for each urothelial tumor grade category, that is, PUNLMP, papillary urothelial carcinoma, low-grade, and high-grade inverted patterns are all acknowledged in their respective sections to have inverted histology.[22] It has been recommended that a tumor should have >80% inverted histology to be diagnosed and terminology such as "papillary urothelial carcinoma, low grade, with predominant (>80%) inverted growth pattern; no evidence of invasion" or "papillary urothelial neoplasm of low malignant potential, exclusive inverted growth, no evidence of invasion." Use of consistent terminology will enable further study of the significance of inverted growth, which is currently limited.[21]

In tumors with inverted papilloma–like growth, the basic configuration is like inverted papilloma, that is, endophytic, expansile growth with or without peripheral palisading of basaloid cells. In contrast to inverted papilloma, inverted urothelial carcinomas usually have a variable proportion of exophytic component; exceptional cases solely consist of urothelial

TABLE 4.1 Analogy for Application of WHO/ISUP System to Inverted Neoplasia

Degree of Atypia	Exophytic Papillary Lesions	Flat Lesions	Endophytic/Inverted Papillary Lesions[a]
None	Papilloma	Normal	Inverted papilloma
Minimal/ absent	PUNLMP	Urothelial hyperplasia	Inverted PUNLMP
Distinct, mild-moderate	Papillary urothelial carcinoma, low grade, noninvasive	Urothelial dysplasia	Inverted papillary urothelial carcinoma, low grade, noninvasive
At least focally severe	Papillary urothelial carcinoma, high grade, noninvasive	Urothelial CIS	Inverted papillary urothelial carcinoma, high grade, noninvasive
At least focally severe	Papillary urothelial carcinoma, high grade, invasive	CIS with invasion	Inverted papillary urothelial carcinoma, high grade, invasive

[a]Inverted lesions may show areas with both exophytic and endophytic growth but should be at least predominantly inverted to be designated as such.

PUNLMP, papillary urothelial neoplasm of low malignant potential.

Adapted by permission from Nature: Amin MB, Smith SC, Reuter VE, et al. Update for the practicing pathologist: The International Consultation on Urologic Disease–European association of urology consultation on bladder cancer. *Mod Pathol.* 2015;28(5):612-630. Copyright © 2014 United States & Canadian Academy of Pathology.

carcinoma with inverted features without an exophytic papillary component. Within inverted carcinomas, the ramifying cords and trabeculae are less uniform, sometimes solid without polarity, and typically consist of large well-circumscribed rounded nests as opposed to anastomosing trabeculae (Table 4.1). If the endophytic component has markedly thickened but otherwise cytologically and architecturally unremarkable cords and the exophytic component is similar, the designation of inverted urothelial neoplasm of low malignant potential is appropriate (Fig. 4.16). As with other urothelial neoplasms, if there is cytologic atypia and depending on the grade, the tumors would be designated as inverted (ie, not with invasion) urothelial carcinoma, low grade, or high grade (Figs. 4.17-4.21). As in broad-front verrucous carcinoma–like growth, inverted papilloma–like destructive invasion may be present in tumors with endophytic growth. In such a case, diagnostic terminology such as invasive high-grade papillary urothelial carcinoma with prominent endophytic/inverted growth pattern may be used.

Rarely, classic inverted papilloma histology may be associated with sizeable areas of inverted low malignant potential tumor or low-grade carcinoma; these tumors should be considered as papillary urothelial

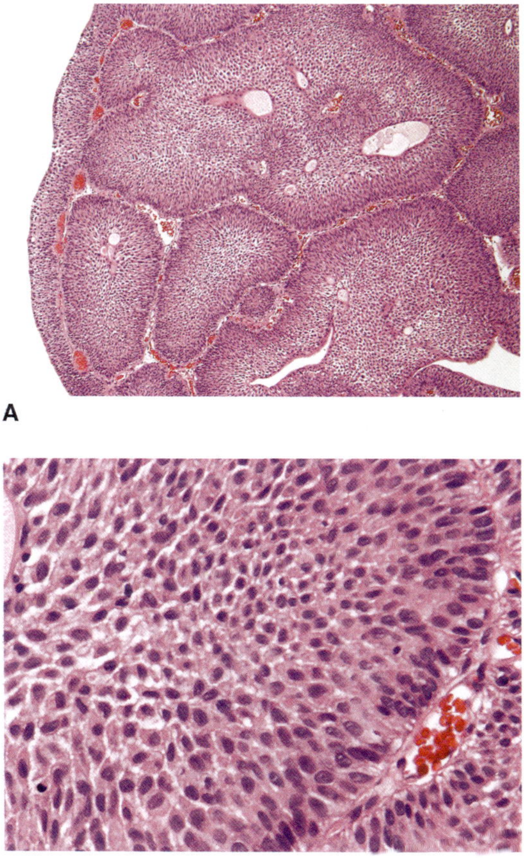

A

B

FIGURE 4.16 Low magnification of PUNLMP with an inverted growth pattern **(A)**. In contrast to inverted urothelial papilloma, there are large rounded nests. Higher magnification shows bland urothelium, many with nuclear grooves **(B)**. The lesion lacks the typical peripheral palisading and central streaming of urothelium seen in inverted papilloma.

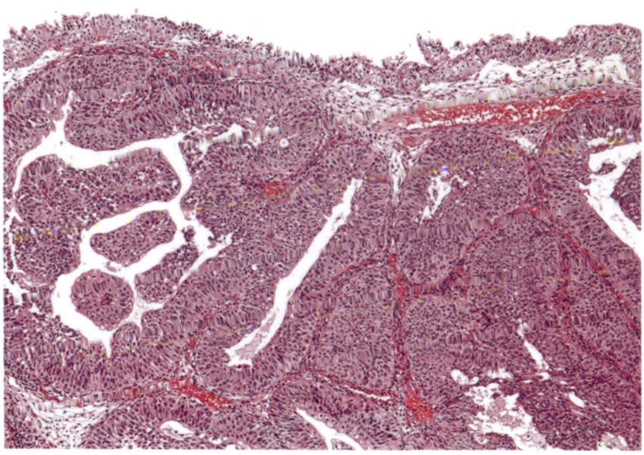

FIGURE 4.17 **Noninvasive low-grade urothelial carcinoma with endophytic cyst formation containing papillary fronds (*left*) as well as inverted nest formation (*right*).**

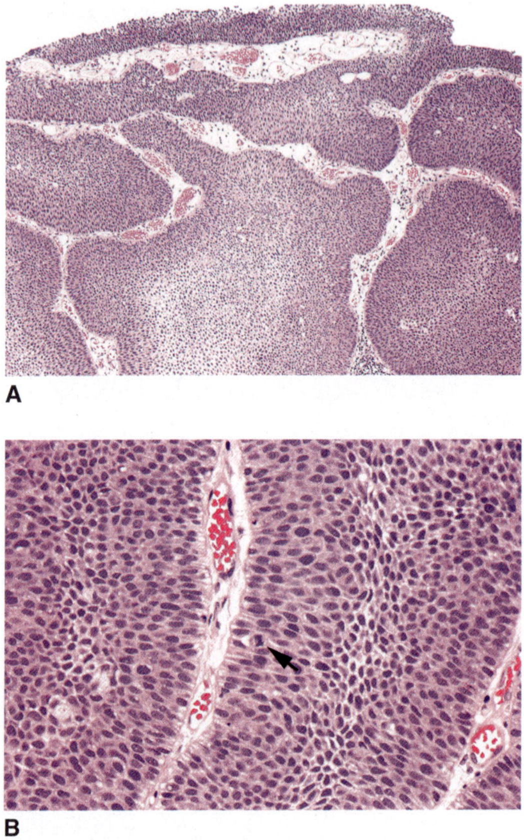

FIGURE 4.18 Noninvasive inverted urothelial carcinoma composed of large irregular nests **(A)**. Higher magnification shows cytology of low-grade carcinoma with scattered hyperchromatic nuclei and mitotic figures (*arrow*) **(B)**.

neoplasm of low malignant potentials (PUNLMPs) or low-grade carcinomas with inverted growth pattern, respectively (eFigs. 4.33-4.42).

The histologic features useful to distinguish inverted papilloma and other urothelial neoplasms with inverted papilloma–like growth are summarized in Table 4.2. Three features are key to the recognition of inverted papilloma: (1) a relatively smooth surface with minimal to absent exophytic component, (2) lesional circumscription with a smooth base without obvious infiltration, and (3) minimal to absent cytologic atypia.[5] In addition, inverted papilloma are not associated with a stromal response, fibrous or otherwise, and the amount of stroma between the inverted papillae is minimal and relatively uniform. A prominent exophytic component, considerable cytologic atypia (equivalent to low-grade or high-grade papillary urothelial carcinoma), irregularity of proliferating nests with solid areas, and obvious invasion would disqualify a lesion as being diagnosed as inverted papilloma. In our opinion, most cases reported as inverted

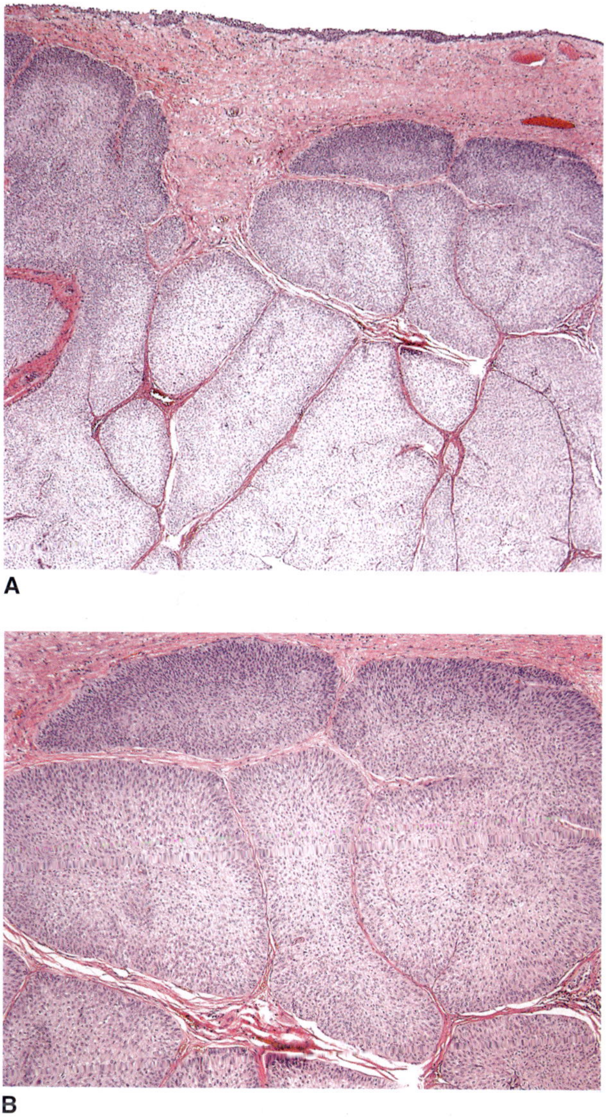

FIGURE 4.19 Noninvasive inverted low-grade urothelial carcinoma composed of large rounded nests as opposed to anastomosing thin cords seen with inverted papilloma (A, B).

papilloma with concurrent urothelial carcinoma represent the inverted pattern of urothelial carcinoma. The differential diagnosis in large fragmented and heavily cauterized tumors may rarely include large nested urothelial carcinoma, carcinoid tumor, and paraganglioma. PUNLMP with inverted growth appears to have rare recurrence.[23] HRAS mutations have been frequently shown in inverted tumors.[16]

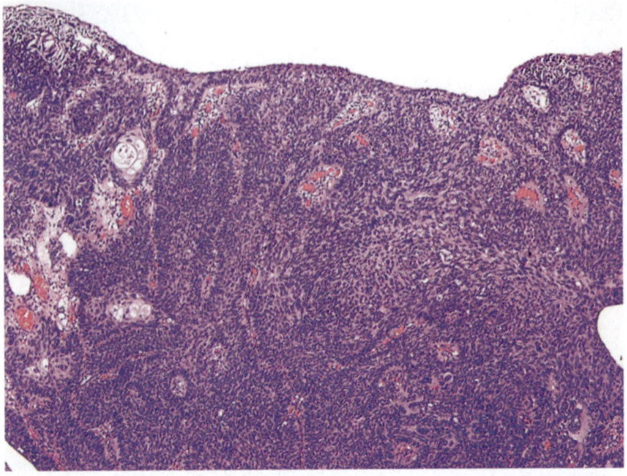

A

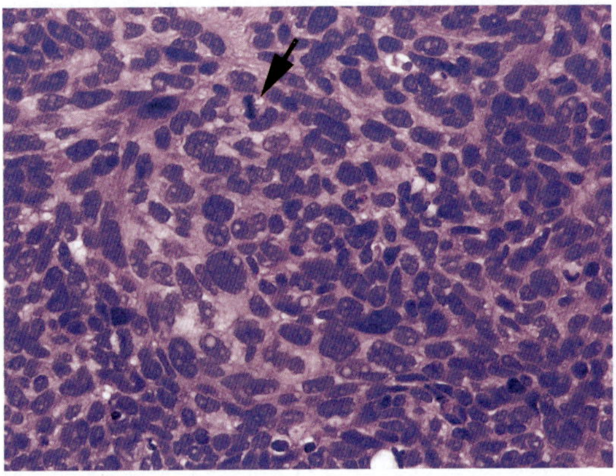

B

FIGURE 4.20 Inverted lesion mimicking inverted papilloma at low magnification **(A)**. At high magnification, cells are overtly malignant with hyperchromasia, pleomorphism, and mitotic figures, diagnostic of noninvasive high-grade urothelial carcinoma with an inverted growth pattern **(B)**.

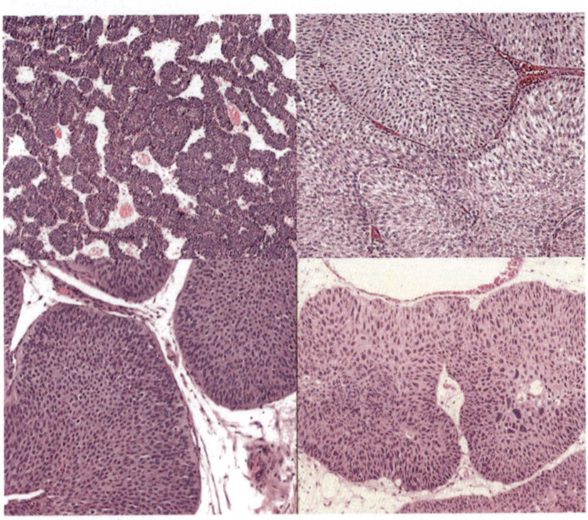

FIGURE 4.21 **Spectrum of noninvasive inverted lesions.** Inverted papilloma (***upper left***), inverted PUNLMP (***upper right***), inverted low-grade urothelial carcinoma (***lower left***), and inverted high-grade urothelial carcinoma (***lower right***).

TABLE 4.2 Differences Between Inverted Papilloma and Urothelial Carcinoma With Inverted Papilloma–Like Growth

	Inverted Papilloma	Urothelial Neoplasms With Inverted Growth (Excluding Inverted Papilloma)
Surface	Smooth dome shaped or focally exophytic, cytologically unremarkable, usually intact surface	Variable, exophytic papillary component
Growth pattern	Endophytic, expansile, sharply delineated lesion	Endophytic, expansile, sharply delineated lesion
	Ramifying cords and trabeculae of even width	Typically large rounded nests. If ramifying cords and trabeculae, irregular width and with transition into solid areas
	Destructive invasion of lamina propria or muscularis propria absent by definition	Invasion into lamina propria or muscle may be present and should be ascertained using criteria for determining invasion
Cytologic features	Orderly polarized cells with tendency to spindle centrally and palisade at the periphery	Maturation, spindling, or palisading variable to absent
	Diffuse, severe cytologic atypia absent	Cytologic features are grade dependent (urothelial neoplasia of low malignant potential–minimal to absent atypia, urothelial carcinoma, low grade or high grade-criteria similar to exophytic lesions)
Biologic potential	Benign, recurrences rare	Recur (usually new occurrences) or progress (depends on grade and stage)

Inverted urothelial neoplasms occur in the bladder most commonly, followed by the urethra; they rarely occur in the upper tracts. Urothelial carcinomas occurring in the renal pelvis and ureter may develop as a manifestation of hereditary nonpolyposis colorectal cancer (HNPCC) syndrome, a disorder in which inactivation or mutations of a number of DNA mismatch genes are present and may be detected by microsatellite instability (MSI).[24] Tumors associated with HNPCC have a greater predilection for inverted growth pattern of urothelial carcinoma, and it has been suggested that the observation of inverted histology in an upper tract tumor is a marker lesion for MSI unstable tumors and patients with Lynch syndrome.[24,25] Approximately 28% of patients with Lynch syndrome develop urothelial carcinoma, and it is currently recommended that urologists should suspect Lynch syndrome for upper tract urothelial carcinoma in a patient <60 years of age; tumors are frequently ureteral in location, with predisposition to bilaterality with female preponderance.[25] MSI testing in inverted lesions of the upper tract is currently not routinely recommended though frequently performed by pathologists or requested by clinicians. Urovysion FISH studies demonstrate chromosomal abnormalities in 72% on inverted carcinomas, as are molecular alterations in FGFR3, TERT promoter, TP53, CDKN1A, PIK3CA, and chromatin-modifying genes.[13,17,26-30] Currently, data regarding biologic potential and outcome are extremely limited, although there is a trend toward inverted tumors to have lower progression rates.[13,23,31]

REFERENCES

1. Kunze E, Schauer A, Schmitt M. Histology and histogenesis of two different types of inverted urothelial papillomas. *Cancer.* 1983;51:348-358.
2. DeMeester LJ, Farrow GM, Utz DC. Inverted papillomas of the urinary bladder. *Cancer.* 1975;36:505-513.
3. Yagi H, Igawa M, Shiina H, et al. Inverted papilloma of the urinary bladder in a girl. *Urol Int.* 1999;63:258-260.
4. Picozzi S, Casellato S, Bozzini G, et al. Inverted papilloma of the bladder: a review and an analysis of the recent literature of 365 patients. *Urol Oncol.* 2013;31:1584-1590.
5. Eiber M, van Oers JM, Zwarthoff EC, et al. Low frequency of molecular changes and tumor recurrence in inverted papillomas of the urinary tract. *Am J Surg Pathol.* 2007;31:938-946.
6. Summers DE, Rushin JM, Frazier HA, Cotelingam JD. Inverted papilloma of the urinary bladder with granular eosinophilic cells. An unusual neuroendocrine variant. *Arch Pathol Lab Med.* 1991;115:802-806.
7. Talmon GA, Khan A, Koerber R, Lele S, Johansson S. A cribriform urothelial neoplasm of the renal pelvis: an adenoid cysticlike variant of inverted urothelial papilloma or florid ureteritis cystica? *Arch Pathol Lab Med.* 2010;134:1557-1559.
8. Patel P, Reikie BA, Maxwell JP, Yilmaz A, Gotto GT, Trpkov K. Long-term clinical outcome of inverted urothelial papilloma including cases with focal papillary pattern: is continuous surveillance necessary? *Urology.* 2013;82:857-860.
9. Sung MT, Eble JN, Wang M, et al. Inverted papilloma of the urinary bladder: a molecular genetic appraisal. *Mod Pathol.* 2006;19:1289-1294.
10. Manel A, Combe M, Devonec M. Inverted papilloma of the pyelo-ureteral junction, current literature data. *Prog Urol.* 2000;10:282-286.
11. Spevack L, Herschorn S, Srigley J. Inverted papilloma of the upper urinary tract. *J Urol.* 1995;153:1202-1204.
12. Ho H, Chen YD, Tan PH, Wang M, Lau WK, Cheng C. Inverted papilloma of urinary bladder: is long-term cystoscopic surveillance needed? A single center's experience. *Urology.* 2006;68:333-336.

13. Jones TD, Zhang S, Lopez-Beltran A, et al. Urothelial carcinoma with an inverted growth pattern can be distinguished from inverted papilloma by fluorescence in situ hybridization, immunohistochemistry, and morphologic analysis. *Am J Surg Pathol.* 2007;31:1861-1867.
14. Kilciler M, Bedir S, Erdemir F, Ors O, Kibar Y, Dayanc M. Evaluation of urinary inverted papillomas: a report of 13 cases and literature review. *Kaohsiung J Med Sci.* 2008;24:25-30.
15. Lott S, Wang M, Zhang S, et al. FGFR3 and TP53 mutation analysis in inverted urothelial papilloma: incidence and etiological considerations. *Mod Pathol.* 2009;22:627-632.
16. McDaniel AS, Zhai Y, Cho KR, et al. HRAS mutations are frequent in inverted urothelial neoplasms. *Hum Pathol.* 2014;45:1957-1965.
17. Isharwal S, Hu W, Sarungbam J, et al. Genomic landscape of inverted urothelial papilloma and urothelial papilloma of the bladder. *J Pathol.* 2019;248:260-265.
18. Amin MB, Gomez JA, Young RH. Urothelial transitional cell carcinoma with endophytic growth patterns: a discussion of patterns of invasion and problems associated with assessment of invasion in 18 cases. *Am J Surg Pathol.* 1997;21:1057-1068.
19. Amin MB, McKenney JK, Paner GP, et al. ICUD-EAU International Consultation on Bladder Cancer 2012: Pathology. *Eur Urol.* 2013;63:16-35.
20. Amin MB, Smith SC, Reuter VE, et al. Update for the practicing pathologist: The International Consultation on Urologic Disease–European Association of Urology Consultation on Bladder Cancer. *Mod Pathol.* 2015;28:612-630.
21. Amin MB, Comperat E, Epstein JI, et al. The Genitourinary Pathology Society Update on classification and grading of flat and papillary urothelial neoplasia with new reporting recommendations and approach to lesions with mixed and early patterns of neoplasia. *Adv Anat Pathol.* 2021;28(4):179-195.
22. Compérat E, Amin MB, Berney DM, et al. What's new in WHO fifth edition–urinary tract. *Histopathology.* 2022;81(4):439-446.
23. Maxwell JP, Wang C, Wiebe N, Yilmaz A, Trpkov K. Long-term outcome of primary papillary urothelial neoplasm of low malignant potential (PUNLMP) including PUNLMP with inverted growth. *Diagn Pathol.* 2015;10:3.
24. Hartmann A, Dietmaier W, Hofstädter F, et al. Urothelial carcinoma of the upper urinary tract: inverted growth pattern is predictive of microsatellite instability. *Hum Pathol.* 2003;34:222-227.
25. Mork M, Hubosky SG, Roupret M, et al. Lynch syndrome: a primer for urologists and panel recommendations. *J Urol.* 2015;194:21-29.
26. Almassi N, Pietzak EJ, Sarungbam J, et al. Inverted urothelial papilloma and urothelial carcinoma with inverted growth are histologically and molecularly distinct entities. *J Pathol.* 2020;250:464-465.
27. Sanguedolce F, Calò B, Chirico M, et al. Distinctive morphological and molecular features of urothelial carcinoma with an inverted growth pattern. *J Pathol Transl Med.* 2021;55(4):239-246.
28. Gayhart MG, Johnson N, Paul A, et al. Universal mismatch repair protein screening in upper tract urothelial carcinoma. *Am J Clin Pathol.* 2020;154(6):792-801.
29. Wang CC, Huang CY, Jhuang YL, Chen CC, Jeng YM. Biological significance of TERT promoter mutation in papillary urothelial neoplasm of low malignant potential. *Histopathology.* 2018;72(5):795-803.
30. Harper HL, McKenney JK, Heald B, et al. Upper tract urothelial carcinomas: frequency of association with mismatch repair protein loss and lynch syndrome. *Mod Pathol.* 2017;30(1):146-156.
31. Arslankoz S, Kulac I, Baydar DE. The influence of inverted growth pattern on recurrence for patients with non-invasive low grade papillary urothelial carcinoma of bladder. *Balkan Med J.* 2017;34(5):464-468.

5

INVASIVE UROTHELIAL CARCINOMA

Invasion in urothelial carcinoma (T1 or higher) may arise at the base of a papillary neoplasm (Ta, noninvasive) or within it. It can also be seen as microinvasive (arbitrarily defined as invasion <2 mm in depth) or invasive disease in association with carcinoma *in situ* (CIS, or CIS with invasion). Approximately 30% of urothelial carcinomas present primarily with invasive disease, and, in some cases, a precursor lesion is not seen, presumably because it has been destroyed by surface ulceration associated with the invasive carcinoma or because the cells have exfoliated into the urine. The morphologic spectrum of invasive urothelial carcinoma is very wide, and numerous variants/subtypes have been described (see Chapter 6). Even the usual or conventional type of urothelial carcinoma spans a range of histology. The occurrence of invasion in bladder carcinoma is one of the most important climacterics in the natural history of the tumor, and the depth of invasion is the quintessential factor impacting prognosis and therapy.[1-5]

USUAL OR CONVENTIONAL TYPE OF UROTHELIAL CARCINOMA

Invasive urothelial carcinoma may present as a polypoid, sessile, ulcerated, or infiltrative lesion in which the neoplastic cells invade the bladder wall as nests, cords, trabeculae, small clusters, or single cells that are often separated by a desmoplastic stroma. The tumor sometimes grows in a more diffuse, sheetlike pattern, but even in these cases, focal nests and clusters are generally present. Occasionally, carcinomas are associated with a pronounced chronic inflammatory cell infiltrate, which partially or substantially obscures the underlying tumor cells. In some instances, the inflammation may appear to be an integral component of the neoplasm and mimic the distinctive lymphoepitheliomalike carcinoma of the bladder (see Chapter 6). The neoplastic cells in typical or conventional patterns of invasive urothelial carcinoma are usually of moderate size and have modest amounts of pale to dense eosinophilic cytoplasm (Fig. 5.1). Sometimes, tumors with a more nestlike architecture, eosinophilic cytoplasm in tumor cells, and prominent stromal vascularity between nests may mimic a paraganglioma (see Chapter 12). In some tumors, the

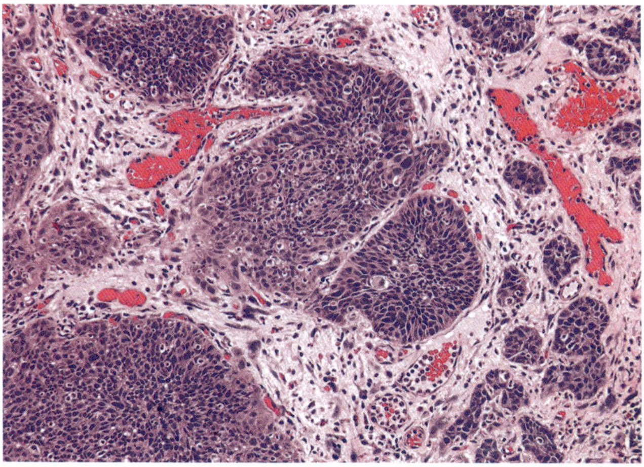

FIGURE 5.1 Irregular nests of urothelial carcinoma with cells having moderate amounts of cytoplasm and pleomorphism.

cytoplasm is more abundant and may be clear or strikingly eosinophilic. The presence of clear cells, with rare exceptions, is focal and should not lead to the diagnosis of clear cell adenocarcinoma, which has a very typical histology. Invasive carcinomas, particularly early and/or with limited invasion into the lamina propria, may be associated with retraction artifact. This finding when conspicuous should not be mistaken for vascular-lymphatic invasion or micropapillary carcinoma, which has distinctive definitional features and prognostic and possibly therapeutic significance (see Chapter 6). Some cases elicit a stromal response, which may occasionally be prominent and elicit a pseudosarcomatous myofibroblastic appearance (not to be mistaken with a biphasic component of sarcomatoid urothelial carcinoma).

Invasive tumors are almost all high grade, although there is a spectrum of some cases exhibiting marked anaplasia; focal tumor giant cell formation may be seen. Typically, most cases show nuclear pleomorphism, markedly irregular cellular borders, and chromatin distribution with frequent mitoses (helpful in the distinction from prostatic adenocarcinoma, which has more monotonous-appearing nuclei and which may secondarily invade the bladder, and paraganglioma involving the bladder, which has spotty endocrine-type atypia). Only a small minority of invasive urothelial carcinomas has a low-grade histology (see Chapter 6 for a description of nested variant of urothelial carcinoma) (Fig. 5.2). In contrast to noninvasive low-grade papillary urothelial carcinoma, nested variant of urothelial carcinoma typically lacks an inflammatory or desmoplastic stromal reaction, usually does not have an overlying papillary component, lacks more irregular shaped nests, and does not consist of small clusters of cells with retraction artifact.[6] However, in these cases, the outcome is not determined by tumor grade but rather by stage.

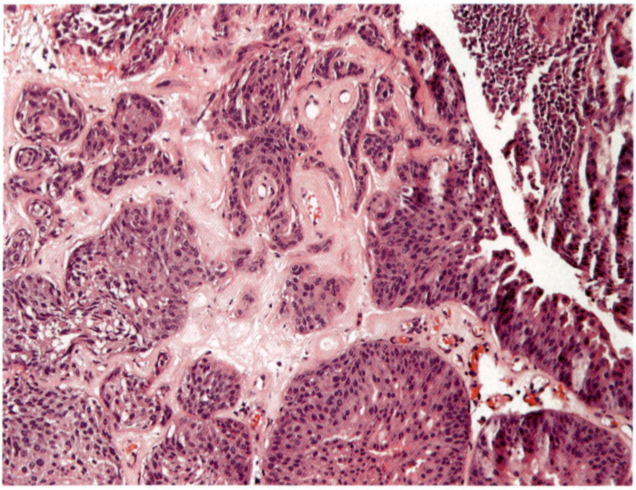

FIGURE 5.2 Invasive low-grade urothelial carcinoma with irregular nests and fibrotic stromal reaction.

UROTHELIAL CARCINOMA WITH DIVERGENT DIFFERENTIATION

Invasive urothelial carcinoma is known for a wide range of histologic manifestation from deceptively bland morphology (unusual) to markedly atypical carcinoma cells (more common). It is important to understand different terms used to describe urothelial carcinoma histology not conforming to typical patterns. The terms "divergent differentiation" and "variant histology" have been variably and sometimes interchangeably used. Divergent differentiation is used when there is differentiation along another histological line/aberrant differentiation, for example, squamous, glandular, and trophoblastic differentiation (pure or admixed with urothelial carcinoma). The term variant is used when process arises fundamentally from a malignancy with urothelial histogenesis/differentiation and where immunohistochemistry and other evidence further supports urothelial malignancy, for example, the nested, micropapillary, clear cell, plasmacytoid, and other variants. In keeping with terminology promoted in the 5th edition of WHO, the term variants is replaced by subtypes.[1,4] Trophoblastic differentiation and subtypes/variants of urothelial carcinoma are described in detail in Chapter 6.

Approximately 10%-20% of urothelial carcinomas contain foci of glandular, and ~30%-40% show variable amounts of squamous differentiation (see Chapters 8 and 9). These numbers likely do not reflect the actual frequency as this information is not consistently or accurately recorded by pathologists. Glandular differentiation is usually in the form of small tubular or glandlike spaces in conventional urothelial carcinoma (urothelial carcinoma with glandlike lumina) or as a histology similar to enteric adenocarcinoma.[7,8] Rare mucin-producing cells in invasive carcinoma or cytoplasmic mucin may be demonstrated in up to 60% of cases by histochemical stains (not recommended), although these features do not qualify for glandular differentiation and do not need to be reported. Rarely, a coexistent signet ring cell or mucinous component may be present.

To designate squamous differentiation, one must see clear-cut evidence of squamous production (intracellular keratin, intercellular bridges, or keratin pearls), and the degree of squamous differentiation, when present, usually parallels the grade of the urothelial carcinoma. While the presence of clear-cut squamous differentiation should be reported, and approximate percentage documented, the mere presence of denser eosinophilic cytoplasm or "squamoid" appearance does not qualify for squamous differentiation and should not be diagnosed (see Chapter 9).

In general, urothelial carcinomas have a relatively nondescript morphology ("patternless pattern"), which when viewed in isolation cannot be differentiated from poorly differentiated carcinomas of other types. Therefore, the presence of divergent differentiation such as squamous or glandular differentiation in a poorly differentiated neoplasm, particularly at metastatic sites and in the context of a bladder primary, should suggest the possibility of urothelial differentiation. To designate a bladder tumor as squamous cell or adenocarcinoma, a pure or almost pure histology of squamous cell carcinoma or adenocarcinoma is required. The presence of some percentage of squamous and glandular differentiation in urothelial carcinomas has generally been thought of as lacking any clinical significance. In stage-matched cases, the outcome of typical urothelial carcinoma is similar to those with divergent differentiation.[9] However, some studies have suggested that these forms of divergent differentiation may be more resistant to chemotherapy or radiation therapy than pure urothelial carcinoma, but this has not been confirmed[10,11]; differing approaches to neoadjuvant therapy have also been proposed but there are no consistent data. Squamous differentiation in biopsies or transurethral resection has been associated with locally advanced disease at cystectomy.[12] From a practical viewpoint, we do make note of prominent squamous or glandular differentiation in urothelial carcinoma by using diagnostic terminology such as "invasive urothelial carcinoma with prominent squamous (40%) and glandular (25%) differentiation," providing some estimate of the amount of differentiation. In cases of metastatic bladder tumor to other sites, knowledge of the presence and percentage of divergent differentiation may be useful to facilitate comparison with the primary.

Recent gene sequencing studies suggest that invasive urothelial carcinoma has unique molecular profiles, for example, basal squamous phenotype (seen in urothelial carcinomas with squamous differentiation) with potentially differing outcomes including poor responsiveness to chemotherapy (see section on "Pertinent molecular aspects in diagnostic pathology"). These tumors more commonly express CK5/6 instead of CK20. The studies are preliminary, and currently, reporting of these subtypes or performing immunostains to diagnose them is not recommended.[4,13-17]

A subset of invasive urothelial carcinomas may exhibit vascular invasion. This parameter should be diagnosed with care because invasive urothelial carcinomas, particularly those with limited or early invasion, frequently show retraction artifact, which mimics vascular-lymphatic invasion. In two studies, only 14% and 40% of cases originally diagnosed with vascular invasion on the basis of morphology could be proven by immunohistochemistry.[18,19] Criteria for recognition of vascular invasion are outlined later in this chapter, and its prognostic significance especially in node-negative carcinomas is uncertain[20] (see Chapter 7 for prognostic significance).

As mentioned before, invasive urothelial carcinoma has a propensity for a myriad of other patterns of subtype/variant morphology (eg, small cell carcinoma, sarcomatoid carcinoma, micropapillary, microcystic, nested, etc.) in ~10% of cases. These are described in detail in Chapter 6.

DIFFERENTIAL DIAGNOSIS OF INFILTRATING UROTHELIAL CARCINOMA

The differential diagnosis of infiltrating urothelial carcinomas includes benign mimics, nonurothelial neoplasms, and urothelial carcinomas (noninvasive) with inverted growth (Chapter 4). Pseudocarcinomatous hyperplasia (Chapter 10) is an important mimic in which squamoid epithelial nests in lamina propria have a jagged irregular appearance simulating invasion. Identification of associated lamina propria hemorrhage and blood vessels with fibrin are useful diagnostic clues, as is the clinical history of prior radiation and/or chemotherapy (which may not be always available or present). Nonurothelial neoplasms mimicking urothelial carcinoma include prostatic adenocarcinoma involving the bladder, gynecological, colorectal, and other visceral malignancies secondarily involving the bladder and paraganglioma.

IMMUNOPROFILE OF INFILTRATING UROTHELIAL CARCINOMA

Immunohistochemistry plays a valuable role in confirming urothelial differentiation in select settings such as (1) confirming urothelial origin in a metastatic tumor in a patient with history of upper urothelial tract or bladder disease; (2) differentiating a bladder primary from high-grade prostatic carcinoma and other high-grade malignancies in the pelvis (colorectal, ovarian, cervical, etc.); (3) proving urothelial differentiation in unusual subtypes of bladder cancer and their accurate distinction from other mimickers; (4) in the differential diagnosis with other epithelioid tumors involving the bladder, for example, paraganglioma, PEComa, epithelioid leiomyosarcoma, etc. While a number of markers are commercially available or evaluated in the literature, only a select few provide clinical diagnostic utility and should be performed based on the differential diagnostic considerations.[17]

Urothelial carcinomas are typically CK7 (87%-100%) and CK20 positive (25%-70%), GATA3 positive (67%-93%), and uroplakin II positive (60%-80%).[21] Uroplakin III is less sensitive and recently fallen out of favor due to the better sensitivity of GATA3 and increased specificity of uroplakin II. It is important to remember that GATA3 may be positive in paraganglioma and nephrogenic adenoma, two important differential diagnostic considerations in bladder neoplasia. PAX 8 may be present in a small subset of urothelial carcinomas, although the staining is not strong or diffuse. p63 and/or p40 (81%-92%), high molecular weight cytokeratin (HMWK), CK5/6, and thrombomodulin are frequently positive in urothelial tumors but lack specificity. S100P is emerging as a useful marker in urothelial tumors (88%-93%), but like GATA3 is positive in several other tumor types.[17,21] Racemase is positive in a high percentage of invasive urothelial carcinomas and has limited role as a differential diagnostic marker in invasive malignancies involving the bladder.

STAGING OF BLADDER CANCER

Stage is the most powerful prognostic indicator in urothelial carcinoma and is a major defining parameter in the management of this disease.[9] The TNM (tumor, node, metastasis) staging system defines T1 tumors as those invading into the lamina propria but not the muscularis propria.[2] Even though several studies have shown that T1 tumors bear a less favorable prognosis than Ta (noninvasive) neoplasms,[22-24] clinically Ta and T1 tumors are usually lumped together by urologists under the term "superficial" bladder tumors, partially because these two stages traditionally have been managed more conservatively. Another possible factor contributing to the clinician's rationale in grouping Ta and T1 tumors as superficial is the pathologists' inability to always accurately recognize lamina propria invasion.[25,26] We strongly discourage the use of the term superficial to describe T1 tumors since contemporary series in which great care was taken to classify Ta and T1 correctly have shown clear differences in progression rates.[26,27] Tumors with involvement of the muscularis propria and beyond (pT2-pT4 tumors) are usually managed with definitive surgical therapy (ie, cystectomy) or radiation therapy, increasingly with neoadjuvant therapy or with adjuvant therapy. Three to seven percent of patients treated by cystectomy will have lymph node metastases, and the clinical outcome varies considerably. Patients with CIS and lymphovascular invasion along with muscularis propria invasion, at primary transurethral resection, tend to have a more adverse outcome.[28]

Traditionally, ~10% of bladder carcinomas, treated by cystectomy, have no evidence of residual disease (pT0). The incidence of pT0 disease is increasing as several high-risk noninvasive bladder cancers may be treated by radical cystectomy. These include patients with high-grade pT1 tumors, multiple recurrent high-grade tumors, and high-grade tumors with concomitant CIS. In addition, NCCN guidelines call for a repeat transurethral resection for high-risk tumors prior to excisional surgery. Systemic neoadjuvant therapy has also increased the percentage of pT0 disease at cystectomy. Currently, there are no universally accepted guidelines on gross dissection of cystectomy specimens without obvious invasive cancer. All mucosal alterations, prior surgical sites and ulcerations submitted in their entirety, and adequate sampling from different areas of the bladder are necessary. Patients with pT0 disease (posttransurethral resection of bladder tumor [TURBT] or neoadjuvant therapy) have markedly improved and overall disease-specific survival compared to cystectomy specimens with residual disease.[29,30] Targeted therapies for anti-FGFR for tumors with FGFR mutations are being increasingly used for refractory cancers.

Before discussing lamina propria (T1) and muscularis propria (T2 and T2+) invasion, it is important to be aware of the type of specimens encountered in bladder pathology and some histologic aspects of the bladder wall that are pertinent for the discussion of invasion.

Most small bladder tumors (usually <1 cm in size) can frequently be excised by cold-cup biopsies. This procedure yields specimens in which the cellular architecture is mostly preserved, and orientation is easier to maintain after embedding. The resulting hematoxylin and eosin sections show the urothelial neoplasm, the lamina propria, and often superficial muscularis propria with orientation maintained, thus facilitating assessment of invasion.[31] Larger tumors (usually >1 cm) usually require hot loop resection (TURBT), in which the urologist attempts to include a generous sample of the underlying muscularis propria to enable adequate pathologic staging. The specimens rendered by this procedure are often fragmented, heavily cauterized, and difficult to orient. Sections from these specimens are complicated by thermal artifact, tangential sectioning, and disruption of the tumor and normal architecture. Changes related to prior TUR may also add to the difficulty. While examining both types of specimens, it is important to note the presence or absence of muscularis propria in the specimen to assess involvement of it by neoplasia and to provide feedback to the urologist regarding adequacy of resection.

The lamina propria is a compact layer of fibrovascular connective tissue. Smooth muscle actin staining has revealed a continuous band of ill-defined, haphazardly oriented, compact spindle cells that are immediately subjacent to the urothelium in all cases. This layer has been referred to as suburothelial band of myofibroblasts. Beneath this layer, in most instances, the lamina propria is further divided by a thin layer of smooth muscle fibers (muscularis mucosae), which may be absent, discontinuous, or rarely complete. Because it is commonly incomplete, it is best to regard the underlying connective tissue, superficial to the muscularis propria, as deep lamina propria rather than submucosa. These anatomic landmarks may be entirely replaced by dense connective tissue at sites of prior biopsy. It was not until the 1980s that the muscularis mucosae layer of the urinary bladder was described[32-34] alerting pathologists and urologists of the importance of recognizing it and differentiating it from the underlying compact smooth muscle bundles of muscularis propria. Muscularis mucosae fibers are usually thin, often discontinuous, wispy, and wavy fascicles of smooth muscle, which are frequently associated with large-caliber blood vessels and surrounded by loose fibroconnective tissue. Most studies have identified some degree of this layer in 94%-100% of cystectomy specimens and in ~18%-83% of specimens from biopsies or TURBT.[26,33-35] Topographical variations in caliber of muscularis mucosae muscle exist between different regions of the bladder and the lamina propria vascular plexus may not be consistently associated with muscularis mucosae muscle. Muscularis mucosae muscle bundles may be thicker (hypertrophic form) or rarely assume the caliber of muscularis propria muscle bundles. This is commonly the case along the wall of bladder diverticula. Distinction is possible by location in the lamina propria and being distinct from deeper muscularis propria muscle.[36] Muscularis propria fascicles, on the other hand, are usually thick and compact, divided into distinct bundles surrounded by perimysium. The muscularis propria has a different morphology in the bladder neck and trigone (see Chapter 1). Occasionally, muscularis mucosae bundles undergo hypertrophy especially after biopsy or at the base of the tumor, and in such situations, the distinction between muscularis mucosae and muscularis propria, especially in biopsy or TURBT specimens, may be difficult. The deep (outer half) muscularis propria often rests on the perivesical fat. The boundary between them is not abrupt. Fat is present in all layers of the bladder beneath the urothelium; the frequency and amount increase from the superficial lamina propria to the deep lamina propria and to the muscularis propria.[37]

DIAGNOSIS OF LAMINA PROPRIA INVASION

Recognition of lamina propria invasion by urothelial carcinoma is occasionally one of the most challenging diagnoses in surgical pathology, and problems with interobserver reproducibility have been documented[28,38] (eFigs. 5.1-5.32). Often faced with distorted, cauterized, and tangentially sectioned specimens, the pathologist should follow strict criteria to diagnose lamina propria invasion (Table 5.1). While evaluating tumors for invasion, it is important to focus on the features discussed in the following paragraphs.

Histologic Grade of Tumor

Lamina propria invasion should be carefully sought in all high-grade papillary carcinomas. Although invasion is not a common finding in low-grade tumors, it is much more common in high-grade lesions. In our experience, more than 90% of pT1 tumors are high grade. Thus, even though clear-cut histologic signs of invasion are required for the diagnosis of invasion into lamina propria, regardless of grade, the level of suspicion should be higher in those cases with a high histologic grade.

TABLE 5.1 Criteria for the Diagnosis of Invasion Into Lamina Propria by Urothelial Carcinoma

Histologic grade
Invasion seen much more frequently, although not exclusively, in high-grade (WHO/ISUP classification) lesions
Invading epithelium
Irregularly shaped nests Single-cell infiltration Irregular or absent basement membrane Tentacular fingerlike projections Invasive component with higher nuclear grade or more cytoplasm (or morphologically different) than overlying noninvasive component (paradoxical differentiation)
Stromal response
Desmoplasia or sclerosis Retraction artifact Inflammation Myxoid stroma Pseudosarcomatous stroma Absent stromal response
Contextual features
Haphazard appearance and irregular spacing Associated with perineural spaces or peritumoral vascular spaces Juxtaposed deeper around blood and between blood vessels or smooth muscle

WHO/ISUP, World Health Organization/International Society of Urological Pathology Consensus Classification of Bladder Tumors.

Characteristics of Invading Epithelium

The invasive front of the neoplasm may show one of several features: single cells or irregularly shaped nests of tumor within the stroma, architectural complexity not conforming to the usual regularity of papillary neoplasms, or an irregular, disrupted, or absent basement membrane (Figs. 5.3 and 5.4). Sometimes, tentacular or fingerlike extensions can be seen arising from the base of the papillary tumor. Frequently, the invading nests appear morphologically different from the cells at the base of the noninvasive component of the tumor, with more abundant cytoplasm and often with a higher degree of pleomorphism (Figs. 5.5-5.7). This phenomenon has been called paradoxical differentiation when seen at other sites such as the uterine cervix. The border between noninvasive carcinoma and the

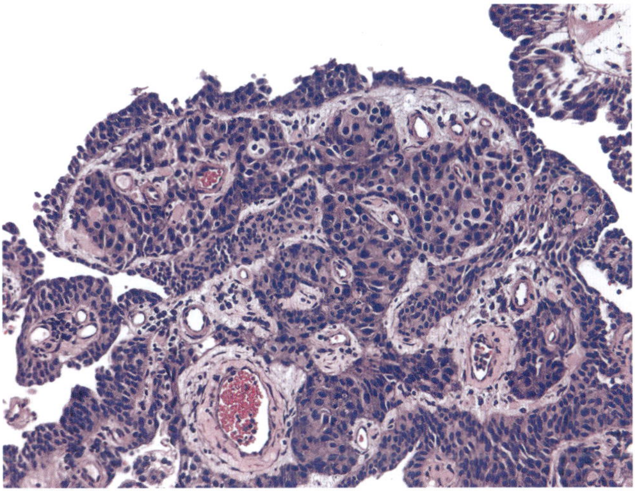

FIGURE 5.3 **Irregular nests of infiltrating urothelial carcinoma in lamina propria.**

underlying stroma will frequently be rimmed by a delicate network of capillaries, which is lacking in invasive nests of tumor.

Stromal Response

The lamina propria may react to invasion in one or more of the following forms:

- Desmoplastic or sclerotic stroma: The stroma may be cellular with spindled fibroblasts and variable collagenization, with or without inflammation.
- Retraction artifact: In some cases, retraction artifact that mimics vascular invasion is seen in tumors invading only superficially into the

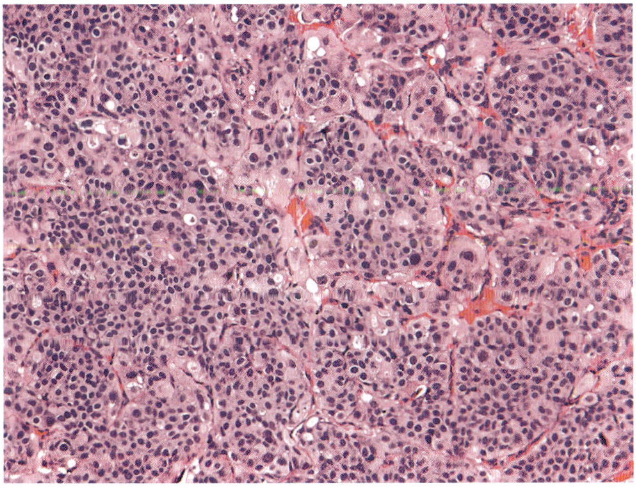

FIGURE 5.4 **Back to back nests of infiltrating urothelial carcinoma.** Nests are too small and crowded to represent CIS in von Brunn nests.

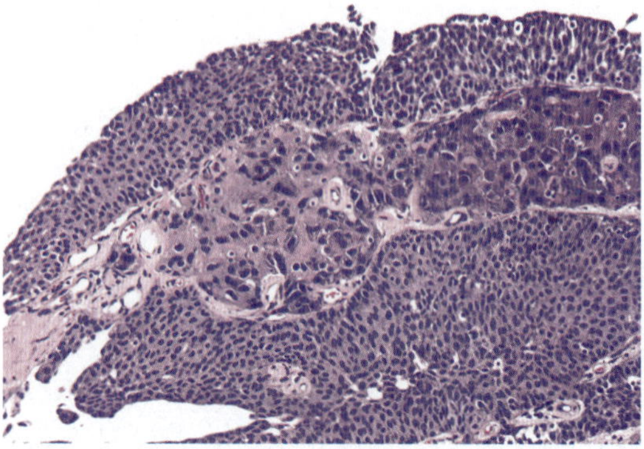

FIGURE 5.5 **Urothelial carcinoma invading the stalk of papillary carcinoma.** Note invasive carcinoma (***center***) has more abundant cytoplasm (paradoxical differentiation) and greater cytological atypia than surrounding noninvasive papillary carcinoma (***top*** and ***bottom***).

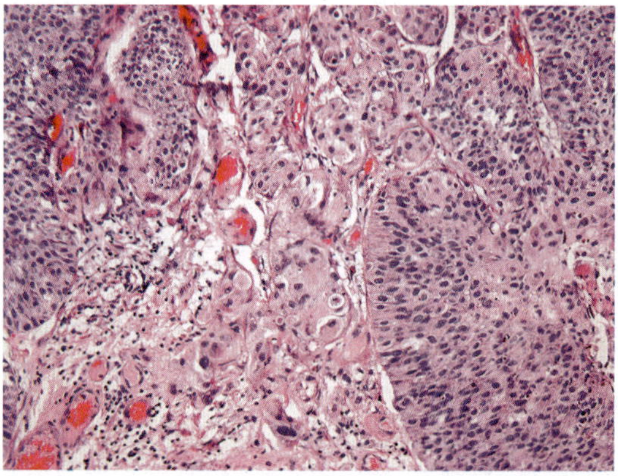

FIGURE 5.6 **Invasive urothelial carcinoma (center) with paradoxical differentiation.** Compare to noninvasive urothelial carcinoma (***right*** and ***far left***).

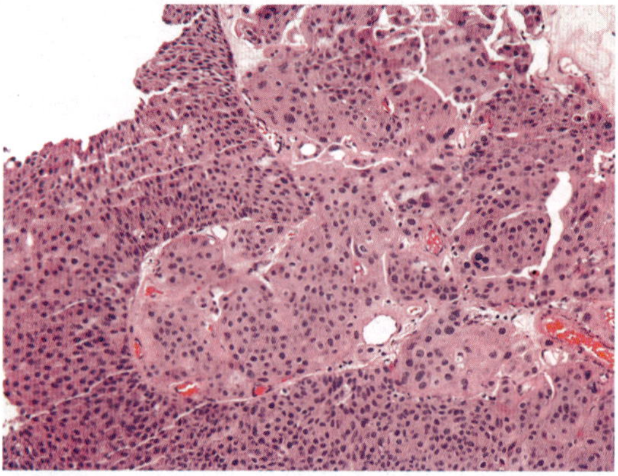

FIGURE 5.7 **Invasive urothelial carcinoma (*center*) with paradoxical differentiation associated with noninvasive papillary urothelial carcinoma (*left* and *bottom*).**

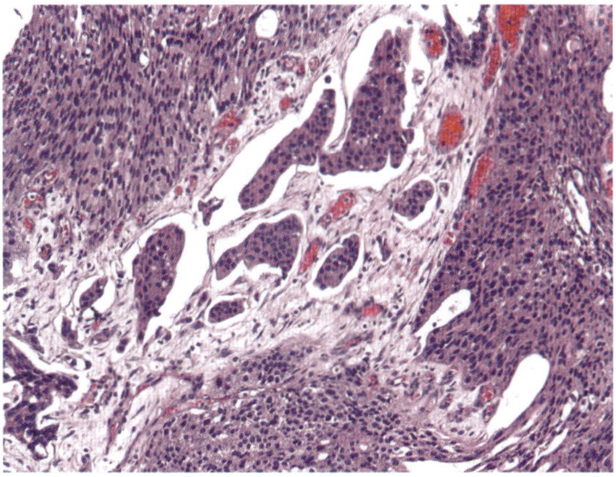

FIGURE 5.8 **Invasive urothelial carcinoma with prominent retraction artifact.**

lamina propria (Figs. 5.8 and 5.9). Often, this finding is focal and, in our opinion, is one of the early signs of invasion into lamina propria. It is especially conspicuous in the micropapillary variant of urothelial carcinoma but may be present in any invasive carcinoma. The presence of this finding alone in an otherwise noninvasive tumor does not warrant the diagnosis of micropapillary carcinoma.

- Inflamed stroma: Invasion may elicit a brisk inflammatory response. The lamina propria is heavily infiltrated by numerous inflammatory cells that may obscure the interface between the epithelium and stroma (Figs. 5.10 and 5.11). This makes recognition of small nests or single-cell invasion difficult to recognize.
- Myxoid stroma: Loose and hypocellular stroma with a myxoid background may occasionally be seen in some cases of invasive urothelial carcinomas (Fig. 5.12). It may rarely be very prominent; in which

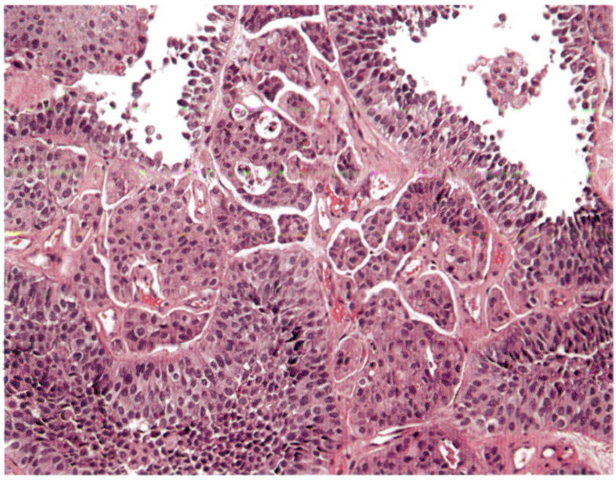

FIGURE 5.9 **Invasive urothelial carcinoma with micropapillary features and retraction artifact.** Tumor invades the stalk of papillary carcinoma.

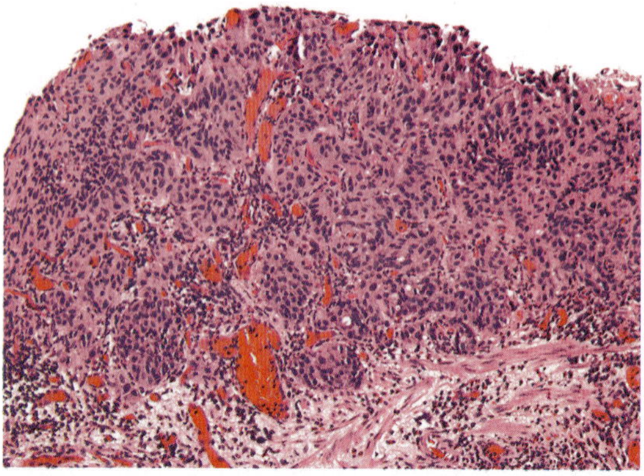

FIGURE 5.10 Crowded nests of urothelial carcinoma invasive up to muscularis mucosae with associated brisk acute inflammatory response.

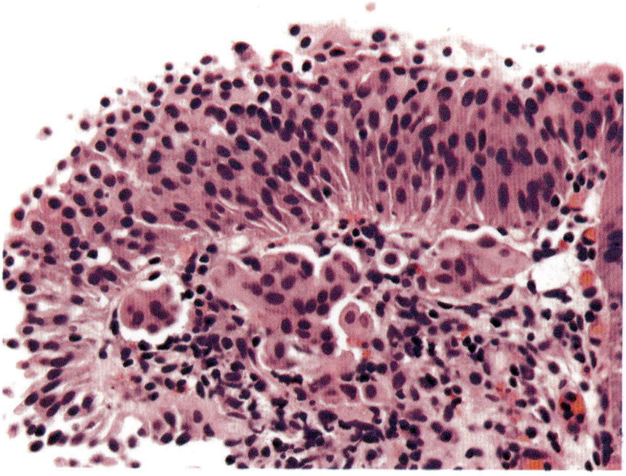

FIGURE 5.11 Microinvasive clusters of urothelial carcinoma with retraction artifact and intense chronic inflammation.

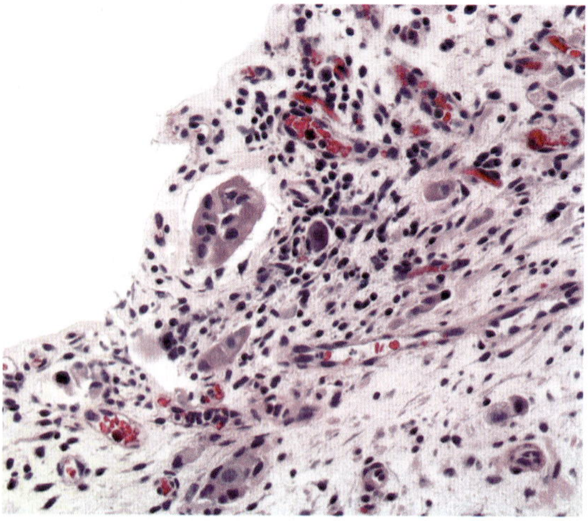

FIGURE 5.12 **Nests and single cells of invasive urothelial carcinoma associated with myxoid and inflamed stroma.** The surface urothelium is denuded.

case, the carcinoma may appear as small- or medium-sized nests and have a filiform morphology, or short cords or individual cells. The myxoid stroma is positive for Alcian blue with and without hyaluronidase, periodic acid-Schiff, and mucicarmine stains.[39]

- Pseudosarcomatous stroma: Sometimes, the tumor induces an exuberant spindle cell response, with proliferation of fibroblasts that may display significant, often alarming, cellular atypia.[40] This feature, although helpful in assessing for invasion, should not be mistaken for the spindle cell component of a biphasic sarcomatoid urothelial cancer (see Chapter 6). The proliferating stroma is usually nonexpansile, being limited to areas around the neoplasm, and is cytologically composed of nuclei that have a degenerate or smudged appearance on high-power examination.
- Absent stromal response: Frequently, the stromal response to invading carcinoma may be absent (Fig. 5.13). This is particularly the case in areas of microinvasion. In these cases, as mentioned earlier, diagnosis of invasion should rely on the characteristics of the invading epithelium.

Histologic Patterns of Lamina Propria Invasion

Lamina propria invasive tumors may be approached from their morphologic perspective according to several patterns/scenarios in which they present.[41] (Figs. 5.14 and 5.15). Awareness of these patterns may be important to the surgical pathologist in order to focus on particular areas of the tumor while assessing for invasion, thus facilitating its recognition, even when it is extremely focal. Not all patterns are associated with clinical significance.

CIS with microinvasion: CIS may be associated with microinvasion (defined as invasion within superficial lamina propria no >2 mm)[41,42] (Figs. 5.16 and 5.17). Invasion is histologically subtle, compounded by the fact that it is clinically not suspected and the obvious histological

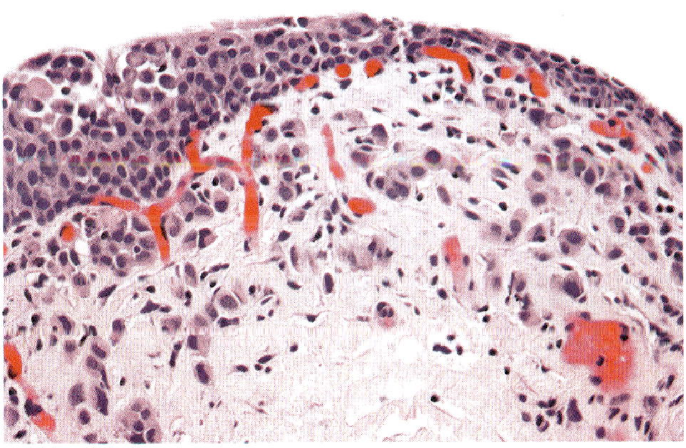

FIGURE 5.13 **Individual cells of infiltrating urothelial carcinoma in lamina propria.** The tumor lacks a stromal response. There is pagetoid involvement by neoplastic cells on the *upper left side*.

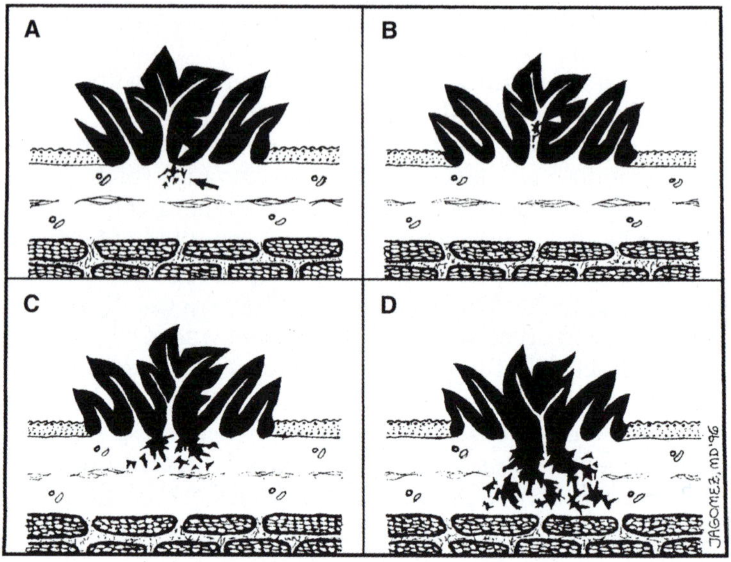

FIGURE 5.14 **A:** Papillary urothelial carcinoma with microinvasion. **B:** Papillary urothelial carcinoma with invasion into stalk. **C:** Papillary urothelial carcinoma with lamina propria invasion (up to muscularis mucosae). **D:** Papillary urothelial carcinoma with lamina propria invasion (beyond the muscularis mucosae). (Reprinted with permission from Amin MB, Gomez JA, Young RH. Urothelial transitional cell carcinoma with endophytic growth patterns: a discussion of patterns of invasion and problems associated with assessment of invasion in 18 cases. *Am J Surg Pathol.* 1997;21(9):1057-1068.)

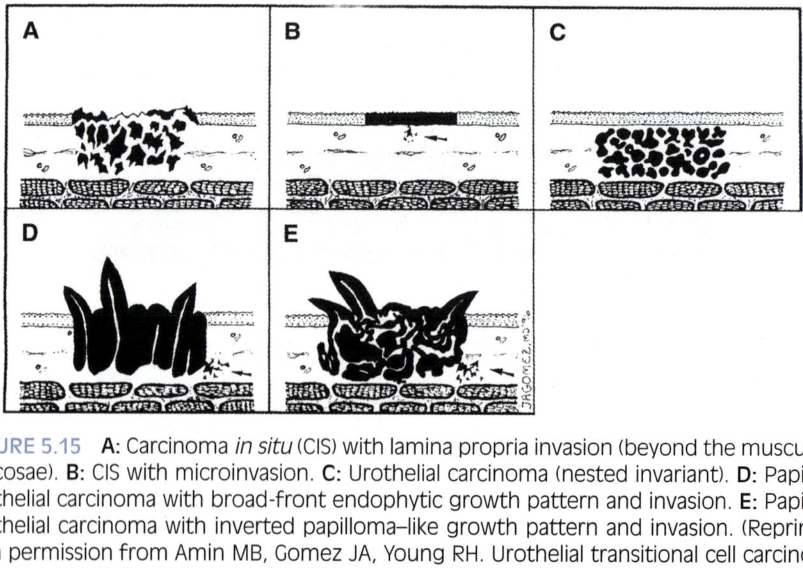

FIGURE 5.15 **A:** Carcinoma *in situ* (CIS) with lamina propria invasion (beyond the muscularis mucosae). **B:** CIS with microinvasion. **C:** Urothelial carcinoma (nested invariant). **D:** Papillary urothelial carcinoma with broad-front endophytic growth pattern and invasion. **E:** Papillary urothelial carcinoma with inverted papilloma–like growth pattern and invasion. (Reprinted with permission from Amin MB, Gomez JA, Young RH. Urothelial transitional cell carcinoma with endophytic growth patterns: a discussion of patterns of invasion and problems associated with assessment of invasion in 18 cases. *Am J Surg Pathol.* 1997;21(9):1057-1068.)

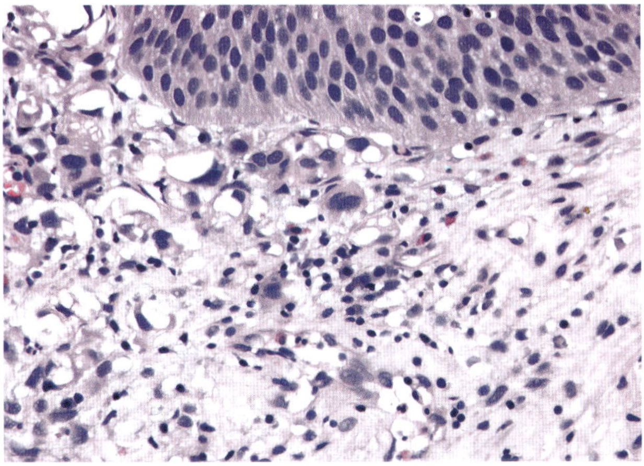

FIGURE 5.16 CIS (*top*) with individual cells of infiltrating urothelial carcinoma in lamina propria.

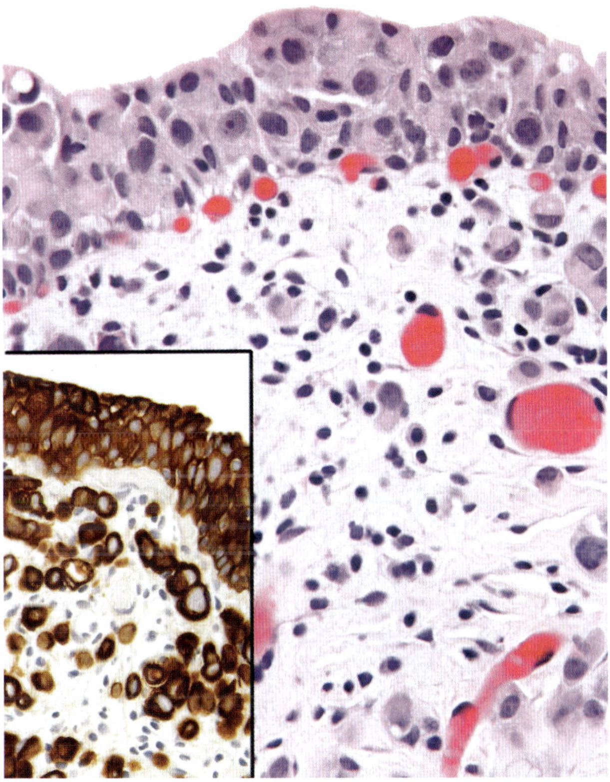

FIGURE 5.17 **CIS with microinvasion.** Cytokeratin immunohistochemistry (**inset**) highlights individual infiltrating carcinoma cells.

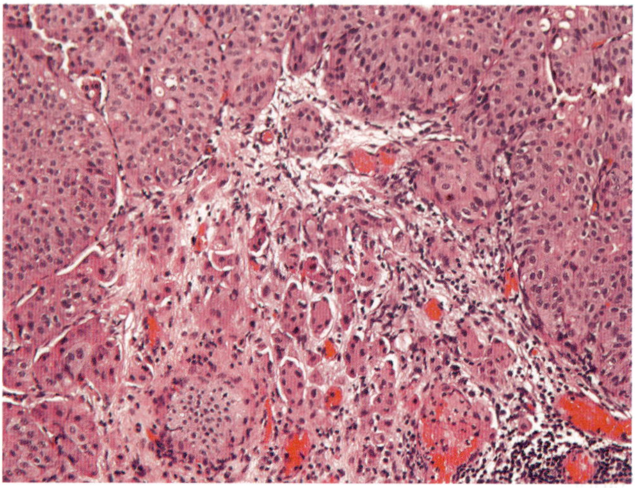

FIGURE 5.18 **Base of papillary urothelial carcinoma (*top*) with small nests of invasive urothelial carcinoma, with retraction artifact.**

abnormality is the CIS. Invasion may be in the form of single cells, clusters, or cords of cells or small nests of cells within the lamina propria. The stroma usually shows an inflammatory or desmoplastic reaction or occasionally shows nests of tumor cells surrounded by retraction artifact.

Papillary urothelial carcinoma with microinvasion (Fig. 5.18): Microinvasion (arbitrarily defines as <2 mm) of papillary tumors can be similarly defined as in cases with CIS and should be mentioned in the diagnosis to document minimal, focal, or early invasion.

Papillary urothelial carcinoma with invasion into stalk (Figs. 5.19 and 5.20): In addition to invading at the base of a papillary carcinoma,

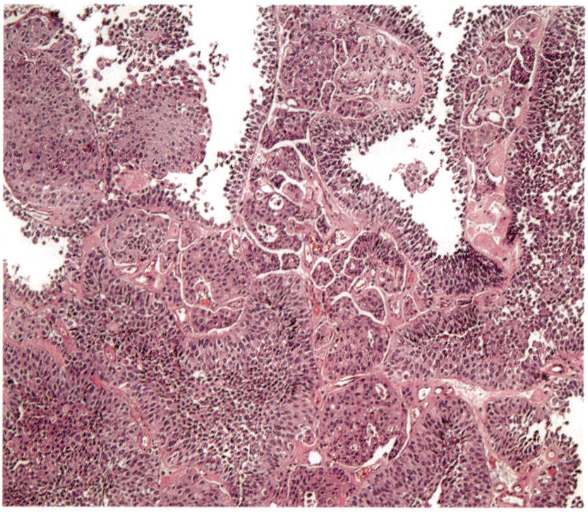

FIGURE 5.19 **Papillary urothelial carcinoma with stalk invasion.** Note prominent retraction artifact surrounding invasive tumor nests.

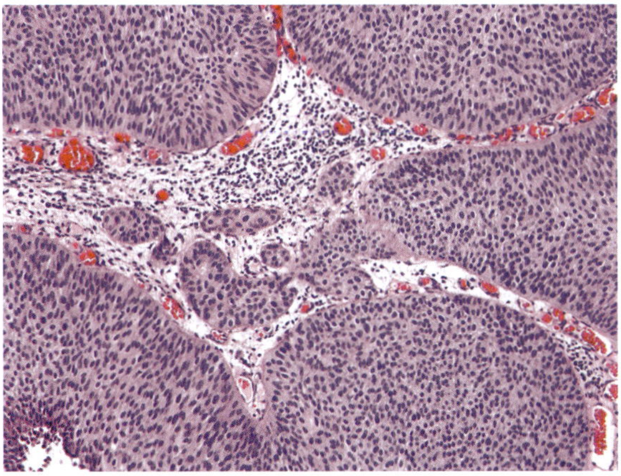

FIGURE 5.20 Small nests of invasive urothelial carcinoma (*center*) within the stalk of papillary carcinoma.

urothelial carcinomas can invade into the stalk of a papillary tumor.[41,43] Appreciation of this pattern requires optimal orientation of the entire or large parts of the papillary tumor, which may not always be the case, especially in TURBT specimens. Paradoxical differentiation and retraction artifact are commonly seen in this setting.

Well-established invasion into underlying lamina propria: In the majority of cases, invasion is seen at the base of the papillary neoplasm (Fig. 5.18). With respect to the muscularis mucosae layer within the lamina propria, invasive tumors may be classified as follows:

- Invasive into lamina propria, but not into muscularis propria (Figs. 5.21 and 5.22)
- Invasive into lamina propria up to muscularis mucosae, but not into muscularis propria
- Invasive into lamina propria beyond muscularis mucosae, but not into muscularis propria
- Urothelial carcinoma with inverted/endophytic or broad-front growth pattern (see Chapter 4)

Problems and Pitfalls in the Diagnosis of T1 Invasion

Diagnosis of lamina propria invasion is often difficult, and the problem is well exemplified in the data from the French Association of Urology Cancer Committee study,[25] which revealed that seven experienced pathologists could agree on lamina propria invasion in only 61% of cases after three assessments. In 10% of cases, no consensus was achieved despite four evaluations. In another study by Abel and colleagues,[26] 15% of lesions initially diagnosed as T1 were down staged to Ta and 22% of urothelial carcinomas diagnosed with muscularis propria invasion were down staged to T1 or Ta by a "dedicated" pathologist. To improve the concordance rates among

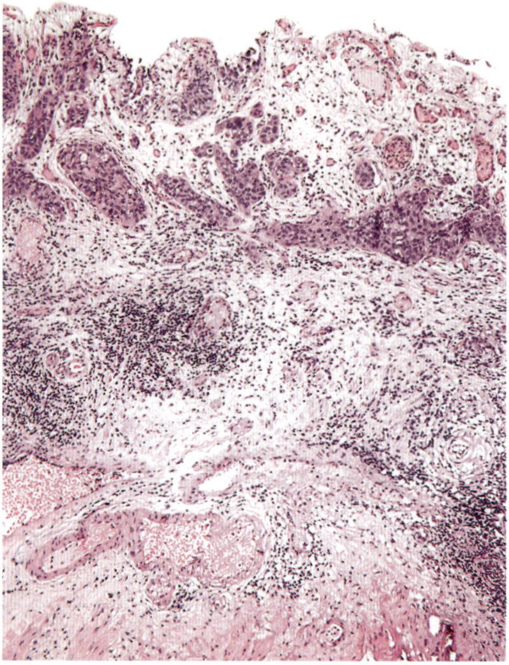

FIGURE 5.21 Nests of urothelial carcinoma associated with myxoid and inflamed stroma invading above the level of the muscularis mucosae, characterized by a horizontal row of dilated vessels (bottom).

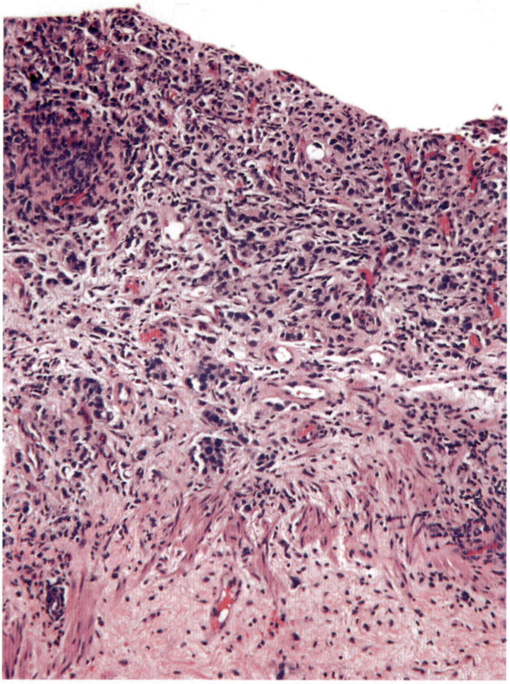

FIGURE 5.22 Nests of urothelial carcinoma invading above small bundle of muscles of the muscularis mucosae (bottom).

TABLE 5.2 Pitfalls in the Diagnosis of Lamina Propria Invasion by Urothelial Carcinoma

Tangential sectioning
Thermal artifact
Obscuring inflammation
Carcinoma *in situ* involving von Brunn nests
Invasion into muscle, indeterminate for muscle type (muscularis mucosae vs muscularis propria)
Invasion into adipose tissue within lamina propria (overdiagnosis of extravesical invasion)
Deceptively bland urothelial carcinomas
• Microcystic variant of urothelial carcinoma (invasive)
• Broad-front or inverted growth, raising the question of invasion
• Nested variant of urothelial carcinoma (invasive)
Overdiagnosis of vascular invasion

Adapted with permission from Jimenez RE, Keane TE, Hardy HT, et al. pT1 Urothelial carcinoma of the bladder: criteria for diagnosis, pitfalls, and clinical implications. *Adv Anat Pathol.* 2000;7(1):13-25.

pathologists, it is imperative to be aware of and understand the possible pitfalls in the diagnosis of lamina propria invasion (Table 5.2). The most common ones follow.

Tangential sectioning and poor orientation: Transurethral resections of bladder tumor specimens are excised in a piecemeal fashion, rendering fragmented specimens that are usually poorly oriented. Furthermore, because of their complex architecture, papillary tumors are inevitably tangentially sectioned in multiple planes, resulting in isolated nests of tumor cells within connective tissue. Smooth, round, and regular contours favor tangential sectioning, whereas irregular, jagged nests with haphazard arrangement favor stromal invasion. Also, if the nests in question have the same cytology as the adjacent noninvasive component, as opposed to more abundant cytoplasm (ie, paradoxical differentiation), one must entertain the possibility of tangential sectioning.

Thermal injury: Thermal injury or cautery artifact produces severely distorted morphology in TURBT specimens and is a frequent source of distress for the pathologist (Figs. 5.23-5.25). Pathologists have no control over this problem, although deeper levels may occasionally display better preserved areas. When this is not helpful, the pathologist should express the inability to render a definitive diagnosis due to thermal effect. Occasionally, we have used the cytokeratin stain to accentuate the presence of infiltrating carcinoma amidst necrotic or poorly preserved tissue. Caution is warranted when interpreting keratin stains as plump myofibroblasts, and smooth muscle bundles may be keratin positive and may be misinterpreted as carcinoma.[44]

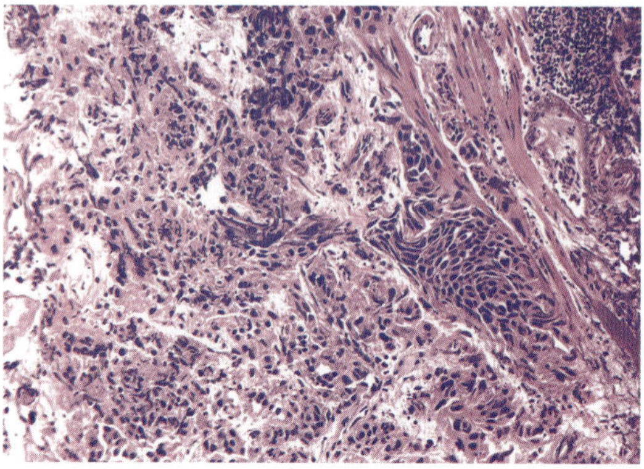

FIGURE 5.23 **Urothelial carcinoma with extensive cautery artifact.**

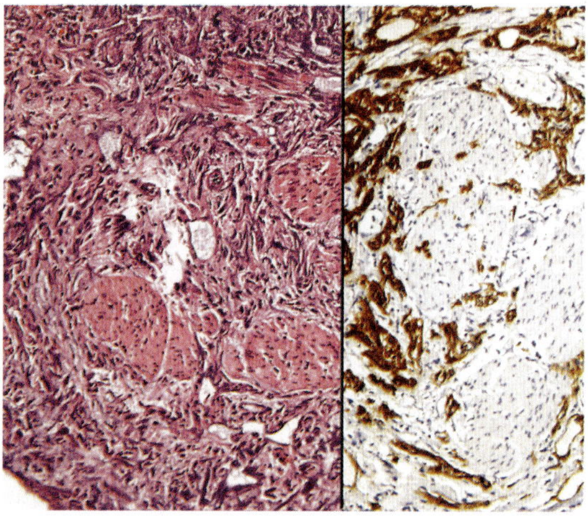

FIGURE 5.24 **Urothelial carcinoma with obscuring artifact (*left*).** Pancytokeratin (***right***) highlights tumor among muscularis propria.

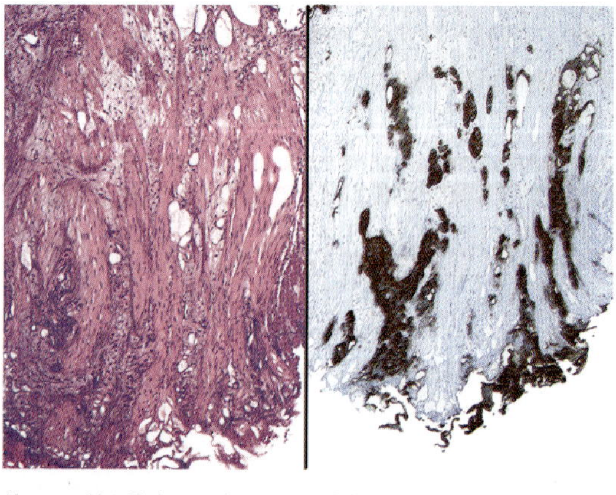

FIGURE 5.25 **Subtle urothelial carcinoma with obscuring artifact (*left*).** Pancytokeratin (***right***) highlights tumor invading muscularis propria.

Obscuring inflammation: Papillary tumors may show variable, often brisk, inflammation at the tumor-stromal interface, which may obscure isolated cells or nests of invasive tumor. If suspicion for tumor is high or if large atypical cells are present in the lamina propria, judicious use of cytokeratin immunostaining may be useful; however, it must be noted that myofibroblasts occasionally stain for keratin and may be misinterpreted as invasive carcinoma.[44]

CIS involving von Brunn nests (see Chapter 2): Flat lesions, when they involve von Brunn nests, may mimic lamina propria invasion by the mere presence of high-grade cells within the lamina propria. This is especially problematic in prominent nests or in those that have been distorted by an inflammatory process.

Muscle invasion indeterminate for type of muscle: In cases of invasive tumor that is juxtaposed to muscle fibers but due to obscuring factors (ie, inflammation, tangential sectioning, cautery artifact, strong desmoplastic response, or poor orientation) or when the caliber of the muscle bundles is such that it is difficult to distinguish between muscularis mucosae or muscularis propria bundles, the pathologist is unable to determine whether the muscle involved belongs to the muscularis mucosae or the muscularis propria (Figs. 5.26 and 5.27). The presence tumor among small muscle bundles adjacent to a linear vascular plexus is consistent with muscularis mucosae invasion (Fig. 5.28). It is recommended that, when faced with this situation, pathologists should clearly state their uncertainty in establishing the depth of invasion rather than commit to a particular type of muscle involvement–muscularis mucosae (T1) or muscularis propria (T2).

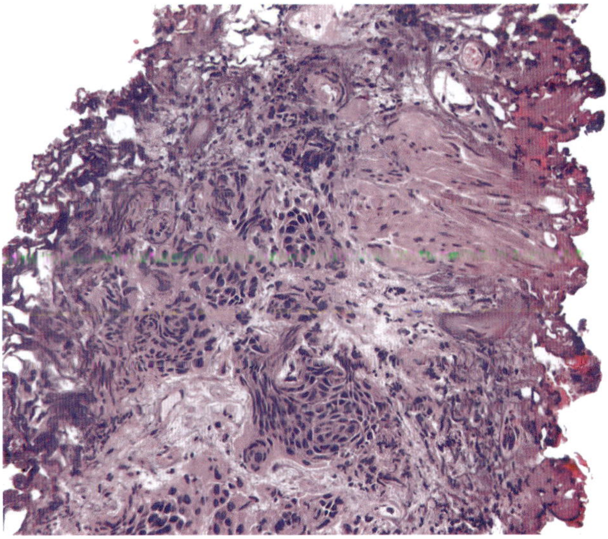

FIGURE 5.26 Muscle invasion indeterminate in size between muscularis propria and muscularis mucosae.

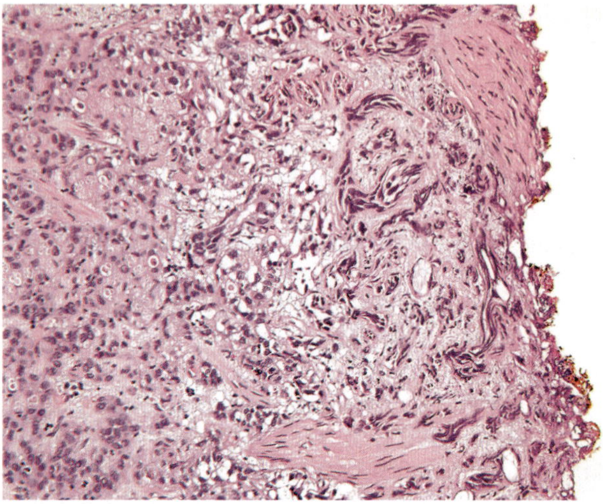

FIGURE 5.27 **Invasive high-grade urothelial carcinoma with medium-sized muscle bundles (*right*) suspicious for muscularis propria invasion, although hyperplastic muscularis mucosae invasion cannot be excluded with certainty.**

This distinction is critical in that muscularis propria invasion is currently regarded as the crossroads between conservative management and definitive therapy. Immunohistochemistry may play a useful role in this setting and the following three markers may be useful.

Desmin: In cases where there is extensive high-grade carcinoma, immunohistochemistry for desmin can highlight numerous muscle bundles, which in the appropriate morphologic context may be too extensive

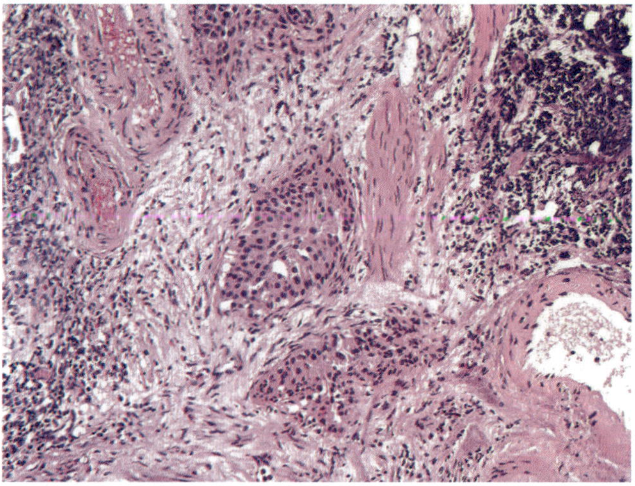

FIGURE 5.28 **Invasive urothelial carcinoma among muscularis mucosae.** Note associated dilated vessels.

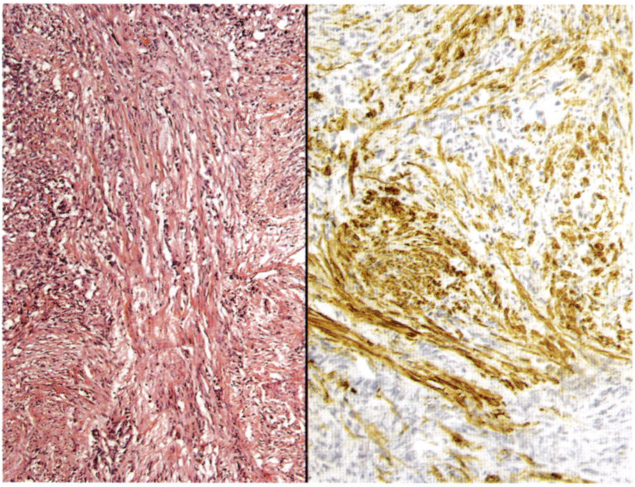

FIGURE 5.29 **Extensive infiltrating high-grade urothelial carcinoma.** It is difficult to distinguish myofibroblastic response to tumor vs partially destroyed muscularis propria (***left***). Desmin immunohistochemistry demonstrates too much muscle to represent muscularis mucosae (***right***). Taking into account the extensive high-grade nature of the tumor and the numerous muscle bundles, it is diagnostic of muscularis propria invasion.

for muscularis mucosae and, therefore, represent muscularis propria partly destroyed by invasive carcinoma (Fig. 5.29). In a recent consensus statement, the utility of desmin to distinguish muscle from desmoplasia and to highlight muscle contours for distinguishing muscularis mucosae from propria was recommended.[17]

Smoothelin, a novel smooth muscle specific contractile protein expressed only by fully differentiated smooth muscle cells, and not by proliferative or noncontractile smooth muscle cells and myofibroblasts, has potential diagnostic utility in the distinction of muscularis mucosae from muscularis propria. When only strong and diffuse immunoreactivity is considered positive, the specificity for muscularis propria is high.[45] Experience in transurethral resections is limited although preliminary experience suggests that staining may be obtained even in the background of cautery artifact (Fig. 5.30). Caution is necessary in overreliance in this immunohistochemical marker alone, and attention is necessary to the staining patterns in control tissues.[46,47] However, there may be overlap in the staining seen with smoothelin in muscularis mucosae and muscularis propria, such that if an internal control of definite muscularis mucosae is not present, the stain may not be useful. In a recent consensus statement, smoothelin was not recommended due to limited and conflicted data.[17,48,49] Smoothelin may be used in diagnostically challenging cases only if there is sufficient experience with control staining and experience with the antibody.

Vimentin is consistently expressed in muscularis mucosae but rarely in muscularis propria. Along with desmin and smoothelin, vimentin staining may have a role in distinguishing subtypes of muscle in the bladder, although data for vimentin in routine bladder specimens are limited.[46]

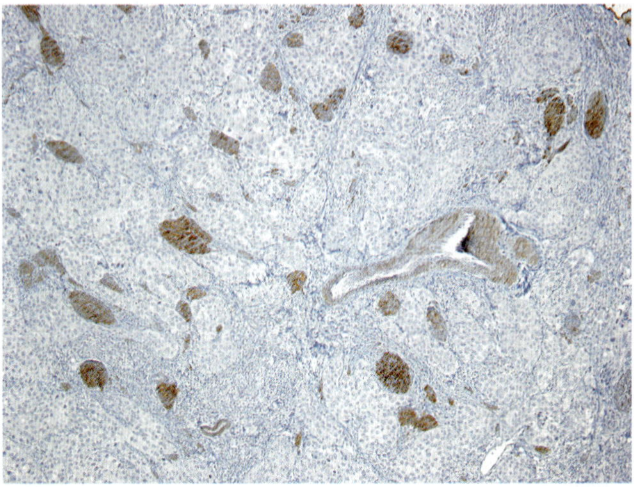

FIGURE 5.30 **Urothelial carcinoma invading between relatively small muscle bundles.** There are too many muscle bundles to represent muscularis mucosae. Immunohistochemistry for smoothelin shows strong staining of the muscle verifying it is muscularis propria.

Invasion into fat does not indicate extravesical spread: Fat may be normally present in the lamina propria; therefore, tumor invasive into fat should not automatically equate to involvement of perivesical fat.[37]

Deceptively bland variants of urothelial carcinomas: When limited to the lamina propria, deceptively bland patterns of invasive urothelial carcinoma may make the recognition of T1 disease extremely difficult (see Chapter 6). For example, microcystic urothelial carcinoma can easily mimic cystitis cystica,[50] and the "nested" pattern may be easily confused with von Brunn nests[51] (see Chapter 1). Recently, a large nested pattern of bladder cancer has also been described (see Chapter 6). Attention should be paid to general features useful in assessing invasion, such as cytologic atypia, infiltrative architecture, desmoplasia, and architectural complexity, especially because they may appear subtle in superficial biopsies.

Overdiagnosis of vascular invasion: As discussed earlier, a peculiar stromal retraction artifact in lamina propria–invasive tumors may mimic vascular invasion. Caution is hence warranted, and strict criteria should be used possibly augmented with immunohistochemistry for vascular and lymphatic markers (Figs. 5.31-5.34, eFigs. 5.33-5.38; Table 5.3).

GRADING OF INVASIVE UROTHELIAL CARCINOMA

By the World Health Organization/International Society of Urological Pathologists (WHO/ISUP) classification, invasive tumors are graded as low grade and high grade. Features indicative of the urothelial character of cells of urothelial carcinoma include the presence of longitudinal nuclear

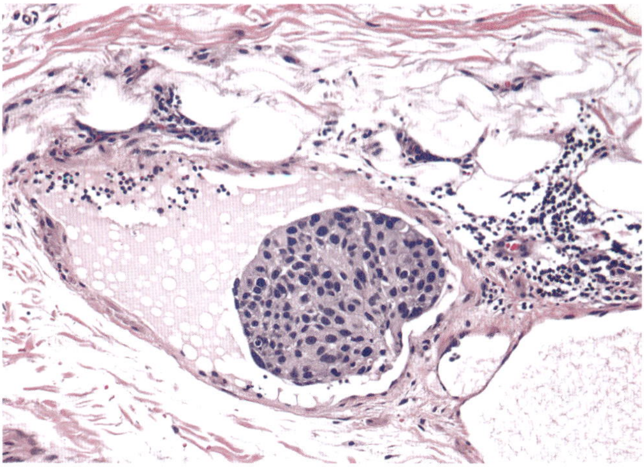

FIGURE 5.31 **Vascular-lymphatic invasion by urothelial carcinoma.** Note vascular channel lined by endothelial cells.

grooves that are often appreciable in low-grade tumors but are rarely seen in high-grade tumors. In clinical practice, most invasive urothelial carcinomas are conventionally graded as high grade, due to the invariably associated high-grade histologic features. In invasive cases, the prognostic value of the histologic grade is not as critical as the key prognostic factor at this point of the disease is the pathologic stage (depth of invasion). Nonetheless, a very small subset of papillary urothelial carcinomas of low grade are associated with invasive cancers of lower appearing histologic

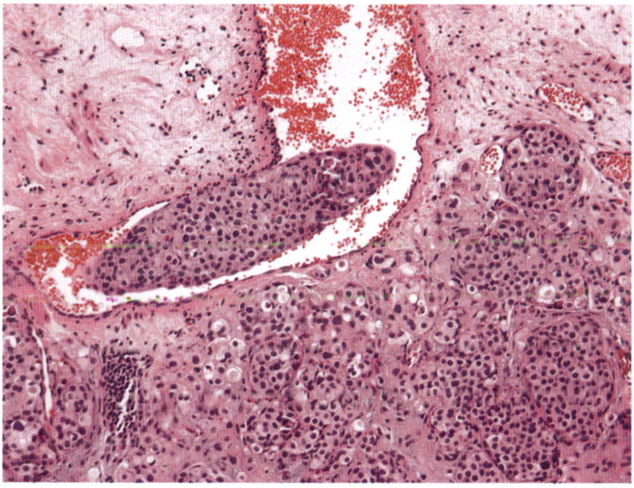

FIGURE 5.32 **Vascular-lymphatic invasion by urothelial carcinoma.** The tumor thrombus is associated with red blood cells and has a different morphology than the surrounding infiltrating tumor, as opposed to what is seen with retraction artifact around invasive tumor.

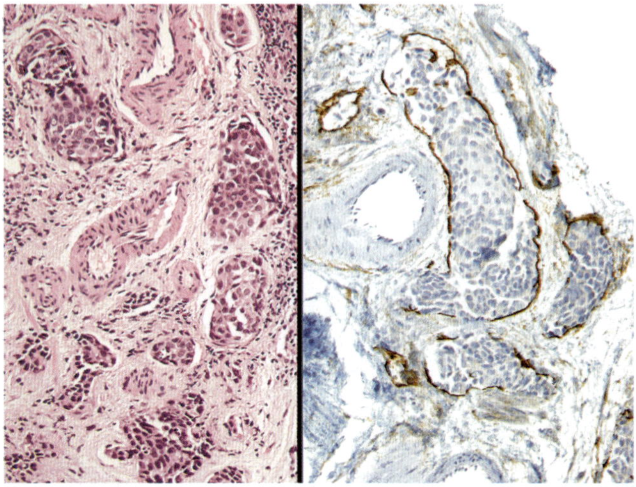

FIGURE 5.33 **Infiltrating urothelial carcinoma where it is difficult to identify vascular invasion on routine stains (*left*).** D2-40 labels lymphatic endothelial cells demonstrating vascular invasion (***right***).

grade, and some deceptively bland subtypes of bladder cancer, for example, nested subtype (Chapter 6) have low-grade features. There is controversy as to the grading of morphologically low-grade invasive urothelial carcinoma. It is the opinion of some experts that all invasive tumors, irrespective of morphology, including deceptively bland subtypes are graded as "high grade" based on their biology. Other experts will diagnose "invasive

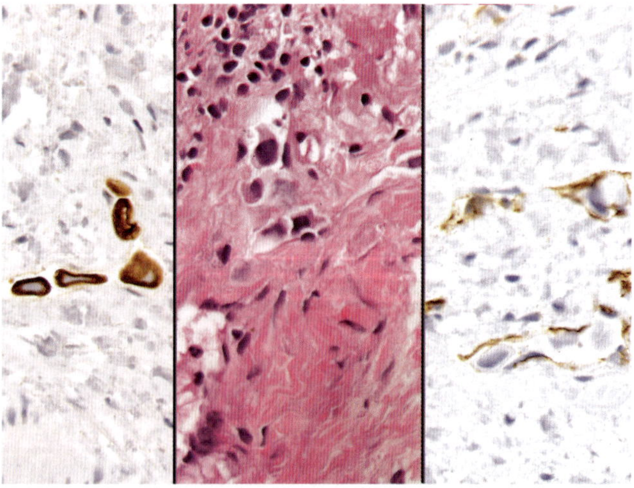

FIGURE 5.34 **Individual cells of infiltrating urothelial carcinoma suspicious for vascular invasion (*center*).** Pancytokeratin labels the carcinoma (***left***) and CD31, the vascular spaces surrounding the tumor (***right***) diagnostic of vascular invasion.

TABLE 5.3 Criteria and Pitfalls for Vascular-Lymphatic Invasion in Urothelial Neoplasms

Criteria for vascular-lymphatic invasion
Presence of unequivocal endothelial lining
Nests attached to wall of lumen containing blood constituents (red blood cells, inflammatory cells, or thrombus)
Nests attached to and conforming to the shape of the vessel
Peritumoral location of vascular invasion (intratumoral invasion not diagnostic by itself)
Tumor cells in the space near large artery or vein (vascular route)
Immunohistochemical confirmation (Erg or CD31)
Pitfalls in recognition of vascular-lymphatic invasion
Pitfall in recognition of endothelial and venular spaces
Retraction of stroma (particularly conspicuous in micropapillary tumors)
Pitfall in recognition of large vessel invasion
Carryover due to fragmentation of neoplasm

Adapted with permission from Jimenez RE, Keane TE, Hardy HT, et al. pT1 Urothelial carcinoma of the bladder: criteria for diagnosis, pitfalls, and clinical implications. *Adv Anat Pathol.* 2000;7(1):13-25.

low-grade urothelial carcinoma" based on the tumor's morphology, yet add a note to the effect of "Invasive urothelial carcinomas that are morphologically low grade are uncommon and have a similar prognosis stage for stage compared to invasive urothelial carcinoma that are morphologically high grade; there are no data to suggest that there should be difference in therapy based on the histological grade of the invasive component."[3]

SUBSTAGING OF T1 DISEASE

Attempts have been made to identify prognostic factors within the category of T1 tumors, but an accurate, easy-to-apply, reproducible method is unavailable. Toward this end, several studies have evaluated the issue of substaging T1 urothelial carcinomas with most using the muscularis mucosae as an anatomic landmark to assess the depth of invasion (tumors above or into muscularis mucosae are T1a; tumors invasive below are T1b).[31,52,53] In the absence of muscularis mucosae (muscularis mucosae is seen in 18%-83% of TURBT specimens only), large vessels have been used as a substitute for muscularis mucosae to designate T1a vs T1b disease. Others have used the depth of invasion in millimeters from the basement membrane[54]; less than one high power filed in content or greatest invasive diameter of 1 mm.[30] Documenting whether the invasion is focal or extensive is strongly recommended, although there are no clear-cut criteria to define them.[55-57]

The aggregate data of many studies indicate that deep lamina propria invasion, whether assessed by the relation of the tumor to the muscularis mucosae or by direct micrometric measurement, identifies a subset of patients with T1 disease with a more adverse prognosis.[31] Tumors invading beyond the muscularis mucosae tend to behave like muscularis propria–invasive (T2) tumors. A recent study has shown differing microarray gene expression profiles between T1a and T1b stages supporting the different biologic differences.[58]

The 1998 WHO/ISUP Consensus Conference Committee as well as the WHO/ISUP classification (including the recent 5th edition of WHO) have recognized and encouraged the need to express some assessment of the degree or extent of invasion in the pathology report.[1,59] The eighth edition of the AJCC staging strongly recommends using any of the above mentioned methods to categorize pT1 disease.[2]

Muscularis Propria (Detrusor Muscle)–Invasive Tumors

Urothelial cancers invading between thick distinct fascicles of muscle bundles of detrusor muscle characterize T2 urothelial cancer (Figs. 5.35-5.40, eFigs. 5.39-5.58). Muscle-invasive carcinoma may or may not elicit a desmoplastic stromal response. In the T-staging system, T2 tumors are divided into those invading the inner half (T2a) and those invading the outer half (T2b). Because TURBT specimens lack orientation with respect to bladder anatomy, substaging of T2 disease should be performed in cystectomy specimens alone. Also, because there is often abundant adipose tissue between muscularis propria bundles, the presence of tumor in adipose tissue in a TURBT specimen does not necessarily equate to perivesical fat involvement. Hence, pathologic staging in TURBT specimens is limited to whether the tumor is Ta, T1, or T2. The distinction between T2a,

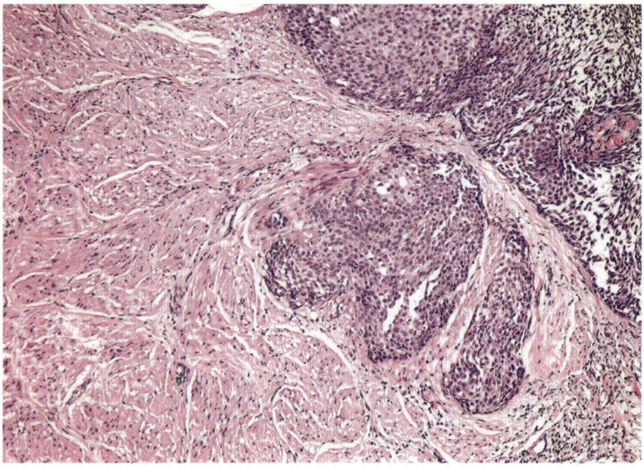

FIGURE 5.35 Large nests of urothelial carcinoma invading muscularis propria.

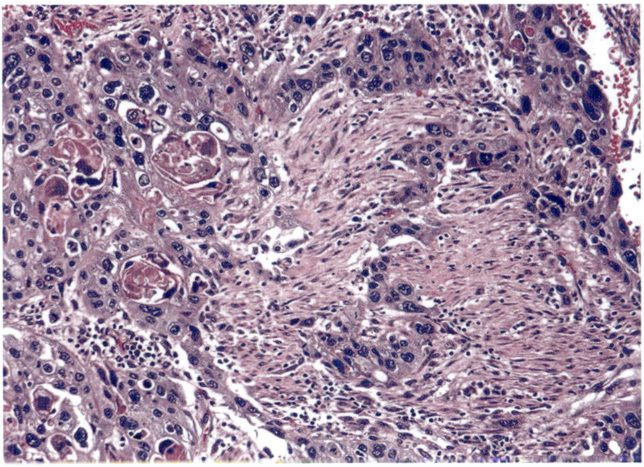

FIGURE 5.36 Pleomorphic urothelial carcinoma partly destroying muscularis propria.

T2b, and pT3 cancer is, hence, performed in cystectomy specimens alone. Because the junction between the muscularis propria layer and perivesical fat is not well demarcated, determining the status of a tumor as pT2b vs pT3a disease is often challenging. Desmoplasia, obscuring inflammation, and admixed lymphovascular invasion compound the dilemma in accurately designating pT3a disease. A interobserver study has documented the variability in diagnosing pT3a disease among experts. In making this determination, an imaginary line may be drawn at low power to demarcate the boundary between the outermost muscle bundles of the bladder wall and perivesical tissue in a cystectomy specimen to determine if the tumor is pT2b or pT3a.[60]

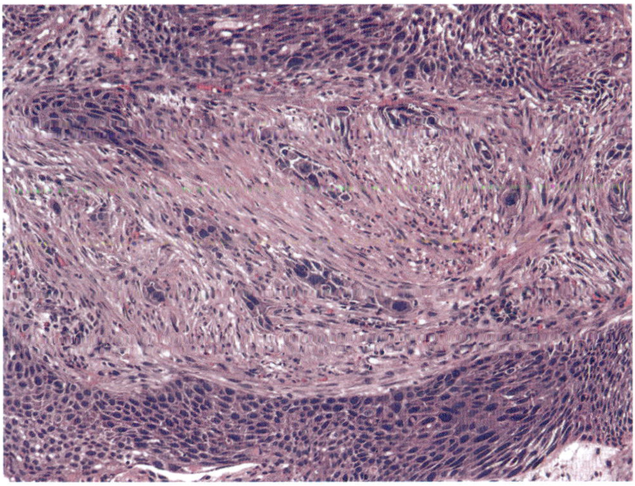

FIGURE 5.37 Pleomorphic urothelial carcinoma extending into muscularis propria.

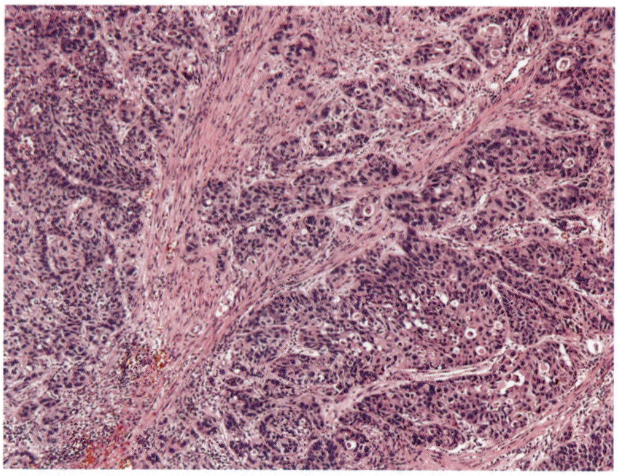

FIGURE 5.38 **Urothelial carcinoma invading muscularis propria.** Although the muscle bundles are partly destroyed, the presence of one relatively large and several smaller bundles of smooth muscle is diagnostic of muscularis propria invasion.

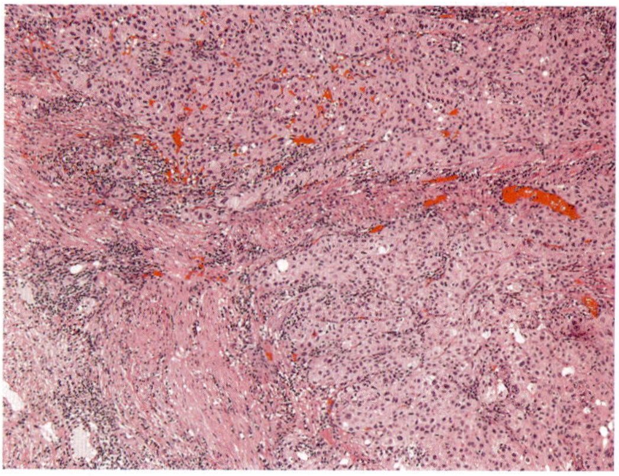

FIGURE 5.39 **Small nests of urothelial carcinoma invading muscularis propria (*left*).**

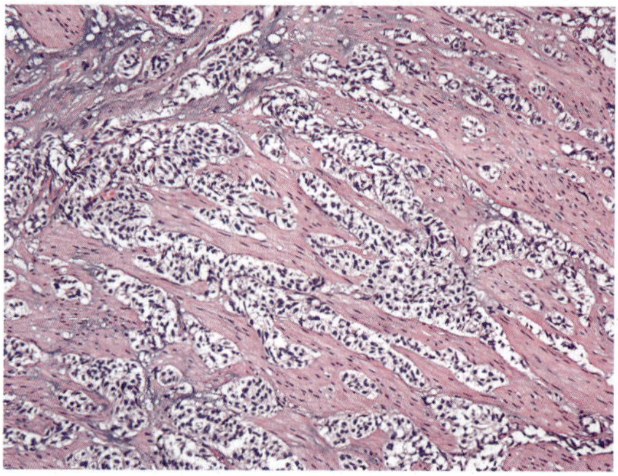

FIGURE 5.40 **Small nests of urothelial carcinoma with clear cytoplasm invading muscularis propria.**

PERTINENT EMERGING MOLECULAR ASPECTS IN DIAGNOSTIC PATHOLOGY

TERT promoter mutations are the most common genetic alteration in urothelial carcinoma across all grades, stages, and most histological subtypes, and some authors have advocated their use as reliable molecular diagnostic biomarker in some clinical settings to distinguish between benign and malignant conditions such as nested subtype from florid von Brunn nests. TERT promoter mutations have also been used to distinguish between urothelial and nonurothelial malignancies (eg, bladder vs prostate or lung).[61-63] In the era of precision medicine, FGFR alterations may be used to determine eligibility for treatment with anti-FGFR agents in refractory tumors. Mutations in ERCC2 and other DNA repair genes have also been used to stratify patients who may benefit from cisplatin-based therapy.[64-66] Assessment of PDL1 immunohistochemistry is used in some institutions and clinical trials as predictors for response to checkpoint inhibitor therapy.[4,5] Six consensus molecular classes of invasive urothelial carcinoma have been defined (luminal papillary, luminal nonspecified, luminal unstable, stroma rich, basal squamous, and neuroendocrine-like)[16]; however, unresolved issues precluding routine clinical use are the inconsistent and unreliable correlation of histology and molecular signatures, and the heterogeneity of concurrent divergent or subtype morphology with representative sampled tissue for molecular testing.

REFERENCES

1. Raspolini MR, Amin MB, Hartmann A, Moch H, Srigley JR. Tumours of the urinary tract: Introduction. In: Comperat EM, Netto GJ, Tsuzki T, eds. WHO classification of tumours. *Urinary and Male Genital Tumours*. International Agency for Research on Cancer; 2022, 5th ed. Chapter 3, Section 5.1.2.1. 2-6.
2. Amin MB, Edge SB, Greene FL, et al., eds. *AJCC Cancer Staging Manual*. 8th ed. Springer; 2017.
3. Amin MB, Comperat E, Epstein JI, et al. The Genitourinary Pathology Society update on classification and grading of flat and papillary urothelial neoplasia with new reporting recommendations and approach to lesions with mixed and early patterns of neoplasia. *Adv Anat Pathol*. 2021;28(4):179-195.
4. Compérat E, Amin MB, Epstein JI, et al. The Genitourinary Pathology Society update on classification of variant histologies, T1 substaging, molecular taxonomy, and immunotherapy and PD-L1 testing implications of urothelial cancers. *Adv Anat Pathol*. 2021;28(4):196-208.
5. Compérat E, Amin MB, Cathomas R, et al. Current best practice for bladder cancer: a narrative review of diagnostics and treatments. *Lancet*. 2022;400(10364):1712-1721.
6. Toll AS, Epstein JI. Invasive low-grade papillary urothelial carcinoma: a clinicopathologic analysis of 41 cases. *Am J Surg Pathol*. 2012;36:1081-1086.
7. Amin MB. Histological variants of urothelial carcinoma: diagnostic, therapeutic and prognostic implications. *Mod Pathol*. 2009;22(suppl 2):S96-S118.
8. Lopez-Beltran A, Martin J, Garcia J, et al. Squamous and glandular differentiation in urothelial bladder carcinomas. Histopathology, histochemistry and immunohistochemical expression of carcinoembryonic antigen. *Histol Histopathol*. 1988;3:63-68.

9. Dalbagni G, Genega E, Hashibe M, et al. Cystectomy for bladder cancer: a contemporary series. *J Urol*. 2001;165:1111-1116.
10. Akdas A, Turkeri L. The impact of squamous metaplasia in transitional cell carcinoma of the bladder. *Int Urol Nephrol*. 1991;23:333-336.
11. Logothetis CJ, Dexeus FH, Chong C, et al. Cisplatin, cyclophosphamide and doxorubicin chemotherapy for unresectable urothelial tumors: the M.D. Anderson experience. *J Urol*. 1989;141:33-37.
12. Kim SP, Frank I, Cheville JC, et al. The impact of squamous and glandular differentiation on survival after radical cystectomy for urothelial carcinoma. *J Urol*. 2012;188:405-409.
13. Cancer Genome Atlas Research Network. Comprehensive molecular characterization of urothelial bladder carcinoma. *Nature*. 2014;507:315-322.
14. Choi W, Czerniak B, Ochoa A, et al. Intrinsic basal and luminal subtypes of muscle-invasive bladder cancer. *Nat Rev Urol*. 2014;11:400-410.
15. Damrauer JS, Hoadley KA, Chism DD, et al. Intrinsic subtypes of high-grade bladder cancer reflect the hallmarks of breast cancer biology. *Proc Natl Acad Sci U S A*. 2014;111:3110-3115.
16. Kamoun A, de Reyniès A, Allory Y, et al. A Consensus molecular classification of muscle-invasive bladder cancer. *Eur Urol*. 2020;77(4):420-433.
17. Amin MB, Trpkov K, Lopez-Beltran A, et al. Best practices recommendations in the application of immunohistochemistry in the bladder lesions: report from the International Society of Urologic Pathology consensus conference. *Am J Surg Pathol*. 2014;38(8):e20-e34.
18. Larsen MP, Steinberg GD, Brendler CB, et al. Use of Ulex europaeus agglutinin I (UEAI) to distinguish vascular and "pseudovascular" invasion in transitional cell carcinoma of bladder with lamina propria invasion. *Mod Pathol*. 1990;3:83-88.
19. Ramani P, Birch BR, Harland SJ, et al. Evaluation of endothelial markers in detecting blood and lymphatic channel invasion in pT1 transitional carcinoma of bladder. *Histopathology*. 1991;19:551-554.
20. Reuter VE. Lymphovascular invasion as an independent predictor of recurrence and survival in node-negative bladder cancer remains to be proven. *J Clin Oncol*. 2005;23: 6450-6451.
21. Smith SC, Mohanty SK, Kunju LP, et al. Uroplakin II outperforms uroplakin III in diagnostically challenging settings. *Histopathology*. 2014;65:132-138.
22. Anderstrom C, Johansson S, Nilsson S. The significance of lamina propria invasion on the prognosis of patients with bladder tumors. *J Urol*. 1980;124:23-26.
23. Kiemeney LA, Witjes JA, Verbeek AL, et al. The clinical epidemiology of superficial bladder cancer. Dutch South-East Cooperative Urological Group. *Br J Cancer*. 1993;67:806-812.
24. Williams JL, Hammonds JC, Saunders N. T1 bladder tumours. *Br J Urol*. 1977;49:663–668.
25. Lamina propria microinvasion of bladder tumors, incidence on stage allocation (pTa vs pT1): recommended approach. Pathologists of the French Association of Urology Cancer Committee. *World J Urol*. 1993;11:161-164.
26. Abel PD, Henderson D, Bennett MK, et al. Differing interpretations by pathologists of the pT category and grade of transitional cell cancer of the bladder. *Br J Urol*. 1988;62:339-342.
27. Sarkis AS, Dalbagni G, Cordon-Cardo C, et al. Nuclear overexpression of p53 protein in transitional cell bladder carcinoma: a marker for disease progression. *J Natl Cancer Inst*. 1993;85:53-59.
28. Cheng L, Montironi R, Davidson DD, et al. Staging and reporting of urothelial carcinoma of the urinary bladder. *Mod Pathol*. 2009;22(suppl 2):S70-S95.
29. Lavery HJ, Stensland KD, Niegisch G, et al. Pathological T0 following radical cystectomy with or without neoadjuvant chemotherapy: a useful surrogate. *J Urol*. 2014;191:898-906.
30. Hansel DE, Amin MB, Comperat E, et al. A contemporary update on pathology standards for bladder cancer: transurethral resection and radical cystectomy specimens. *Eur Urol*. 2013;63:321-332.

31. Jimenez RE, Keane TE, Hardy HT, et al. pT1 urothelial carcinoma of the bladder: criteria for diagnosis, pitfalls, and clinical implications. *Adv Anat Pathol.* 2000;7:13-25.
32. Dixon JS, Gosling JA. Histology and fine structure of the muscularis mucosae of the human urinary bladder. *J Anat.* 1983;136:265-271.
33. Keep JC, Piehl M, Miller A, et al. Invasive carcinomas of the urinary bladder. Evaluation of tunica muscularis mucosae involvement. *Am J Clin Pathol.* 1989;91:575-579.
34. Ro JY, Ayala AG, el-Naggar A. Muscularis mucosa of urinary bladder. Importance for staging and treatment. *Am J Surg Pathol.* 1987;11:668-673.
35. Platz CE, Cohen MB, Jones MP, et al. Is microstaging of early invasive cancer of the urinary bladder possible or useful? *Mod Pathol.* 1996;9:1035-1039.
36. Paner GP, Ro JY, Wojcik EM, et al. Further characterization of the muscle layers and lamina propria of the urinary bladder by systematic histologic mapping: implications for pathologic staging of invasive urothelial carcinoma. *Am J Surg Pathol.* 2007;31:1420-1429.
37. Philip AT, Amin MB, Tamboli P, et al. Intravesical adipose tissue: a quantitative study of its presence and location with implications for therapy and prognosis. *Am J Surg Pathol.* 2000;24:1286-1290.
38. Amin MB, Murphy WM, Reuter VE. Controversies in the pathology of transitional cell carcinoma of the urinary bladder. Part II. In: Rosen PP, Fechner RE, eds. *Reviews of Pathology*. ASCP Press; 1997:72–100.
39. Tavora F, Epstein JI. Urothelial carcinoma with abundant myxoid stroma. *Hum Pathol.* 2009;40(10):1391-1398.
40. Young RH, Wick MR. Transitional cell carcinoma of the urinary bladder with pseudosarcomatous stroma. *Am J Clin Pathol.* 1988;90:216-219.
41. Amin MB, Gomez JA, Young RH. Urothelial transitional cell carcinoma with endophytic growth patterns: a discussion of patterns of invasion and problems associated with assessment of invasion in 18 cases. *Am J Surg Pathol.* 1997;21:1057-1068.
42. McKenney JK, Gomez JA, Desai S, et al. Morphologic expressions of urothelial carcinoma in situ: a detailed evaluation of its histologic patterns with emphasis on carcinoma in situ with microinvasion. *Am J Surg Pathol.* 2001;25:356-362.
43. Pagano F, Pegoraro V, Prayer-Galetti T, et al. Prognosis of bladder cancer. II. The fate of patients with T1b transitional cell bladder cancer. *Eur Urol.* 1987;13:305-309.
44. Tamas EF, Epstein JI. Detection of residual tumor cells in bladder biopsy specimens: pitfalls in the interpretation of cytokeratin stains. *Am J Surg Pathol.* 2007;31:390-397.
45. Paner GP, Shen SS, Lapetino S, et al. Diagnostic utility of antibody to smoothelin in the distinction of muscularis propria from muscularis mucosae of the urinary bladder: a potential ancillary tool in the pathologic staging of invasive urothelial carcinoma. *Am J Surg Pathol.* 2009;33:91-98.
46. Council L, Hameed O. Differential expression of immunohistochemical markers in bladder smooth muscle and myofibroblasts, and the potential utility of desmin, smoothelin, and vimentin in staging of bladder carcinoma. *Mod Pathol.* 2009;22:639-650.
47. Paner GP, Brown JG, Lapetino S, et al. Diagnostic use of antibody to smoothelin in the recognition of muscularis propria in transurethral resection of urinary bladder tumor (TURBT) specimens. *Am J Surg Pathol.* 2010;34:792-799.
48. Mihai IM, Olteanu GE, Herman D, et al. Analysis of tumor depth invasion with anti-smoothelin antibody in equivocal transurethral resection of urinary bladder tumor surgical specimens. *Int J Surg Pathol.* 2021;29(1):54-63.
49. Miyamoto H, Sharma RB, Illei PB, et al. Pitfalls in the use of smoothelin to identify muscularis propria invasion by urothelial carcinoma. *Am J Surg Pathol.* 2010;34:418-422.
50. Young RH, Zukerberg LR. Microcystic transitional cell carcinomas of the urinary bladder. A report of four cases. *Am J Clin Pathol.* 1991;96:635-639.

51. Drew PA, Furman J, Civantos F, et al. The nested variant of transitional cell carcinoma: an aggressive neoplasm with innocuous histology. *Mod Pathol.* 1996;9:989-994.
52. Holmang S, Hedelin H, Anderstrom C, et al. The importance of the depth of invasion in stage T1 bladder carcinoma: a prospective cohort study. *J Urol.* 1997;157:800-803. discussion 4.
53. Younes M, Sussman J, True LD. The usefulness of the level of the muscularis mucosae in the staging of invasive transitional cell carcinoma of the urinary bladder. *Cancer.* 1990;66:543-548.
54. Cheng L, Weaver AL, Neumann RM, et al. Substaging of T1 bladder carcinoma based on the depth of invasion as measured by micrometer: a new proposal. *Cancer.* 1999;86: 1035-1043.
55. Raspollini MR, Montironi R, Mazzucchelli R, et al. pT1 high-grade bladder cancer: histologic criteria, pitfalls in the assessment of invasion, and substaging. *Virchows Arch Int J Pathol.* 2020;477(1):3-16.
56. Hu Z, Mudaliar K, Quek ML, et al. Measuring the dimension of invasive component in pT1 urothelial carcinoma in transurethral resection specimens can predict time to recurrence. *Ann Diagn Pathol.* 2014;18(2):49-52.
57. Bertz S, Denzinger S, Otto W, et al. Substaging by estimating the size of invasive tumour can improve risk stratification in pT1 urothelial bladder cancer-evaluation of a large hospital-based single-centre series. *Histopathology.* 2011;59(4):722-732.
58. Descotes F, Dessen P, Bringuier PP, et al. Microarray gene expression profiling and analysis of bladder cancer supports the sub-classification of T1 tumours into T1a and T1b stages. *BJU Int.* 2014;113:333-342.
59. Epstein JI, Amin MB, Reuter VR, et al. The World Health Organization/International Society of Urological Pathology consensus classification of urothelial (transitional cell) neoplasms of the urinary bladder. Bladder Consensus Conference Committee. *Am J Surg Pathol.* 1998;22:1435-1448.
60. Ananthanarayanan V, Pan Y, Tretiakova M, et al. Influence of histologic criteria and confounding factors in staging equivocal cases for microscopic perivesical tissue invasion (pT3a): an interobserver study among genitourinary pathologists. *Am J Surg Pathol.* 2014;38:167-175.
61. Zhong M, Tian W, Zhuge J, et al. Distinguishing nested variants of urothelial carcinoma from benign mimickers by TERT promoter mutation. *Am J Surg Pathol.* 2015;39(1): 127-131.
62. Pietzak EJ, Bagrodia A, Cha EK, et al. Next-generation sequencing of nonmuscle invasive bladder cancer reveals potential biomarkers and rational therapeutic targets. *Eur Urol.* 2017;72(6):952-959.
63. Isharwal S, Audenet F, Drill E, et al. Prognostic value of TERT Alterations, mutational and copy number alterations burden in urothelial carcinoma. *Eur Urol Focus.* 2019;5(2):201-204.
64. Pal SK, Rosenberg JE, Hoffman-Censits JH, et al. Efficacy of BGJ398, a fibroblast growth factor receptor 1-3 inhibitor, in patients with previously treated advanced urothelial carcinoma with FGFR3 alterations. *Cancer Discov.* 2018;8(7):812-821.
65. Loriot Y, Necchi A, Park SH, et al. Erdafitinib in Locally Advanced or metastatic urothelial carcinoma. *N Engl J Med.* 2019;381(4):338-348.
66. Van Allen EM, Mouw KW, Kim P, et al. Somatic ERCC2 mutations correlate with cisplatin sensitivity in muscle-invasive urothelial carcinoma. *Cancer Discov.* 2014;4(10): 1140-1153.

6

HISTOLOGIC SUBTYPES OF UROTHELIAL CARCINOMA

With increasing experience with urothelial carcinomas at the light microscopic level, the spectrum of microscopic forms of urothelial carcinoma has been expanded to include several unusual histologic subtypes, which have been incorporated in the new WHO classification.[1] Invasive urothelial carcinoma is known for a wide range of histologic manifestation from deceptively bland morphology (unusual) to markedly atypical carcinoma cells (more common). It is important to understand different terms used to describe urothelial carcinoma histology not conforming to typical patterns. The terms "divergent differentiation" and "variant histology" have been variably and sometimes interchangeably used. Divergent/aberrant differentiation is used when there is differentiation along another histological line, for example, squamous, glandular, and trophoblastic differentiation (pure or admixed with urothelial carcinoma) (see Chapter 5). The term variant is used when process arises fundamentally from a malignancy with urothelial histogenesis/differentiation and where immunohistochemistry and other evidence further supports urothelial malignancy, for example, the nested, micropapillary, clear cell, plasmacytoid, and other variants. In keeping with terminology promoted in the fifth edition of WHO, the term variants (reserved for genetic alterations) is replaced by subtypes and it is the focus of this chapter.[1-5] By definition, they arise from the surface urothelium and are urothelial in nature. The recognition of histologic subtypes is important because (1) some types may be associated with a different clinical outcome, and some of them have been incorporated into risk stratification models[6,7]; (2) some may have a different therapeutic approach and are incorporated in treatment decision algorithms such as the NCCN guidelines[6-10]; or (3) awareness of the unusual pattern may be critical in avoiding diagnostic misinterpretations. We generally recommend following two general rules when dealing with histologic subtypes. First, the subtype histology should be documented in the pathology reports because metastatic tumors usually continue to exhibit the distinctive histologic pattern, and knowledge of the subtype histology facilitates association of the metastasis to the primary tumor. Second, because the pattern of

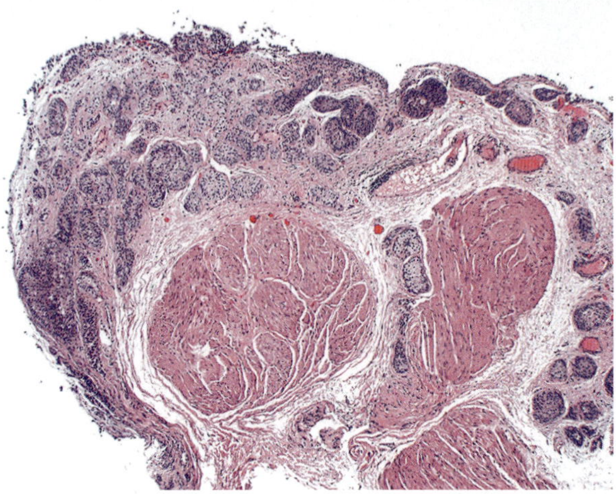

FIGURE 6.1 Nested variant of urothelial carcinoma with extension of nests into muscularis propria.

the neoplasm deviates from the conventional form, the possibility that this "unusual" morphology represents a metastasis should be considered and ruled out.

DECEPTIVELY BENIGN VARIANTS OF UROTHELIAL CARCINOMA

Some urothelial carcinomas have histologic variants that mimic nonneoplastic conditions such as cystitis cystica, proliferative von Brunn nests, nephrogenic adenoma, and inverted papilloma.[11-14] Awareness of these variants (nested [small and large nested], urothelial carcinoma with small

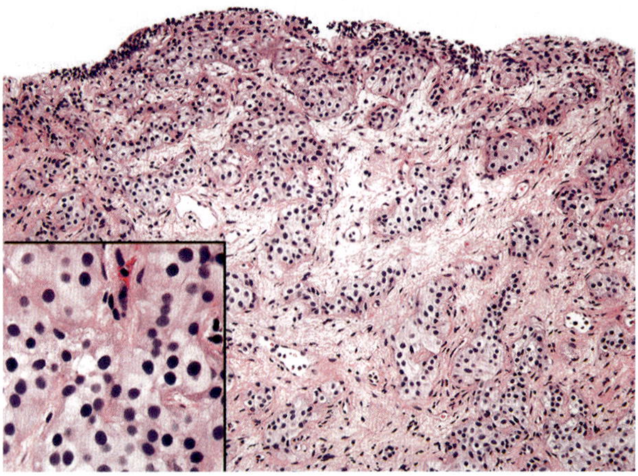

FIGURE 6.2 **Nested variant of urothelial carcinoma.** The nests are too small and crowded to represent von Brunn nests. ***Inset*** shows bland cytology.

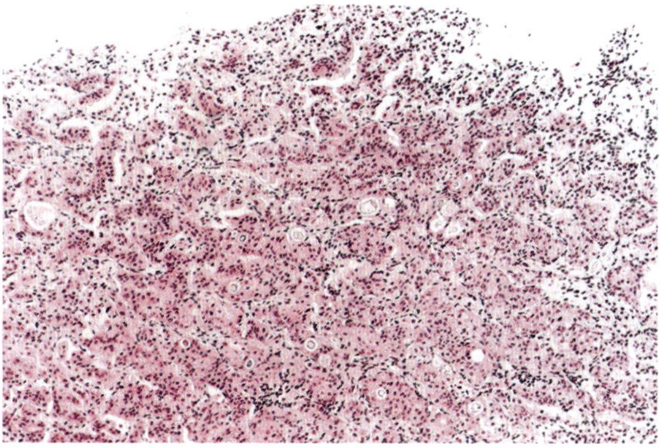

FIGURE 6.3 **Nested variant of urothelial carcinoma.** The nests are too small and crowded with complex architecture to represent von Brunn nests.

tubules, microcystic urothelial carcinoma, and inverted papilloma–like growth pattern) is important because limited sampling, particularly in cystoscopic biopsy specimens, could lead to an underdiagnosis of malignancy.[11-16]

Nested Variant of Urothelial Carcinoma

From a pathologist's perspective, the nested variant should appropriately be recognized as a malignant process, particularly in superficial biopsies. This rare subtype, characterized by a nested, deceptively bland pattern, may be composed of small nests or, as recently described, large nests ("large nested variant of urothelial carcinoma").

The nested pattern (referring to carcinomas with small nested pattern) has distinct patterns in the superficial and deep portions. In superficial biopsy samples and transurethral resectates, the superficial component appears as discrete nests, occasionally with tubules or even microcysts[11-19] (Figs. 6.1-6.9, eFigs. 6.1-6.18). The nests are tightly packed, often confluent,

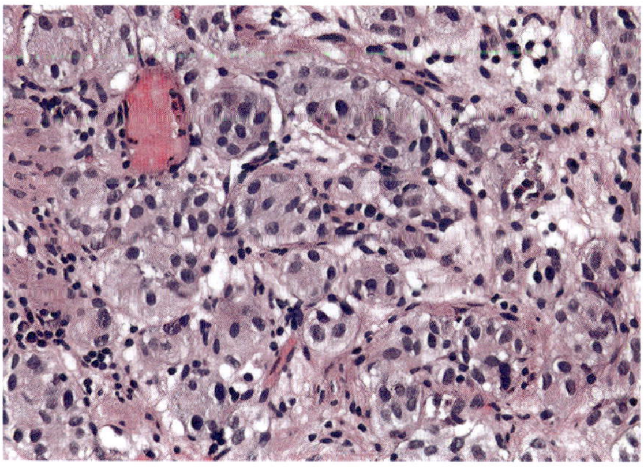

FIGURE 6.4 Nested variant of urothelial carcinoma (higher magnification of Fig. 6.3).

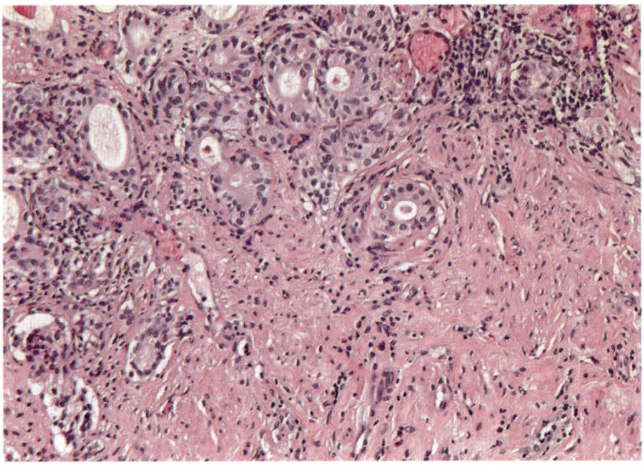

FIGURE 6.5 **Nested variant of urothelial carcinoma with focal tubule formation (higher magnification of Fig. 6.3).**

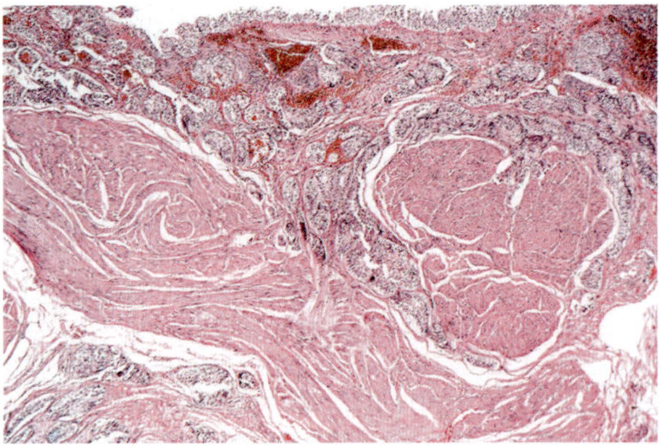

FIGURE 6.6 **Nested variant of urothelial carcinoma.** Tumor invades muscularis propria.

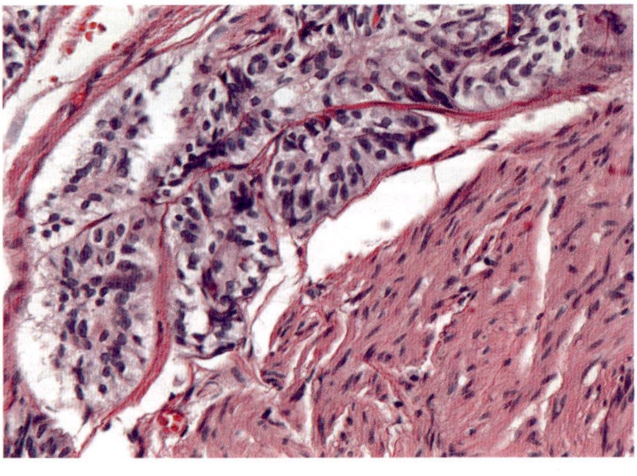

FIGURE 6.7 **Nested variant of urothelial carcinoma.** Tumor invades muscularis propria (higher magnification of Fig. 6.6).

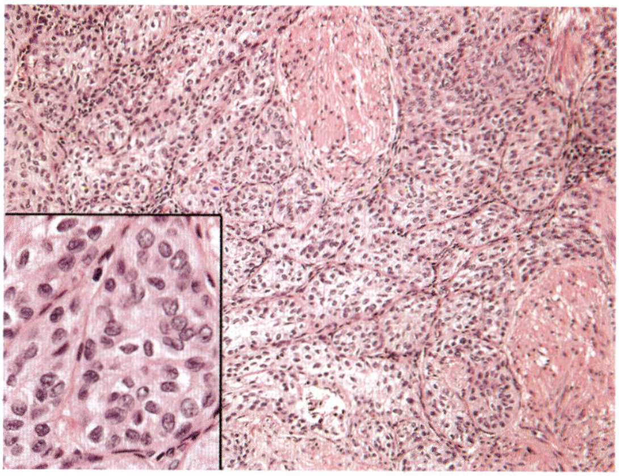

FIGURE 6.8 Nested variant of urothelial carcinoma with extension of nests into muscularis propria. *Inset* shows bland cytology.

and haphazardly arranged with little or no intervening stroma. Most nests have a relatively bland cytological appearance, but at least some have more atypical nuclei and larger nucleoli. A desmoplastic stromal response is lacking, which contributes to its "nonmalignant" appearance. Overlying papillary carcinoma or recognizable flat *in situ* disease is usually not evident[20]; a variable component of conventional urothelial carcinoma may be present.[21] The architectural complexity, confluence, and anastomosis between the nests are features that are particularly helpful in distinguishing carcinoma from von Brunn nests or other benign conditions. Proliferative von Brunn nests extend to a uniform level within the lamina propria creating a sharp, linear border at the base that contrasts with the irregular, infiltrative base of nested carcinoma. In the ureter and renal pelvis, von

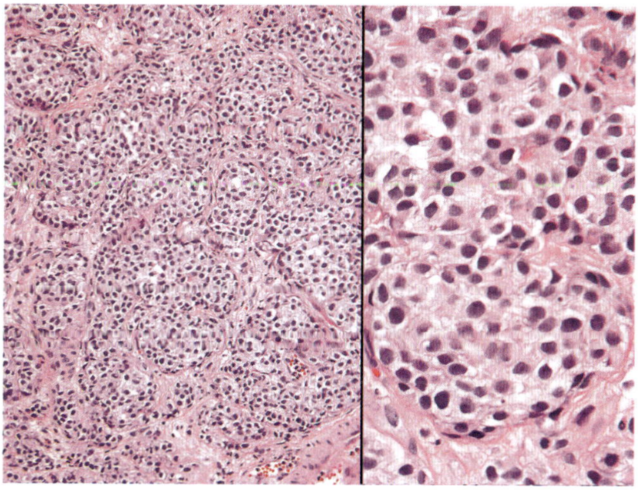

FIGURE 6.9 Nested variant of urothelial carcinoma with crowded almost back-to-back proliferation of small nests (higher magnification [*right*]).

Brunn nests tend to be smaller and more crowded than in the bladder, closely mimicking nested carcinoma (Figs. 1.17 and 1.18). However, von Brunn nests in these sites still have a lobular or linear arrangement with a sharp border at the base. Also, nested variant of urothelial carcinoma is exceedingly rare in the ureter and renal pelvis, and a diagnosis of nested carcinoma at these sites should be made with great caution on biopsy and only in the presence of a cystoscopic filling defect or an obstructive mass lesion. In contrast to nested carcinoma of the urinary bladder, nested carcinoma in the upper urothelial tract is (1) more frequently associated with an overlying papillary urothelial carcinoma, (2) more commonly has a large nested pattern, and (3) appears to behave less aggressively.[22]

In the deeper portion of nested variant of urothelial carcinoma, the neoplasm usually shows greater cytological atypia and an irregular infiltrative pattern. These tumors are frequently muscle invasive and, despite their innocuous histology, are paradoxically associated with aggressive clinical outcome including metastasis and death. Even with therapy, 70% of patients with adequate follow-up died within 4-40 months of diagnosis.[11-14,17-19] Nested carcinomas tend to present as locally advanced tumors; however, stage for stage their prognosis is similar to urothelial tumors of similar stage.[21] For this reason, we believe that a bladder cancer with only pure to predominant histology where the deceptively bland histology raised other differential diagnostic considerations should be reported as nested carcinoma. If there is a conspicuous and obvious component of high-grade invasive urothelial carcinoma, we do not believe that the diagnosis of nested carcinoma should be made. Invasion of the muscularis propria, despite the bland nuclear features, is diagnostic of carcinoma and is the most definitive distinguishing feature. Unfortunately, in some superficial biopsies or those complicated by extensive cautery artifact, it may be difficult to categorize lesions as unequivocally benign or malignant. In such cases, it is important to correlate the microscopic findings with the clinical impression of the urologist, as the presence of a mass lesion would indicate the need for additional sampling to ascertain for the presence of a more aggressive lesion.

Another differential diagnostic consideration is nephrogenic adenoma (metaplasia) with a more solid appearance.[12] The problem is compounded when the nephrogenic adenoma has an "infiltrative" growth at the base. The marked variation or occasional large nests, nuclear atypia in deeper aspects, stromal reaction, and muscularis propria invasion argue for a nested carcinoma diagnosis. Nephrogenic adenoma may show other coexisting patterns (tubules, papillary, signet ring, cystic) and often contains stroma that is edematous and inflamed. Adding to the diagnostic conundrum is the positivity for PAX8 in high percentage of nephrogenic adenoma and ~50% of the nested subtype of bladder cancer.[23] Posttreatment pseudocarcinomatous hyperplasia (Chapter 10) is an important mimic in which squamoid epithelial nests in lamina propria have a jagged irregular appearance, simulating invasion. Several other tumors primarily or secondarily involving the urinary bladder may have a nested pattern including paraganglioma, carcinoid tumor, prostatic adenocarcinoma, melanoma, and alveolar soft part sarcoma.[24] In this differential diagnostic context, once the diagnosis of neoplasia is made, the issue is the distinction of urothelial vs nonurothelial nature of the different nested tumors and their distinction from one another by using an appropriately constructed immunohistochemical panel. Immunohistochemical studies indicate that the nested variant shares many characteristics with invasive urothelial carcinoma including positivity for GATA3, S100P, uroplakin 2, and cytokeratins 7 and 20 and for p63 and high molecular weight cytokeratin (HMWCK).[25-30] The nested variant shows loss or absence of immunoreactivity for cyclin-dependent kinase inhibitors p21 and p27 and positivity for tumor suppressor gene *p53*, which have been associated with poor prognosis in conventional urothelial carcinoma, although these tests are not in routine clinical use.[26] There have been studies supporting MIB-1 as a useful marker in the distinction from benign proliferative lesions, although it must be noted that some cases of nested variant may have low MIB-1 proliferation index and some proliferative lesions may have higher rates.[26,31] This variability and range of immunostaining for MIB-1 has precluded us from using p53 or MIB-1 immunohistochemistry as a diagnostic adjunct for such cases. FISH studies in paraffin-embedded tissues may be helpful to distinguish nested carcinoma from von Brunn nests.[32] although this testing is also not readily available. Identification of *TERT* promoter mutation (suggesting malignant process) can help in difficult TURBT cases.[1] Molecularly, the nested subtype of bladder cancer correlates with the luminal subtype in the 6-tier molecular classification (Chapter 5) and have low frequency of FGFR mutations.[15,33]

Large Nested Variant of Urothelial Carcinoma

Urothelial carcinomas may occasionally present with a large nested morphology that may simulate an inverted urothelial tumor or when present in fragmented transurethral resection fragments pose considerable challenges in terms of recognition of invasion. The tumors are composed of broad nests of tumor with bland cytological features that are randomly and haphazardly arranged and are present deep in the bladder wall, including between muscle bundles of muscularis propria (Fig. 6.10). Upon closer inspection, a slightly greater degree of nuclear atypia is invariably present (helpful if the differential is with von Brunn nests with atypia). While evaluating for invasion vs inverted or verrucous carcinoma–like growth, the presence of tumor between muscularis propria is virtually diagnostic of muscle-invasive carcinoma. Except for urachal rests and the intramural segment of the ureter, benign urothelial proliferations or lesions do not involve the muscularis propria. Desmoplasia, while unusual, may be present in large nested urothelial carcinomas and is of further value in confirming invasion when present. In contrast to the small nested pattern, a

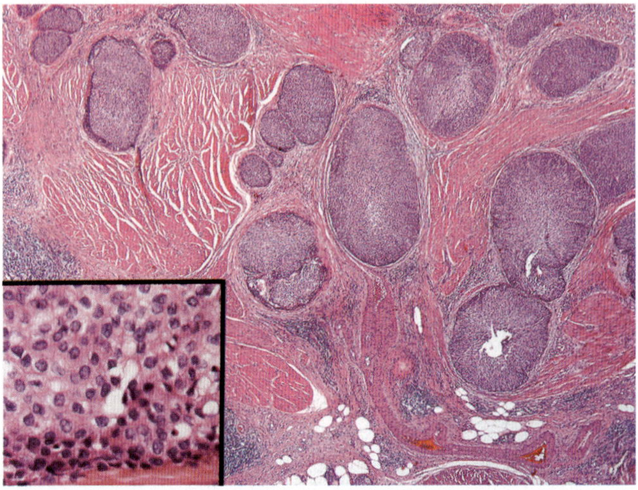

FIGURE 6.10 Large nested urothelial carcinoma with irregular large nests of urothelium invading the muscularis propria associated with moderate stromal response. *Inset* shows very bland cytology.

surface urothelial component may be recognized in some of these cases. Seventy percent of patients present with muscle invasive tumors, and 58% have extravesical disease or nodal involvement. One-fifth of patients recur or metastasize, and 24% died of disease.[34,35]

Urothelial Carcinoma With Small Tubules

Some urothelial carcinomas may have a prominent component of small-sized to medium-sized, round to elongated tubules that may be misdiagnosed as nephrogenic adenoma (metaplasia), cystitis glandularis, or müllerianosis[14] (Figs. 6.11-6.16). The tubules, however, are lined by urothelial cells in contrast to the cuboidal, columnar, or occasionally flattened cells that line the tubules of nephrogenic adenoma. The small caliber of tubules and random infiltrative pattern contrast with the overall organized arrangement of cystitis cystica or glandularis. Transition to areas of nested subtype is common. The cytological features are invariably low grade, but the recognition of carcinoma is based on diffusely infiltrative architecture, considerable variation of tubular shape with haphazard organization, and the frequent presence of muscle invasion. The biologic significance of this pattern is uncertain, but some of these cases occur in conjunction with the nested pattern and may result in an aggressive behavior. The differential diagnosis with an extension of a prostatic carcinoma is often also a consideration but easily handled by immunohistochemistry for prostate-specific and urothelial markers.[36] Like the nested variant, the chief reason for awareness of this morphologic variant of urothelial carcinoma is not to mistake it in superficial biopsies as a benign glandular proliferative les ion.[5,11,18,19,23,25,26,37]

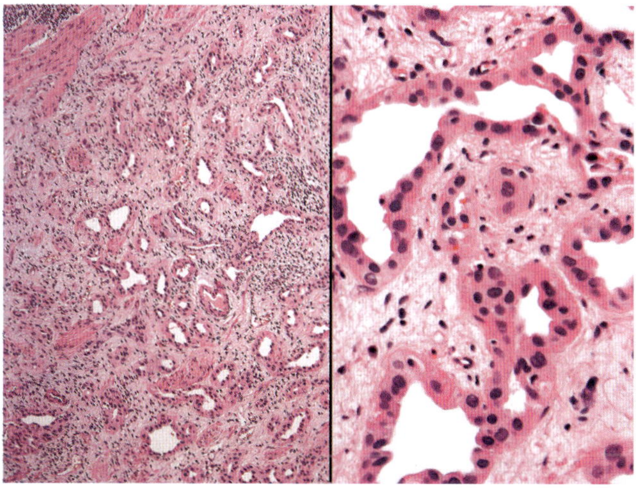

FIGURE 6.11 Tubular variant of urothelial carcinoma invading muscularis propria (higher magnification [*right*]).

Microcystic Urothelial Carcinoma

This is yet another deceptively benign form of urothelial carcinoma and is exemplified by the formation of numerous microcysts, which may lead to the misdiagnosis of cystitis cystica upon superficial examination or in limited biopsy specimens[38-40] (Figs. 6.17 and 6.18). The pattern is characterized by prominent widespread cystic change of variable size within nests of urothelial carcinoma or within urothelial carcinoma with glandular differentiation. The cysts are round to oval and 1-2 mm in size and contain secretions that may be targetoid. The cyst lining is most commonly

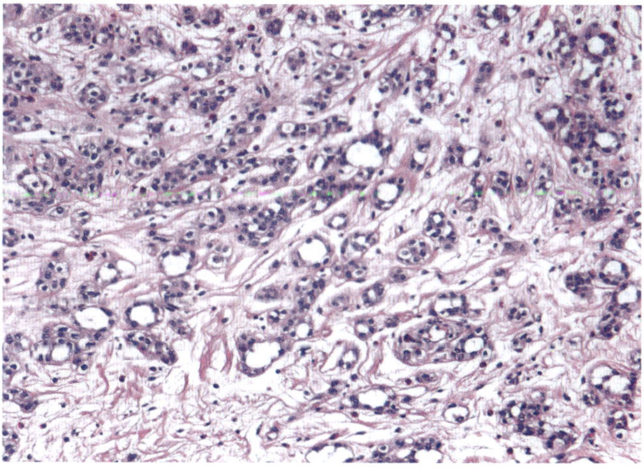

FIGURE 6.12 **Urothelial carcinoma with small tubules.** This pattern may accompany the nested variant.

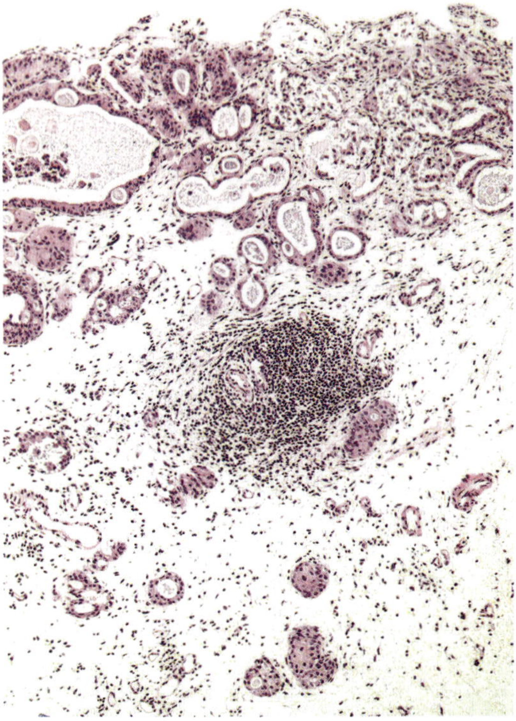

FIGURE 6.13 **Nested variant of urothelial carcinoma with tubule formation.** Note irregular proliferation of nests and tubules in inflamed, edematous stroma.

urothelial and is usually focally glandular (columnar); larger cysts may possess a flattened epithelium or a denuded lining. Cytological blandness is present by definition, and the most critical feature in distinguishing this carcinoma type from benign conditions is the variation, often dramatic, in

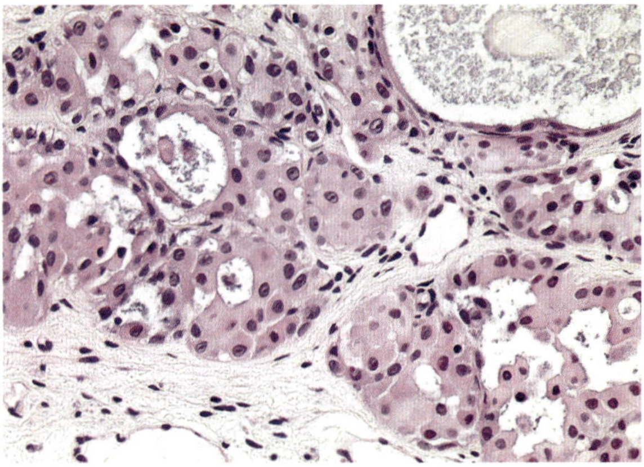

FIGURE 6.14 **Nested variant of urothelial carcinoma with moderate atypia (higher magnification of Fig. 6.13).** Although the cytologic features appear "low grade" on low power, this high-power illustration shows diagnostic features of malignancy.

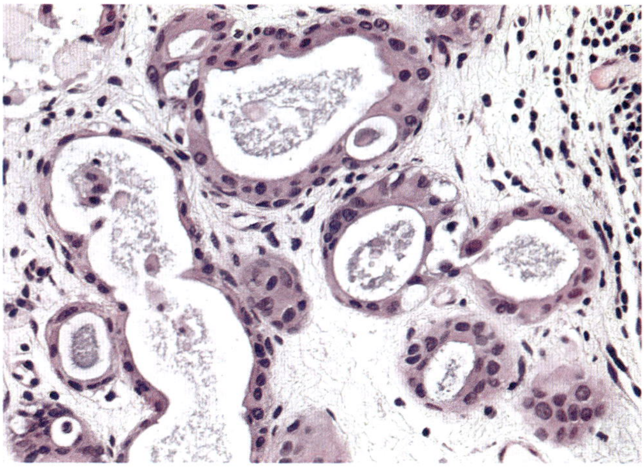

FIGURE 6.15 Nested variant of urothelial carcinoma with tubule formation (higher magnification of Fig. 6.13).

size and shape of the epithelial formations and the relatively haphazard infiltrative growth into the wall of the urinary bladder. There is no striking biologic significance associated with this pattern, except that it represents a potentially serious diagnostic pitfall, particularly in limited samples.[38,40,41] Once again, the nested, small tubule, and microcystic subtypes may coexist in the same lesion.[14] The chief differential diagnostic considerations are from cystitis cystica et glandularis and von Brunn nests, which overall tend to have a very organized appearance and lack the overt size variation that typifies microcystic carcinoma.[38-40,42] Studies have reported positivity for

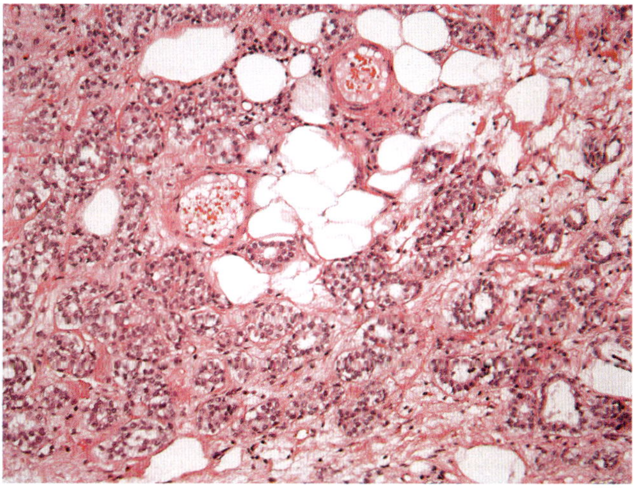

FIGURE 6.16 Nested variant of urothelial carcinoma with tubule formation invading adipose tissue.

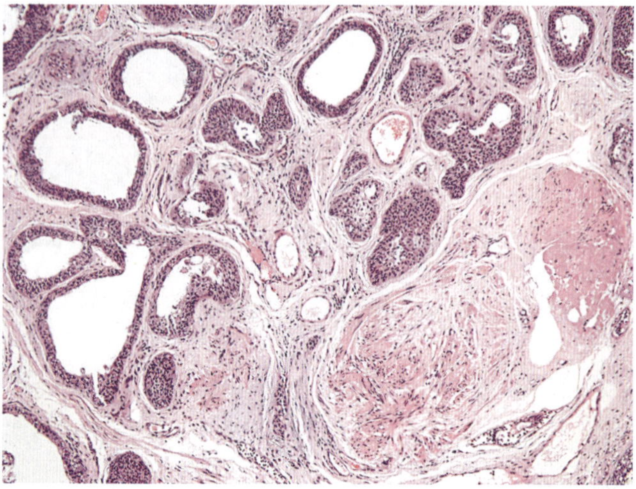

FIGURE 6.17 Microcystic urothelial carcinoma.

GATA3, CK20, CK7, S100P, p63, and HMWCK in these tumors.[29,41] Identification of *TERT* promoter mutation (suggesting malignancy) has been employed in difficult TURBT cases when the differential includes benign conditions.[43] The outcome of microcystic urothelial carcinoma is like conventional urothelial carcinoma of similar stage.[43]

INVERTED PAPILLOMA–LIKE GROWTH PATTERN OF UROTHELIAL CARCINOMA

This form of urothelial carcinoma is associated with two diagnostic concerns: (1) distinction from inverted papilloma (see Chapter 4) and (2)

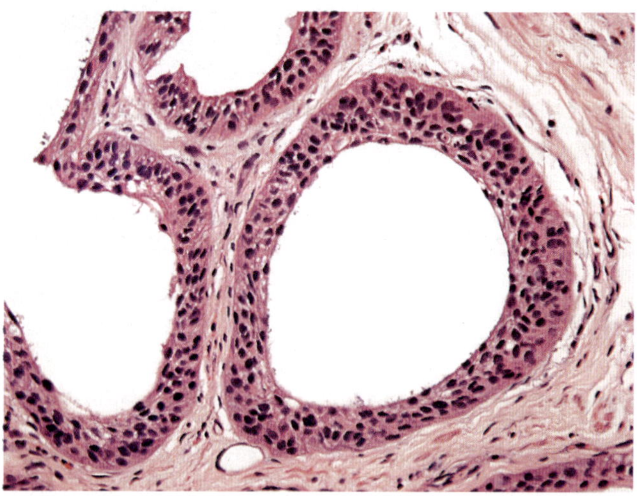

FIGURE 6.18 Microcystic urothelial carcinoma (higher magnification of Fig. 6.17).

difficulty in assessing invasion (see Chapter 5).[44,45] Distinction from the inverted papilloma requires attention to the architectural and cytologic features of the lesion. Urothelial carcinomas with inverted growth usually have thicker columns, with irregularity in width of the columns or transition of cords and columns into large rounded nests. The characteristic orderly maturation, spindling, and peripheral palisading seen in inverted papilloma are generally absent or inconspicuous in urothelial carcinomas with inverted growth. The amount of stroma between the epithelial columns and cords can be quite variable from area to area. Unequivocal stromal invasion into the lamina propria or muscularis propria rules out the diagnosis of inverted papilloma, as does the presence of appreciable exophytic papillary architecture. Furthermore, cytological atypia is an important feature for the diagnosis of carcinoma; thus, carcinomas with inverted growth, like their exophytic counterparts, may be classified as low grade or high grade. Inverted urothelial carcinoma may or may not be associated with destructive invasion (see Chapter 5 for criteria for invasion). The distinction of inverted papilloma vs carcinoma is usually based on routine light microscopic evaluation. However, a study has investigated and proposed a role for ancillary techniques including immunohistochemistry (p53, Ki-67, CK20 all show statistically significant higher expression in carcinomas as compared to urothelial papillomas) and UroVysion FISH studies (chromosomal abnormalities absent in urothelial papilloma and present in urothelial carcinoma).[46] These tests are currently not recommended for clinical use until further studies validate the results. Once invasive urothelial carcinoma is recognized (and inverted papilloma or noninvasive carcinoma is ruled out), this subtype may not be separately diagnosed in the pathology report as it is merely a descriptive category without prognostic significance meant only to draw awareness to noninvasive mimics. Identification of *TERT* promoter mutation (to support malignancy) has been advocated in difficult TURBT cases in the literature, although we do not resort to this testing in our practice.[43]

MICROPAPILLARY SUBTYPE OF UROTHELIAL CARCINOMA

This histologic subtype of urothelial carcinoma has a micropapillary architecture that is reminiscent of the papillary configuration seen in ovarian papillary serous tumors.[47-51] This rare histologic subtype comprises 0.6%-1% of urothelial carcinomas and shows a definite male predominance (male-to-female ratio 5:1) that is higher than in conventional urothelial carcinoma (3:1). In a recent Surveillance, Epidemiology and End Results (SEER) registry (2001-2016) study of 210 491 patients of all stages, 518 (0.2%) harbored micropapillary histology.[52] More than 95% of these tumors are muscle invasive at the time of presentation. Histologically, the micropapillary component of these tumors may be encountered in (1) the noninvasive component, (2) the invasive component, and (3) metastasis. This

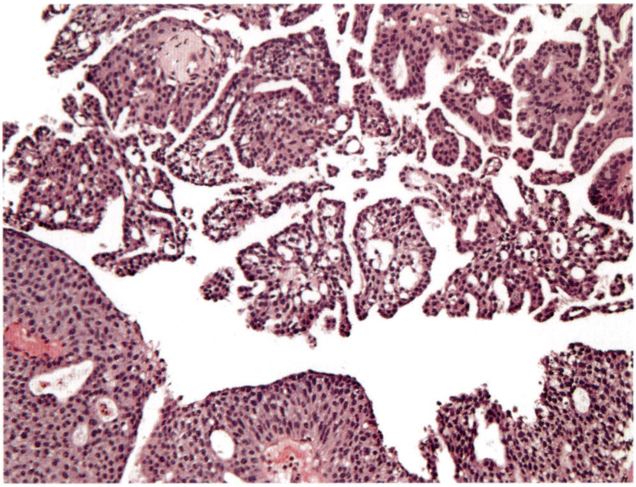

FIGURE 6.19 Noninvasive urothelial carcinoma with micropapillary features (*top*) compared to usual papillary urothelial carcinoma (*bottom*).

pattern may be focal, extensive (>90%), or exclusive. Urothelial carcinoma *in situ* (urothelial CIS) is demonstrable in >50% of the cases, and concurrent glandular differentiation is known to occur. Six histologic features of the micropapillary component are noteworthy. First, micropapillary carcinoma has two distinct patterns. On the surface, it forms slender, delicate filiform processes, rarely with a fibrovascular core (Figs. 6.19-6.22, eFigs. 6.19-6.22). When cut in cross sections, these papillae appear as glomeruloid bodies, sometimes with reversed polarity or palisading of cells. When micropapillary features are only present in the noninvasive component, the tumor should not be called micropapillary carcinoma. Cases described as urothelial carcinoma with villoglandular features (endometrioid carcinoma or enteric carcinoma–like appearance of urothelial carcinoma cells) frequently have micropapillary features in the noninvasive component.[53,54]

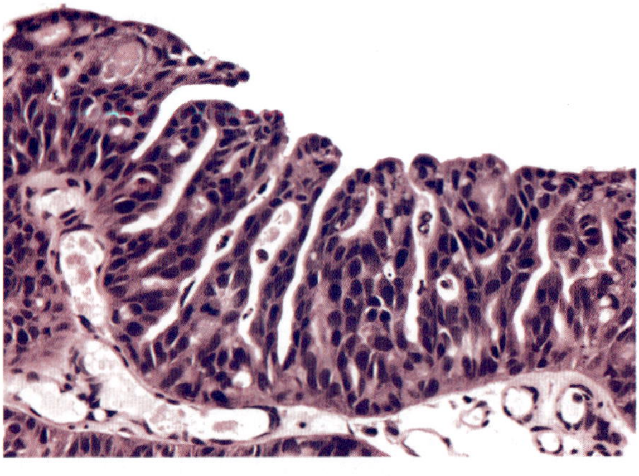

FIGURE 6.20 Urothelial CIS with micropapillary features.

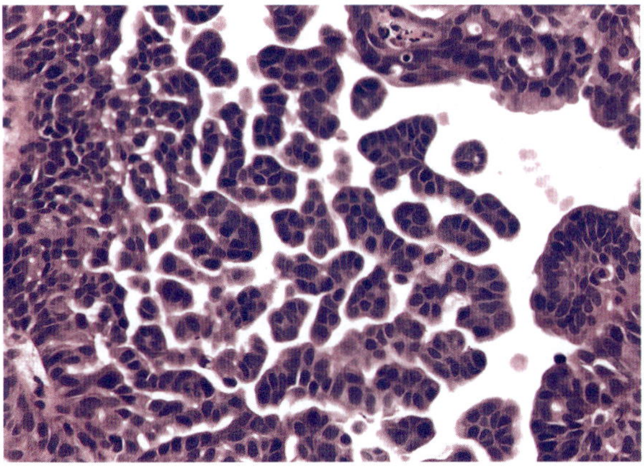

FIGURE 6.21 Noninvasive urothelial carcinoma with micropapillary features.

Alternatively, they could be designated as either "CIS with micropapillary features" or "high-grade noninvasive papillary urothelial carcinoma with micropapillary features." When diagnosing these noninvasive subtype morphologies in the absence of invasive carcinoma, we specifically add in the report: "There is no invasive micropapillary urothelial carcinoma" to clarify the diagnosis and to prevent overtreatment. In the invasive component and in all metastatic sites, the tumor cells are arranged in small tight nests or balls (Figs. 6.23-6.28, eFigs. 6.23-6.36); the absence of vascular cores allows for the recognition of micropapillae. Second, the presence of epithelial ring forms tumor cells resulting from intracytoplasmic vacuolation. Third, psammoma bodies, a feature of ovarian papillary serous neoplasia, are exquisitely rare in micropapillary urothelial carcinoma. Fourth, the tumor cells in the invasive and metastatic components are aggregated in lacunae, which mimic vascular invasion. This feature is intriguing and extremely characteristic of invasive micropapillary carcinoma. The presence of multiple nests within the same lacunar space is very helpful to

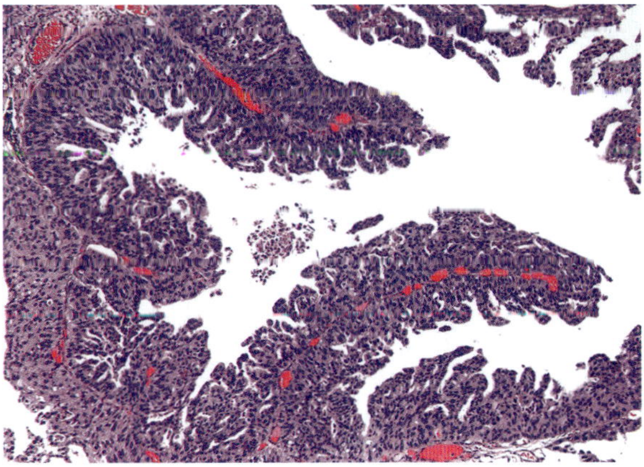

FIGURE 6.22 Noninvasive urothelial carcinoma with micropapillary features.

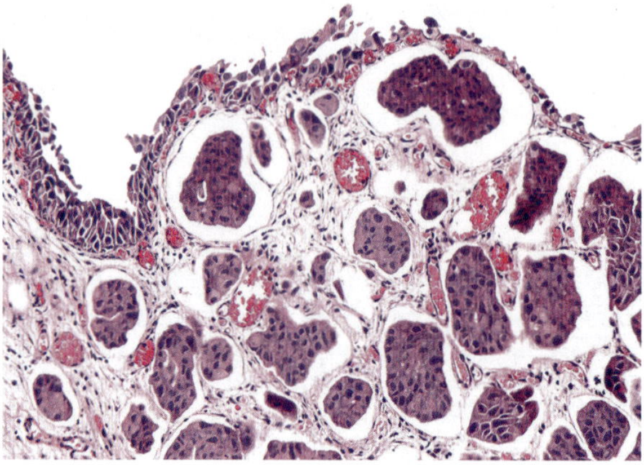

FIGURE 6.23 **Invasive micropapillary carcinoma beneath urothelium, mimicking vascular invasion.** There are numerous blood vessels that are uninvolved in-between invasive carcinoma.

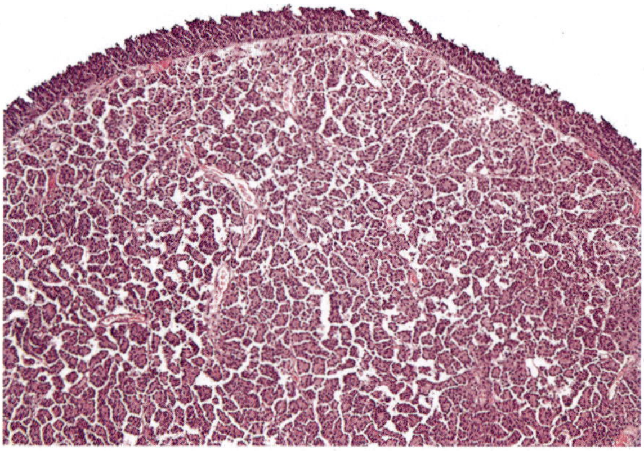

FIGURE 6.24 **Invasive micropapillary carcinoma beneath urothelium.**

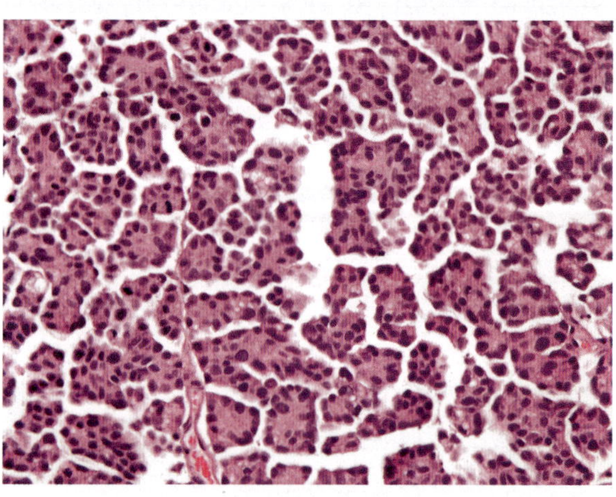

FIGURE 6.25 **Invasive micropapillary urothelial carcinoma (higher magnification of Fig. 6.24).**

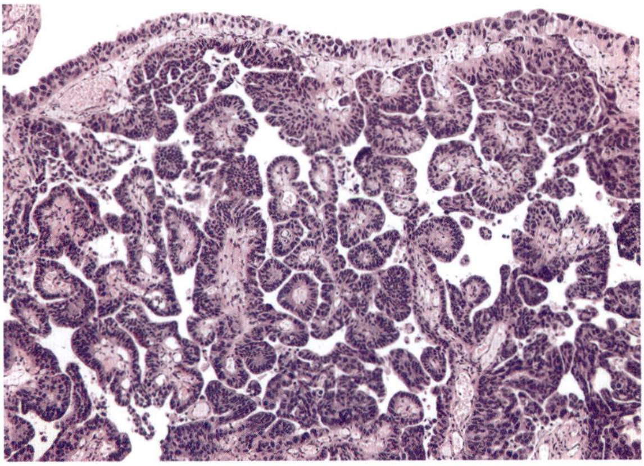

FIGURE 6.26 Invasive micropapillary urothelial carcinoma composed of thin cords lacking fibrovascular stalks admixed with conventional papillary urothelial carcinoma.

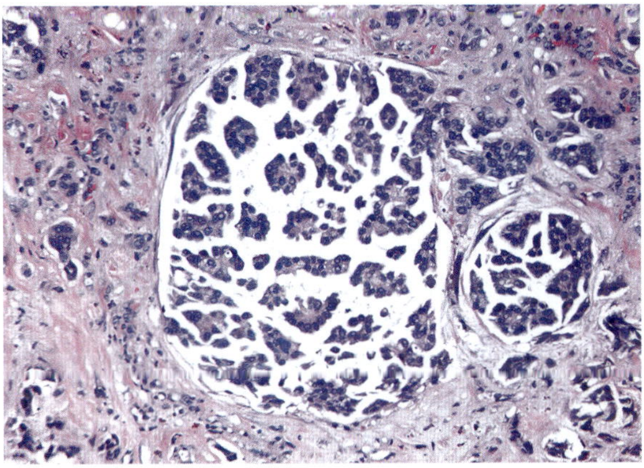

FIGURE 6.27 Invasive micropapillary urothelial carcinoma with adjacent usual invasive urothelial carcinoma.

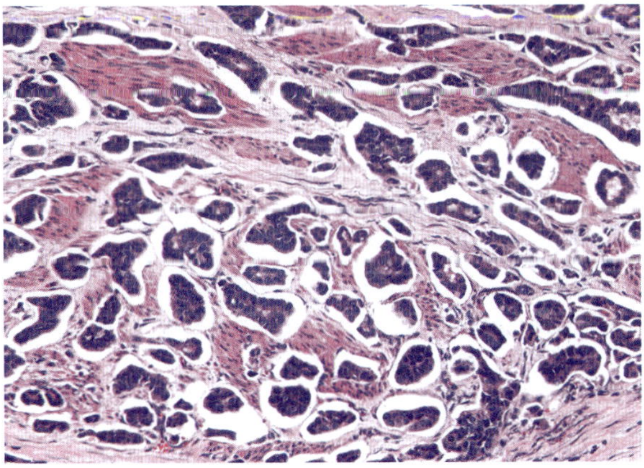

FIGURE 6.28 Invasive micropapillary urothelial carcinoma in muscularis propria.

distinguish this pattern from retraction artifact around invasive carcinoma, which may be quite prominent in some usual or conventional urothelial carcinomas. The spaces may be lined focally by flattened spindled cells or may be devoid of any lining. In most instances, there is no host response to the tumor cells that merely seem to reside in hollow spaces at various random intervals within the tumor.[50] This pattern of lacunae containing neoplastic cells is also seen in the metastatic sites. Awareness that lacunae of micropapillary urothelial carcinoma may mimic vascular invasion is important so that one does not overdiagnose the presence of vascular invasion. Fifth, micropapillary carcinoma always demonstrates a high nuclear grade (high grade by WHO/ISUP classification), although some areas within a neoplasm may parallel low-grade urothelial carcinoma. Sixth, most reported cases with micropapillary carcinoma show at least focal unequivocal vascular invasion. Like urothelial carcinomas, the tumors are often positive for CK7, CK20, uroplakin 2, GATA3, S100P, p63, and HMWCK.[28,29,55] Leu-M1, CEA, and Ca antigen 125 may be focally positive, in keeping with glandular differentiation that may be concurrent. While most micropapillary urothelial carcinomas are muscle invasive at presentation, a small subset of urothelial carcinoma with micropapillary features may be only noninvasive[56] or invasive limited to the lamina propria.[57] Noninvasive urothelial carcinoma with micropapillary features may also be associated with urothelial CIS (conventional flat histology) or invasive micropapillary carcinoma (see Chapter 2).

- There are several important reasons for recognizing the micropapillary variant of urothelial carcinoma: These tumors are high grade and high stage and are almost always associated with vascular invasion. Recent studies have shown that the percentage of micropapillary histology identified in transurethral resection specimens predicts stage- and disease-specific survival, or both[58-60] and in a recent large study, as little as 10% of micropapillary component was deemed to be significant and recommended to be reported.[58] Noninvasive urothelial carcinoma with micropapillary features needs to be distinguished from invasive micropapillary carcinoma, as the former is not associated with an adverse prognosis.
- Micropapillary carcinoma has a higher DNA index than conventional urothelial carcinoma (limited cases examined),[50] and because metastatic sites of tumors with micropapillary histology are predominantly composed of micropapillary carcinoma, it is likely that this unique configuration of urothelial carcinoma connotes a more aggressive clone of neoplastic cells. The presence of micropapillary histology in metastatic sites forces one to consider the possibility of urothelial carcinoma, especially if the micropapillary configuration is encountered in the peritoneum, abdominal lymph nodes, or mesentery of a male patient with an unknown primary or in a female patient with no apparent abnormality of the gynecologic tract.[48-51] One of the authors

(MBA) has seen two cases presenting in supraclavicular lymph nodes of male patients.

- The high association of micropapillary carcinoma with muscle-invasive disease should make the pathologist look diligently for muscle invasion if it is not readily apparent. If the biopsy is superficial and lacks muscularis propria, a second biopsy should be considered. If the biopsy is superficial and lacks muscularis propria, there should be a suggestion for a rebiopsy and reevaluation for staging. There are recent data that suggest that for micropapillary carcinomas presenting as early-stage disease, there is limited response to immunotherapy such that one leading group has advocated for early cystectomy for pTa and pT1 tumors with micropapillary histology,[61,62] although this recommendation remains controversial since it has not been substantiated in other studies.[57,63,64] Documentation of metastatic disease prior to cystectomy has also led to advocating for neoadjuvant chemotherapy in these cases. Other groups have argued the need for an aggressive approach in cases with limited micropapillary component, absence of concurrent CIS, and lack of muscularis propria invasion.[57,59] The prognosis for invasive micropapillary carcinoma in general is uniformly unfavorable due to high local invasiveness, presentation with high-stage disease, and lymph node metastasis; the 5- and 10-year survival rate in the largest study was 51% and 24%, respectively.[65] However, this poor prognosis is similar to that which is reported in high-grade, high-stage urothelial carcinoma of the usual type as well as pure adenocarcinomas and small cell carcinomas of the urinary bladder.[66-68]
- Promising for this disease due to the high proclivity for metastatic disease is the recent documentation of high prevalence of *ERBB2*, the Her-2 oncogene, which may be amplified or mutated providing a potential therapeutic target. *ERBB2* abnormalities are not restricted to the micropapillary variant and may be seen in typical invasive urothelial carcinomas.[69,70]

Invasive urothelial carcinoma of the usual type may demonstrate retraction artifact, which is usually focal and in more superficial areas of invasion; the mere presence of retraction is not diagnostic of micropapillary urothelial carcinoma component. The presence of multiple nests of cells within the same retraction space with epithelial ring forms strongly favors micropapillary carcinoma histology. The main differential diagnosis in women is with a metastatic papillary serous carcinoma, especially if the tumor is originally discovered in the peritoneum, abdominal lymph nodes, and mesentery or as a carcinoma of unknown origin. Other sites of carcinomas with micropapillary histology are the lung and breast, and rarely the pancreas and salivary glands. Clinical/radiographic correlation is usually required, but the possibility of a bladder primary may be suggested if there is no obvious primary tumor at another anatomic site. Identification of an admixed urothelial carcinoma of more typical morphology would be helpful.[55,60] In a bladder tumor, pure micropapillary histology may raise concern for a primary adenocarcinoma of the bladder. However, the micropapillary architecture is due to neoplastic urothelial cells in a micropapillary configuration and not true glandular differentiation, as also supported by immunohistochemistry (GATA3, and uroplakin 2 positivity).[29,30] In primary adenocarcinoma of the bladder, there is a greater variability of gland shape and size and range of differentiation in contrast to the typically uniform appearance of micropapillary component of urothelial carcinoma.[48-51,60,65,71-76] In a study of micropapillary carcinomas from the bladder, ovary, lung, and breast, the following immunohistochemical panel was recommended: CK20 and uroplakin 2 (positive in some the bladder), PAX8 or WT-1 (positive in the ovary), TTF-1 (positive in the lung), and mammaglobin (positive in the breast).[58] In terms of the 6-tier molecular classification (briefly outlined in Chapter 5), micropapillary urothelial carcinoma is of the luminal nonspecified subtype.[33]

LYMPHOEPITHELIOMALIKE CARCINOMA

Tumors with this histology are so termed because of their striking morphologic resemblance to the undifferentiated nasopharyngeal carcinoma or lymphoepithelioma[77] (Figs. 6.29-6.31, eFigs. 6.37-6.49). They have also been reported at multiple sites including the prostate, breast, cervix, skin, lung, thymus, stomach, and salivary glands.[77] The neoplastic cells are large and arranged in sheets, cords, or trabeculae with syncytia of cells containing vesicular nuclei, prominent nucleoli, and numerous mitoses.[77-81] Aggregates of tumor cells may be mistaken for plump endothelial cells. The *sine qua non* for the diagnosis of this histologic pattern of urothelial

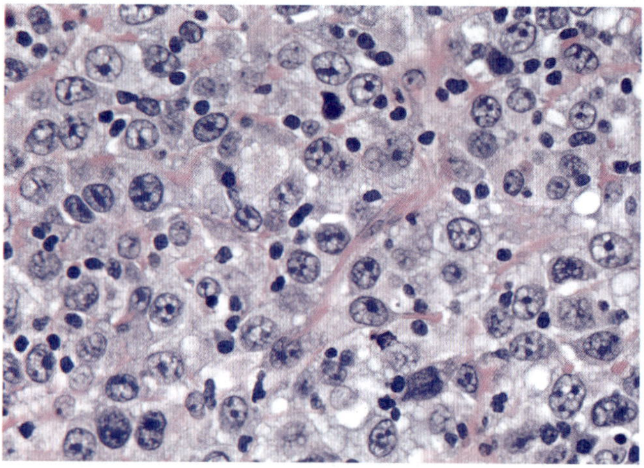

FIGURE 6.29 Lymphoepitheliomalike carcinoma.

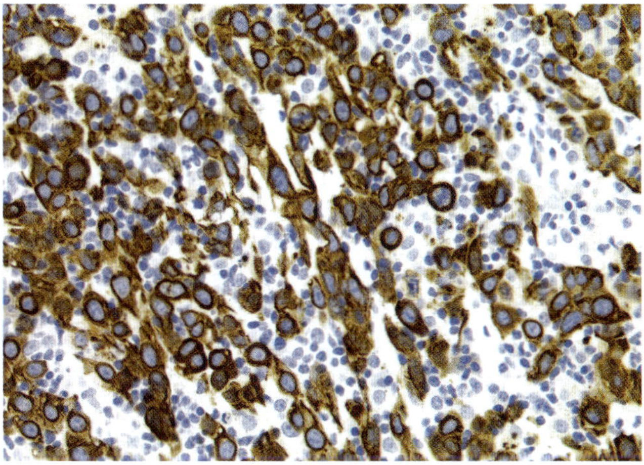

FIGURE 6.30 **Lymphoepitheliomalike carcinoma.** Keratin stain highlights epithelial tumor cells.

carcinoma is the presence of a prominent lymphoid infiltrate, although an admixture of other inflammatory cells including plasma cells and eosinophils is not uncommon. The relationship to EBV (by immunohistochemistry and *in situ* hybridization) has been well explored with no documented association.[81-83]

The tumors may occur in a pure form, or the lymphoepitheliomalike histology may be predominant or focal. CIS may be present elsewhere in the bladder. The tumor cells are positive for cytokeratin, CK7, p63, and HMWCK and are rarely positive for CK20; they variably express

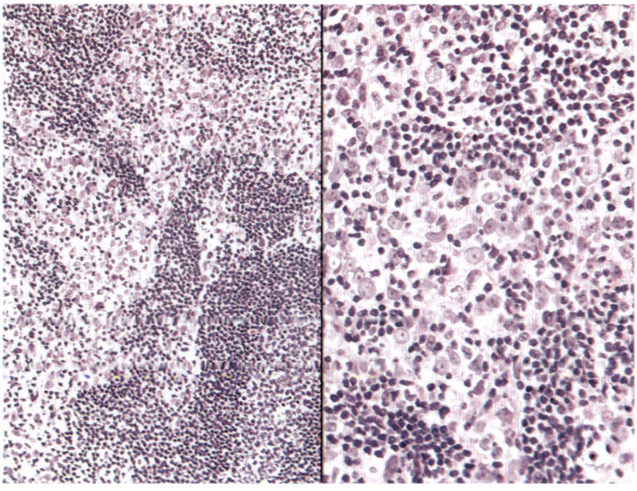

FIGURE 6.31 **Lymphoepitheliomalike carcinoma with nesting pattern.** Low power (***left***) and high power (***right***).

GATA3.[29] Relatively few series and cases of this subtype of urothelial carcinoma have been reported, but the aggregate data suggest that when these tumors occur in a pure form, they are more responsive to systemic chemotherapy, providing the potential to salvage bladder function.[77-80] It is unclear if this difference in response to systemic therapy remains with more modern chemotherapy. When mixed with conventional urothelial carcinoma, their outcome is similar to that for conventional urothelial carcinoma and depends on the stage of the associated conventional urothelial carcinoma. The differential diagnosis includes malignant lymphoma and, in limited and crushed biopsies, marked chronic cystitis.[84] High-grade urothelial carcinoma of the usual type should not be termed lymphoepitheliomalike merely because of a brisk inflammatory infiltrate. The syncytial arrangement and typical cytology are essential for the diagnosis of lymphoepitheliomalike carcinoma, which, as mentioned, in its purest form may be treated differently than the usual or conventional invasive carcinoma. A majority of reported tumors are muscle-invasive carcinomas (pT2 or higher), and when admixed with conventional urothelial carcinoma, their outcome is similar to that for conventional urothelial carcinoma and depends on the stage of the associated conventional urothelial carcinoma. Some studies have shown that tumors with a predominant lymphoepitheliomalike histology have a more favorable prognosis compared to those with only a focal component of this histology. In a large series, cases treated with cystectomy had a 5-year actuarial survival rate of 59% (62% for pure and 57% for mixed); in comparison, the 5-year recurrence-free rate of usual muscle-invasive bladder cancer treated by cystectomy was similar and in the range of 65%-68%.[77,79-81,85] Tumors are enriched for PDL1 expression. These findings are consistent with the known sensitivity of LELC tumors to chemotherapy and support the potential of immune checkpoint inhibitors as a therapeutic option.[86,87] In terms of the 6-tier molecular classification (briefly outlined in Chapter 5), lymphoepitheliomalike urothelial carcinoma is of the basal squamous molecular type.[33]

SARCOMATOID CARCINOMA (CARCINOSARCOMA)

Although rare, sarcomatoid carcinoma is more common than primary sarcoma of the urinary bladder. By definition, this is a tumor showing both a malignant spindle cell component and a malignant epithelial component, although the latter may only be identifiable immunohistochemically[88-91] (Figs. 6.32-6.39, eFigs. 6.50-6.71). The spindle cell component is usually high grade with nondescript architecture (often resembling pleomorphic high-grade sarcoma). The sarcomatoid areas may merge with foci of overlying CIS or with invasive urothelial carcinoma, squamous cell carcinoma, adenocarcinoma, or small cell carcinoma. Heterologous differentiation (carcinosarcoma) may be in the form of rhabdomyosarcoma, osteosarcoma, angiosarcoma, chondrosarcoma, or liposarcoma. The prognostic

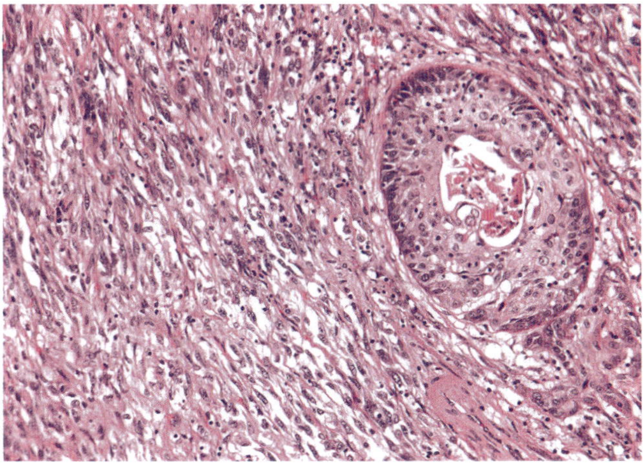

FIGURE 6.32 Sarcomatoid carcinoma with nests of squamous carcinoma surrounded by undifferentiated sarcomatoid component.

significance of heterologous differentiation is controversial, while some studies show no difference, in others the presence of one or more heterologous components has been suggested to impart a more adverse behavior.[92-95] Data reported to the SEER registry and analyzed for outcome strictly on the basis of ICD-O-3 histologic code showed that sarcomatoid carcinoma and carcinosarcoma patients did worse than high-grade urothelial carcinoma, and when separated, carcinosarcoma patients did worse than sarcomatoid carcinoma cases.[92] A potential well-known shortcoming of analyzing data from large publicly reported databases is that the

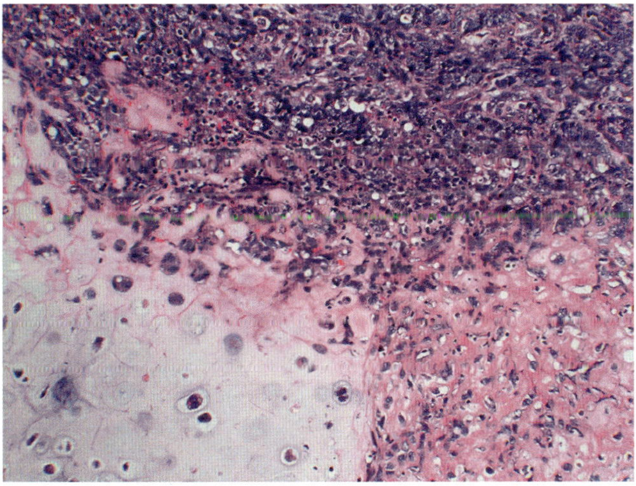

FIGURE 6.33 Sarcomatoid carcinoma (epithelial component not shown) with heterologous cartilaginous differentiation.

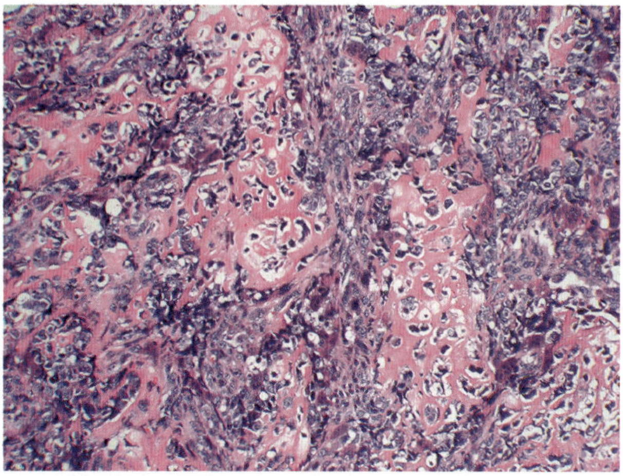

FIGURE 6.34 Sarcomatoid carcinoma (epithelial component not shown) with heterologous osteoblastic differentiation.

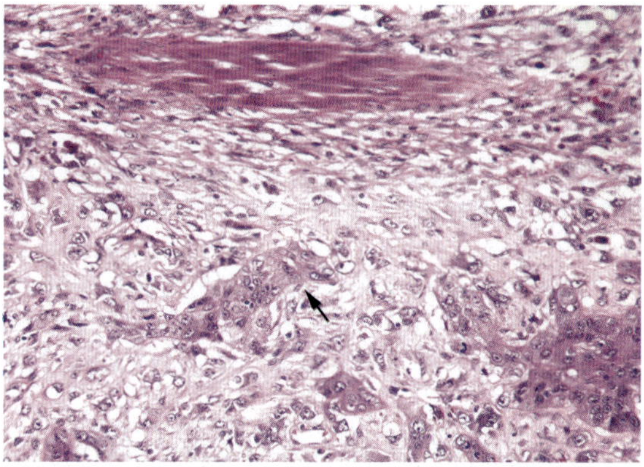

FIGURE 6.35 Sarcomatoid carcinoma showing focal nests of carcinoma (*arrow*).

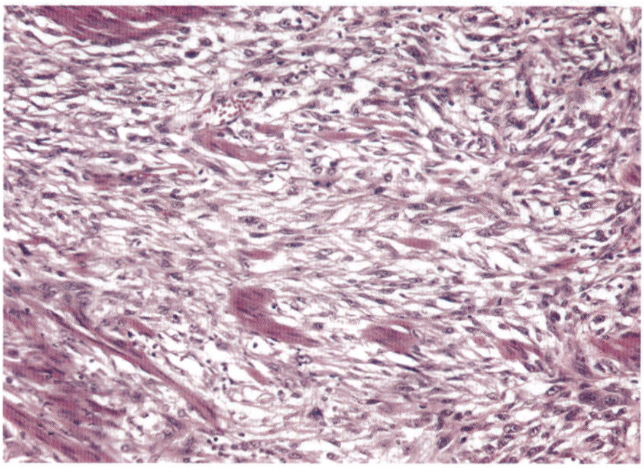

FIGURE 6.36 Sarcomatoid carcinoma (same case as in Fig. 6.35) mostly composed of undifferentiated malignant spindle cells. Tumor infiltrates muscularis propria.

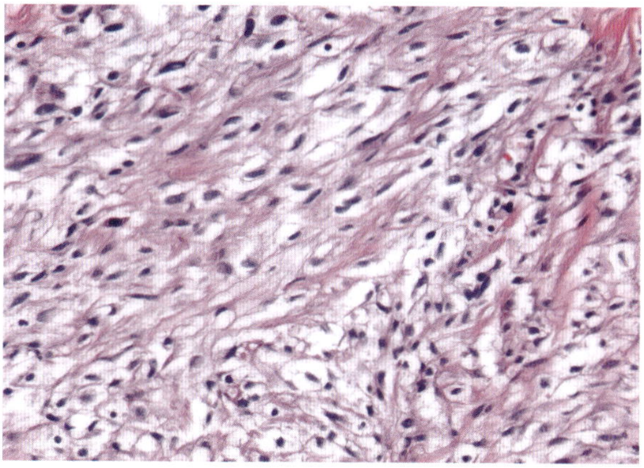

FIGURE 6.37 Sarcomatoid carcinoma (higher magnification of Fig. 6.35).

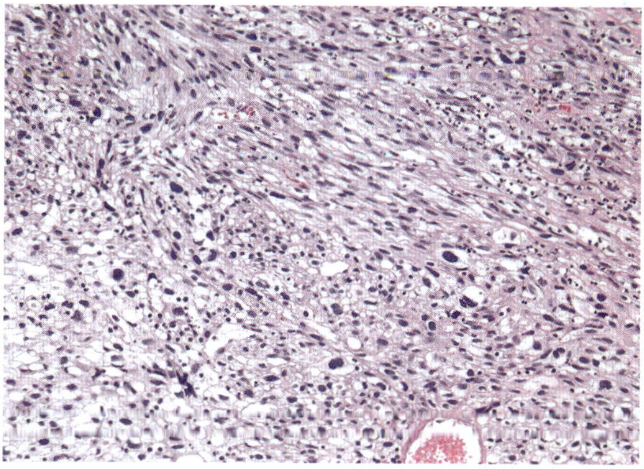

FIGURE 6.38 Sarcomatoid carcinoma composed entirely of sarcomatous-appearing cells.

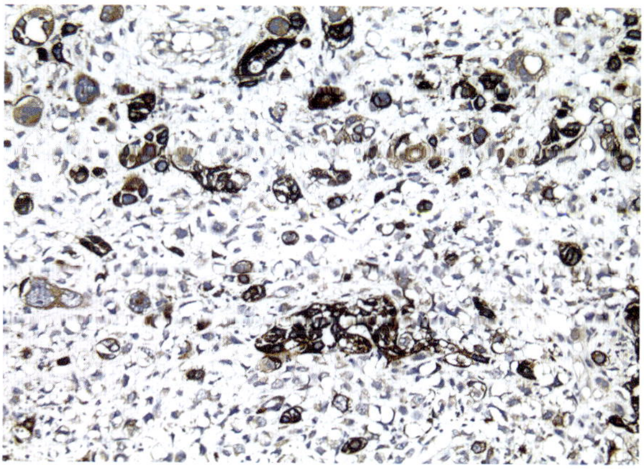

FIGURE 6.39 Sarcomatoid carcinoma (higher magnification of Fig. 6.38) with keratin positivity documenting epithelial differentiation.

cases are not centrally reviewed by a group of dedicated pathologists and differing criteria and nomenclature may be used by pathologists. It is still recommended by the WHO that sarcomatoid carcinoma is the preferred terminology for these lesions and that carcinosarcoma be used as a synonym rather than recognized as a distinct entity. Radiation and cyclophosphamide therapy are known risk factors.[96,97]

Grossly, many tumors present as polypoid masses. The sarcomatoid areas (obvious sarcomatoid overgrowth) may merge with foci of urothelial carcinoma, squamous cell carcinoma, adenocarcinoma, or small cell carcinoma and most commonly resemble a high-grade sarcoma, not otherwise specified high-grade sarcoma histology. In the absence of an obvious invasive urothelial carcinoma or other epithelial differentiation, the history of prior urothelial carcinoma, the coexistence of urothelial CIS, or strong cytokeratin immunoreactivity is helpful in making the diagnosis of sarcomatoid carcinoma over a primary sarcoma. The epithelial elements are consistently positive for cytokeratin, but the reactivity in the malignant spindle cell component varies. The spindle cell component is consistently positive for vimentin and may express specific markers corresponding to specific mesenchymal differentiation if present. The cytological atypia present in these lesions and the concurrent presence of neoplastic epithelial elements should exclude inflammatory myofibroblastic tumor (IMT)/pseudosarcomatous myofibroblastic proliferation.[98,99] The immunohistochemical profile of sarcomatoid carcinoma includes positivity for pancytokeratin, HMWCK, epithelial membrane antigen (EMA), CK5/6, and p63. Frequent (>80% cases) vimentin positivity in the epithelial cells and GATA positivity have been reported in the spindle cells along with p63, p40, CK5/6, or HMWCK.[88,91,100] Smooth muscle actin is only variably positive at best, and Alk-1 is negative (markers that are more frequently expressed in leiomyosarcoma and IMT, respectively).[101] Depending on the differential diagnostic setting when there is a pure spindle cell morphology, recently a panel of up to six markers has been recommended in spindle cell lesions of the bladder and includes pancytokeratin, p63, HMWCK (or cytokeratin 5/6), Alk-1, smooth muscle actin, and desmin.[93] In order to diagnose sarcomatoid carcinoma in a predominantly spindle cell tumor, at least one of the following must be identified: (1) epithelial differentiation on H&E; (2) expression of keratins, most often focal CK 34βE12 or CK5/6 in the sarcomatous component; or (3) GATA3 expression in the sarcomatous component.

A subset of sarcomatoid carcinomas have a markedly myxoid stroma that may result in some cases of sarcomatoid carcinoma ("myxoid and sclerosing sarcomatoid urothelial carcinoma") being diagnosed as IMTs.[89] The presence of a malignant epithelial component rules out the diagnosis of a primary sarcoma as well as IMT. Finally, sarcomatoid carcinoma should be distinguished from the rare carcinoma with metaplastic, benign-appearing bone or cartilage in the stroma or from carcinoma associated with an unusual degenerative yet atypical appearing stromal reaction (pseudosarcomatous stromal reaction) (see Chapter 11 on Mesenchymal Tumors).[102,103] Primary leiomyosarcoma and urothelial carcinoma with pseudoangiosarcomatous histology (see below) are also in the differential. In the former, a biphasic pattern is lacking, usually with evidence of a smooth muscle differentiation by histology. In the latter, there is potential for misinterpreting pseudoangiosarcomatous histology for heterologous differentiation. Almost all sarcomatoid carcinomas present at a high stage and have a poor prognosis.[88-91] There are no standardized clinical management paradigms for sarcomatoid carcinoma, and adjuvant therapy tends to vary from institution to institution and may be different from therapy for a primary sarcoma such as a leiomyosarcoma. Limited data have shown downstaging (pT0 at cystectomy) for almost half the patients in one center's experience.[61] An estimated 70% of patients die within 2 years of diagnosis.[88-92,103-106] Compared to patients with urothelial carcinomas alone, these patients are at a greater risk for death even after adjusting for stage at presentation.[88-92,102-107] The survival of patients with sarcomatoid urothelial carcinoma is particularly poor, with a reported 5-year cancer-specific survival of 28% and a median overall survival of 14 months.[108] Tumors are enriched for PDL1 expression and in terms of the 6-tier molecular classification (briefly outlined in Chapter 5); sarcomatoid urothelial carcinomas evolve from progression of the basal squamous molecular type with acquisition of *p53*, *RB1*, *PI3CA* gene mutations.[15]

SMALL CELL CARCINOMA

The gross features of this tumor are not characteristic, and tumors may appear sessile, nodular, ulcerated, polypoid, or infiltrative. They are, however, usually very large and arise from any region within the bladder, including in diverticula. Morphologically, this tumor is identical to undifferentiated small cell carcinoma of the lung but is more frequently admixed in ~40%-50% of the cases with an epithelial component of urothelial carcinoma including CIS, squamous cell carcinoma or adenocarcinoma, and rarely even a sarcomatoid component (Figs. 6.40-6.42, eFigs. 6.72-6.82). Molecular genetic evidence suggests a common clonal relationship for small cell carcinoma and coexistent urothelial carcinoma. The tumor usually has a patternless pattern of diffuse growth, though occasionally and focally, some nesting may be present. The cells have scant cytoplasm and consequently show nuclear crowding and molding. Nucleoli are inconspicuous, and the chromatin is finely stippled. Geographic necrosis, frequent mitoses, and frequent apoptotic bodies are indicative of its high proliferation rate. Tumors are positive for chromogranin A and synaptophysin (>60% of cases) and frequently show a dotlike positivity for pancytokeratin. TTF-1 may be positive in ~40% of the cases.[109] Insulinoma-associated protein 1 (INMS1) is a promising new marker with high percentage of positivity in small cell carcinoma.[15] The tumors are infrequently positive for GATA3, uroplakin 2, and CK20.[29,30,110,111] Comparative genomic hybridization

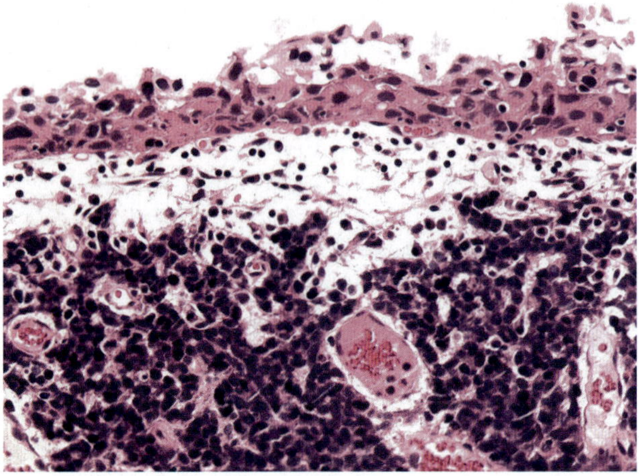

FIGURE 6.40 Small cell carcinoma with overlying squamous cell carcinoma *in situ*.

studies show frequent genomic alterations including deletions of 10q, 4q, 5q, and 13q and gain of 8p, 5p, 6p, and 13q.[112] Methylation studies show similar rates in pure small cell carcinoma and small cell carcinoma concurrent with urothelial carcinoma.[113] *TERT* promoter mutation is more commonly seen in small cell carcinoma of bladder origin than in those that arise at other sites.[114] In terms of the 6-tier molecular classification, lymphoepitheliomalike urothelial carcinoma is of the neuroendocrinelike molecular type.[32] Small cell neuroendocrine carcinoma has a very low rate of PD-L1 expression, making checkpoint immune therapy a less likely therapeutic option in these patients compared to typical urothelial carcinoma. The genetic landscape of small cell carcinoma is better understood in terms of

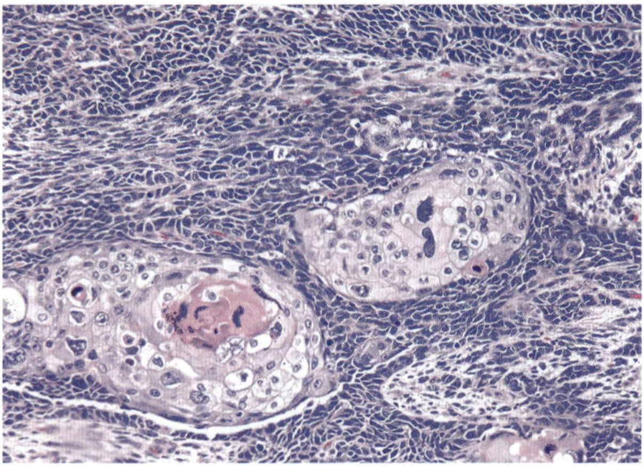

FIGURE 6.41 Small cell carcinoma and squamous cell carcinoma.

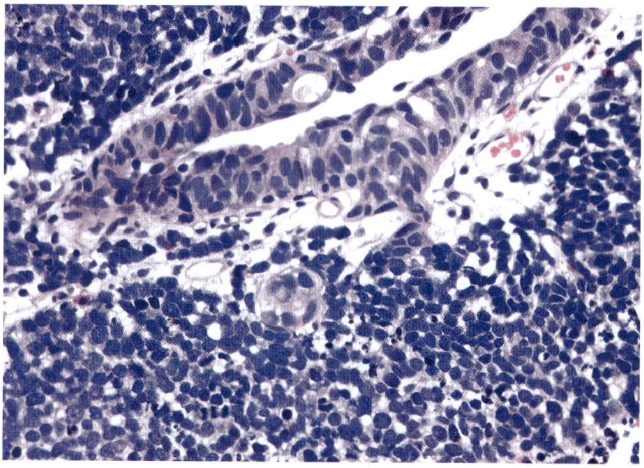

FIGURE 6.42 Small cell carcinoma with associated urothelial carcinoma.

driver mutations, markers for immunotherapy, stem cell modulation, and novel drug candidates; these remain investigational at this time.[115]

Small cell carcinoma may be mistaken for malignant lymphoma, poorly differentiated urothelial carcinoma with scant cytoplasm, and even inflammation in a crushed, cauterized, superficial, or scant specimen. Metastasis from the lung or extension from adjacent viscera must be ruled out by clinicopathologic correlation as immunohistochemistry offers limited assistance. TTF-1 may be expressed in small cell carcinomas of any anatomic site and does not indicate a lung origin, and PSA is usually negative in prostatic small cell carcinomas.[109,116] If the tumor is not felt to be a typical primary bladder neoplasm at presentation, attention to the morphology of the accompanying epithelial component such as prostatic or urothelial histology, if present, would be useful to determine the primary site. GATA3, p63, and HMWCK positivity favors a urothelial small cell carcinoma, and ERG positivity by FISH or IHC favors a prostatic origin, although these markers are not consistently expressed in these tumors. Another significant diagnostic pitfall is alveolar rhabdomyosarcoma, which may rarely involve the bladder and has a predilection to occur in adults. It may occur either in a pure form or as a component of heterologous differentiation in a sarcomatoid carcinoma. These tumors have significant overlap with small cell carcinoma as the classic "alveolar" morphology may not be appreciated and the tumor may present with an almost exclusive round cell primitive appearance. The tumors are positive for desmin, myogenin, and MyoD1 and negative for keratin. The morphologic overlap is compounded by synaptophysin immunoreactivity in alveolar rhabdomyosarcomas.[117]

The vast majority of patients (94%) with small cell carcinoma of the bladder present with muscle-invasive disease, and ~67% patients develop systemic metastases during the disease course. Metastatic sites include the lymph nodes, liver, bone, lung, and brain. An important reason for the accurate recognition of a small cell carcinoma component is that it is recognized as a systemic disease and apparently has response to newer chemotherapy protocols (cisplatin- and etoposide-based therapy), which, in combination with surgical resection, have shown encouraging results including reports of long-term survivors. It is difficult to compare outcome between different series as different therapeutic strategies, including surgery alone, neoadjuvant and adjuvant chemotherapy, radiation therapy, etc., have been variably employed.[118,119] The mean survival is 6-34.9 months, and the reported 5-year survival rate ranges from 8% to 40%; patients presenting with organ-confined disease have a more favorable survival.[82,109,116,118-128] Data from the National Cancer Database show a 3-year overall survival of 53% for patients with clinically localized disease treated with neoadjuvant chemotherapy followed by radical cystectomy.[129] In another large single institution experience, the 5-year disease-specific survival of patients undergoing cystectomy alone was 36% compared to 78% in those receiving chemotherapy, underscoring the importance of accurate histopathologic classification of small cell carcinoma.[130]

Other Neuroendocrine Tumors

The range of neuroendocrine tumors in the bladder includes well-differentiated neuroendocrine tumor (carcinoid), small cell carcinoma, large cell neuroendocrine carcinoma, and mixed patterns.[131] Neuroendocrine tumors outside of small cell carcinoma are extraordinarily rare.[132-137]

Tumors with the typical histology of well-differentiated neuroendocrine tumor are distinctly rare, and <20 cases have been reported.[135,138-141] They are discussed in Chapter 12. In the rare event that carcinoid morphology is seen in addition to a small cell carcinoma histology, the diagnosis of small cell carcinoma is made.

In contrast to small cell carcinoma, large cell neuroendocrine carcinomas have a more discernable architecture (nests, trabeculae, organoid, and palisaded) and have prominent nucleoli, and criteria for their pulmonary counterparts should be used in the bladder. Large cell neuroendocrine carcinomas of the bladder may be pure (rare) or admixed with components of urothelial, glandular, squamous, or small cell carcinoma. CK20 and TTF-1 positivity is reported in these tumors along with requisite expression of markers for neuroendocrine differentiation (synaptophysin, chromogranin, and CD56). It is important not to overcall a poorly differentiated urothelial carcinoma as large cell neuroendocrine carcinoma without comprehensive morphologic and immunohistochemical support. The outcome of large cell neuroendocrine carcinoma appears to be similar to small cell carcinoma with most reported cases having early metastases and a fatal outcome.[81,104,116,118-127,130-138,142-146] In a recent large single institutional study of 22 cases, most large cell neuroendocrine carcinomas of the bladder and upper tract expressed neuroendocrine markers including synaptophysin, chromogranin, CD56, TTF1, and INSM1. They were negative for common urothelial markers, including HMWCK, p40/p63, CK20, and had variable GATA3 staining. Patient survival was adversely associated with high cancer stage, and pure large cell neuroendocrine carcinomas showed worse survival than mixed neuroendocrine carcinomas. Compared with small cell carcinoma at similar stages, large cell neuroendocrine carcinoma had a worse prognosis only when patients developed metastatic disease.[147]

UROTHELIAL CARCINOMA WITH PSEUDOANGIOSARCOMATOUS FEATURES

In contrast to high-grade squamous cell carcinomas that occasionally show acantholysis, urothelial carcinomas may uncommonly have prominent acantholysis and discohesion within tumor nests resulting superficially in an appearance similar to a vasoformative tumor.[148] The pattern may raise consideration of sarcomatoid urothelial carcinoma with angiosarcomatous differentiation or, if prominent, an angiosarcoma of the bladder. In a series of seven cases, the percentage of pseudoangiosarcomatous features varied from 35% to 85% of the bladder cancer; in all cases, urothelial differentiation was confirmed by CK7 and CK20 and GATA3 immunohistochemistry in the acantholytic areas. Cases were associated with a high tumor stage at cystectomy, admixed with other aggressive carcinoma variant morphologies, and consequently associated with a poor outcome.[149]

UROTHELIAL CARCINOMA WITH UNUSUAL CYTOPLASMIC FEATURES

Plasmacytoid Urothelial Carcinoma

In the past few years, urothelial carcinomas with a striking resemblance to plasma cells have been described.[150-161] A series of 10 cases mimicking lobular carcinoma of the breast, the so-called discohesive variant, shares many features with the plasmacytoid variant, although the most distinctive feature of cases in this series was the arrangement of tumor cells in a single cell discohesive single cell file pattern.[162] Some experts consider that these tumors are in the spectrum of undifferentiated noncohesive carcinomas, which include nonmucinous carcinoma with signet ring cell and rhabdoid features as well as tumor cells that resemble infiltrating lobular carcinoma of the breast (Figs. 6.43 and 6.44, eFigs. 6.83-6.87). The neoplastic cells are usually discohesive and set in a loose, myxoid stroma. A plasmacytoid histology may be seen in a variety of bladder neoplasms including malignant lymphomas, plasmacytomas, malignant melanoma, metastatic carcinoma including lobular and gastric adenocarcinoma, paraganglioma, rhabdomyosarcoma, and urothelial carcinoma. The correct diagnosis may not always be difficult if adequate tissue exhibiting

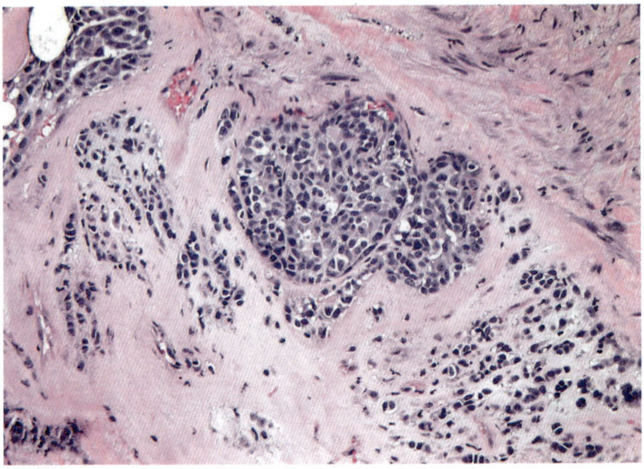

FIGURE 6.43 Plasmacytoid urothelial carcinoma.

more typical patterns diagnostic of a particular neoplasm is available for histologic examination. Plasmacytoid urothelial carcinoma cells overlap in their morphology with signet-ring carcinoma cells, but notably, they lack the extracellular mucin found in signet-ring adenocarcinomas. Small biopsies occasionally show only the plasmacytoid pattern and may closely mimic a plasmacytoma or lymphoma. Immunohistochemistry may be required in this setting, and demonstration of cytokeratin reactivity confirms the diagnosis of carcinoma. A broad panel including cytokeratin, leukocyte common antigen, and/or T- and B-cell markers and S100 protein may be necessary if the initial differential diagnosis is

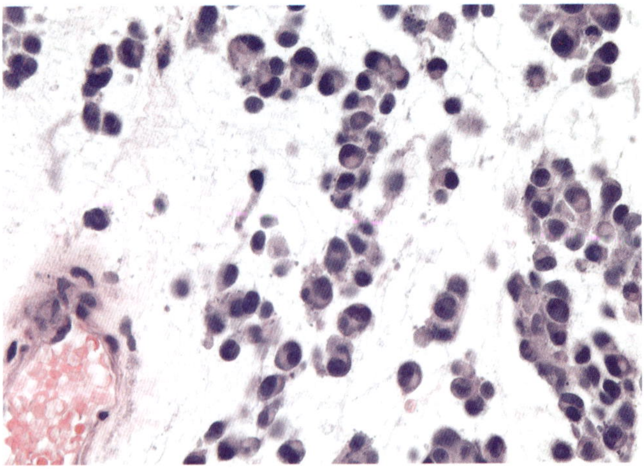

FIGURE 6.44 Plasmacytoid urothelial carcinoma (higher magnification of Fig. 6.43). Epithelial nature of tumor was highlighted by positive keratin stains (not shown).

wide. In the differential with metastatic carcinoma, plasmacytoid carcinomas are positive for cytokeratins 7 and 20, GATA3, S100P, p40, and uroplakin 2. They may occasionally commonly express CD138, so this marker should not be used in isolation as evidence of a plasma cell neoplasm.[29,30,155,158] MUM1 is typically negative.[43] Plasmacytoid carcinoma is characterized by somatic mutations of *CDH1* (resulting in loss of E-cadherin expression), akin to lobular breast carcinoma and signet ring gastric cancer.[163]

A recent large meta-analysis has shown that the plasmacytoid histology in bladder cancer is an independent adverse prognostic indicator for overall survival.[164] The prognosis of tumors with this morphology is uniformly poor with most patients having advanced stage at presentation and metastatic disease progression. Association with margin positivity and peritoneal spread (peritoneal carcinomatosis) is also known as poor response to neoadjuvant therapy.[165-168]

Urothelial Carcinoma With Rhabdoid Features

Urothelial carcinomas may also rarely have focal areas showing rhabdoid features: a population of large, relatively discohesive cells with distinct cell borders, large vesicular nuclei, prominent nucleoli, and eosinophilic cytoplasmic inclusions (Fig. 6.45, eFigs. 6.88-6.90). Less than a dozen cases have been reported in adults.[169-171] Most cases have features of conventional urothelial carcinoma at least focally; concurrent CIS, small cell, and sarcomatoid histology have been reported. As noted above, some experts consider that these tumors are in the spectrum of undifferentiated noncohesive carcinomas, which includes nonmucinous carcinoma with signet ring cell, rhabdoid, and plasmacytoid features, as well as tumor cells that resemble infiltrating lobular carcinoma of the breast.

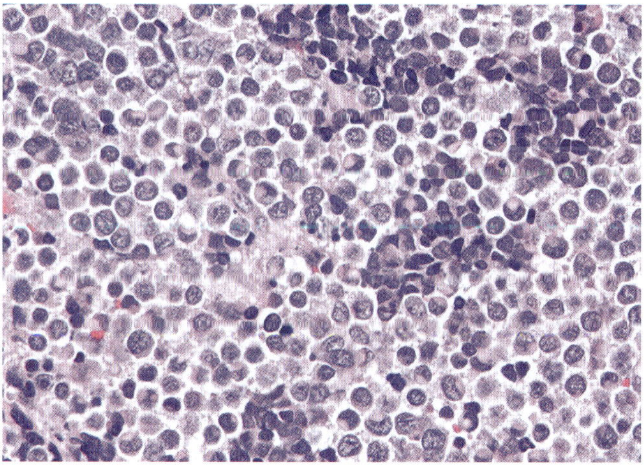

FIGURE 6.45 Rhabdoid urothelial carcinoma.

The differential diagnosis includes more entities when the tumor has a homogeneous rhabdoid phenotype. The main distinction is from a true malignant extrarenal rhabdoid tumor, which is a pathogenetically unrelated sarcoma occurring in the pediatric population. Although there are two case reports of "true" malignant rhabdoid tumors of the bladder in young patients, their existence is controversial. Both malignant rhabdoid tumors that have a characteristic mutation or deletion of the INI1 gene at chromosome 22q11 and urothelial carcinoma with rhabdoid features may have INI1 loss by immunohistochemistry.[172] From a practical standpoint, bladder tumors with a rhabdoid morphology in adults are almost always poorly differentiated urothelial carcinomas with rhabdoid features. The prognosis of these tumors is poor and characterized by an aggressive clinical course.

Urothelial Carcinoma With Clear Cytoplasm (Glycogen Rich)

Reports have cumulatively described ~35 cases of urothelial carcinomas with glycogen-rich, clear cytoplasm (Figs. 6.46 and 6.47, eFigs. 6.91-6.93).[173-180] These carcinomas are typically high grade, so the differential diagnosis includes clear cell adenocarcinoma and metastatic renal cell carcinoma. PEComa (smooth muscle actin and HMB45 positive) involving the bladder may also be in the differential. Focal clear cell change may be seen in any urothelial carcinoma of the usual type, and the change may be more common in areas with thermal injury. Clear cell change can rarely be more prominent (noteworthy when >50% of the tumor). The finding has no known prognostic impact, although a recent study of 10 cases (30%-90% clear cell change) showed tumors to be of high grade with 60% demonstrating PAX8 positivity (an immunohistochemical diagnostic

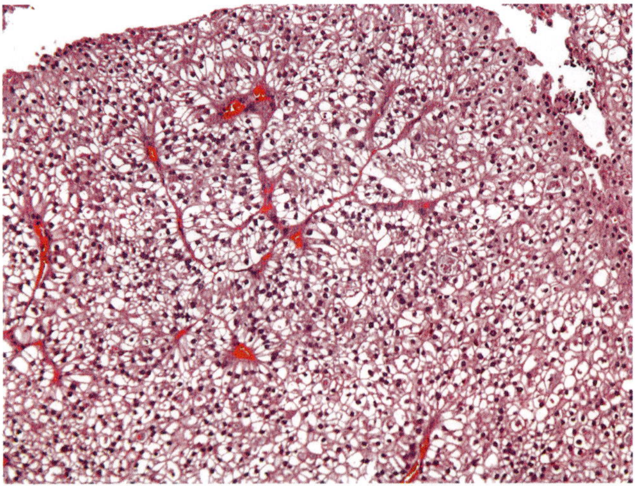

FIGURE 6.46 Noninvasive papillary urothelial carcinoma with clear cytoplasm.

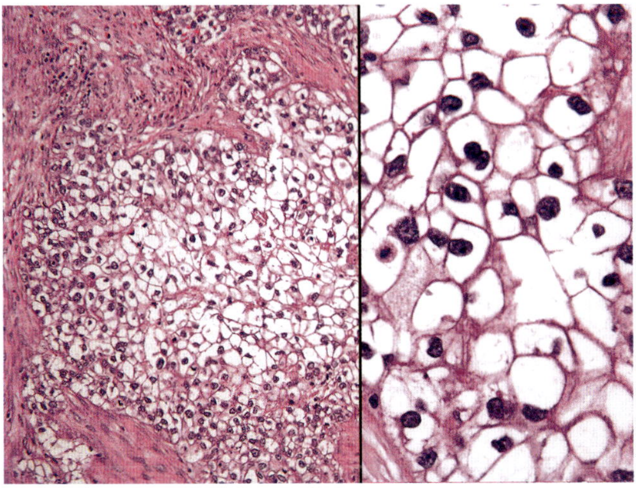

FIGURE 6.47 Invasive urothelial carcinoma with clear cytoplasm (higher magnification [*right*]).

pitfall).[180] Clear cell adenocarcinomas of the bladder more frequently occur in women and typically have a combination of morphologic patterns within the same tumor including solid, papillary, or tubulocystic architectural arrangement; the papillae are lined by a single epithelial layer with a hyalinized core. The cytoplasm may be eosinophilic or clear, and the cells may have a hobnail appearance. In contrast, poorly differentiated urothelial carcinomas with clear cell features have a more sheetlike growth pattern and often have more characteristic appearing areas, at least focally, of urothelial carcinoma with conventional morphology. They are positive for GATA3, S100P, p63, and CK7 and CK20[28]; PAX8 positivity may be seen in both tumor types and should be interpreted with caution. Metastatic renal cell carcinoma can usually be excluded based on clinical grounds (presence of renal mass). In the one reported series of seven cases of renal cell carcinoma metastatic to bladder, all patients had metastasis in multiple organs; no patient had isolated bladder metastasis.[181] It is conceivable though that a vesical involvement may be the initial manifestation of renal cell carcinoma. Morphologically, the presence of a well-developed alveolar or nested pattern with intervening interconnecting septa containing a lattice arrangement of capillaries and admixed mature lymphocytes should greatly raise suspicion of a renal primary. Given the infidelity of PAX8 in this differential, positivity for RCC antigen and negative reaction for cytokeratins 7 and 20 provide immunohistochemical support for the diagnosis of renal cell carcinoma[182] over urothelial carcinoma. Prostatic carcinomas typically involve the muscularis propria and may spare the lamina propria and the lining mucosa as it directly invades the bladder wall from the prostate. Even the high-grade and high-stage prostatic adenocarcinomas most typically show more homogenous nuclear features with prominent nucleoli. Appreciation of a multitude of patterns including cribriform, small acinar and solid, and the cytological tinctorial appearances such as clear, eosinophilic, and foamy pattern may be useful. Pleomorphism and frequent mitoses are unusual for prostate carcinoma. Immunoreactivity with PSA supports a prostatic carcinoma. Most urothelial carcinomas are positive for p63, p40, and HMWCK, markers that are usually negative in prostate carcinomas.[26,55,183] Newer prostate-specific markers including NKX3.1, P501S, and prostate-specific membrane antigens are useful in cases where the above stains are all negative.[184] While it is important for pathologists to be aware that urothelial carcinomas may have prominent clear cell change, the prognostic utility is uncertain due to rarity of cases.

Lipid-Rich Urothelial Carcinoma

Rare urothelial carcinomas may have large carcinoma cells with optically clear empty multivacuolated cells resembling lipoblasts (Fig. 6.48).[1] The lipid-rich cellular areas comprise from <10% to up to 50% of the tumor, and when prominent, they raise the possibility of a signet ring component (glandular differentiation) or heterologous liposarcomatous elements of a sarcomatoid carcinoma. Less than 10 cases are reported in which the presence of lipid has convincingly been proven by histochemistry, and hence, the term lipoid variant has been proposed.[185] The cells are S100 protein negative. The background urothelial carcinoma is invariably high grade and invasive. The absence of intracellular mucin by special stains may aid in the distinction from a signet ring cell component but is rarely necessary when one puts this unusual observation in the context of the morphology of the entire invasive carcinoma. The demonstration of cytokeratin reactivity should resolve the diagnosis of carcinoma in the most difficult case. Less than 40 cases have been reported, and in a large study of 27 patients,

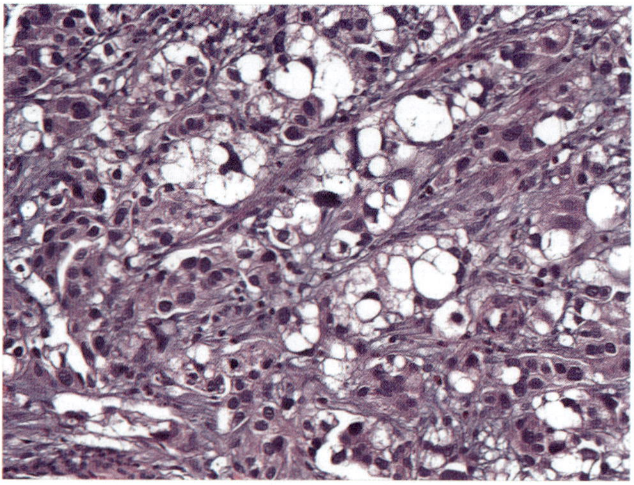

FIGURE 6.48 Lipid-rich urothelial carcinoma.

60% were dead of disease in 58 months[186]; other recent anecdotal reports document such change in high-stage tumors with poor prognosis.[187,188]

UROTHELIAL CARCINOMA WITH TROPHOBLASTIC DIFFERENTIATION

According to the nomenclatural approach in this chapter, and in keeping with the latest WHO, trophoblastic differentiation is considered to be divergent differentiation than a subtype of urothelial carcinoma. More than 30 cases of urothelial carcinoma with areas of trophoblastic differentiation have been reported, and a small subset has had symptoms related to excess human chorionic gonadotropin production including gynecomastia.[189-193] Although some of the early reports have described tumors that apparently were composed solely of tissue resembling choriocarcinoma, most tumors reported in the last three decades or so have been composed of a mixture of urothelial carcinoma with trophoblastic elements.

For purposes of reviewing clinical significance, we divide this group of neoplasms into three categories: (1) urothelial carcinoma with scattered syncytiotrophoblasts, (2) urothelial carcinoma with choriocarcinomatous differentiation or pure choriocarcinoma, and (3) urothelial carcinoma with immunohistochemical expression of β-hCG, but no recognizable trophoblasts (Figs. 6.49-6.52, eFigs. 6.94-6.100). One recently reported case, however, was associated with an isochromosome 12p, a specific genetic marker found in germ cell tumors of any histologic type.[194]

Immunohistochemistry can often detect human chorionic gonadotropin in typical urothelial carcinoma and some variants, including

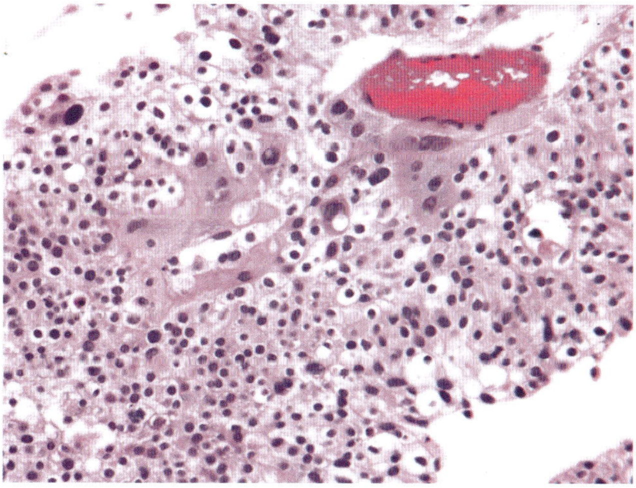

FIGURE 6.49 **Noninvasive papillary urothelial carcinoma with trophoblastic differentiation.** Note scattered syncytiotrophoblasts.

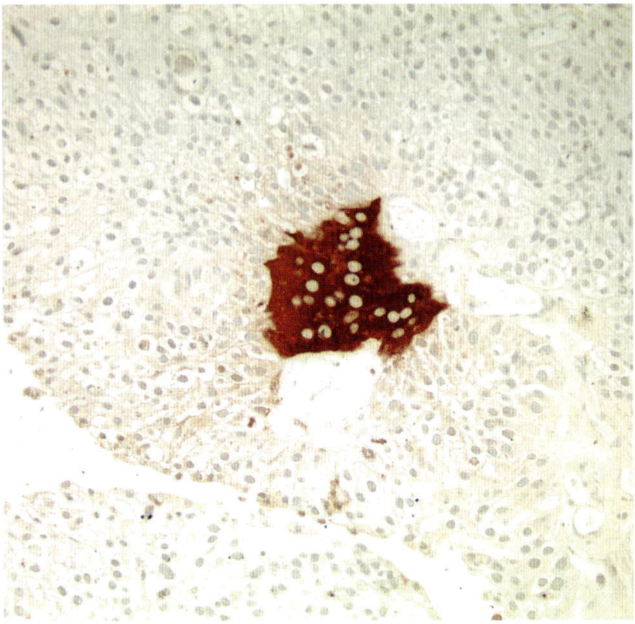

FIGURE 6.50 Scattered syncytiotrophoblasts as highlighted by stains for hCG (same case as Fig. 6.49).

micropapillary and plasmacytoid variant.[160] This is more common in high-grade carcinoma (~33% of cases) and may be seen in 22%-76% of metastatic tumors.[195,196] Areas with positive staining may be juxtaposed to identical areas without demonstrable staining. The presence of syncytiotrophoblasts has been associated with a poor prognosis; in most cases,

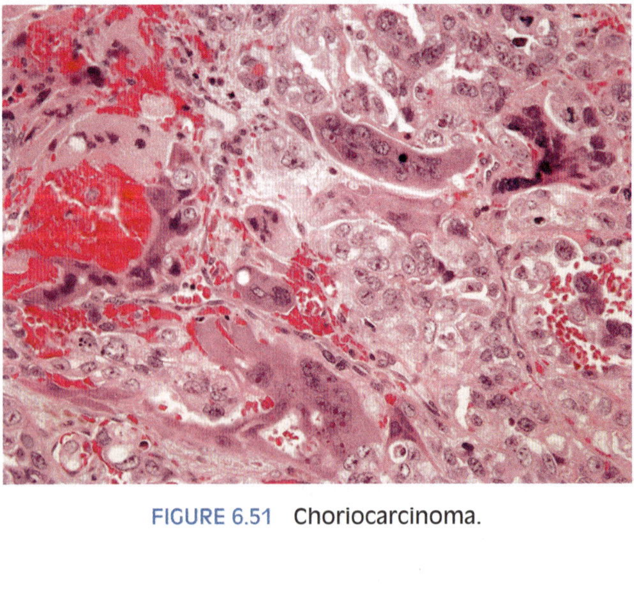

FIGURE 6.51 Choriocarcinoma.

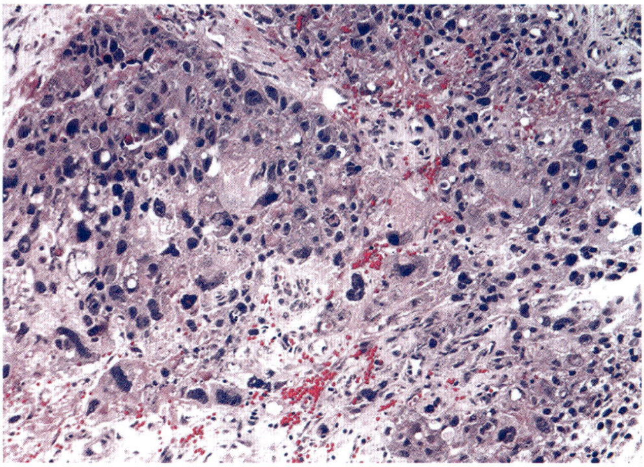

FIGURE 6.52 **Anaplastic urothelial carcinoma associated with markedly elevated serum hCG level.** The tumor lacks cytotrophoblasts and syncytiotrophoblasts necessary for diagnosis of choriocarcinoma.

<12 months has elapsed between the presentation and death. For this reason, the presence of elements with trophoblastic morphology and some estimate as to their quantity has been suggested to be reported. Also, elevated urine or serum β-hCG in these patients offers a marker for response to therapy.[192,196] In a recent study of 859 cases of urothelial carcinoma of the bladder and 65 cases of the upper tract, trophoblastic differentiation was seen in 5.9% and 10.2% tumors, respectively. Trophoblastic differentiation was significantly associated with higher risk of recurrence, progression, and patient death, and diffuse expression of β-hCG predicted a worse prognosis. Although serum β-hCG is a potential marker for monitoring recurrence and a potential prognostic marker, currently immunostaining or serum monitoring with β-hCG is not recommended.[197] In the largest pathology series of 16 cases (only cases with syncytiotrophoblasts or accompanying choriocarcinoma were included), most tumors presented at a high stage and were associated with poor clinical outcomes.[198] It does appear that choriocarcinomatous differentiation has a higher risk of metastatic disease and tumor-related death. Because of its rarity, the utility of germ cell therapy for vesical choriocarcinoma has not been fully addressed; initial cases reported a poor response, but there are reports of good clinical responses to germ cell therapy in rare patients with pure choriocarcinomas.[193] Whether or not pure choriocarcinoma of the bladder represents a tumor with better chemosensitivity is unknown. The possibility of a metastatic choriocarcinoma should always be excluded clinically before the diagnosis of a primary vesical choriocarcinoma is accepted; involution of testicular tumors is well known, and small, residual testicular scars may be the only clinical sign of primary disease.

UROTHELIAL CARCINOMA WITH UNUSUAL STROMAL REACTIONS

Pseudosarcomatous Stroma

Urothelial carcinomas may have a pseudosarcomatous stromal response in the primary or metastatic sites[103] (Fig. 6.53, eFig. 6.101). In these cases, the stroma contains atypical mesenchymal cells that are similar to those seen in giant cell cystitis. The chief reason for their awareness is that they should not be misinterpreted as the biphasic component of sarcomatoid carcinoma. The superficially very atypical appearing spindle cells often have abundant eosinophilic cytoplasm and pleomorphic hyperchromatic nuclei yet having the appearance of degenerative atypia. The spindle cell component lacks mitotic activity or an expansile growth, and there is a lack of morphologic transition between the spindle cells and the carcinoma cells. This lesion is different from urothelial carcinoma with myxoid stroma, in which atypical cells are absent (eFigs. 7.35-7.37). The nonexpansile nature of the stromal proliferation and close relationship to the edge of the invasive carcinoma with bland cytological features is usually diagnostic. Caution is warranted in application of cytokeratin immunohistochemistry as there may be focal or occasionally brisk cytokeratin positivity, which may be diagnostically misleading.

With Chordoid or Myxoid/Mucinous Features

A unique subtype of urothelial carcinoma, reminiscent of chordoma, extraskeletal mesenchymal chondrosarcoma, myoepithelioma, or yolk sac tumor has been described as "urothelial carcinoma with chordoid features".[199] Although conventional invasive urothelial carcinoma is invariably present, the striking arrangement in other areas of tumors cells arranged in cords with a prominent myxoid stroma may pose diagnostic challenges

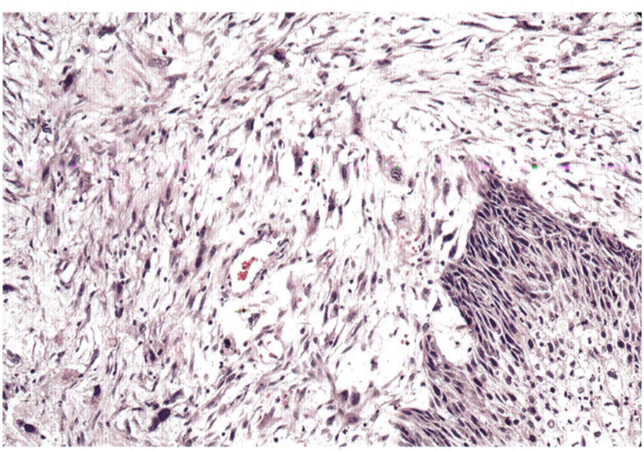

FIGURE 6.53 Carcinoma with pseudosarcomatous stroma.

in the appropriate recognition of the tumor as a form of urothelial carcinoma. The tumor cells are positive for urothelial-associated markers, p63, and HMWCK and are negative for myoepithelial markers–calponin and glial fibrillary acid protein and glypican 3 (positive in yolk sac tumor) and brachyury (chordoma). Reported cases are high-stage tumors associated with metastasis and death due to disease.[199]

More typical invasive urothelial carcinoma may also be associated with mucinous/myxoid features (Fig. 6.54). Given the presence of an abundant extracellular myxoid matrix, there is a potential to misdiagnose urothelial carcinomas with myxoid stroma as a mucinous adenocarcinoma, such as from the prostate, intestine, or bladder. The histogenesis and corresponding designation of these cases are controversial. Some experts consider that they should be designated as *urothelial carcinoma with abundant myxoid stroma*, given the absence of overt glandular epithelium. However, others favor that the myxoid matrix represents mucinous secretions from the urothelial carcinoma, whereby they should be designated as *urothelial carcinoma with mucinous features*. In the one study on this variant, there was positivity for MUC2, MUC5, and CEA in the invasive urothelial carcinoma associated with the myxoid matrix.[200] Further support that the myxoid material in the current study could be epithelial in origin is that its histochemical characteristics were similar to that reported in adenocarcinomas of the bladder, showing histochemical properties of neutral and acid mucosubstances, with positive Alcian blue at pH 2.5, positive mucicarmine, and positive PAS. Mucinous/myxoid urothelial carcinomas show a range of aggressiveness. An unusual feature is the presence of invasive low-grade urothelial carcinoma or associated low-grade papillary urothelial carcinoma in ~50% of the cases.

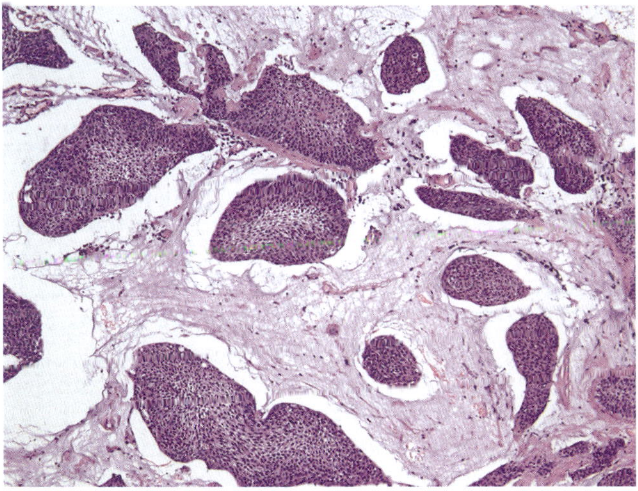

FIGURE 6.54 Infiltrating low-grade urothelial carcinoma with mucinous/myxoid stroma.

TABLE 6.1 Urothelial Carcinoma With Giant Cells

Giant cell carcinoma
Sarcomatoid carcinoma with anaplastic spindle cell giant cells
High-grade urothelial carcinoma with syncytiotrophoblasts and/or choriocarcinomatous elements
Urothelial carcinoma with osteoclastlike stromal response
Osteoclast-rich undifferentiated carcinoma
Urothelial carcinoma with treatment-associated giant cells (post-BCG or posttransurethral resection)

Osseous or Cartilaginous Metaplasia

The stroma of urothelial carcinomas or their metastases may rarely undergo osseous or cartilaginous metaplasia. This feature should not be mistaken for heterologous differentiation in a sarcomatoid carcinoma.[3,102]

Osteoclast-Type Giant Cells

Giant cells resembling osteoclasts are occasionally present in the stroma of bladder carcinoma. They are histiocytic in nature, are immunoreactive for histiocytic rather than epithelial markers, and have no prognostic significance. On rare occasions, these may be prominent and may resemble "osteoclastomas of the bladder," most cases of which we believe fall into the spectrum of osteoclast-rich poorly differentiated carcinoma of the bladder. Giant cells may be seen in several different settings in bladder pathology. Table 6.1 summarizes these conditions.

OSTEOCLAST-RICH POORLY DIFFERENTIATED CARCINOMA OF THE URINARY BLADDER

"Giant cell tumors" or "osteoclastomalike giant cell tumors" of the pancreas, gall bladder, liver, breast, salivary gland, thyroid, skin, lung, intestines, larynx, and female genital tract have been reported. Less than 30 cases of a similar spectrum have been reported in the bladder, most as case reports, with one series of six cases.[201-207] The tumors are composed of mononuclear cells (frequently positive for epithelial markers), osteoclastlike giant cells (CD68, CD51, CD54 positive), and recognizable usual urothelial neoplasia (CIS, papillary or invasive carcinoma) in varying proportions (Figs. 6.55 and 6.56, eFigs. 6.102-6.110).[202] Urothelial CIS is the most commonly found urothelial component in the two large reported series,[207] and a conventional invasive urothelial tumor may be difficult to find. Some areas may be entirely composed of histology similar to giant cell tumors of the bone, while other areas may show single cells or aggregates of mononuclear cells with a spectrum of atypia including marked

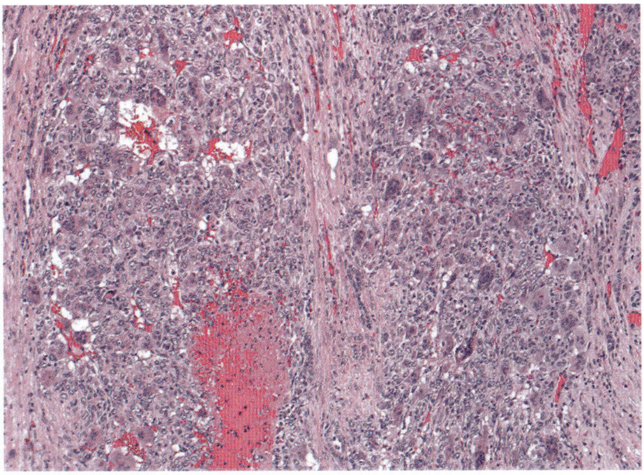

FIGURE 6.55 Undifferentiated urothelial carcinoma with osteoclastic giant cells.

pleomorphism, which are distinct from the nuclei of the osteoclastlike giant cells. These mononuclear cells may stain for pancytokeratin, EMA, CAM 5.2, and cytokeratin 7, and rarely for S100 protein, actin, desmin, and p53.[202] Although these tumors have several histologic features of their skeletal counterparts including areas with blood-filled cysts mimicking aneurysmal bone cyst, we believe them to be poorly differentiated carcinomas that are rich in osteoclasts because of the cytokeratin and GATA3 positivity, concurrent presence of high-grade urothelial neoplasia, and matched p53 positivity in mononuclear cells and urothelial tumor cells. In the series of six cases, four of five patients with follow-up died of disease, three with documented metastasis.[202] A large majority of patients reported in case reports who have adequate follow-up have also had documented metastatic disease or death.[202-207]

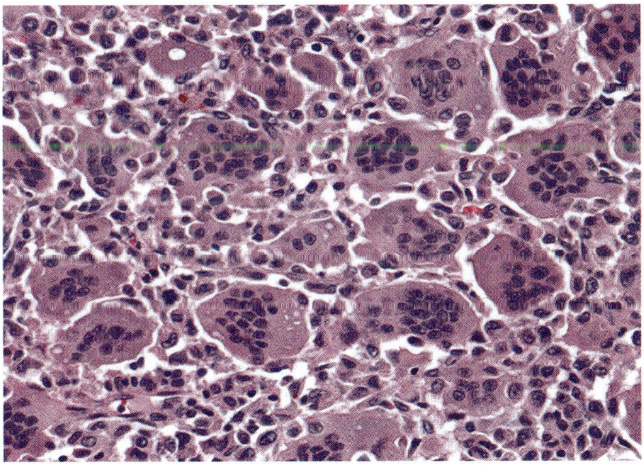

FIGURE 6.56 Undifferentiated urothelial carcinoma with osteoclastic giant cells.

GIANT CELL CARCINOMA/POORLY DIFFERENTIATED CARCINOMA

This is an undifferentiated carcinoma of the bladder that occasionally may be composed predominantly or purely of poorly differentiated, large, cohesive pleomorphic, multinucleated, and multinucleated anaplastic cells with abundant eosinophilic or amphophilic cytoplasm[3,4,208] (Fig. 6.57, eFigs. 6.111 and 6.112). The tumor cells often contain multiple nucleoli and are similar to giant cell carcinomas seen in the lung and in other parts of the body. This high-grade component may comprise 20%-100% of the tumor. Necrosis and muscularis propria invasion are typically present. The high degree of nuclear anaplasia helps differentiate giant cell carcinoma from the osteoclast-type giant cells that may be seen in urothelial carcinoma. Outcome data are limited, but based on few reported cases, the prognosis is poor in keeping with its poorly differentiated to undifferentiated histology; check point inhibitor therapy may be promising.[209] Other giant cells that may be seen with urothelial carcinoma include syncytiotrophoblastic giant cells or foreign body giant cells secondary to previous biopsy or resection (Table 6.1).

Uncommonly, an epithelial tumor is found in the urinary bladder and consists of sheets of nondescript undifferentiated cells without squamous, urothelial, or glandular differentiation. Some authorities would classify these cases as large cell undifferentiated carcinoma (Figs. 6.58 and 6.59, eFigs. 6.113 and 6.114). Others may prefer to denote these lesions as high-grade urothelial carcinoma, given that this is the most common cancer within the bladder and that this pattern of tumor most likely represents the most poorly differentiated manifestation of usual urothelial carcinoma. There are currently no studies to determine whether there are any biologic differences in prognosis or treatment between high-grade urothelial carcinoma and "large cell undifferentiated" carcinoma. Until such data exist, either term used to describe such a lesion is appropriate.

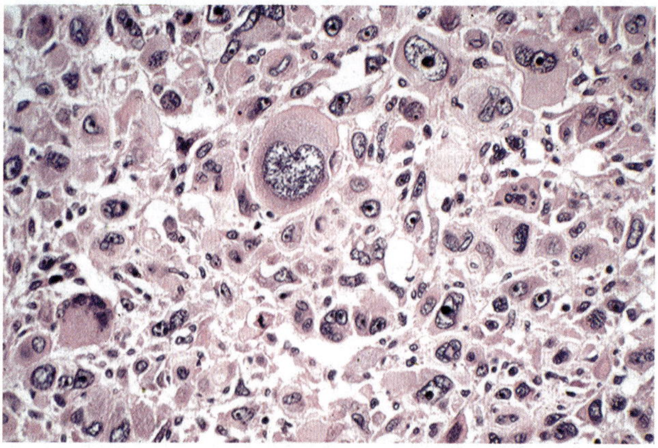

FIGURE 6.57 Pleomorphic giant cell carcinoma.

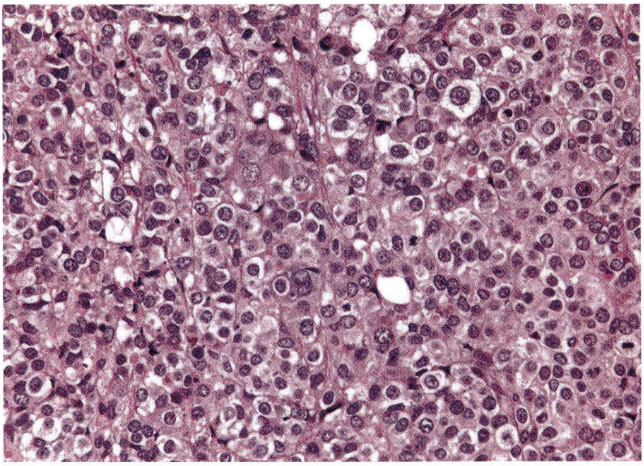

FIGURE 6.58 Large cell undifferentiated carcinoma.

REPORTING RECOMMENDATIONS AND SUMMARY

It has been shown that histologic subtypes of bladder cancer are underreported in clinical practice.[210,211] Almost all subtypes of urothelial carcinoma discussed in this chapter have been described in the urinary bladder and in the upper tract. From the wide histologic spectrum of invasive urothelial carcinoma described, it is amply apparent that urothelial neoplasia has ability to manifest itself with several subtype histologies and divergent differentiation. While nested or microcystic, micropapillary or inverted urothelial carcinoma are histogenetically urothelial in nature, it may some of the more undifferentiated forms (eg, small cell or sarcomatoid carcinoma) arise from a common stem cell abnormality. It is important that surgical pathologists be aware of this potential for subtype manifestation, as the correct characterization of the tumors have shown to have diagnostic, therapeutic, or

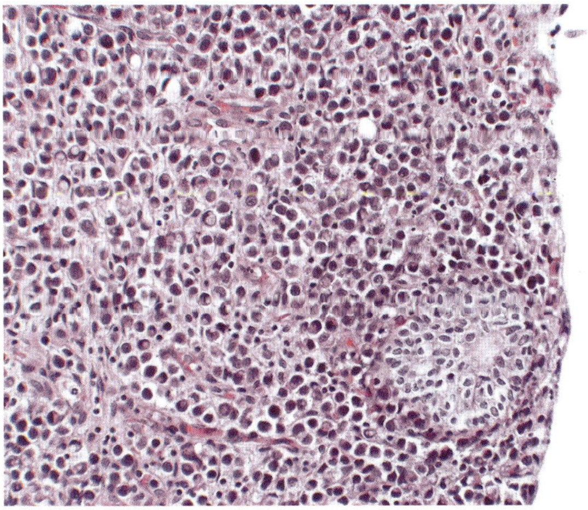

FIGURE 6.59 Lymphomalike large cell undifferentiated carcinoma.

prognostic implications, which could significantly impact management. It is also not uncommon that tumors with subtype histology show multiple patterns and divergent differentiation within the same tumor such as sarcomatoid, small cell, squamous, and glandular differentiation. The Genitourinary Pathology Society (GUPS) has recently made the following recommendations in reporting subtype histology. It is not clear as to how much subtype histology impacts prognosis or treatment decisions. However, when multiple histologies are encountered, it is recommended to routinely provide the relative percentage of each of the different components [ie, invasive high-grade urothelial carcinoma (50%), sarcomatoid differentiation (30%), small cell carcinoma (20%)]. Divergent differentiation and subtype morphology should be recorded both in transurethral resections and in radical cystectomy specimens, and any significant difference in the morphologic patterns seen between the two specimens during clinicopathologic correlation should ideally be reconciled in the final cystectomy report.[15]

Several subtype histologies appear to inherently define "high-risk" bladder cancer in both nonmuscle invasive and muscle invasive (see Chapter 7 on Prognostic Factors). In the appropriate clinicopathologic setting, some would advocate for early cystectomy for T1 disease and consider neoadjuvant chemotherapy for T2-T4 disease in some subtypes.[6,212] Treatment algorithms for resectable urothelial carcinoma of the bladder contain subtype histology as a stratifying feature, and this information has been incorporated into clinical treatment algorithms for resectable urothelial carcinoma including the National Comprehensive Cancer Network (NCCN) Clinical Practice Guidelines for Bladder Cancer.[6,61] In the future, it is possible that treatment strategies will be tailored based on the particular genomic or immunogenic profile of a tumor (see Chapter 7), which in part can be inferred by the subtype histology. Since many subtypes are clinically aggressive and may present at metastatic sites in which case the unusual subtype histology may not readily facilitate relationship with bladder cancer, comparison with the histology of the bladder primary, if available, and/or immunohistochemical support is often necessary to arrive at the correct diagnosis.

REFERENCES

1. Raspolini MR, Amin MB, Hartmann A, Moch H, Srigley JR. Tumours of the urinary tract: introduction. In: Comperat EM, Netto GJ, Tsuzki T, eds. *WHO classification of tumours. Urinary and Male Genital Tumours.* 5th ed. International Agency for Research on Cancer; 2022:2-3. Chapter 3, Section 5.0.0.1.
2. Amin MB. Histological variants of urothelial carcinoma: diagnostic, therapeutic and prognostic implications. *Mod Pathol.* 2009;22(Suppl 2):S96-S118.
3. Amin MB, Murphy WM, Reuter VE, et al. A symposium on controversies in the pathology of transitional cell carcinomas of the urinary bladder. Part I. *Anat Pathol Chic Ill Annu.* 1996;1:1-39.
4. Eble JN, Young RH. Carcinoma of the urinary bladder: a review of its diverse morphology. *Semin Diagn Pathol.* 1997;14(2):98-108.

5. Nigwekar P, Amin MB. The many faces of urothelial carcinoma: an update with an emphasis on recently described variants. *Adv Anat Pathol.* 2008;15(4):218-233.
6. National Comprehensive Cancer Network. Bladder Cancer (version 2.2022). https://www.nccn.org/guidelines/guidelines-process/transparency-process-and-recommendations
7. Shah JB, McConkey DJ, Dinney CPN. New strategies in muscle-invasive bladder cancer: on the road to personalized medicine. *Clin Cancer Res.* 2011;17(9):2608-2612.
8. Soave A, Schmidt S, Dahlem R, et al. Does the extent of variant histology affect oncological outcomes in patients with urothelial carcinoma of the bladder treated with radical cystectomy? *Urol Oncol.* 2015;33(1):21.e1-21.e9.
9. Seisen T, Compérat E, Léon P, Roupret M. Impact of histological variants on the outcomes of nonmuscle invasive bladder cancer after transurethral resection. *Curr Opin Urol.* 2014;24(5):524-531.
10. Xylinas E, Rink M, Robinson BD, et al. Impact of histological variants on oncological outcomes of patients with urothelial carcinoma of the bladder treated with radical cystectomy. *Eur J Cancer 1990.* 2013;49(8):1889-1897.
11. Murphy WM, Deana DG. The nested variant of transitional cell carcinoma: a neoplasm resembling proliferation of Brunn's nests. *Mod Pathol.* 1992;5(3):240-243.
12. Oliva E, Young RH. Nephrogenic adenoma of the urinary tract: a review of the microscopic appearance of 80 cases with emphasis on unusual features. *Mod Pathol.* 1995;8(7):722-730.
13. Talbert ML, Young RH. Carcinomas of the urinary bladder with deceptively benign-appearing foci. A report of three cases. *Am J Surg Pathol.* 1989;13(5):374-381.
14. Young RH, Oliva E. Transitional cell carcinomas of the urinary bladder that may be underdiagnosed. A report of four invasive cases exemplifying the homology between neoplastic and non-neoplastic transitional cell lesions. *Am J Surg Pathol.* 1996;20(12):1448-1454.
15. Compérat E, Amin MB, Epstein JI, et al. The Genitourinary Pathology Society Update on classification of variant histologies, T1 substaging, molecular taxonomy, and immunotherapy and PD-L1 testing implications of urothelial cancers. *Adv Anat Pathol.* 2021;28(4):196-208.
16. Lobo N, Shariat SF, Guo CC, et al. What is the significance of variant histology in urothelial carcinoma? *Eur Urol Focus.* 2020;6(4):653-663.
17. Cardillo M, Reuter VE, Lin O. Cytologic features of the nested variant of urothelial carcinoma: a study of seven cases. *Cancer.* 2003;99(1):23-27.
18. Drew PA, Furman J, Civantos F, Murphy WM. The nested variant of transitional cell carcinoma: an aggressive neoplasm with innocuous histology. *Mod Pathol.* 1996;9(10):989-994.
19. Holmäng S, Johansson SL. The nested variant of transitional cell carcinoma—a rare neoplasm with poor prognosis. *Scand J Urol Nephrol.* 2001;35(2):102-105.
20. Amin MB, Young RH. Intraepithelial lesions of the urinary bladder with a discussion of the histogenesis of urothelial neoplasia. *Semin Diagn Pathol.* 1997;14(2):84-97.
21. Beltran AL, Cheng L, Montironi R, et al. Clinicopathological characteristics and outcome of nested carcinoma of the urinary bladder. *Virchows Arch Int J Pathol.* 2014;465(2):199-205.
22. Fatima A, Russell DH, Epstein JI. Nested subtype of urothelial carcinoma in the upper urinary tract: a series of 15 cases. *Am J Surg Pathol.* 2014;2(2):102-110.
23. Legesse T, Matoso A, Epstein JI. PAX8 positivity in nested variant of urothelial carcinoma: a potential diagnostic pitfall. *Hum Pathol.* 2019;94:11-15.
24. Amin MB, Patel RM, Oliveira P, et al. Alveolar soft-part sarcoma of the urinary bladder with urethral recurrence: a unique case with emphasis on differential diagnoses and diagnostic utility of an immunohistochemical panel including TFE3. *Am J Surg Pathol.* 2006;30(10):1322-1325.

25. Dhall D, Al-Ahmadie H, Olgac S. Nested variant of urothelial carcinoma. *Arch Pathol Lab Med.* 2007;131(11):1725-1727.
26. Lin O, Cardillo M, Dalbagni G, et al. Nested variant of urothelial carcinoma: a clinicopathologic and immunohistochemical study of 12 cases. *Mod Pathol.* 2003;16(12): 1289-1298.
27. McKenney JK, Amin MB. The role of immunohistochemistry in the diagnosis of urinary bladder neoplasms. *Semin Diagn Pathol.* 2005;22(1):69-87.
28. Zhai QJ, Black J, Ayala AG, Ro JY. Histologic variants of infiltrating urothelial carcinoma. *Arch Pathol Lab Med.* 2007;131(8):1244-1256.
29. Paner GP, Annaiah C, Gulmann C, et al. Immunohistochemical evaluation of novel and traditional markers associated with urothelial differentiation in a spectrum of variants of urothelial carcinoma of the urinary bladder. *Hum Pathol.* 2014;45(7):1473-1482.
30. Smith SC, Mohanty SK, Kunju LP, et al. Uroplakin II outperforms uroplakin III in diagnostically challenging settings. *Histopathology.* 2014;65(1):132-138.
31. Volmar KE, Chan TY, De Marzo AM, Epstein JI. Florid von Brunn nests mimicking urothelial carcinoma: a morphologic and immunohistochemical comparison to the nested variant of urothelial carcinoma. *Am J Surg Pathol.* 2003;27(9):1243-1252.
32. Epstein JI, Amin MB, Reuter VE. *Biopsy Interpretation of the Bladder.* Lippincott Williams & Wilkins; 2012:368.
33. Sjödahl G, Lauss M, Lövgren K, et al. A molecular taxonomy for urothelial carcinoma. *Clin Cancer Res.* 2012;18(12):3377-3386.
34. Compérat E, McKenney JK, Hartmann A, et al. Large nested variant of urothelial carcinoma: a clinicopathological study of 36 cases. *Histopathology.* 2017;71(5):703-710.
35. Cox R, Epstein JI. Large nested variant of urothelial carcinoma: 23 cases mimicking von Brunn nests and inverted growth pattern of noninvasive papillary urothelial carcinoma. *Am J Surg Pathol.* 2011;35(9):1337-1342.
36. Huang Q, Chu PG, Lau SK, Weiss LM. Urothelial carcinoma of the urinary bladder with a component of acinar/tubular type differentiation simulating prostatic adenocarcinoma. *Hum Pathol.* 2004;35(6):769-773.
37. Neşe N, Kandiloğlu AR, Atesçi YZ. Nested variant of transitional cell carcinoma with osseous metaplasia of the urinary bladder: a case report and review of published reports. *Int J Urol.* 2007;14(4):365-367.
38. Young RH, Zukerberg LR. Microcystic transitional cell carcinomas of the urinary bladder. A report of four cases. *Am J Clin Pathol.* 1991;96(5):635-639.
39. Paz A, Rath-Wolfson L, Lask D, et al. The clinical and histological features of transitional cell carcinoma of the bladder with microcysts: analysis of 12 cases. *Br J Urol.* 1997;79(5):722-725.
40. Leroy X, Leteurtre E, De La Taille A, et al. Microcystic transitional cell carcinoma: a report of 2 cases arising in the renal pelvis. *Arch Pathol Lab Med.* 2002;126(7):859-861.
41. Lopez Beltran A, Montironi R, Cheng L. Microcystic urothelial carcinoma: morphology, immunohistochemistry and clinical behaviour. *Histopathology.* 2014;64(6):872-879.
42. Sari A, Uyaroglu MA, Ermete M, et al. Microcystic urothelial carcinoma of the urinary bladder metastatic to the penis. *Pathol Oncol Res.* 2007;13(2):170-173.
43. Lopez-Beltran A, Henriques V, Montironi R, et al. Variants and new entities of bladder cancer. *Histopathology.* 2019;74(1):77-96.
44. Amin MB, Gómez JA, Young RH. Urothelial transitional cell carcinoma with endophytic growth patterns: a discussion of patterns of invasion and problems associated with assessment of invasion in 18 cases. *Am J Surg Pathol.* 1997;21(9):1057-1068.
45. Terai A, Tamaki M, Hayashida H, et al. Bulky transitional cell carcinoma of bladder with inverted proliferation. *Int J Urol.* 1996;3(4):316-319.

46. Jones TD, Zhang S, Lopez-Beltran A, et al. Urothelial carcinoma with an inverted growth pattern can be distinguished from inverted papilloma by fluorescence in situ hybridization, immunohistochemistry, and morphologic analysis. *Am J Surg Pathol.* 2007;31(12):1861-1867.

47. Maranchie JK, Bouyounes BT, Zhang PL, et al. Clinical and pathological characteristics of micropapillary transitional cell carcinoma: a highly aggressive variant. *J Urol.* 2000;163(3):748-751.

48. Vera J, Marigil M, García MD, et al. Micropapillary bladder carcinoma. *Virchows Arch Int J Pathol.* 2002;441(4):412-413.

49. Johansson SL, Borghede G, Holmäng S. Micropapillary bladder carcinoma: a clinicopathological study of 20 cases. *J Urol.* 1999;161(6):1798-1802.

50. Amin MB, Ro JY, el-Sharkawy T, et al. Micropapillary variant of transitional cell carcinoma of the urinary bladder. Histologic pattern resembling ovarian papillary serous carcinoma. *Am J Surg Pathol.* 1994;18(12):1224-1232.

51. Ylagan LR, Humphrey PA. Micropapillary variant of transitional cell carcinoma of the urinary bladder: a report of three cases with cytologic diagnosis in urine specimens. *Acta Cytol.* 2001;45(4):599-604.

52. Deuker M, Stolzenbach LF, Collà Ruvolo C, et al. Micropapillary versus urothelial carcinoma of the urinary bladder: stage at presentation and efficacy of chemotherapy across all stages–a SEER-based study. *Eur Urol Focus.* 2021;7(6):1332-1338.

53. Sangoi AR, Cox RM, Higgins JP, et al. Non-invasive papillary urothelial carcinoma with "micropapillary" architecture: clinicopathological study of 18 patients emphasising clinical outcomes. *Histopathology.* 2020;77(5):728-733.

54. Lim M, Adsay NV, Grignon D, Osunkoya AO. Urothelial carcinoma with villoglandular differentiation: a study of 14 cases. *Mod Pathol.* 2009;22(10):1280-1286.

55. Parker DC, Folpe AL, Bell J, et al. Potential utility of uroplakin III, thrombomodulin, high molecular weight cytokeratin, and cytokeratin 20 in noninvasive, invasive, and metastatic urothelial (transitional cell) carcinomas. *Am J Surg Pathol.* 2003;27(1):1-10.

56. Amin A, Epstein JI. Noninvasive micropapillary urothelial carcinoma: a clinicopathologic study of 18 cases. *Hum Pathol.* 2012;43(12):2124-2128.

57. Spaliviero M, Dalbagni G, Bochner BH, et al. Clinical outcome of patients with T1 micropapillary urothelial carcinoma of the bladder. *J Urol.* 2014;192(3):702-707.

58. Compérat E, Roupret M, Yaxley J, et al. Micropapillary urothelial carcinoma of the urinary bladder: a clinicopathological analysis of 72 cases. *Pathology (Phila).* 2010;42(7):650-654.

59. Gaya JM, Palou J, Algaba F, et al. The case for conservative management in the treatment of patients with non-muscle-invasive micropapillary bladder carcinoma without carcinoma in situ. *Can J Urol.* 2010;17(5):5370-5376.

60. Samaratunga H, Khoo K. Micropapillary variant of urothelial carcinoma of the urinary bladder; a clinicopathological and immunohistochemical study. *Histopathology.* 2004;45(1):55-64.

61. Black PC, Brown GA, Dinney CPN. The impact of variant histology on the outcome of bladder cancer treated with curative intent. *Urol Oncol.* 2009;27(1):3-7.

62. Kamat AM, Gee JR, Dinney CPN, et al. The case for early cystectomy in the treatment of nonmuscle invasive micropapillary bladder carcinoma. *J Urol.* 2006;175(3 Pt 1):881-885.

63. Fairey AS, Daneshmand S, Wang L, et al. Impact of micropapillary urothelial carcinoma variant histology on survival after radical cystectomy. *Urol Oncol.* 2014;32(2):110-116.

64. Wang JK, Boorjian SA, Cheville JC, et al. Outcomes following radical cystectomy for micropapillary bladder cancer versus pure urothelial carcinoma: a matched cohort analysis. *World J Urol.* 2012;30(6):801-806.

65. Kamat AM, Dinney CPN, Gee JR, et al. Micropapillary bladder cancer: a review of the University of Texas M. D. Anderson Cancer Center experience with 100 consecutive patients. *Cancer.* 2007;110(1):62-67.
66. International Bladder Cancer Nomogram Consortium; Bochner BH, Kattan MW, Vora KC. Postoperative nomogram predicting risk of recurrence after radical cystectomy for bladder cancer. *J Clin Oncol.* 2006;24(24):3967-3972.
67. Rogers CG, Palapattu GS, Shariat SF, et al. Clinical outcomes following radical cystectomy for primary nontransitional cell carcinoma of the bladder compared to transitional cell carcinoma of the bladder. *J Urol.* 2006;175(6):2048-2053.
68. Shariat SF, Karakiewicz PI, Palapattu GS, et al. Outcomes of radical cystectomy for transitional cell carcinoma of the bladder: a contemporary series from the Bladder Cancer Research Consortium. *J Urol.* 2006;176(6 Pt 1):2414-2422.
69. Amin MB, Smith SC, Reuter VE, et al. Update for the practicing pathologist: The International Consultation On Urologic Disease-European association of urology consultation on bladder cancer. *Mod Pathol.* 2015;28(5):612-630.
70. Compérat E, Amin MB, Cathomas R, et al. Current best practice for bladder cancer: a narrative review of diagnostics and treatments. *The Lancet.* 2022;400(10364): 1712-1721.
71. Charfi S, Moussa A, Njim L, et al. Micropapillary bladder carcinoma. *Progres En Urol J Assoc Francaise.* 2006;16(5):607-609.
72. Holmäng S, Thomsen J, Johansson SL. Micropapillary carcinoma of the renal pelvis and ureter. *J Urol.* 2006;175(2):463-466.
73. Alvarado-Cabrero I, Sierra-Santiesteban FI, Mantilla-Morales A, Hernández-Hernandez DM. Micropapillary carcinoma of the urothelial tract. A clinicopathologic study of 38 cases. *Ann Diagn Pathol.* 2005;9(1):1-5.
74. Dhouib RS, Abbes I, Mrad K, et al. Micropapillary transitional cell carcinoma of the urinary bladder: report of two cases. *Pathologica.* 2005;97(5):338-340.
75. Munakata S, Tahara H, Kojima K, Kishimoto T. Micropapillary urothelial carcinoma of the renal pelvis: report of a case and review of the literature. *Med Sci Monit.* 2007;13(4):CS47-CS52.
76. Perez-Montiel D, Hes O, Michal M, Suster S. Micropapillary urothelial carcinoma of the upper urinary tract: clinicopathologic study of five cases. *Am J Clin Pathol.* 2006;126(1):86-92.
77. Amin MB, Ro JY, Lee KM, Ordóñez NG, et al. Lymphoepithelioma-like carcinoma of the urinary bladder. *Am J Surg Pathol.* 1994;18(5):466-473.
78. Holmäng S, Borghede G, Johansson SL. Bladder carcinoma with lymphoepithelioma-like differentiation: a report of 9 cases. *J Urol.* 1998;159(3):779-782.
79. Ward JN, Dong WF, Pitts WR. Lymphoepithelioma-like carcinoma of the bladder. *J Urol.* 2002;167(6):2523-2524.
80. Lopez-Beltrán A, Luque RJ, Vicioso L, et al. Lymphoepithelioma-like carcinoma of the urinary bladder: a clinicopathologic study of 13 cases. *Virchows Arch Int J Pathol.* 2001;438(6):552-557.
81. Tamas EF, Nielsen ME, Schoenberg MP, Epstein JI. Lymphoepithelioma-like carcinoma of the urinary tract: a clinicopathological study of 30 pure and mixed cases. *Mod Pathol.* 2007;20(8):828-834.
82. Choong NWW, Quevedo JF, Kaur JS. Small cell carcinoma of the urinary bladder. The Mayo Clinic experience. *Cancer.* 2005;103(6):1172-1178.
83. Gulley ML, Amin MB, Nicholls JM, et al. Epstein-Barr virus is detected in undifferentiated nasopharyngeal carcinoma but not in lymphoepithelioma-like carcinoma of the urinary bladder. *Hum Pathol.* 1995;26(11):1207-1214.

84. Zukerberg LR, Harris NL, Young RH. Carcinomas of the urinary bladder simulating malignant lymphoma. A report of five cases. *Am J Surg Pathol.* 1991;15(6):569-576.
85. Dinney CP, Ro JY, Babaian RJ, Johnson DE. Lymphoepithelioma of the bladder: a clinicopathological study of 3 cases. *J Urol.* 1993;149(4):840-841.
86. Manocha U, Kardos J, Selitsky S, et al. RNA Expression profiling of lymphoepithelioma-like carcinoma of the bladder reveals a basal-like molecular subtype. *Am J Pathol.* 2020;190(1):134-144.
87. Necchi A, Raggi D, Gallina A, et al. Updated results of PURE-01 with preliminary activity of neoadjuvant pembrolizumab in patients with muscle-invasive bladder carcinoma with variant histologies. *Eur Urol.* 2020;77(4):439-446.
88. Lopez-Beltran A, Pacelli A, Rothenberg HJ, et al. Carcinosarcoma and sarcomatoid carcinoma of the bladder: clinicopathological study of 41 cases. *J Urol.* 1998;159(5):1497-1503.
89. Jones EC, Young RH. Myxoid and sclerosing sarcomatoid transitional cell carcinoma of the urinary bladder: a clinicopathologic and immunohistochemical study of 25 cases. *Mod Pathol.* 1997;10(9):908-916.
90. Torenbeek R, Blomjous CE, de Bruin PC, et al. Sarcomatoid carcinoma of the urinary bladder. Clinicopathologic analysis of 18 cases with immunohistochemical and electron microscopic findings. *Am J Surg Pathol.* 1994;18(3):241-249.
91. Ikegami H, Iwasaki H, Ohjimi Y, et al. Sarcomatoid carcinoma of the urinary bladder: a clinicopathologic and immunohistochemical analysis of 14 patients. *Hum Pathol.* 2000;31(3):332-340.
92. Wright JL, Black PC, Brown GA, et al. Differences in survival among patients with sarcomatoid carcinoma, carcinosarcoma and urothelial carcinoma of the bladder. *J Urol.* 2007;178(6):2302-2306.
93. Amin MB, Trpkov K, Lopez-Beltran A, Grignon D; Members of the ISUP Immunohistochemistry in Diagnostic Urologic Pathology Group. Best practices recommendations in the application of immunohistochemistry in the bladder lesions: report from the International Society of Urologic Pathology consensus conference. *Am J Surg Pathol.* 2014;38(8):e20-e34.
94. Sanfrancesco J, McKenney JK, Leivo MZ, et al. Sarcomatoid urothelial carcinoma of the bladder: Analysis of 28 cases with emphasis on clinicopathologic features and markers of epithelial-to-mesenchymal transition. *Arch Pathol Lab Med.* 2016;140(6):543-551.
95. Cheng L, Zhang S, Alexander R, et al. Sarcomatoid carcinoma of the urinary bladder: the final common pathway of urothelial carcinoma dedifferentiation. *Am J Surg Pathol.* 2011;35(5):e34-e46.
96. Mukhopadhyay S, Shrimpton AE, Jones LA, et al. Carcinosarcoma of the urinary bladder following cyclophosphamide therapy: evidence for monoclonal origin and chromosome 9p allelic loss. *Arch Pathol Lab Med.* 2004;128(1):e8-e11.
97. Lopez-Beltran A, Luque RJ, Mazzucchelli R, et al. Changes produced in the urothelium by traditional and newer therapeutic procedures for bladder cancer. *J Clin Pathol.* 2002;55(9):641-647.
98. Harik LR, Merino C, Coindre JM, et al. Pseudosarcomatous myofibroblastic proliferations of the bladder: a clinicopathologic study of 42 cases. *Am J Surg Pathol.* 2006;30(7):787-794.
99. Montgomery EA, Shuster DD, Burkart AL, et al. Inflammatory myofibroblastic tumors of the urinary tract: a clinicopathologic study of 46 cases, including a malignant example inflammatory fibrosarcoma and a subset associated with high-grade urothelial carcinoma. *Am J Surg Pathol.* 2006;30(12):1502-1512.
100. Lopez-Beltran A, Escudero AL, Cavazzana AO, et al. Sarcomatoid transitional cell carcinoma of the renal pelvis. A report of five cases with clinical, pathological, immunohistochemical and DNA ploidy analysis. *Pathol Res Pract.* 1996;192(12):1218-1224.

101. Westfall DE, Folpe AL, Paner GP, et al. Utility of a comprehensive immunohistochemical panel in the differential diagnosis of spindle cell lesions of the urinary bladder. *Am J Surg Pathol.* 2009;33(1):99-105.
102. Gazaigne J, Mozziconacci JG, Provendier B, et al. Sarcomatoid carcinoma of the bladder with major osseous metaplasia. *Prog Urol.* 1998;8:1051-1053.
103. Young RH, Wick MR. Transitional cell carcinoma of the urinary bladder with pseudosarcomatous stroma. *Am J Clin Pathol.* 1988;90(2):216-219.
104. Sung MT, Wang M, MacLennan GT, et al. Histogenesis of sarcomatoid urothelial carcinoma of the urinary bladder: evidence for a common clonal origin with divergent differentiation. *J Pathol.* 2007;211(4):420-430.
105. Acikalin MF, Kabukcuoglu S, Can C. Sarcomatoid carcinoma of the renal pelvis with giant cell tumor-like features: case report with immunohistochemical findings. *Int J Urol.* 2005;12(2):199-203.
106. Reuter VE. Sarcomatoid lesions of the urogenital tract. *Semin Diagn Pathol.* 1993;10(2):188-201.
107. Peyromaure M, Beuzeboc P, Chekulaev D, et al. Sarcomatoid carcinoma with heterologous osteoid differentiation. *Prog Urol.* 2006;16:378-380.
108. Wang J, Wang FW, Lagrange CA, et al. Clinical features of sarcomatoid carcinoma (carcinosarcoma) of the urinary bladder: analysis of 221 cases. *Sarcoma.* 2010;2010:454792.
109. Agoff SN, Lamps LW, Philip AT, et al. Thyroid transcription factor-1 is expressed in extrapulmonary small cell carcinomas but not in other extrapulmonary neuroendocrine tumors. *Mod Pathol.* 2000;13(3):238-242.
110. Buza N, Cohen PJ, Hui P, Parkash V. Inverse p16 and p63 expression in small cell carcinoma and high-grade urothelial cell carcinoma of the urinary bladder. *Int J Surg Pathol.* 2010;18(2):94-102.
111. Bezerra SM, Lotan TL, Faraj SF, et al. GATA3 expression in small cell carcinoma of bladder and prostate and its potential role in determining primary tumor origin. *Hum Pathol.* 2014;45(8):1682-1687.
112. Terracciano L, Richter J, Tornillo L, et al. Chromosomal imbalances in small cell carcinomas of the urinary bladder. *J Pathol.* 1999;189(2):230-235.
113. Abbosh PH, Wang M, Eble JN, et al. Hypermethylation of tumor-suppressor gene CpG islands in small-cell carcinoma of the urinary bladder. *Mod Pathol.* 2008;21(3):355-362.
114. Zheng X, Zhuge J, Bezerra SM, et al. High frequency of TERT promoter mutation in small cell carcinoma of bladder, but not in small cell carcinoma of other origins. *J Hematol Oncol.* 2014;7:47.
115. Kouba EJ, Cheng L. Understanding the genetic landscape of small cell carcinoma of the urinary bladder and implications for diagnosis, prognosis, and treatment: a review. *JAMA Oncol.* 2017;3(11):1570-1578.
116. Wang W, Epstein JI. Small cell carcinoma of the prostate. A morphologic and immunohistochemical study of 95 cases. *Am J Surg Pathol.* 2008;32(1):65-71.
117. Paner GP, McKenney JK, Epstein JI, Amin MB. Rhabdomyosarcoma of the urinary bladder in adults: predilection for alveolar morphology with anaplasia and significant morphologic overlap with small cell carcinoma. *Am J Surg Pathol.* 2008;32(7):1022-1028.
118. Bex A, de Vries R, Pos F, et al. Long-term survival after sequential chemoradiation for limited disease small cell carcinoma of the bladder. *World J Urol.* 2009;27(1):101-106.
119. Bex A, Nieuwenhuijzen JA, Kerst M, et al. Small cell carcinoma of bladder: a single-center prospective study of 25 cases treated in analogy to small cell lung cancer. *Urology.* 2005;65(2):295-299.
120. Pan CX, Yang XJ, Lopez-Beltran A, et al. c-kit Expression in small cell carcinoma of the urinary bladder: prognostic and therapeutic implications. *Mod Pathol.* 2005;18(3):320-323.

121. Sved P, Gomez P, Manoharan M, et al. Small cell carcinoma of the bladder. *BJU Int.* 2004;94(1):12-17.
122. Abrahams NA, Moran C, Reyes AO, Siefker-Radtke A, Ayala AG. Small cell carcinoma of the bladder: a contemporary clinicopathological study of 51 cases. *Histopathology.* 2005;46(1):57-63.
123. Mukesh M, Cook N, Hollingdale AE, Ainsworth NL, Russell SG. Small cell carcinoma of the urinary bladder: a 15-year retrospective review of treatment and survival in the Anglian Cancer Network. *BJU Int.* 2009;103(6):747-752.
124. Cheng L, Pan CX, Yang XJ, et al. Small cell carcinoma of the urinary bladder: a clinicopathologic analysis of 64 patients. *Cancer.* 2004;101(5):957-962.
125. Mills SE, Wolfe JT, Weiss MA, et al. Small cell undifferentiated carcinoma of the urinary bladder. A light-microscopic, immunocytochemical, and ultrastructural study of 12 cases. *Am J Surg Pathol.* 1987;11(8):606-617.
126. Mangar SA, Logue JP, Shanks JH, et al. Small-cell carcinoma of the urinary bladder: 10-year experience. *Clin Oncol (R Coll Radiol).* 2004;16(8):523-527.
127. Weiss MA. Small-cell carcinoma of the urinary tract. Important prognostic and therapeutic implications. *Arch Pathol Lab Med.* 1993;117(3):237-238.
128. Jung K, Ghatalia P, Litwin S, et al. Small-cell carcinoma of the bladder: 20-year single-institution retrospective review. *Clin Genitourin Cancer.* 2017;15(3):e337-e343.
129. Patel SG, Stimson CJ, Zaid HB, et al. Locoregional small cell carcinoma of the bladder: clinical characteristics and treatment patterns. *J Urol.* 2014;191(2):329-334.
130. Sweeney P, Millikan R, Donat M, et al. Is there a therapeutic role for post-chemotherapy retroperitoneal lymph node dissection in metastatic transitional cell carcinoma of the bladder? *J Urol.* 2003;169(6):2113-2117.
131. Vakar-Lopez F, True LD. How wide is the spectrum of neuroendocrine carcinoma of the urinary bladder? *Am J Clin Pathol.* 2007;128(5):723-725.
132. Alijo Serrano F, Sánchez-Mora N, Angel Arranz J, et al. Large cell and small cell neuroendocrine bladder carcinoma: immunohistochemical and outcome study in a single institution. *Am J Clin Pathol.* 2007;128(5):733-739.
133. Evans AJ, Al-Maghrabi J, Tsihlias J, et al. Primary large cell neuroendocrine carcinoma of the urinary bladder. *Arch Pathol Lab Med.* 2002;126(10):1229-1232.
134. Hailemariam S, Gaspert A, Komminoth P, et al. Primary, pure, large-cell neuroendocrine carcinoma of the urinary bladder. *Mod Pathol.* 1998;11(10):1016-1020.
135. Martignoni G, Eble JN. Carcinoid tumors of the urinary bladder. Immunohistochemical study of 2 cases and review of the literature. *Arch Pathol Lab Med.* 2003;127(1):e22-e24.
136. McCabe JE, Das S, Dowling P, et al. Oncocytic carcinoid tumour of the bladder. *J Clin Pathol.* 2005;58(4):446-447.
137. Murali R, Kneale K, Lalak N, Delprado W. Carcinoid tumors of the urinary tract and prostate. *Arch Pathol Lab Med.* 2006;130(11):1693-1706.
138. Akimov OV, Chukin SE. Malignant carcinoid of the urinary bladder. *Arkh Patol.* 2002;64(1):41-42.
139. Chen YB, Epstein JI. Primary carcinoid tumors of the urinary bladder and prostatic urethra: a clinicopathologic study of 6 cases. *Am J Surg Pathol.* 2011;35(3):442-446.
140. Baydar DE, Tasar C. Carcinoid tumor in the urinary bladder: unreported features. *Am J Surg Pathol.* 2011;35(11):1754-1757.
141. Zozumi M, Nakai M, Matsuda I, et al. Primary carcinoid tumor of the urinary bladder with prominent subnuclear eosinophilic granules. *Pathol Res Pract.* 2012;208(2):109-112.
142. Dundr P, Pesl M, Povýsil C, et al. Large cell neuroendocrine carcinoma of the urinary bladder with lymphoepithelioma-like features. *Pathol Res Pract.* 2003;199(8):559-563.

143. Martín IJP, Vilar DG, Aguado JM, et al. Large cell neuroendocrine carcinoma of the urinary bladder. Bibliographic review. *Arch Esp Urol.* 2011;64(2):105-113.
144. Hata S, Tasaki Y. A case of the large cell neuroendocrine carcinoma of the urinary bladder. *Case Rep Med.* 2013;2013:804136.
145. Colarossi C, Pino P, Giuffrida D, et al. Large cell neuroendocrine carcinoma (LCNEC) of the urinary bladder: a case report. *Diagn Pathol.* 2013;8:19.
146. Sari A, Ermete M, Sadullahoğlu C, et al. Large cell neuroendocrine carcinoma of urinary bladder; case presentation. *Turk Patoloji Derg.* 2013;29(2):138-142.
147. Wang G, Yuan R, Zhou C, et al. Urinary large cell neuroendocrine carcinoma: a clinicopathologic analysis of 22 cases. *Am J Surg Pathol.* 2021;45(10):1399-1408.
148. Yıldız P, Behzatoğlu K, Hacıhasanoğlu E, et al. Histological, immunohistochemical features and pathogenesis of pseudoangiosarcomatous urothelial carcinoma. *Ann Diagn Pathol.* 2017;30:17-20.
149. Paner GP, Cox RM, Richards K, et al. Pseudoangiosarcomatous urothelial carcinoma of the urinary bladder. *Am J Surg Pathol.* 2014;38(9):1251-1259.
150. Ro JY, Shen SS, Lee HI, et al. Plasmacytoid transitional cell carcinoma of urinary bladder: a clinicopathologic study of 9 cases. *Am J Surg Pathol.* 2008;32(5):752-757.
151. Sahin AA, Myhre M, Ro JY, et al. Plasmacytoid transitional cell carcinoma. Report of a case with initial presentation mimicking multiple myeloma. *Acta Cytol.* 1991;35(3):277-280.
152. Kohno T, Kitamura M, Akai H, et al. Plasmacytoid urothelial carcinoma of the bladder. *Int J Urol.* 2006;13(4):485-486.
153. Zhang XM, Elhosseiny A, Melamed MR. Plasmacytoid urothelial carcinoma of the bladder. A case report and the first description of urinary cytology. *Acta Cytol.* 2002;46(2):412-416.
154. Fritsche HM, Burger M, Denzinger S, et al. Plasmacytoid urothelial carcinoma of the bladder: histological and clinical features of 5 cases. *J Urol.* 2008;180(5):1923-1927.
155. Mai KT, Park PC, Yazdi HM, et al. Plasmacytoid urothelial carcinoma of the urinary bladder report of seven new cases. *Eur Urol.* 2006;50(5):1111-1114.
156. Gaafar A, Garmendia M, de Miguel E, et al. Plasmacytoid urothelial carcinoma of the urinary bladder. A study of 7 cases. *Actas Urol Esp.* 2008;32:806-810.
157. Sato K, Ueda Y, Kawamura K, et al. Plasmacytoid urothelial carcinoma of the urinary bladder: a case report and immunohistochemical study. *Pathol Res Pract.* 2009;205(3):189-194.
158. Nigwekar P, Tamboli P, Amin MB, Osunkoya AO, Ben-Dor D, Amin MB. Plasmacytoid urothelial carcinoma: detailed analysis of morphology with clinicopathologic correlation in 17 cases. *Am J Surg Pathol.* 2009;33(3):417-424.
159. Soylu A, Aydin NE, Yilmaz U, et al. Urothelial carcinoma featuring lipid cell and plasmacytoid morphology with poor prognostic outcome. *Urology.* 2005;65(4):797.
160. Shimada K, Nakamura M, Ishida E, Konishi N. Urothelial carcinoma with plasmacytoid variants producing both human chorionic gonadotropin and carbohydrate antigen 19–9. *Urology.* 2006;68(4):891.e7-891.e10.
161. Coyne JD, Sim E. Urothelial neoplasia with plasmacytoid morphology. *Histopathology.* 2006;48(2):200-201.
162. Baldwin L, Lee AHS, Al-Talib RK, Theaker JM. Transitional cell carcinoma of the bladder mimicking lobular carcinoma of the breast: a discohesive variant of urothelial carcinoma. *Histopathology.* 2005;46(1):50-56.
163. Al-Ahmadie HA, Iyer G, Lee BH, et al. Frequent somatic CDH1 loss-of-function mutations in plasmacytoid variant bladder cancer. *Nat Genet.* 2016;48(4):356-358.
164. Kim DK, Kim JW, Ro JY, et al. Plasmacytoid variant urothelial carcinoma of the bladder: a systematic review and meta-analysis of clinicopathological features and survival outcomes. *J Urol.* 2020;204(2):215-223.

165. Kaimakliotis HZ, Monn MF, Cheng L, et al. Plasmacytoid bladder cancer: variant histology with aggressive behavior and a new mode of invasion along fascial planes. *Urology.* 2014;83(5):1112-1116.

166. Dayyani F, Czerniak BA, Sircar K, et al. Plasmacytoid urothelial carcinoma, a chemosensitive cancer with poor prognosis, and peritoneal carcinomatosis. *J Urol.* 2013;189(5):1656-1661.

167. Ricardo-Gonzalez RR, Nguyen M, et al. Plasmacytoid carcinoma of the bladder: a urothelial carcinoma variant with a predilection for intraperitoneal spread. *J Urol.* 2012;187(3):852-855.

168. Diamantopoulos LN, Khaki AR, Grivas P, et al. Plasmacytoid urothelial carcinoma: response to chemotherapy and oncologic outcomes. *Bladder Cancer Amst Neth.* 2020;6(1):71-81.

169. Abello A, Delto JC, Wagner AA, Das AK. An unusual presentation of metastatic urothelial bladder carcinoma with rhabdoid features presenting as obstructive uropathy. *Urology.* 2018;115:33-35.

170. Kumar S, Kumar D, Cowan DF. Transitional cell carcinoma with rhabdoid features. *Am J Surg Pathol.* 1992;16(5):515-521.

171. Parwani AV, Herawi M, Volmar K, et al. Urothelial carcinoma with rhabdoid features: report of 6 cases. *Hum Pathol.* 2006;37(2):168-172.

172. Sirohi D, Ohe C, Smith SC, Amin MB. SWI/SNF-deficient neoplasms of the genitourinary tract. *Semin Diagn Pathol.* 2021;38(3):212-221.

173. Gilcrease MZ, Delgado R, Vuitch F, Albores-Saavedra J. Clear cell adenocarcinoma and nephrogenic adenoma of the urethra and urinary bladder: a histopathologic and immunohistochemical comparison. *Hum Pathol.* 1998;29(12):1451-1456.

174. Kotliar SN, Wood CG, Schaeffer AJ, Oyasu R. Transitional cell carcinoma exhibiting clear cell features. A differential diagnosis for clear cell adenocarcinoma of the urinary tract. *Arch Pathol Lab Med.* 1995;119(1):79-81.

175. Oliva E, Amin MB, Jimenez R, Young RH. Clear cell carcinoma of the urinary bladder: a report and comparison of four tumors of mullerian origin and nine of probable urothelial origin with discussion of histogenesis and diagnostic problems. *Am J Surg Pathol.* 2002;26(2):190-197.

176. Sun K, Huan Y, Unger PD. Clear cell adenocarcinoma of urinary bladder and urethra: another urinary tract lesion immunoreactive for P504S. *Arch Pathol Lab Med.* 2008;132(9):1417-1422.

177. Sung MT, Zhang S, MacLennan GT, et al. Histogenesis of clear cell adenocarcinoma in the urinary tract: evidence of urothelial origin. *Clin Cancer Res.* 2008;14:1947-1955.

178. Knez VM, Barrow W, Lucia MS, et al. Clear cell urothelial carcinoma of the urinary bladder: a case report and review of the literature. *J Med Case Reports.* 2014;8:275.

179. Zhang Y, Huang J, Feng H, Tang Y. Primary multiple clear cell variant urothelial carcinomas of urinary bladder: a rare case report. *Int J Clin Exp Pathol.* 2014;7(6):3385-3388.

180. Mai KT, Bateman J, Djordjevic B, et al. Clear cell urothelial carcinoma. *Int J Surg Pathol.* 2017;25(1):18-25.

181. Sim SJ, Ro JY, Ordonez NG, et al. Metastatic renal cell carcinoma to the bladder: a clinicopathologic and immunohistochemical study. *Mod Pathol.* 1999;12(4):351-355.

182. Gupta R, Balzer B, Picken M, et al. Diagnostic implications of transcription factor Pax 2 protein and transmembrane enzyme complex carbonic anhydrase IX immunoreactivity in adult renal epithelial neoplasms. *Am J Surg Pathol.* 2009;33(2):241-247.

183. Di Como CJ, Urist MJ, Babayan I, et al. p63 expression profiles in human normal and tumor tissues. *Clin Cancer Res.* 2002;8(2):494-501.

184. Sheridan T, Herawi M, Epstein JI, Illei PB. The role of P501S and PSA in the diagnosis of metastatic adenocarcinoma of the prostate. *Am J Surg Pathol.* 2007;31(9):1351-1355.

185. Leroy X, Gonzalez S, Zini L, Aubert S. Lipoid-cell variant of urothelial carcinoma: a clinicopathologic and immunohistochemical study of five cases. *Am J Surg Pathol.* 2007;31(5):770-773.

186. Lopez-Beltran A, Amin MB, Oliveira PS, et al. Urothelial carcinoma of the bladder, lipid cell variant: clinicopathologic findings and LOH analysis. *Am J Surg Pathol.* 2010;34(3):371-376.

187. Chaudhary K, Pareek T, Sharma A, Thirunavukkarasu B. Lipid-rich variant of urothelial carcinoma: a lethal enigma. *BMJ Case Rep.* 2021;14(3):e240593.

188. Patel A, Velilla RE, Shurbaji MS. Lipid-rich variant of urothelial carcinoma presenting as the dominant morphology in a recurrent tumor after local therapy. *Am J Case Rep.* 2018;19:478-481.

189. Dirnhofer S, Koessler P, Ensinger C, et al. Production of trophoblastic hormones by transitional cell carcinoma of the bladder: association to tumor stage and grade. *Hum Pathol.* 1998;29(4):377-382.

190. Iles RK, Chard T. Human chorionic gonadotropin expression by bladder cancers: biology and clinical potential. *J Urol.* 1991;145(3):453-458.

191. Iles RK, Jenkins BJ, Oliver RT, et al. Beta human chorionic gonadotrophin in serum and urine. A marker for metastatic urothelial cancer. *Br J Urol.* 1989;64(3):241-244.

192. Martin JE, Jenkins BJ, Zuk RJ, et al. Human chorionic gonadotrophin expression and histological findings as predictors of response to radiotherapy in carcinoma of the bladder. *Virchows Arch A Pathol Anat Histopathol.* 1989;414(3):273-277.

193. Sievert K, Weber EA, Herwig R, et al. Pure primary choriocarcinoma of the urinary bladder with long-term survival. *Urology.* 2000;56(5):856.

194. Rodriguez E, Mathew S, Reuter V, et al. Cytogenetic analysis of 124 prospectively ascertained male germ cell tumors. *Cancer Res.* 1992;52(8):2285-2291.

195. Iles RK. Ectopic hCGbeta expression by epithelial cancer: malignant behaviour, metastasis and inhibition of tumor cell apoptosis. *Mol Cell Endocrinol.* 2007;260-262:264-270.

196. Douglas J, Sharp A, Chau C, et al. Serum total hCGβ level is an independent prognostic factor in transitional cell carcinoma of the urothelial tract. *Br J Cancer.* 2014;110(7):1759-1766.

197. Cheng HL, Chou LP, Tsai HW, et al. Urothelial carcinoma with trophoblastic differentiation: reappraisal of the clinical implication and immunohistochemically features. *Urol Oncol.* 2021;39(10):732.e17-732.e23.

198. Przybycin CG, McKenney JK, Nguyen JK, et al. Urothelial carcinomas with trophoblastic differentiation, including choriocarcinoma: clinicopathologic series of 16 cases. *Am J Surg Pathol.* 2020;44(10):1322-1330.

199. Cox RM, Schneider AG, Sangoi AR, et al. Invasive urothelial carcinoma with chordoid features: a report of 12 distinct cases characterized by prominent myxoid stroma and cordlike epithelial architecture. *Am J Surg Pathol.* 2009;33(8):1213-1219.

200. Tavora F, Epstein JI. Urothelial carcinoma with abundant myxoid stroma. *Hum Pathol.* 2009;40(10):1391-1398.

201. Amir G, Rosenmann E. Osteoclast-like giant cell tumour of the urinary bladder. *Histopathology.* 1990;17(5):413-418.

202. Baydar D, Amin MB, Epstein JI. Osteoclast-rich undifferentiated carcinomas of the urinary tract. *Mod Pathol.* 2006;19(2):161-171.

203. Garcia Garcia F, Garcia Ligero J, Martinez Diaz F, et al. Bladder carcinoma with osteoclast-type giant cells. A case with a rare presentation. Review of the literature. *Actas Urol Esp.* 2003;27:317-320.

204. Krüger S, Johannisson R, Kausch I, Feller AC. Papillary urothelial bladder carcinoma associated with osteoclast-like giant cells. *Int Urol Nephrol.* 2005;37(1):61-64.

205. O'Connor RC, Hollowell CMP, Laven BA, et al. Recurrent giant cell carcinoma of the bladder. *J Urol.* 2002;167(4):1784.

206. Zukerberg LR, Armin AR, Pisharodi L, Young RH. Transitional cell carcinoma of the urinary bladder with osteoclast-type giant cells: a report of two cases and review of the literature. *Histopathology.* 1990;17(5):407-411.

207. Satturwar S, Parwani AV, Thomas R, Bastacky S, Dhir R, Quiroga-Garza GM. The osteoclast-type giant cell rich carcinoma of urinary bladder: a case series. *Pathol Res Pract.* 2022;239:154164.

208. Samaratunga H, Delahunt B. Recently described and unusual variants of urothelial carcinoma of the urinary bladder. *Pathology (Phila).* 2012;44(5):407-418.

209. Nezu K, Kakoi N, Tezuka F, Ota S. Successful treatment of metastatic bladder pleomorphic giant cell carcinoma with pembrolizumab. *IJU Case Rep.* 2021;4(4):200-203.

210. Shah RB, Montgomery JS, Montie JE, Kunju LP. Variant (divergent) histologic differentiation in urothelial carcinoma is under-recognized in community practice: impact of mandatory central pathology review at a large referral hospital. *Urol Oncol.* 2013;31(8):1650-1655.

211. Amin MB, McKenney JK, Paner GP, et al. ICUD-EAU International Consultation on Bladder Cancer 2012: pathology. *Eur Urol.* 2013;63(1):16-35.

212. Willis DL, Porten SP, Kamat AM. Should histologic variants alter definitive treatment of bladder cancer? *Curr Opin Urol.* 2013;23(5):435-443.

7

MORPHOLOGIC, PROGNOSTIC, AND PREDICTIVE FACTORS AND REPORTING OF BLADDER CANCER

The traditional morphologic, prognostic, and predictive factors for bladder cancer vary according to the type of bladder cancer presentation in the patient: noninvasive papillary tumors, primary urothelial carcinoma *in situ* (CIS), or invasive urothelial carcinoma.[1-5] Therefore, the prognostic factors are discussed separately for each category; they are summarized in Table 7.1. In the European Association of Urology guidelines and the NCCN guidelines (which have adopted the American Urology Association and Society for Urologic Oncology [AUA/SUO] guidelines), Ta, T1, and CIS lesions are combined in the recommendations for non–muscle-invasive bladder cancer[4,6] (Table 7.2). Additionally, clinical parameters (eg, comorbid disease) as well as clinical features (initial response and duration of response to intravesical BCG, increased frequency of recurrence, and short interval between recurrences), patient age, and sex (female) influence progression in grade and stage.[3-5,7]

NONINVASIVE PAPILLARY TUMORS

Histologic Grade

Histologic grade of the papillary tumor (Chapter 3) is a powerful prognostic factor for recurrence and progression in noninvasive tumors. Urothelial papilloma has the lowest risk for either recurrence or progression, whereas papillary urothelial neoplasm of low malignant potential has a risk for recurrence but still has a very low risk for progression. Invasion is not seen in association with these tumors, and patients with papilloma and neoplasms of low malignant potential have essentially a normal age-related life expectancy (see Chapter 3). Risk of progression in grade, stage, and mortality increases from low-grade carcinomas to high-grade carcinomas. High-grade disease is critical for management and therapeutic decisions in the recent NCCN guidelines for noninvasive tumors.[2,6] Invasion must be diligently looked for in high-grade noninvasive tumors.

TABLE 7.1 Adverse Morphologic Prognostic and Predictive Factors of Bladder Cancer

Noninvasive papillary urothelial carcinoma
High histologic grade
Large tumor size (≥3 cm)
Multifocality (number of tumors)
Associated CIS
Bladder neck involvement (emerging)
Prior recurrence
Female sex
Patient age (>70)
Urothelial CIS
Multifocality (number of tumors)
Not primary (*de novo*)
Female sex
Failure to respond to typical therapy
Involvement of prostatic urethra
Invasive urothelial carcinoma
Increased depth of invasion in bladder wall (pT stage)
Lymph node involvement (pN stage)
Involvement of prostate gland and seminal vesicles
Aggressive histologic subtypes
Increased histologic grade
Vascular-lymphatic invasion
Positive surgical margins (perivesicle, vaginal cuff and urethral)
Multifocality and CIS of urethra or ureters
Increased time from diagnosis to surgery (controversial)
Maximum tumor size
Patient age (>70)
Female sex

Size of Tumor

Large tumors (>3 cm) are at an increased risk for recurrence and progression.[3-5,8-11]

Multifocality and Number of Tumors

Patients with multifocal tumors in the bladder and involving other regions of the urothelial tract (ureters and urethra) are at increased risk for recurrence, progression, or death due to disease.[9,12,13] The number of tumors has been shown to correlate with higher risk of recurrence.[3-5,10,14,15]

TABLE 7.2 AUA/SUO Risk Stratification for Non–Muscle-Invasive Bladder Cancer

Low Risk	Intermediate Risk	High Risk
Papillary urothelial neoplasm of low malignant potential	*Papillary low-grade urothelial carcinoma (any)* • *pT1* • *>3 cm* • *Multifocal* • *Recurrence within 1 year*	*Papillary high-grade urothelial carcinoma (any)* • *Associated CIS* • *T1* • *>3 cm* • *Multifocal*
Noninvasive low-grade papillary urothelial carcinoma • *≤3 cm* *&* • *Solitary*	*Papillary high-grade urothelial carcinoma (any)* • *pTa* • *≤3 cm* • *Solitary*	*Very high-risk features (any)* • *BCG unresponsive* • *Lymphovascular invasion* • *Variant histologies* • *Prostatic urethral invasion*

Adopted with permission from Chang SS, Boorjian SA, Chou R, et al. Diagnosis and treatment of non-muscle invasive bladder cancer: AUA/SUO guideline. *J Urol.* 2016;196(4):1021-1029. Copyright © 2016 by American Urological Association Education and Research, Inc.

Clinical Parameters

Clinical history of prior recurrence, patient age >70, and female sex has been associated with bladder cancer recurrence in non–muscle-invasive bladder cancer.[3-5,15]

Urothelial Carcinoma *In Situ* in Nonpapillary Mucosa

Although the impact of the presence of dysplasia in the nonpapillary urothelium is controversial as a prognostic factor and at best may represent a marker of urothelial instability, the presence of urothelial CIS is a known adverse prognostic factor in terms of recurrence and progression.[3-5,16,17] CIS most commonly occurs in papillary tumors concurrently or develops secondarily during surveillance during intravesical management.

UROTHELIAL CARCINOMA *IN SITU*

Patients with primary (*de novo*) CIS are more likely to have no evidence of disease (62% vs 45%) and are less likely to progress (28% vs 59%) or die of disease (7% vs 45%) as compared to patients who have CIS in association with high-grade papillary carcinoma,[18] although the data are not conclusive. Patients with CIS often respond to intravesical installation of BCG, but virtually all will experience tumor recurrence over time. Patients with multifocal disease, those with involvement of the prostatic urethra, and those who fail to respond to intravesical therapy have a worse outcome.[1,3-5,16,17,19,20] Patients with CIS are also at a significant risk to develop metachronous upper tract urothelial carcinoma with potential for aggressive behavior, high risk of recurrence, and death from cancer after nephroureterectomy such that surveillance of the upper tract and lower tract in the setting of bladder CIS is recommended.[3-5,14]

INVASIVE UROTHELIAL CARCINOMA

Depth of Invasion in Bladder Wall

Once a urothelial carcinoma is invasive, the most seminal prognostic factor is the American Joint Committee on Cancer/International Union against Cancer pathologic stage[21-24] (Table 7.3). The pT system of staging has excellent correlation with prognosis and distinguishes distinct prognostic groups. Tumors invasive into the lamina propria (pT1) have a better survival than tumors invasive into the muscularis propria (pT2), with poor survival for tumors with extravesicular extension (pT3, pT4).[1,25-28] Although substaging of urothelial tumors (pTla–tumors invasive up to muscularis mucosae, pTlb–tumors invasive into or beyond muscularis mucosae) has shown prognostic value in multiple studies (T1b showing higher rates of progression (58% vs 36%) and death from disease (46% vs 23%) than T1a,[29] it is not always easy to substage using this criterion due to fragmentation and lack of orientation in TURBT specimens.[30] Chapter 5 outlines the diagnostic criteria, pitfalls, and reporting recommendations for T1 disease. In T1 disease, several other substaging strategies have been proposed to improve outcome prediction.[31-33] One strategy separates T1 disease into that above the muscularis mucosae (T1a), below the muscularis mucosae but above the venous plexus (T1b), and beyond the venous plexus (T1c) or separates microinvasive (T1m) disease from more deeply invasive disease (T1e).[31,34] Whereas T1a and T1b corresponded to a 5-year survival rate of 75%, T1c disease was associated with a 5-year survival rate of only 11%, more akin to outcomes in T2 disease.[35] A maximum diameter of invasive carcinoma of <1 high-power field vs ≥1 high-power fields (irrespective of direction), and a cutoff of 1 mm maximum invasive diameter have all also been shown to be associated with prognosis.[22,36] The eighth edition of the AJCC staging manual and the WHO (2022) continue to encourage T1 substaging by depth and/or extent of subepithelial tissue invasion without specifying a method, as an ideal method that is reproducible and prognostically valuable is still to be determined.[22,24,37,38] Assessment of the depth of invasion in lamina propria should be performed independently on the initial, and if available on the repeat TUR specimens; aggregate data during clinicopathologic correlation allow complete information regarding the depth of lamina propria for optimal management considerations.

TABLE 7.3 American Joint Committee on Cancer Staging System for Bladder Cancer, Eighth Edition (2017)

Primary tumor (T)[a]	
TX	Primary tumor cannot be assessed
T0	No evidence of primary tumor
Ta	Noninvasive papillary carcinoma
Tis	Urothelial CIS: "flat tumor"
T1	Tumor invades lamina propria (subepithelial connective tissue)
T2	Tumor invades muscularis propria
T2a	Tumor invades superficial muscularis propria (inner half)
T2b	Tumor invades deep muscularis propria (outer half)
T3	Tumor invades perivesicle tissue
T3a	Microscopically
T3b	Macroscopically (extravesicular mass)
T4	Tumor invades any of the following: prostatic stroma, seminal vesicles, uterus, vagina, pelvic wall, or abdominal wall
T4a	Tumor invades prostatic stroma, uterus, or vagina
T4b	Tumor invades pelvic wall or abdominal wall
Regional lymph nodes (N)	
Regional lymph nodes are those within the true pelvis; all others are distant nodes	
NX	Lymph nodes cannot be assessed
N0	No lymph node metastasis
N1	Single regional lymph node metastasis in the true pelvis (hypogastric, obturator, external iliac, or presacral lymph node)
N2	Multiple regional lymph node metastasis in the true pelvis (hypogastric, obturator, external iliac, or presacral lymph node)
N3	Lymph node metastasis to the common iliac lymph nodes
Distant metastasis (M)	
M0	No distant metastasis
M1	Distant metastasis
M1 a	Distant metastasis limited to lymph nodes below the common iliac
M1 b	No lymph node distant metastasis

[a]The suffix "m" should be added to the appropriate T category to indicate multiple tumors. The suffix "is" may be added to any T to indicate the presence of associated carcinoma *in situ*.

Used with permission of the American College of Surgeons. Urinary bladder. In: Amin MB, Edge SB, Greene FL, et al., eds. *AJCC Cancer Staging Manual*. 8th ed. Springer; 2017:757-766.

On transurethral resection specimens, substaging of the muscularis propria invasion cannot and should not be performed. This principle also applies for involvement of perivesicle fat. For muscularis propria–invasive tumors, the prognostic significance of tumors invading the inner half (pT2a) vs those invading the outer half is not that clear as some investigators report an overall similar outcome[24,39,40]; while others have found prognostic relevance. In a study of patients with pT2N0 disease, there was worse prognosis in pT2b patients over pT2a patients (5-year recurrence free survival: 85.9% vs 37.5%, 5-year cancer specific survival: 84.8% vs 59.6%). Furthermore, in this study, proportional hazards regression showed that pT2 substaging was the only independent risk factor of recurrence and cancer specific death.[41] Tumor size (largest tumor dimension) may also be a predictor of cancer-specific survival in these patients,[42] but there is subjectivity in measurement of this parameter. For tumors invading perivesicle soft tissue, subdivision into pT3a–microscopic extravesical invasion, vs pT3b–gross extravesical extension, is controversial, although studies suggest that grossly recognized tumor at margin is an adverse prognostic factor.[43,44] Chapter 5 outlines the diagnostic issues and problems related to interpretation of pT2 and pT3 disease in cystectomy specimens.

Lymph Node Involvement

Lymph node status after cystectomy is a critical prognostic factor as patients with regional spread of tumor (node positive) have a poor prognosis. Approximately 25% of patients (pre neoadjuvant therapy era) undergoing lymph node dissection at cystectomy have nodal metastasis. The 5-year recurrence-free survival of patients is 35%, and the 5-year overall survival is 31%. Immunohistochemical detection of micrometastasis has no established prognostic value.[45] The extent of lymphadenectomy, number of total lymph nodes removed (at least 15-20), and number of positive nodes and aggregate of metastatic lymph node diameter have been reported as predictors of outcome after radical cystectomy.[3,14,24,46,47] Extranodal extension has also shown to be a prognostic factor, though data on prognostic utility are inconsistent.

Involvement of Prostate Gland and Seminal Vesicles

The prostate ducts and acini and seminal vesicular epithelium may be involved by urothelial carcinoma extending along the luminal aspect (mucosal spread of CIS). When urothelial carcinoma involves the prostate as part of a multifocal process involving the prostatic urethra or prostatic ducts and acini, the AJCC staging system for "prostatic urethra" from the urethra staging system should be employed and not the staging system for the bladder.[48,49] Invasive bladder cancer present in the bladder should be separately staged using the "urinary bladder" staging system (Table 7.3).

Involvement of prostate by CIS of prostate ducts and acini predicts a high recurrence on a stage-adjusted basis but is not equivalent to pT4 disease of bladder cancer (direct invasion of bladder cancer into the prostate or seminal vesicles). Involvement of prostatic stroma from direct extension from a transmurally invasive bladder cancer indicates pT4 disease using the bladder staging system; it is associated with dismal prognosis.[48,50,51] When tumor invades the prostatic stroma secondary to urothelial carcinoma involving prostatic ducts and acini, the staging designation is pT2 using the urethra staging system (prostatic urethra section); the disease process is usually microscopic but portends a very poor prognosis.[3,48,52,53]

Histologic Type

It is important to specify if the invasive tumor in the bladder has conventional infiltrating urothelial carcinoma morphology (Chapter 5), the most common histology, seen in ~90% of cases, or whether it has mixed histology (divergent differentiation or with subtype morphology).[22,54,55] Management implications of histologic subtype of urothelial carcinoma vary from possible indication for early cystectomy, need and/or type of neoadjuvant or adjuvant chemotherapy, or immunotherapy, and prognostic risk stratification (see Chapter 6). It is also important to specify when an invasive carcinoma is a pure squamous cell carcinoma or adenocarcinoma. The prognostic impact of squamous differentiation and pure squamous cell carcinoma and glandular differentiation and pure adenocarcinoma is described in Chapters 8 and 9. In cases with mixed histologies of divergent differentiation or subtypes, it is important for the pathologist to report the differing histologies encountered in TURBT and cystectomy specimens, providing approximate percentages of the different components as a percentage of the total invasive carcinoma. Divergent differentiation/subtype morphology should be recorded both in transurethral resections and in radical cystectomy specimens, and any significant difference in the morphologic patterns seen between the two specimens for a particular patient should ideally be reconciled in the final cystectomy report.[22]

Histologic Grade

Once the tumor is invasive, the importance of histologic grade is extremely controversial and not shown to be of great value.[22,56,57] Our approach to grading invasive tumors and the issue of high grade vs the exceptionally rare low-grade invasive urothelial tumors with reporting recommendation is provided in Chapter 5.

Vascular-Lymphatic Invasion

Recent studies have reiterated the importance of this feature.[58,59] Initially, there was controversy regarding the significance of vascular-lymphatic invasion as retraction artifact around a tumor was often overdiagnosed as such. Unequivocal invasion into endothelium-lined spaces has been shown to be significant in univariate and multivariate analysis to correlate with increasing T classification, higher tumor grade, disease recurrence, and presence of lymph node metastasis; in node-negative patients, it has shown to correlate with overall survival.[58,60-63] In transurethral resection specimens, lymphovascular invasion is an important prognosticator and guides therapy.[59,64] The aggregate data support diligently evaluating for and reporting vascular-lymphatic invasion in TURBT and cystectomy specimens. Routine immunohistochemistry for its detection is not recommended.

Surgical Margin Status

Presence of invasive carcinoma at the resection margin (perivesicle soft tissue, vaginal cuff and urethral) is an adverse prognostic parameter, primarily for local recurrence.[65] The incidence of positive soft tissue margins in large series is ~4%, and this feature is associated with poor survival. In one study, the 5-year cancer-specific survival rates were 32% and 72% for those with and without positive margins.[66,67] No patient with positive margins survived 10 years.[24,68,69]

MULTIFOCALITY AND CARCINOMA *IN SITU* OF URETHRA OR URETERS

Patients with multifocal high-grade papillary or invasive tumors or multifocal CIS are at an increased risk for recurrence. Presence of CIS at the urethral margin at cystoprostatectomy is prognostically important and may be an indication for urethrectomy, although this remains controversial. Since many patients are offered a continent diversion at the time of cystectomy, it is common for the urethral margin to be submitted to frozen section analysis.[70] In patients with pT0 disease (ie, no residual cancer in the cystectomy specimen), the presence of CIS in the transurethral resection is an adverse prognostic factor. The number of tumors also has been shown to correlate with a higher risk of recurrence.[15] In analyses including all patients, concomitant CIS associated with ureteral involvement did not show significant differences in mortality or recurrence-free survival. On subanalysis of studies restricted to patients with organ confined bladder cancer at radical cystectomy, concomitant CIS was associated with worse recurrence-free survival and greater cancer-specific mortality.[24,70]

Other Factors: Tumor Location and Clinical Parameters

Tumor location (trigone, bladder neck, and prostatic urethra) has been associated with decreased survival.[70,71] Clinical features including increased age (>70 years) and female sex have been shown to have worse outcomes.[72] Delay in definitive surgical treatment from the time of diagnosis may have potential impact on survival.[14]

EMERGING PROGNOSTIC AND PREDICTIVE MOLECULAR MARKERS

There are several molecular and chromosomal markers (eg, loss of chromosome 9, loss of material on chromosome 17, p53, retinoblastoma tumor suppressor gene status, cell cycle regulation markers including p21 and cell adhesion, angiogenesis, and cell migration–related markers such as E-cadherin, vascular endothelial growth factor, etc.) that have been traditionally described in bladder cancer.[30,73,74] In recent years, tumor mutation burden, molecular subtypes, immune, mutational, or gene expression signatures have all been well studied with promising results as prognosticators or predictors of therapy. In Chapter 5, the section on "Pertinent emerging molecular aspects in diagnostic pathology" summarizes molecular markers that are variably employed at the clinical level in some practices.

Data from the Cancer Genome Atlas show that genetic alterations are common in bladder cancer and rank bladder cancer as the third highest mutated cancer.[75,76] APOBEC mutagenesis is dominant, particularly *APOBEC3*. The *ERCC2* mutations are the second most common mutational signature. *ERCC2* mutations (as well as other genes involved in DNA damage response and repair) are associated with improved response to cisplatin-based chemotherapy, immunotherapy, and radiation therapy for advanced urothelial carcinoma. The most identified clinically relevant genetic alterations from ~300 cases of advanced bladder cancer include cyclin-dependent kinase inhibitor 2A (CDKN2A, 34%), FGFR3 (21%), phosphatidylinositol 3-kinase catalytic subunit alpha (PIK3CA, 20%), and ERBB2 (17%).[77]

RNA expression profiling with some corroborative immunohistochemical protein expression has led to several molecular classification schemes with significant overlap. To simplify and unify the terminology for these subtypes from the different classification schema, a recent consensus clustering was proposed by the Bladder Cancer Molecular Taxonomy Group, based on re-analysis of the data from six independent classification systems on muscle invasive bladder cancer.[78] The molecular subtypes include luminal papillary, luminal nonspecified, luminal unstable, stroma rich, basal squamous, and neuroendocrine-like tumor classes. The consensus classification schema attempts to correlate different underlying oncogenic mechanisms, infiltration by immune and stromal cells, histologic characteristics, and clinical outcome between these molecular subtypes.

The genitourinary pathology society has recently summarized the role of molecular markers in the context of recommendations for diagnostic pathology.[22] They reiterate that morphologically distinct areas within a primary tumor, or between a primary tumor vs metastases, may demonstrate similar or different molecular subtypes. Due to lack of data or uncertainty of the optimal sample for molecular testing, it is currently not recommended to perform molecular subtyping, either by expression profiling or immunohistochemistry for the routine workup of bladder cancer

TABLE 7.4 Elements to be Included in Bladder Cancer Surgical Pathology Reports
Biopsy/transurethral resection
Essential
Histologic type (eg, urothelial, squamous cell and subtype and divergent morphology/subtype in urothelial carcinoma)
Histologic grade (WHO/ISUP for urothelial carcinoma)
Pathologic stage (T) (only Ta, T1, or T2)
- Extent of invasion in lamina propria invasive tumors
Presence or absence of muscularis propria
Presence or absence of urothelial carcinoma *in situ* (CIS)
Unequivocal vascular-lymphatic invasion
Optional
Configuration of tumor (eg, papillary, ulcerative, solid)
Urothelial dysplasia
Other benign or proliferative, inflammatory, or therapy-related changes
Cystoprostatectomy/anterior exenteration
Essential
Histologic type (eg, urothelial, squamous cell, adenocarcinoma, and subtype and divergent morphology in urothelial carcinoma)
Histologic grade (WHO/ISUP for urothelial carcinoma)
Pathologic stage (pT and pN status)–staging system for carcinoma of urinary bladder
Presence or absence of urothelial CIS
Tumor focality (single, multifocal)
Unequivocal vascular-lymphatic invasion
Involvement of prostate (AJCC staging system for prostatic urethra in urethral carcinoma staging)
Direct extension
Involvement of prostatic ducts and acini without stromal invasion
Involvement of prostatic ducts and acini with stromal invasion
Direct involvement of adjacent viscera (exenteration specimen)
Margins of excision for CIS (mention all negative and positive margins)
Margins of excision for invasive carcinoma (mention all negative and positive margins)
Optional
Location
Tumor size
Configuration of tumor (eg, papillary, flat, ulcerative, solid)
Urothelial dysplasia
Other benign or proliferative, inflammatory, or therapy-related changes

ISUP, International Society of Urological Pathology; WHO, World Health Organization; AJCC, American Joint Commission on Cancer.

samples. Until further data emerge, molecular classification may be determined either considering the individual case need or institutional or clinical trial protocols. In terms of recommendations for immunotherapy and PD-L1 testing, potential biomarkers of response to immune checkpoint inhibitors include PD-L1 status as assessed by immunohistochemistry, tumor mutation burden, molecular subtype, and immune cell gene signature. PD-L1 expression status by immunohistochemistry is the most used biomarker in urothelial carcinoma in the clinical setting, primarily due to its availability, applicability, and fast turnaround time. However, interpretation of PD-L1 is challenging due to variation in antibodies and their performance, staining methodology, tumor heterogeneity, and interobserver reproducibility. The European Urology guidelines state that there is insufficient evidence to use molecular markers in routine clinical practice.[79] Molecular genomic testing and molecular testing for immune checkpoint inhibitors (companion diagnostic testing or analysis for *FGFR3* or *FGFR2* genetic alterations) have been suggested for consideration in metastatic urothelial bladder cancer in the NCCN guidelines.[2]

REPORTING OF BLADDER CANCER

The elements that should be included in the surgical pathology report must have prognostic significance and should be important for patient management. Checklists for reporting bladder cancer have been developed by the College of American Pathologists, the Association of Directors of Anatomic and Surgical Pathology; standardized nomenclature for data to be reported and collected internationally has been advocated by the International Collaboration on Cancer Reporting (ICCR).[22,24,80-84] Table 7.4 summarizes the essential elements to be reported in biopsy and transurethral resection and in radical cystectomy and cystoprostatectomy specimens.

REFERENCES

1. Reuter VE. Bladder. Risk and prognostic factors–a pathologist's perspective. *Urol Clin North Am.* 1999;26(3):481-492.
2. National Comprehensive Cancer Network. *Bladder Cancer (version 2.2022).* Accessed November 23, 2022. https://www.nccn.org/guidelines/guidelines-process/transparency-process-and-recommendations/GetFileFromFileManager?fileManagerId=13485
3. Witjes JA, Bruins HM, Cathomas R, et al. European Association of Urology guidelines on muscle-invasive and metastatic bladder cancer: summary of the 2020 guidelines. *Eur Urol.* 2021;79(1):82-104.
4. Babjuk M, Burger M, Capoun O, et al. European Association of Urology guidelines on non-muscle-invasive bladder cancer (Ta, T1, and carcinoma in situ). *Eur Urol.* 2022;81(1):75-94.
5. Sylvester RJ, Rodríguez O, Hernández V, et al. European Association of Urology (EAU) prognostic factor risk groups for non-muscle-invasive bladder cancer (NMIBC) incorporating the WHO 2004/2016 and WHO 1973 classification systems for grade: an update from the EAU NMIBC Guidelines Panel. *Eur Urol.* 2021;79(4):480-488.
6. Chang SS, Boorjian SA, Chou R, et al. Diagnosis and treatment of non-muscle invasive bladder cancer: AUA/SUO guideline. *J Urol.* 2016;196(4):1021-1029.

7. Shariat SF, Karakiewicz PI, Palapattu GS, et al. Outcomes of radical cystectomy for transitional cell carcinoma of the bladder: a contemporary series from the Bladder Cancer Research Consortium. *J Urol.* 2006;176(6 Pt 1):2414-2422. discussion 2422.
8. Heney NM, Ahmed S, Flanagan MJ, et al. Superficial bladder cancer: progression and recurrence. *J Urol.* 1983;130(6):1083-1086.
9. Millán-Rodríguez F, Chéchile-Toniolo G, Salvador-Bayarri J, et al. Multivariate analysis of the prognostic factors of primary superficial bladder cancer. *J Urol.* 2000;163(1):73-78.
10. Isharwal S, Konety B. Non-muscle invasive bladder cancer risk stratification. *Indian J Urol.* 2015;31(4):289-296.
11. Busato Júnior WFS, Almeida GL, Ribas CAPM, et al. EORTC risk model to predict progression in patients with non-muscle-invasive bladder cancer: is it safe to use in clinical practice? *Clin Genitourin Cancer.* 2016;14(2):176-182.
12. Lutzeyer W, Rübben H, Dahm H. Prognostic parameters in superficial bladder cancer: an analysis of 315 cases. *J Urol.* 1982;127(2):250-252.
13. Millán-Rodríguez F, Chéchile-Toniolo G, Salvador-Bayarri J, et al. Upper urinary tract tumors after primary superficial bladder tumors: prognostic factors and risk groups. *J Urol.* 2000;164(4):1183-1187.
14. Youssef RF, Lotan Y. Predictors of outcome of non-muscle-invasive and muscle-invasive bladder cancer. *ScientificWorldJournal.* 2011;11:369-381.
15. Cambier S, Sylvester RJ, Collette L, et al. EORTC Nomograms and risk groups for predicting recurrence, progression, and disease-specific and overall survival in non-muscle-invasive stage Ta-T1 urothelial bladder cancer patients treated with 1-3 years of maintenance Bacillus Calmette-Guérin. *Eur Urol.* 2016;69(1):60-69.
16. Bono AV, Benvenuti C, Damiano G, Lovisolo J. Results of transurethral resection and intravesical doxorubicin prophylaxis in patients with T1G3 bladder cancer. *Urology.* 1994;44(3):329-334. discussion 334-335.
17. Nixon RG, Chang SS, Lafleur BJ, Smith JA, Cookson MS. Carcinoma in situ and tumor multifocality predict the risk of prostatic urethral involvement at radical cystectomy in men with transitional cell carcinoma of the bladder. *J Urol.* 2002;167(2 Pt 1):502-505.
18. Orozco RE, Martin AA, Murphy WM. Carcinoma in situ of the urinary bladder. Clues to host involvement in human carcinogenesis. *Cancer.* 1994;74(1):115-122.
19. Nese N, Gupta R, Bui MHT, Amin MB. Carcinoma in situ of the urinary bladder: review of clinicopathologic characteristics with an emphasis on aspects related to molecular diagnostic techniques and prognosis. *J Natl Compr Canc Netw.* 2009;7(1):48-57.
20. Librenjak D, Novaković ZS, Milostić K. Carcinoma in situ of urinary bladder: incidence, treatment and clinical outcomes during ten-year follow-up. *Acta Clin Croat.* 2012;51(2):201-207.
21. Paner GP, Stadler WM, Hansel DE, et al. Updates in the Eighth Edition of the tumor-node-metastasis staging classification for urologic cancers. *Eur Urol.* 2018;73(4):560-569.
22. Compérat E, Amin MB, Epstein JI, et al. The Genitourinary Pathology Society update on classification of variant histologies, T1 substaging, molecular taxonomy, and immunotherapy and PD-L1 testing implications of urothelial cancers. *Adv Anat Pathol.* 2021;28(4):196-208.
23. Amin MB, Edge SB, Greene FL, et al., eds. *AJCC Cancer Staging Manual.* 8th ed. Springer; 2017:757-766. Chapter 62.
24. Compérat E, Oszwald A, Wasinger G, et al. Updated pathology reporting standards for bladder cancer: biopsies, transurethral resections and radical cystectomies. *World J Urol.* 2022;40(4):915-927.
25. Pagano F, Bassi P, Galetti TP, et al. Results of contemporary radical cystectomy for invasive bladder cancer: a clinicopathological study with an emphasis on the inadequacy of the tumor, nodes and metastases classification. *J Urol.* 1991;145(1):45-50.
26. Richie JP, Skinner DG, Kaufman JJ. Radical cystectomy for carcinoma of the bladder: 16 years of experience. *J Urol.* 1975;113(2):186-189.

27. Stein JP, Lieskovsky G, Cote R, et al. Radical cystectomy in the treatment of invasive bladder cancer: long-term results in 1,054 patients. *J Clin Oncol.* 2001;19(3):666-675.
28. Giacalone NJ, Shipley WU, Clayman RH, et al. Long-term outcomes after bladder-preserving tri-modality therapy for patients with muscle-invasive bladder cancer: an updated analysis of the Massachusetts General Hospital Experience. *Eur Urol.* 2017;71(6):952-960.
29. Holmäng S, Hedelin H, Anderström C, et al. The importance of the depth of invasion in stage T1 bladder carcinoma: a prospective cohort study. *J Urol.* 1997;157(3):800-803. discussion 804.
30. Jimenez RE, Keane TE, Hardy HT, Amin MB. pT1 urothelial carcinoma of the bladder: criteria for diagnosis, pitfalls, and clinical implications. *Adv Anat Pathol.* 2000;7(1):13-25.
31. van Rhijn BWG, van der Kwast TH, Alkhateeb SS, et al. A new and highly prognostic system to discern T1 bladder cancer substage. *Eur Urol.* 2012;61(2):378-384.
32. Brimo F, Wu C, Zeizafoun N, et al. Prognostic factors in T1 bladder urothelial carcinoma: the value of recording millimetric depth of invasion, diameter of invasive carcinoma, and muscularis mucosa invasion. *Hum Pathol.* 2013;44(1):95-102.
33. Hu Z, Mudaliar K, Quek ML, et al. Measuring the dimension of invasive component in pT1 urothelial carcinoma in transurethral resection specimens can predict time to recurrence. *Ann Diagn Pathol.* 2014;18(2):49-52.
34. van Rhijn BWG, Liu L, Vis AN, et al. Prognostic value of molecular markers, sub-stage and European Organisation for the Research and Treatment of Cancer risk scores in primary T1 bladder cancer. *BJU Int.* 2012;110(8):1169-1176.
35. Younes M, Sussman J, True LD. The usefulness of the level of the muscularis mucosae in the staging of invasive transitional cell carcinoma of the urinary bladder. *Cancer.* 1990;66(3):543-548.
36. Chang WC, Chang YH, Pan CC. Prognostic significance in substaging of T1 urinary bladder urothelial carcinoma on transurethral resection. *Am J Surg Pathol.* 2012;36(3):454-461.
37. Asimakopoulos AD, Colalillo G, Telesca R, et al. T1 Bladder cancer: comparison of the prognostic impact of two substaging systems on disease recurrence and progression and suggestion of a novel nomogram. *Front Surg.* 2021;8:704902.
38. Kardoust Parizi M, Enikeev D, Glybochko PV, et al. Prognostic value of T1 substaging on oncological outcomes in patients with non-muscle-invasive bladder urothelial carcinoma: a systematic literature review and meta-analysis. *World J Urol.* 2020;38(6):1437-1449.
39. Girgin C, Sezer A, Delibaş M, et al. Impact of the level of muscle invasion in organ-confined bladder cancer. *Urol Int.* 2007;78(2):145-149.
40. Yu RJ, Stein JP, Cai J, et al. Superficial (pT2a) and deep (pT2b) muscle invasion in pathological staging of bladder cancer following radical cystectomy. *J Urol.* 2006;176(2):493-498. discussion 498-499.
41. Gakis G, Schilling D, Renninger M, et al. Comparison of the new American Joint Committee on Cancer substratification in node-negative pT2 urothelial carcinoma of the bladder: analysis of patient outcomes in a contemporary series. *BJU Int.* 2011;107(6):919-923.
42. Cheng L, Neumann RM, Scherer BG, et al. Tumor size predicts the survival of patients with pathologic stage T2 bladder carcinoma: a critical evaluation of the depth of muscle invasion. *Cancer.* 1999;85(12):2638-2647.
43. Quek ML, Stein JP, Clark PE, et al. Microscopic and gross extravesical extension in pathological staging of bladder cancer. *J Urol.* 2004;171(2 Pt 1):640-645.
44. Ananthanarayanan V, Pan Y, Tretiakova M, et al. Influence of histologic criteria and confounding factors in staging equivocal cases for microscopic perivesical tissue invasion (pT3a): an interobserver study among genitourinary pathologists. *Am J Surg Pathol.* 2014;38(2):167-175.
45. Yang XJ, Lecksell K, Epstein JI. Can immunohistochemistry enhance the detection of micrometastases in pelvic lymph nodes from patients with high-grade urothelial carcinoma of the bladder? *Am J Clin Pathol.* 1999;112(5):649-653.

46. Stephenson AJ, Gong MC, Campbell SC, et al. Aggregate lymph node metastasis diameter and survival after radical cystectomy for invasive bladder cancer. *Urology.* 2010;75(2):382-386.
47. Herr HW. Extent of pelvic lymph node dissection during radical cystectomy: where and why! *Eur Urol.* 2010;57(2):212-213.
48. Patel AR, Cohn JA, Abd El Latif A, et al. Validation of new AJCC exclusion criteria for subepithelial prostatic stromal invasion from pT4a bladder urothelial carcinoma. *J Urol.* 2013;189(1):53-58.
49. Wang G, McKenney JK. Urinary bladder pathology: World Health Organization classification and American Joint Committee on Cancer Staging Update. *Arch Pathol Lab Med.* 2019;143(5):571-577.
50. Esrig D, Freeman JA, Elmajian DA, et al. Transitional cell carcinoma involving the prostate with a proposed staging classification for stromal invasion. *J Urol.* 1996;156(3):1071-1076.
51. Ro JY, Ayala AG, el-Naggar A, Wishnow KI. Seminal vesicle involvement by in situ and invasive transitional cell carcinoma of the bladder. *Am J Surg Pathol.* 1987;11(12):951-958.
52. Sobin LH, Gospodarowicz MK, Wittekind C. International Union against Cancer. *TNM Classification of Malignant Tumours.* 7th ed. Wiley-Blackwell; 2009.
53. Oliva IV, Smith SL, Chen Z, Osunkoya AO. Urothelial carcinoma of the bladder with transmural and direct prostatic stromal invasion: does extent of stromal invasion significantly impact patient outcome? *Hum Pathol.* 2011;42(1):51-56.
54. Lobo N, Shariat SF, Guo CC, et al. What is the significance of variant histology in urothelial carcinoma? *Eur Urol Focus.* 2020;6(4):653-663.
55. Guo CC, Al-Ahmadie HA, Flaig TW, et al. Contribution of bladder cancer pathology assessment in planning clinical trials. *Urol Oncol.* 2021;39(10):713-719.
56. Amin MB, Smith SC, Reuter VE, et al. Update for the practicing pathologist: the International Consultation on Urologic Disease-European Association of Urology consultation on bladder cancer. *Mod Pathol.* 2015;28(5):612-630.
57. Jimenez RE, Gheiler E, Oskanian P, et al. Grading the invasive component of urothelial carcinoma of the bladder and its relationship with progression-free survival. *Am J Surg Pathol.* 2000;24(7):980-987.
58. Mari A, Kimura S, Foerster B, et al. A systematic review and meta-analysis of lymphovascular invasion in patients treated with radical cystectomy for bladder cancer. *Urol Oncol.* 2018;36(6):293-305.
59. Werntz RP, Smith ZL, Packiam VT, et al. The Impact of lymphovascular invasion on risk of upstaging and lymph node metastasis at the time of radical cystectomy. *Eur Urol Focus.* 2020;6(2):292-297.
60. Heney NM, Proppe K, Prout GR, et al. Invasive bladder cancer: tumor configuration, lymphatic invasion and survival. *J Urol.* 1983;130(5):895-897.
61. Shipley WU, Rose MA, Perrone TL, et al. Full-dose irradiation for patients with invasive bladder carcinoma: clinical and histological factors prognostic of improved survival. *J Urol.* 1985;134(4):679-683.
62. Quek ML, Stein JP, Nichols PW, et al. Prognostic significance of lymphovascular invasion of bladder cancer treated with radical cystectomy. *J Urol.* 2005;174(1):103-106.
63. Reuter VE. Lymphovascular invasion as an independent predictor of recurrence and survival in node-negative bladder cancer remains to be proven. *J Clin Oncol Off J Am Soc Clin Oncol.* 2005;23(27):6450-6451.
64. Cho KS, Seo HK, Joung JY, et al. Lymphovascular invasion in transurethral resection specimens as predictor of progression and metastasis in patients with newly diagnosed T1 bladder urothelial cancer. *J Urol.* 2009;182(6):2625-2630.
65. Neuzillet Y, Soulie M, Larre S, et al. Positive surgical margins and their locations in specimens are adverse prognosis features after radical cystectomy in non-metastatic carcinoma invading bladder muscle: results from a nationwide case-control study. *BJU Int.* 2013;111(8):1253-1260.

66. Cheng L, Montironi R, Davidson D, Lopez-Beltran A. Staging and reporting of urothelial carcinoma of the urinary bladder. *Mod Pathol.* 2009;22(suppl 2):S70-S95.
67. Cheng L, Weaver AL, Leibovich BC, et al. Predicting the survival of bladder carcinoma patients treated with radical cystectomy. *Cancer.* 2000;88(10):2326-2332.
68. Tilki D, Svatek RS, Karakiewicz PI, et al. Characteristics and outcomes of patients with pT4 urothelial carcinoma at radical cystectomy: a retrospective international study of 583 patients. *J Urol.* 2010;183(1):87-93.
69. Saint F, Masson-Lecomte A. Achieving disease free distal ureteral margin at the time of radical cystectomy: why and for whom? (An overview of literature). *Progres En Urol J Assoc Francaise Urol Soc Francaise Urol.* 2021;31(6):303-315.
70. Kimura S, Mari A, Foerster B, et al. Prognostic value of concomitant carcinoma in situ in the radical cystectomy specimen: a systematic review and meta-analysis. *J Urol.* 2019;201(1):46-53.
71. Dutta R, Abdelhalim A, Martin JW, et al. Effect of tumor location on survival in urinary bladder adenocarcinoma: a population-based analysis. *Urol Oncol.* 2016;34(12):531.e1-531.e6.
72. Kang M, Kim HS, Jeong CW, et al. Prognostic factors for conditional survival in patients with muscle-invasive urothelial carcinoma of the bladder treated with radical cystectomy. *Sci Rep.* 2015;5:12171.
73. Ehdaie B, Theodorescu D. Molecular markers in transitional cell carcinoma of the bladder: new insights into mechanisms and prognosis. *Indian J Urol.* 2008;24(1):61-67.
74. Têtu B. Diagnosis of urothelial carcinoma from urine. *Mod Pathol.* 2009;22(suppl 2): S53-S59.
75. Alexandrov LB, Nik-Zainal S, Wedge DC, et al. Signatures of mutational processes in human cancer. *Nature.* 2013;500(7463):415-421.
76. Cancer Genome Atlas Research Network. Comprehensive molecular characterization of urothelial bladder carcinoma. *Nature.* 2014;507(7492):315-322.
77. Ross JS, Wang K, Khaira D, et al. Comprehensive genomic profiling of 295 cases of clinically advanced urothelial carcinoma of the urinary bladder reveals a high frequency of clinically relevant genomic alterations. *Cancer.* 2016;122(5):702-711.
78. Kamoun A, de Reyniès A, Allory Y, et al. A consensus molecular classification of muscle-invasive bladder cancer. *Eur Urol.* 2020;77(4):420-433.
79. Compérat E, Amin MB, Cathomas R, et al. Current best practice for bladder cancer: a narrative review of diagnostics and treatments. *Lancet.* 2022;400(10364):1712-1721.
80. Amin MB, Srigley JR, Grignon DJ, et al. Updated protocol for the examination of specimens from patients with carcinoma of the urinary bladder, ureter, and renal pelvis. *Arch Pathol Lab Med.* 2003;127(10):1263-1279.
81. Murphy WM, Crissman JD, Johansson SL, Ayala AG. Recommendations for the reporting of urinary bladder specimens that contain bladder neoplasms. *Mod Pathol.* 1996;9(7):796-798.
82. Compérat E, Babjuk M, Algaba F, et al. SIU-ICUD on bladder cancer: pathology. *World J Urol.* 2019;37(1):41-50.
83. Compérat E, Srigley JR, Brimo F, et al. Dataset for the reporting of carcinoma of the bladder-cystectomy, cystoprostatectomy and diverticulectomy specimens: recommendations from the International Collaboration on Cancer Reporting (ICCR). *Virchows Arch Int J Pathol.* 2020;476(4):521-534.
84. College of American Pathologists. Cancer Protocol templates (internet). 2021. https://www.cap.org/protocols-and-guidelines/cancer-reporting-tools/cancer-protocol-templates

8

GLANDULAR LESIONS

CYSTITIS GLANDULARIS (INTESTINAL TYPE)

In some cases, the epithelial lining of Brunn nests and cystitis cystica undergo glandular metaplasia, giving rise to what is called cystitis glandularis.[1,2] The cells become cuboidal or columnar and mucin secreting, taking on the appearance of intestinal-type goblet cells. This variant is called cystitis glandularis with intestinal metaplasia (Figs. 8.1-8.4, eFigs. 8.1-8.19). The change may be focal or may diffusely replace the lining urothelium, both presenting as flat or minimally elevated or otherwise distorted mucosa. Some cases of intestinal metaplasia may be associated with abundant mucin extravasation and may present as symptomatic mass lesions. Although there is overlap between some examples of intestinal metaplasia and well-differentiated adenocarcinoma in some of the histological features (dissecting mucin, infiltration of muscularis propria, reactive atypia, and mitoses), the degree and extent of these findings differ between the two conditions.[3,4] In contrast to the extensive mucinous pools seen in some adenocarcinomas, florid intestinal metaplasia has only focal areas of mucin extravasation and is devoid of neoplastic cells within mucin pools. Whereas adenocarcinomas typically show extensive and deep muscularis propria invasion, intestinal metaplasia is usually confined to the lamina propria and muscularis propria involvement if present is typically limited and superficial (Fig. 8.5). Although rare bladder adenocarcinomas may show bland cytology, which in our experience often represent metastases from the pancreas, most will have areas of the tumor with overt cytological atypia. The atypia seen in intestinal metaplasia is negligible, and mitoses, although frequent in adenocarcinoma, are found only rarely in intestinal metaplasia. The cells lining the colonic-type glands are cytologically bland, while those seen in bladder adenocarcinoma are more akin to what is seen in intestinal-type or mucinous adenocarcinoma of the colon. Other less well-differentiated cases of adenocarcinoma may contain signet cells embedded in mucin and necrosis, findings that are not found in intestinal metaplasia. Long-term follow-up of cases of intestinal metaplasia has confirmed a benign behavior.[5] Exceptionally, isolated glands of

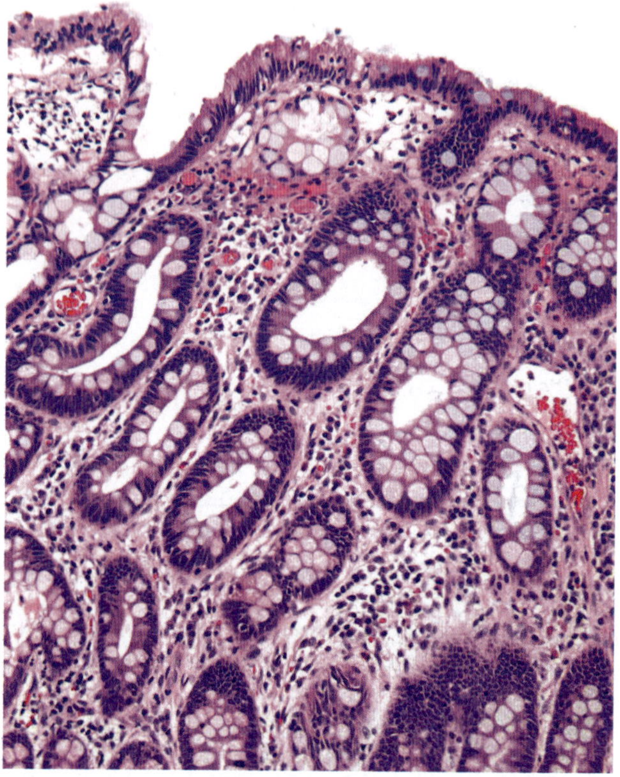

FIGURE 8.1 Cystitis glandularis, intestinal type.

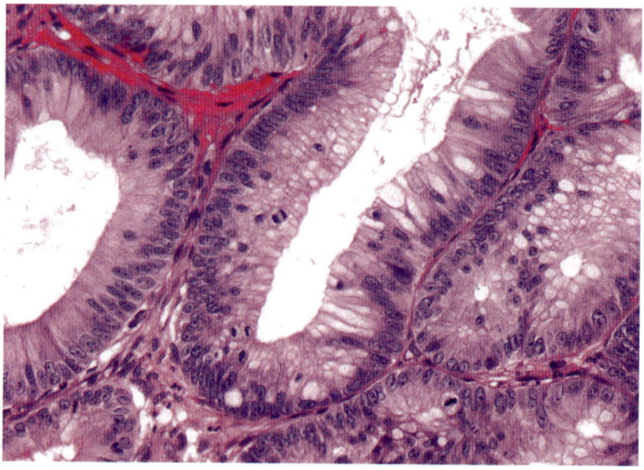

FIGURE 8.2 Cystitis glandularis, intestinal type with adenomatous changes.

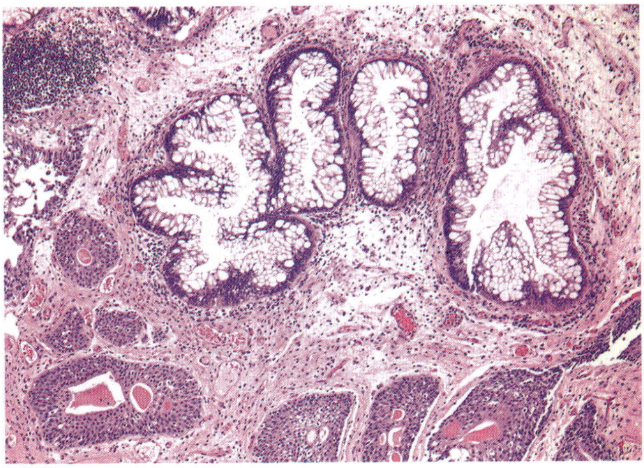

FIGURE 8.3 **Cystitis glandularis, intestinal type.** Note nonintestinal type cystitis cystica and glandularis (***bottom***).

intestinal metaplasia may show moderate dysplasia, in an analogous fashion to those seen in a colonic adenoma; the significance of this finding is unknown, although close follow-up is warranted (Fig. 8.6).[6] In this setting, if the lesion is extensive on the initial transurethral resection, it may be prudent to suggest that the area be re-resected. In a significant portion of cases, dysplasia may be present concurrent with adenocarcinoma.[6]

Glandular metaplasia may also occur within surface urothelium, usually as a response to chronic inflammation or irritation, such as in cases of bladder exstrophy.[7,8] The epithelium is composed of tall columnar cells with mucin-secreting goblet cells, strikingly similar to benign colonic or small intestinal epithelium in which one might identify even Paneth cells.

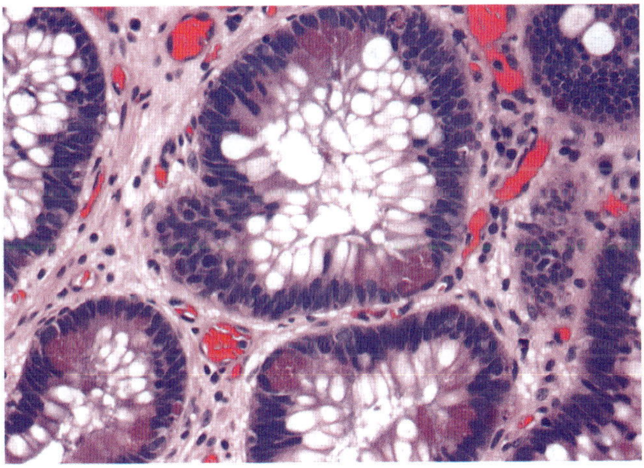

FIGURE 8.4 Cystitis glandularis, intestinal type with Paneth cell–like metaplasia.

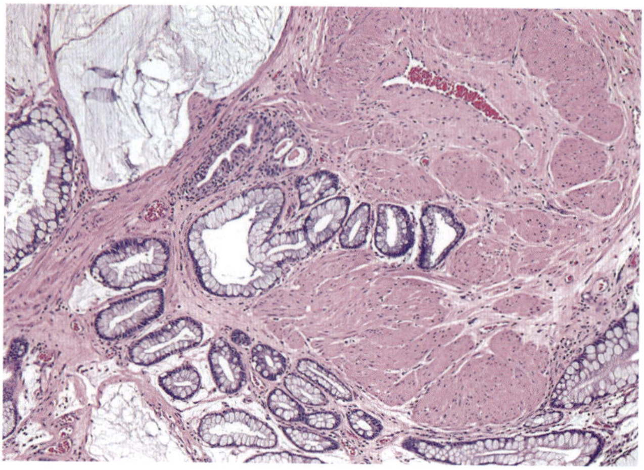

FIGURE 8.5 Cystitis glandularis, intestinal type with extracellular mucinous pools dissecting muscularis propria.

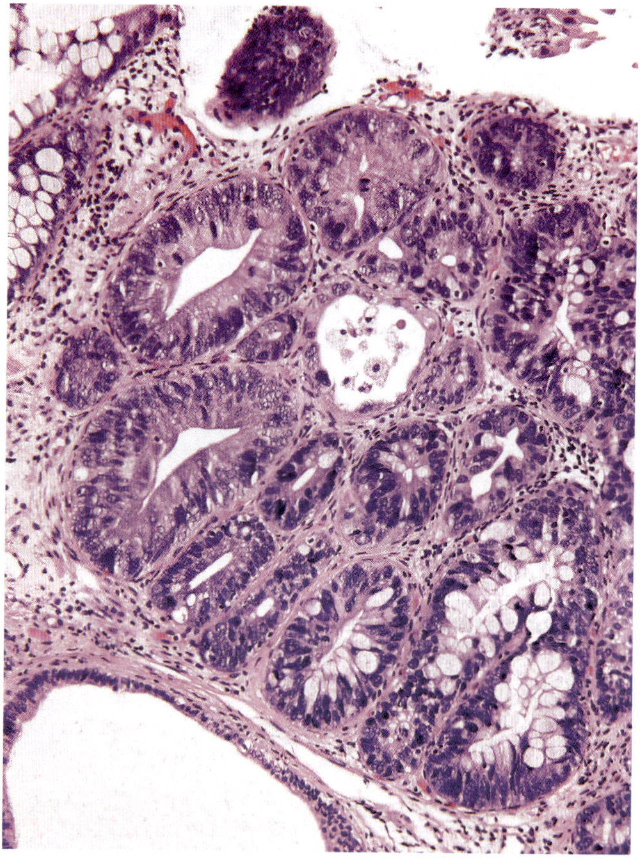

FIGURE 8.6 Cystitis glandularis, intestinal type with adenomatous change.

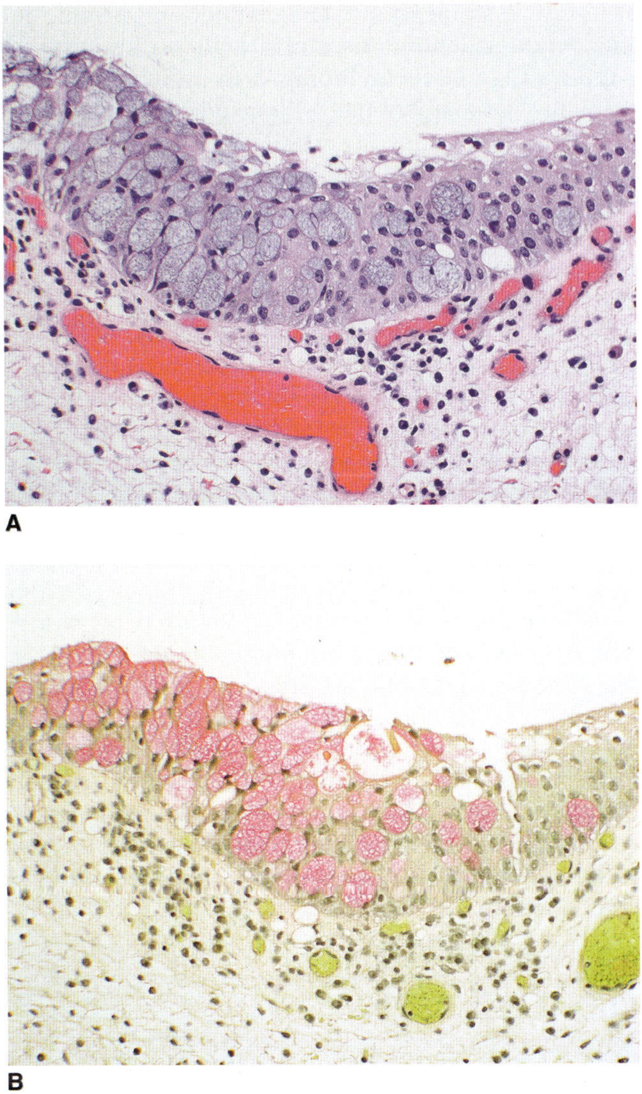

FIGURE 8.7 A: Mucinous metaplasia within surface urothelium. B: Mucicarmine stain.

Rarely will mucinous metaplasia occur within the surface urothelium in the absence glandular differentiation (Fig. 8.7A and B).

VILLOUS ADENOMA

The way to conceptualize glandular lesions occurring in the bladder and urethra is that they are analogous to glandular lesions seen in the intestinal tract both in term of types of lesion and their morphology. The full spectrum of lesions may be seen in the bladder and urethra including villous adenoma, villous adenoma with in situ adenocarcinoma, villous adenoma with infiltrating adenocarcinoma, and infiltrating adenocarcinoma unassociated with villous adenoma. Villous adenomas and adenocarcinomas in the bladder occur in one of several scenarios. They may arise within the urachus such that they are seen at the dome or anterior wall of the bladder, where they may present as a painful suprapubic mass. Another setting in which glandular lesions arise in the bladder or diverticulum is from a process of neometaplasia in which they may occur anywhere but typically near the trigone.

For both villous adenoma and adenocarcinoma of the bladder, there is a male predominance. Patients with villous adenoma or adenocarcinoma may either present with nonspecific findings or occasionally present with mucosuria. If the lesion is pure villous adenoma with or without in situ adenocarcinoma and the lesion is entirely resected, then the prognosis is excellent.[9-13] However, if the lesion has been only subtotally removed especially in the setting of coexistent *in situ* adenocarcinoma, the tumors have the potential to progress to infiltrating adenocarcinoma. As infiltrating adenocarcinoma is frequently present with villous adenoma, it necessitates thorough sampling of any lesion diagnosed by biopsy as villous adenoma. The diagnosis of villous adenoma should be reserved for cases in which the villous projections are lined by intestinal-type epithelium, which exhibits typical adenomatous features (Figs. 8.8-8.12, eFigs. 8.20-8.36). Nuclei may be enlarged and multilayered with abundant apically located cytoplasm. Mitoses are unapparent or few and regular. Cytologic and architectural features of intramucosal carcinoma are absent. Caution is warranted in making a diagnosis of villous adenoma in a small biopsy sample as a surface villous histology may be seen in villous adenoma as well as villous adenoma associated with adenocarcinoma in which the

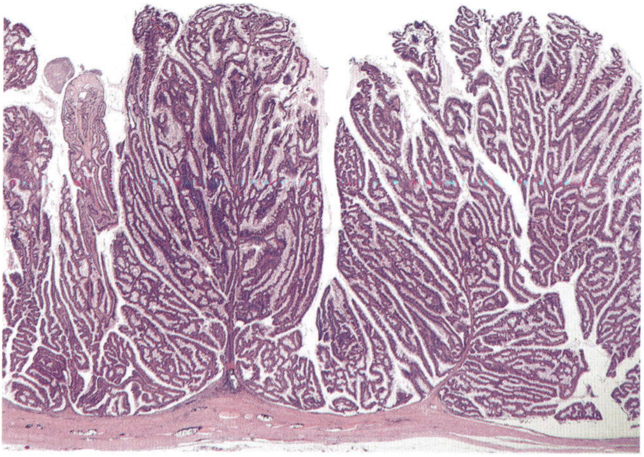

FIGURE 8.8 Villous adenoma.

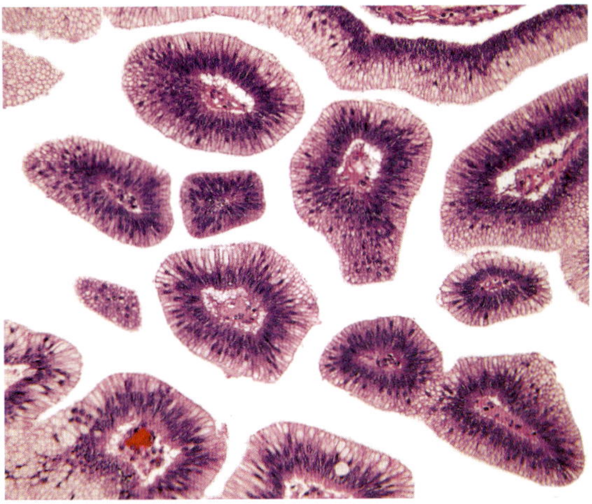

FIGURE 8.9 Higher magnification of villous adenoma.

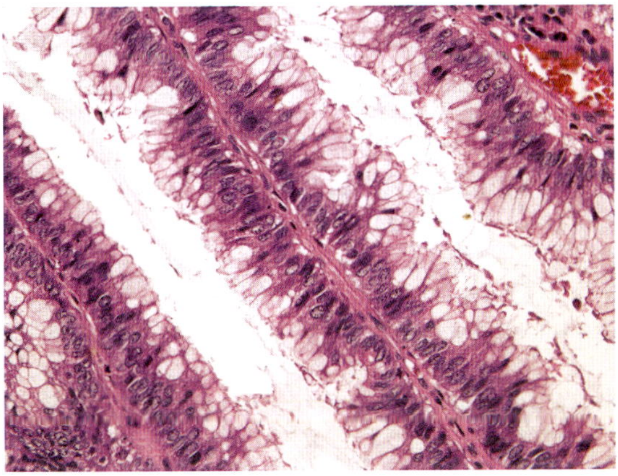

FIGURE 8.10 Villous adenoma.

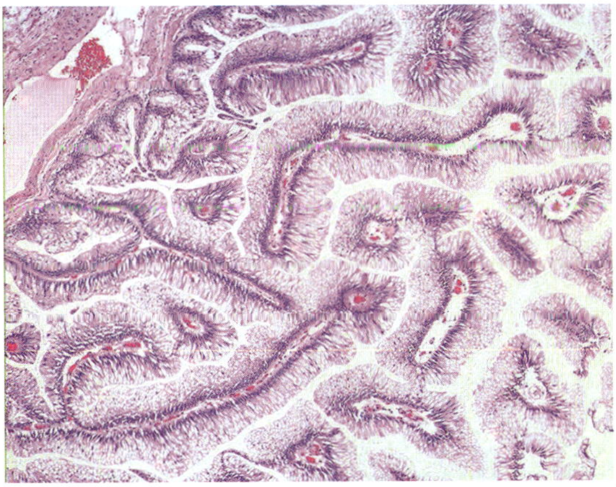

FIGURE 8.11 Villous adenoma.

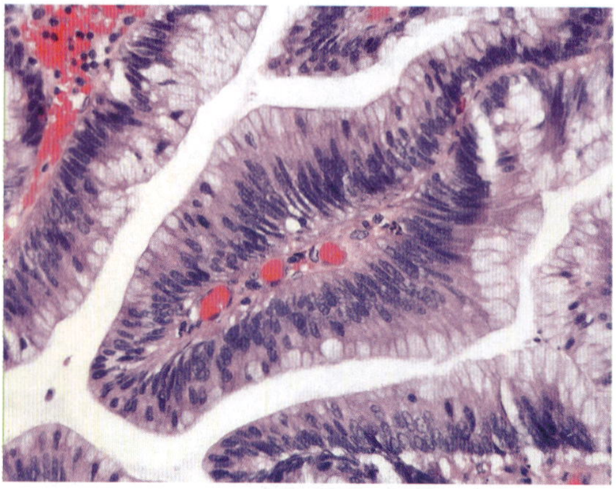

FIGURE 8.12 Villous adenoma.

latter is not sampled. Colonic/rectal adenocarcinomas can invade the bladder mimicking a primary villous adenoma of the bladder, especially on limited biopsy material. Therefore, it is prudent to include a comment in the pathology report that while the lesion is probably a primary villous adenoma of the bladder, spread from an intestinal neoplasm should be clinically excluded. Interestingly, adenocarcinomas of bladder and urachal origin have molecular signatures akin to those seen in colonic primaries with enrichment of *KRAS*, *TP53*, and *PIK3CA* alterations, whereas TERT promoter and FGFR3 mutations are rare.[14] Thus, performing next-generation sequencing of these samples to establish histogenesis may not be informative.

In addition to *in situ* or invasive adenocarcinoma, urinary tract villous adenomas have been found in association with squamous cell carcinoma, flat *in situ* urothelial carcinoma, noninvasive papillary urothelial carcinoma, infiltrating urothelial carcinoma, and sarcomatoid urothelial carcinoma of the bladder. Associated urothelial carcinoma elements are not always discrete from villous adenomas but often merge imperceptibly with them. These findings indicate that glandular lesions of the urothelium, whether benign or malignant, arise through a process of metaplasia/neometaplasia and are a manifestation of the morphologic plasticity of the urothelium.

CARCINOMA *IN SITU* (CIS) WITH GLANDULAR DIFFERENTIATION

Noninvasive papillary urothelial carcinomas may have glandlike lumina, a common finding that should not be confused with adenocarcinoma (Figs. 8.13 and 8.14). In other cases, the noninvasive component, whether

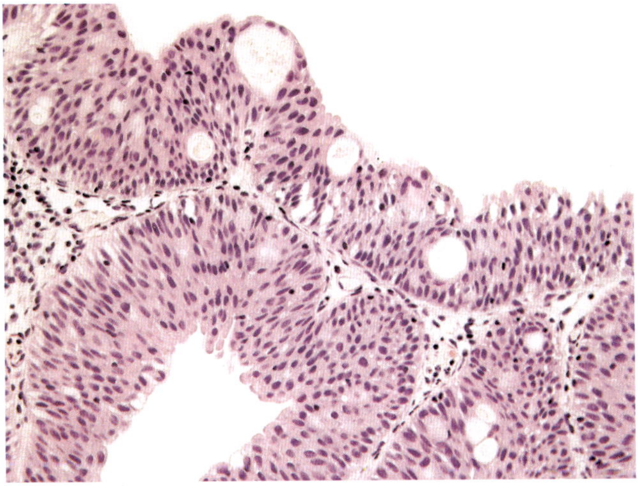

FIGURE 8.13 Noninvasive papillary urothelial carcinoma with glandlike lumina.

flat or papillary, may exhibit unequivocal glandular features (Figs. 8.15-8.19, eFigs. 8.37-8.54). Chan and Epstein described a series of 19 cases of noninvasive urothelial carcinomas with glandular differentiation (referred to as "*in situ* adenocarcinoma") of the bladder unaccompanied by infiltrating adenocarcinoma.[15] In fact, the invasive component, when present, was likely to be urothelial carcinoma of the usual type. These lesions are best referred to as *CIS with glandular differentiation*. CIS with glandular differentiation has a high incidence of association with usual CIS and specific subtypes of prognostically poor invasive carcinomas, such as small cell and

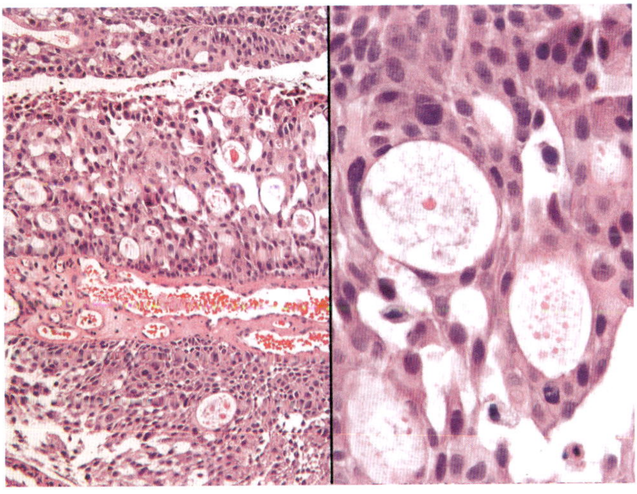

FIGURE 8.14 Noninvasive papillary urothelial carcinoma with glandlike lumina (higher magnification [right]).

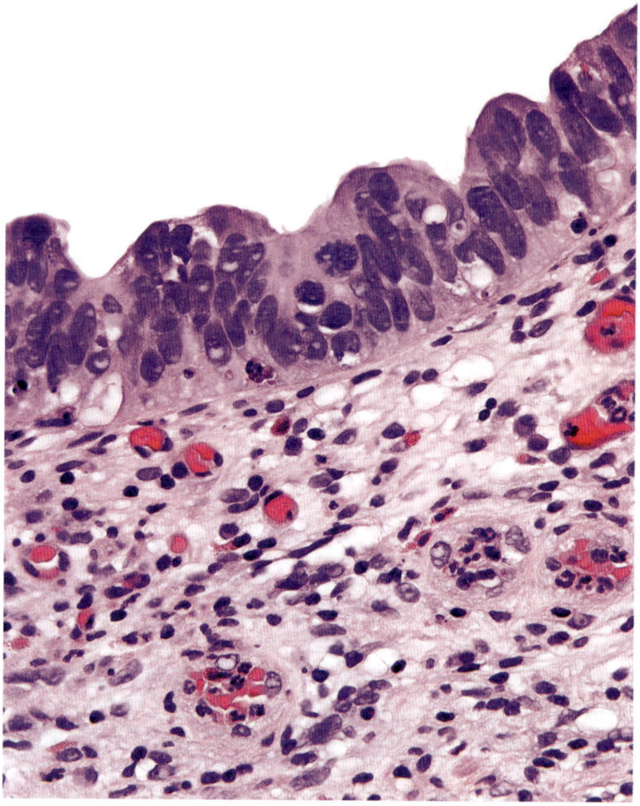

FIGURE 8.15 CIS with glandular differentiation, flat pattern.

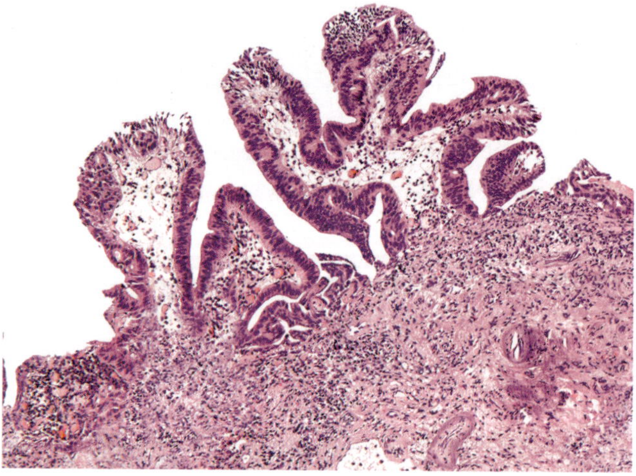

FIGURE 8.16 CIS with glandular differentiation, papillary pattern composed of simple and branching fronds.

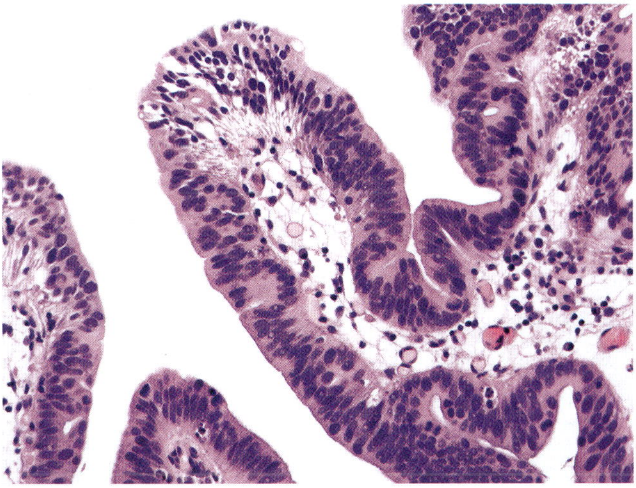

FIGURE 8.17 **Higher magnification of Figure 8.16 shows glandular differentiation with columnar nuclei and apical cytoplasm.** The nuclei still retain some of the features of CIS cells (ie, hyperchromatic enlarged cells without prominent nucleoli).

micropapillary urothelial carcinoma. In a more recent larger study from the same group, CIS with glandular differentiation consisted of one or more patterns, including papillary, glandular, cribriform, and flat. Half of the cases were associated with usual CIS or high-grade papillary urothelial carcinoma. Of those cases that subsequently progressed to invasion, none did so as adenocarcinoma but rather as small cell carcinoma or poorly differentiated urothelial carcinoma.[16] These data confirm that this disease is a morphologic variant of urothelial carcinoma *in situ* and that divergent

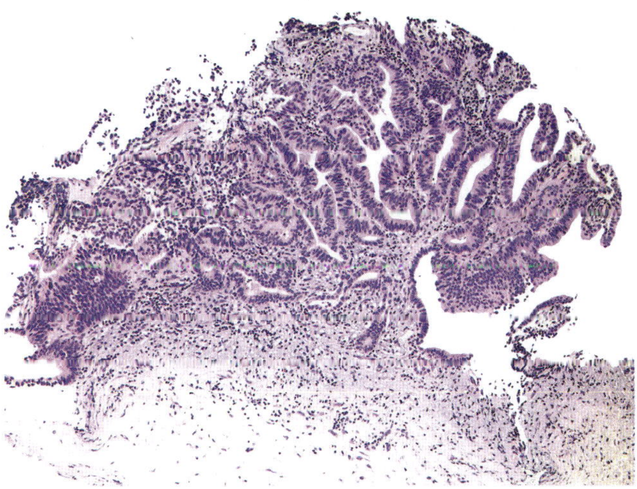

FIGURE 8.18 **CIS with glandular differentiation, complex papillary pattern.**

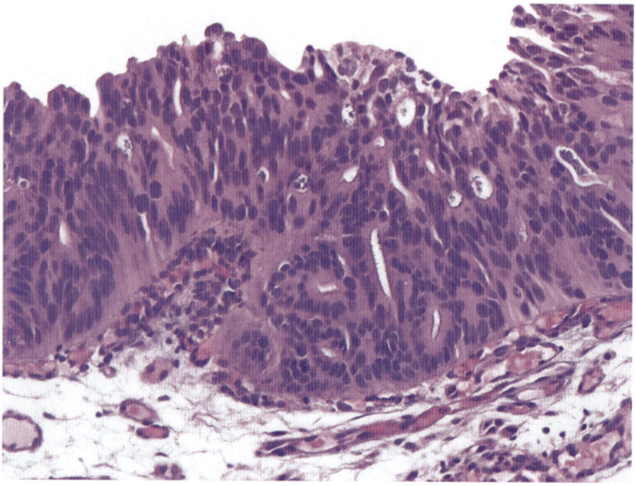

FIGURE 8.19 CIS with glandular differentiation, cribriform pattern.

differentiation in urothelial carcinoma, whether invasive or not, is usually associated with aggressive clinical behavior. The only situation where the term "adenocarcinoma *in situ*" is used is when associated with intestinal metaplasia or a villous adenoma. Otherwise, precursor glandular lesions with atypia should be referred to as either noninvasive papillary urothelial carcinoma or CIS with glandular differentiation. Occasionally, the flat mucosa of CIS may show a micropapillary architecture (this pattern has no prognostic significance or association with micropapillary urothelial carcinoma).

INFILTRATING ADENOCARCINOMA

Primary pure adenocarcinomas of the bladder are rare, representing no more than 2.5% of all malignant vesical neoplasms. By definition, the tumor should be composed entirely, or virtually entirely, of glandular elements. With the exception of the extremely rare examples of adenocarcinomas that arise from müllerian or mesonephric remnants located within the wall of the urinary bladder, they arise through a process of divergent differentiation in urothelial carcinoma.[17-24] They constitute up to 90% of carcinomas associated with bladder exstrophy. The tumor is also more frequently encountered in a setting of schistosomiasis. Shaaban et al.[25] and el-Mekresh et al.[26] reported series of 93 and 185 cases, respectively, of vesical adenocarcinoma arising in this setting. Adenocarcinomas can arise anywhere on the bladder surface, although a large percentage originates from the trigone and posterior wall. A major clinical difference as compared to usual urothelial carcinomas is that two-thirds of adenocarcinomas are single discrete lesions, while "usual" urothelial carcinoma tend to be multifocal.[27,28] Grossly, the tumors can be papillary, nodular, or

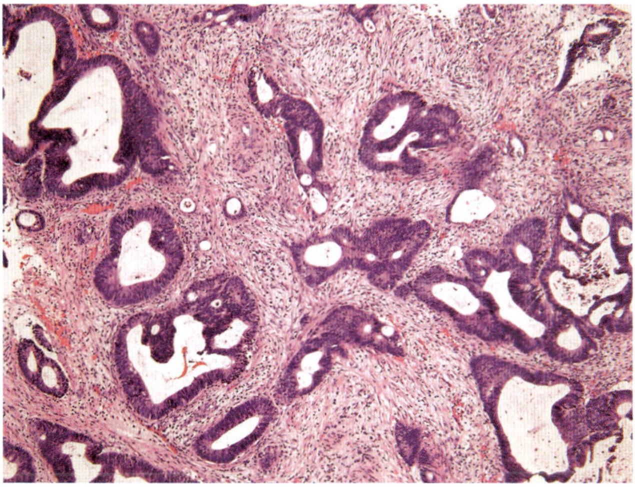

FIGURE 8.20 Infiltrating adenocarcinoma, enteric type.

flat and ulcerated. Microscopically, the tumor is most often composed of colonic-type glandular epithelium (enteric morphology) and often contains abundant extracellular mucin (Figs. 8.20-8.22, eFigs. 8.55-8.68). However, some tumors are very cellular, cytologically less well differentiated, and do not contain extracellular mucin. We have seen rare examples with hepatoid or even yolk sac differentiation, the latter associated with serum elevation of alpha-fetoprotein (Fig. 8.23). Regardless of the histologic pattern, cystitis cystica et glandularis or surface glandular metaplasia is commonly present in the adjacent benign urothelium. Rarely, they may be associated with villous adenoma of the bladder. Most adenocarci-

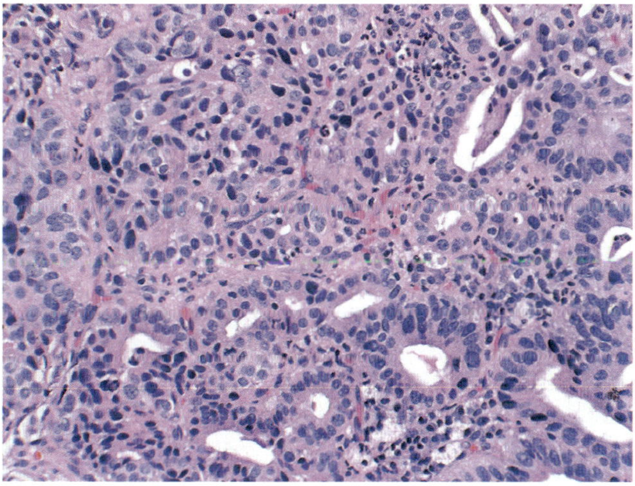

FIGURE 8.21 Infiltrating adenocarcinoma, NOS pattern.

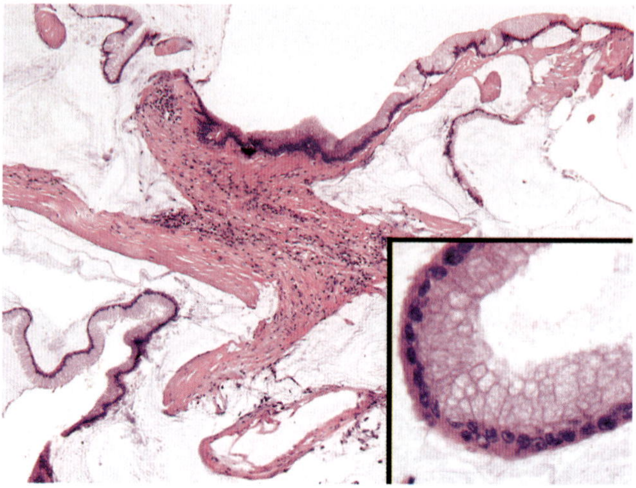

FIGURE 8.22 **Infiltrating adenocarcinoma, colloid type, with abundant extracellular mucinous secretions.** Note relatively bland cytology (***inset***).

nomas have infiltrated deeply at the time of initial diagnosis and are associated with a poor prognosis. Recent data suggest that, in its pure form, adenocarcinoma arising in the bladder has a worse prognosis than usual urothelial carcinoma even after adjusting for pathologic stage, lymph node status, and the presence of lymphovascular invasion.[29] Whether this finding is due to the fact that adenocarcinoma differentiation is resistant to systemic therapies directed at usual urothelial carcinoma remains to be proven. However, what has been well established is that tumors with mixed histologic features that include glandular differentiation have similar clinical outcome than pure urothelial carcinoma, when stratified by pathologic stage.[30-32]

In the differential diagnosis, one must first consider the possibility of secondary adenocarcinoma involving the bladder either by metastasis or by direct invasion. Theoretically, it should be important to identify in situ carcinoma, although this is rarely possible on TUR specimens due to ulceration of the overlying urothelium or to incomplete sampling. Furthermore, secondary tumors such as colonic adenocarcinoma with invasion of the bladder wall may colonize the urothelium, mimicking *in situ* disease. Tumors that directly invade the bladder and mimic primary vesical adenocarcinoma include those arising in the rectum, prostate, appendix, and endometrium.[27,28,33] The only unequivocal way to establish such a tumor as a primary vesical neoplasm is to see a transition to usual urothelial carcinoma. For this reason, we have routinely added the following disclaimer to our pathology report of the biopsy specimen... "*we would accept as primary at this site if a metastasis or direct extension from an adjacent organ can be ruled out clinically.*" The treating clinician is in the best position to evaluate the patient and consider other primary sites. Rarely prostatic

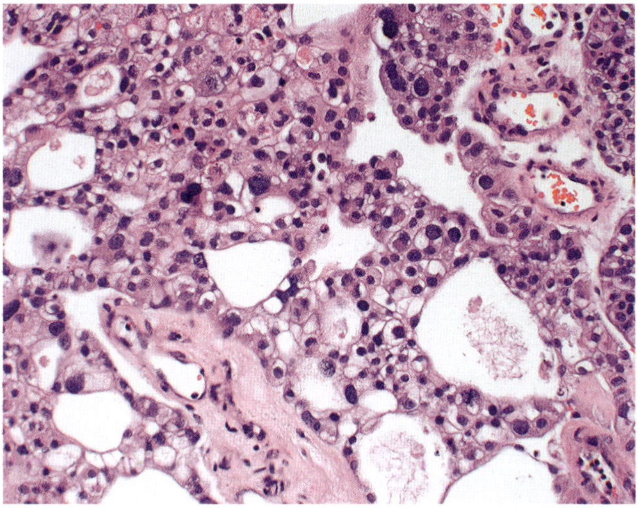

A

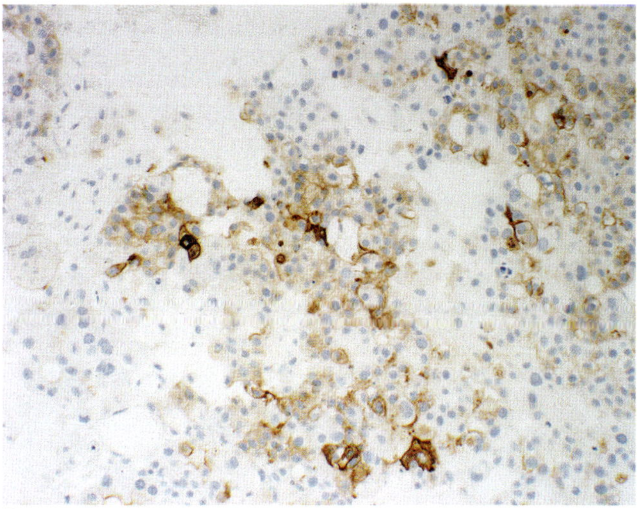

B

FIGURE 8.23 A: Adenocarcinoma with yolk sac differentiation. B: Glypican 3 immunohistochemical stain.

ductal carcinomas may secondarily involve the bladder and mimic a primary carcinoma.

Urothelial carcinomas may also be associated with abundant myxoid stroma mimicking a primary or secondary adenocarcinoma.[34] In urothelial carcinoma with myxoid stroma, the infiltrating component has urothelial rather than glandular features, and the tumor cells consists of cords and nests of cells embedded in a myxoid stroma, which is positive for

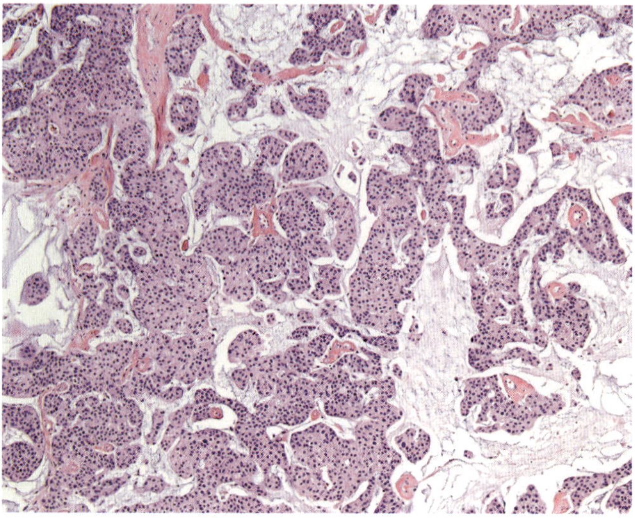

FIGURE 8.24 Small- and medium-sized nests of invasive urothelial carcinoma admixed with extracellular myxoid matrix.

mucicarmine, periodic acid-Schiff (PAS), and Alcian blue with and without hyaluronidase (Figs. 8.24 and 8.25). Infiltrating urothelial carcinoma with glandlike lumina should also be distinguished from adenocarcinoma (Fig. 8.26).

Immunohistochemistry may aid in establishing primary site.[35-39] Urothelial carcinoma of the usual type is likely to express CK7 and CK20 as well as 34βE12, p63 (clone 4A4), GATA3, and thrombomodulin. Carcinomas with glandular differentiation are quite likely to lose expression of some or all of these markers with the exception of CK20. In addition,

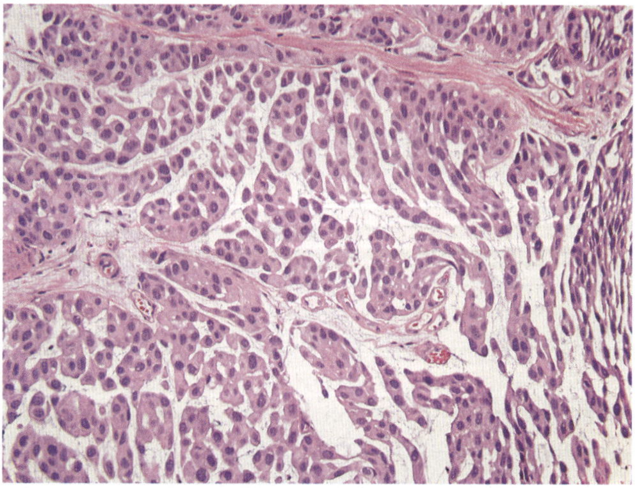

FIGURE 8.25 Cords of invasive urothelial carcinoma admixed with myxoid stroma.

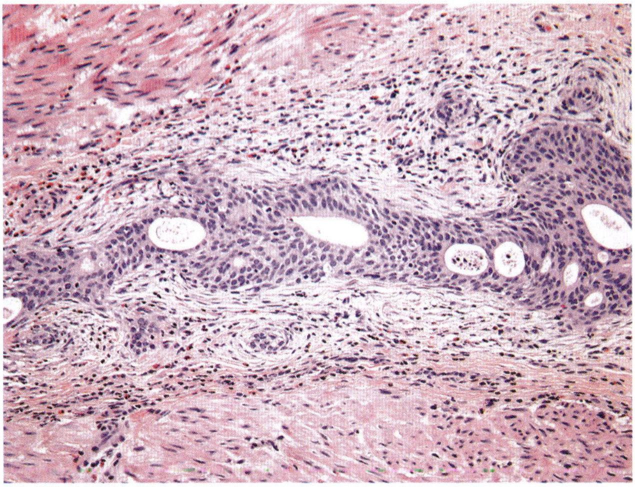

FIGURE 8.26 Invasive urothelial carcinoma with glandlike lumina.

they are likely to neoexpress CDX2 and β-catenin, the latter in a cytoplasmic rather than a nuclear distribution. In contrast, colonic adenocarcinoma will usually express CK20 diffusely but not CK7. β-Catenin is usually expressed in a nuclear distribution, and thrombomodulin is universally negative. SATB2 is not helpful as it is frequently present in primary adenocarcinomas of colon and of the bladder. Immunohistochemistry for CEA and villin is not useful in solving this differential diagnosis. Coexpression of CK7 and GATA3 in combination with lack of nuclear β-catenin immunoreactivity strongly favors urothelial over colonic origin.[40] Uroplakin III is a highly sensitive maker for urothelial origin but suffers from low sensitivity. A recently described monoclonal antibody directed to uroplakin II is said to be more sensitive yet retain a similar level of specificity.[41,42] However, in our experience, this marker is rarely useful when you need it most; poorly differentiated and metastatic disease.

Plasmacytoid (including signet-ring cell carcinoma of the bladder without mucin extravasation) is a rare subtypes of urothelial carcinoma[43-47] (Figs. 8.27-8.30, eFigs. 8.69-8.78). It is not uncommon to see signet ring cells within mucinous carcinomas, but we reserve the term signet-ring cell carcinoma for those tumors composed almost entirely of signet ring cells with intracytoplasmic mucin including those with a minor component of cells cytologically similar to mammary lobular carcinoma.

Contemporary thinking suggests that signet ring cell, plasmacytoid, lobularlike carcinoma, and rhabdoid variants of urothelial carcinoma are belonging to the same spectrum of tumors and are likely to represent the same disease. In fact, virtually, all cases of signet-ring cell carcinoma contain a variable (and sometimes predominant) number of cells with plasmacytoid, rhabdoidlike, or lobularlike features, while occasional signet ring cells may be present in both plasmacytoid and rhabdoidlike variants

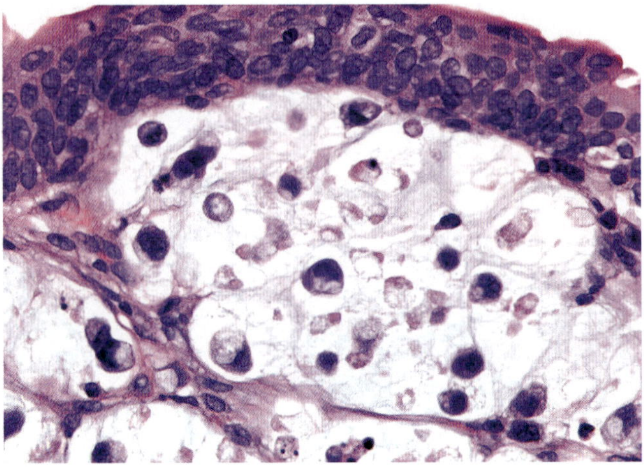

FIGURE 8.27 Adenocarcinoma of the bladder with extracellular mucin-containing signet ring cells.

of urothelial carcinoma. Other shared features of these loosely cohesive tumors include a diffuse pattern of infiltration, advanced stage at presentation, poor clinical outcome, and shared molecular abnormalities.[48-52]

Confirming origin in the bladder by finding carcinoma in situ may be very difficult, particularly on biopsy specimens. It is not unusual to find a dense layer of signet ring cells within the lamina propria directly below a denuded basement membrane (so-called cambium layer). These tumors tend to infiltrate the bladder wall diffusely giving it an indurated and thickened quality similar to the "linitis plastica" seen in gastric signet-ring cell

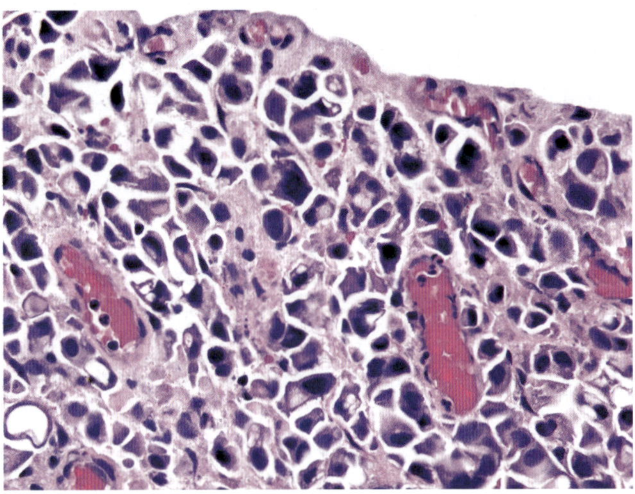

FIGURE 8.28 Adenocarcinoma of the bladder, signet-ring cell type (some poorly differentiated cells show plasmacytoid features).

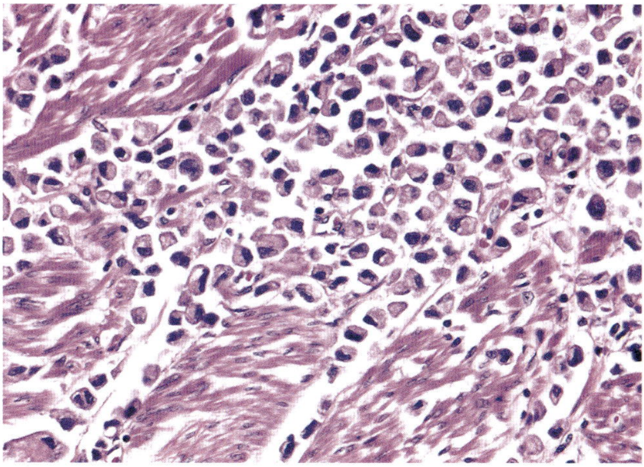

FIGURE 8.29 Adenocarcinoma of the bladder, signet-ring cell type infiltrating muscularis propria (some poorly differentiated cells show plasmacytoid features).

carcinomas. The tumor also commonly infiltrates extensively throughout adjacent soft tissue, making primary resection for cure virtually impossible. Because of their advanced stage at presentation and poor prognosis, it is important to make the diagnosis on the TUR specimen, if at all possible.[51,53] In the differential diagnosis, one must rule out direct extension, usually from a rectal carcinoma, or metastasis from the stomach or lobular carcinoma of the breast, or other organs.[54] Prostate carcinomas with a similar morphology are with rare exception composed of signet-ring–like cells with empty clear vacuoles, which do not usually stain for mucin.

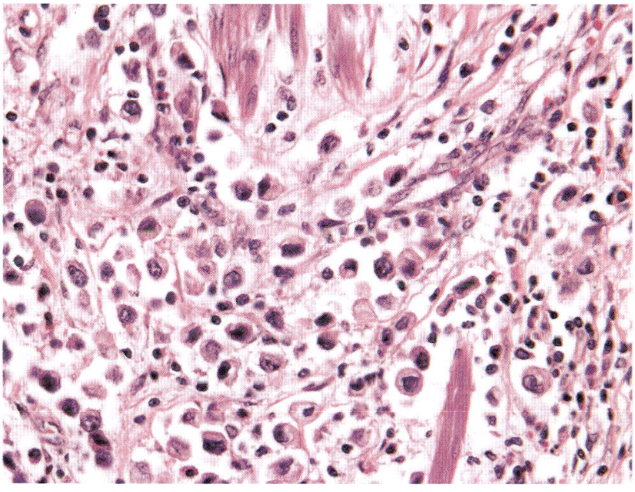

FIGURE 8.30 Adenocarcinoma of the bladder, signet-ring cell type (some poorly differentiated cells show plasmacytoid features).

Mucinous adenocarcinomas of the prostate typically reveal cords of epithelium and cribriform glands with bland cytology floating in mucin[55,56] (see Chapter 13).

URACHAL CARCINOMA

The urachus is a thick tubelike structure, which is formed in the embryo as the allantois involutes (eFigs. 8.51 and 8.52). It extends from the bladder dome to the umbilicus. After birth, it becomes a fibrous cord called the median umbilical ligament. If remnants of the allantois (endoderm) remain within the ligament, they may develop into cysts as well as epithelial neoplasms. Such remnants have been found in 25%-35% of bladders at the time of autopsy, usually in the dome but also along the anterior and rarely along the posterior bladder wall.[57] The epithelial lining usually is urothelial, but in 33% of cases, it will have undergone glandular metaplasia (Figs. 8.31 and 8.32). Neoplasms arising from the urachal remnant are usually adenocarcinomas, and they account for as much as 22%-35% of vesical glandular neoplasms.[58,59] Most adenocarcinomas have enteric features and are mucinous; some may have a papillary or signet-ring cell component.[60,61] Squamous cell, "usual" urothelial carcinomas, and anaplastic carcinomas also arise from the urachus.[62] Rare cases of villous adenomas of the urachus have been reported, sometimes associated with mucosuria, suggesting communication with the bladder lumen.[63] As previously stated, it is interesting that urachal adenocarcinoma, similar to those that arise in the bladder, are characterized by mutations commonly seen in colonic primaries rather than those that are characteristic of urothelial carcinoma,[14] despite the fact that they arise from the surface epithelium at these sites.

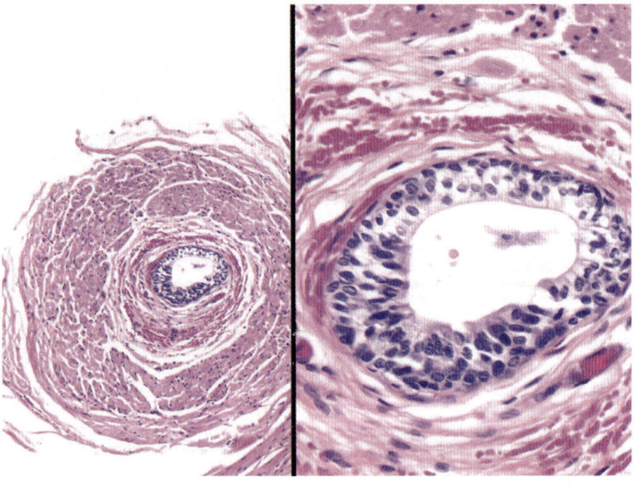

FIGURE 8.31 Urachal remnant lined by normal urothelium (higher magnification [right]).

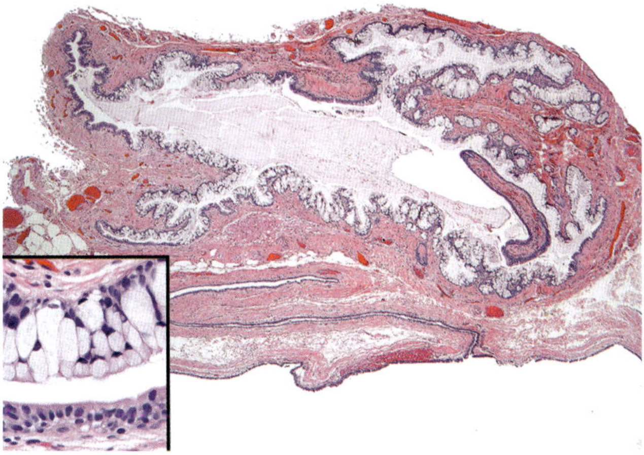

FIGURE 8.32 **Dilated urachal remnant replaced by glandular metaplasia.** *Inset* shows part of urachal remnant lined by urothelium (*bottom*) with most lined by intestinal epithelium with goblet cells.

Because the urachus is usually found along the free surface of the bladder, urachal carcinomas are frequently amenable to partial cystectomy. Since the entire length of the median umbilical ligament may harbor urachal remnants, which may develop carcinoma synchronously or metachronously, the surgery of choice should include *en bloc* resection of the entire length of the ligament including the umbilicus.[64,65] The bladder is usually only partially resected owing to the unifocality of the tumor. However, complete excision with negative margins is mandatory since local recurrence is a common complication. The most important prognostic factor is pathologic stage at the time of surgery.[61,65-67] Given the fact that urachal carcinomas may arise within urachal remnants in the bladder wall or in perivesical soft tissue along the dome of the bladder, staging of urachal carcinoma differs from those that arise from the bladder surface, the most common staging system used being that proposed by Sheldon,[61,66,67] although a staging system proposed by investigators at the Mayo Clinic is also useful in predicting outcome.[68] Complete resection and negative margins are other important prognostic factors.

While most glandular neoplasms of the urachus are invasive adenocarcinoma, there is a subset of tumors with a predominant mucinous and cystic morphology resembling mucinous tumors of the ovary. There are several criteria that must be met to establish the diagnosis of urachal carcinoma. The bladder involvement by tumor should be localized to an area usually at or near the dome, in relation to the medial umbilical ligament. The overlying bladder urothelium may be ulcerated but no in situ carcinoma or glandular metaplasia should be present (other than cystitis glandularis). Very often, this issue is difficult to address because the overlying epithelium is ulcerated or previously biopsied. Rarely will the urachal tumor communicate directly with bladder surface. Occasionally, urachal remnants will be found, characterized by cystic structures of variable size lined by urothelium or benign glandular epithelium. A metastatic tumor should be ruled out clinically.

The differential diagnosis includes metastatic adenocarcinoma and primary adenocarcinoma arising from the bladder surface. The latter is usually associated with an intraluminal mass, and the diagnosis is established by finding *in situ* carcinoma or extensive glandular metaplasia of the adjacent urothelium. Since these features are rarely seen on a TURBT specimen of an ulcerated lesion, we include the following note in the pathology report of any solitary glandular lesion involving the dome of the bladder; "*we would accept as primary at this site, including the possibility of urachal origin, if a metastasis or direct extension from an adjacent organ has been ruled out.*" Immunohistochemistry may help in the differential diagnosis since these tumors rarely express nuclear immunoreactivity for β-catenin, whereas most will express markers commonly seen in tumors of urothelial origin such as CK7, 34βE12, etc.[61] Urachal tumors are similar to primary adenocarcinomas of the bladder in their immunohistochemical profile. CK7, CDX2, and SATB2 may be positive; occasionally, CK20 is positive. Lack of TERT mutations and presence of RAS mutations favor urachal over primary bladder carcinoma.[69,70]

Ultimately, the urologist is in the best position to make the determination as to whether the adenocarcinoma is primary to the bladder or spread from another site.

Mucinous cystic neoplasms of the urachus are distinctly rare and only one large series has been reported.[68] Due to the resemblance of these tumors to those occurring in the ovary, the authors have used nomenclature similar to that for ovarian mucinous cystic neoplasms (mucinous cystadenoma, mucinous cystic tumor of low malignant potential, with intraepithelial carcinoma, and with microscopic or frank invasion).[71] An alternative is to use terminology used for mucinous cystic tumors seen in the appendix. Mucinous cystadenomas may be associated with extravasated mucin, but if the mucin is acellular, then the lesion is still benign (Fig. 8.33). The entire category of mucinous cystic neoplasms of the urachus that are not associated with frank invasion have a favorable prognosis.

CARCINOMAS WITH DIVERGENT DIFFERENTIATION

Urothelial carcinomas, particularly high-grade tumors, may show divergent differentiation (Figs. 8.34 and 8.35, eFigs. 8.79 and 8.80). This feature is seen primarily in invasive tumors but may occasionally be present with in situ disease. The entire spectrum of histologic variants may be encountered accompanying "usual" invasive urothelial carcinoma, mostly in cases

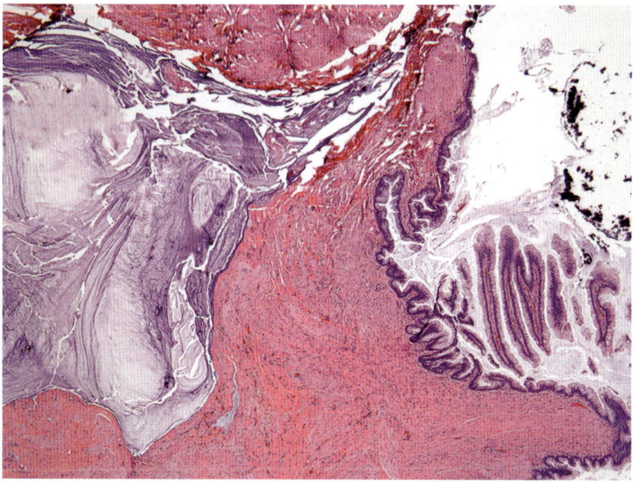

FIGURE 8.33 Mucinous cystadenoma of the urachus with mucin extravasation.

of high-grade and high-stage disease, including squamous, glandular, small cell, and sarcomatoid differentiation, among others. In a series of bladder carcinomas from the Memorial Sloan-Kettering Cancer Center (MSKCC), some form of divergent differentiation was seen in 27% of cystectomy specimens.[30] On pathologic re-review, a similar percentage of cases were found to have divergent differentiation at the Mayo Clinic.[32] The incidence of divergent differentiation on transurethral resection is lower, ~7%. However, these incidences may be overrepresented compared to other institutions, as the case material from tertiary care centers tends to have a greater proportion of advanced disease. When divergent differentiation is

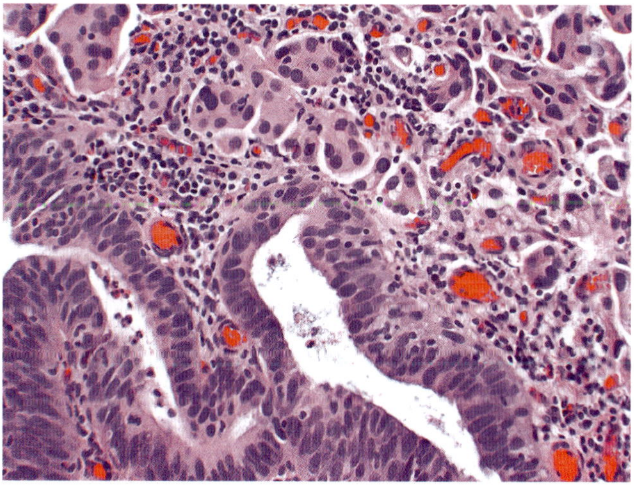

FIGURE 8.34 Urothelial carcinoma with glandular differentiation.

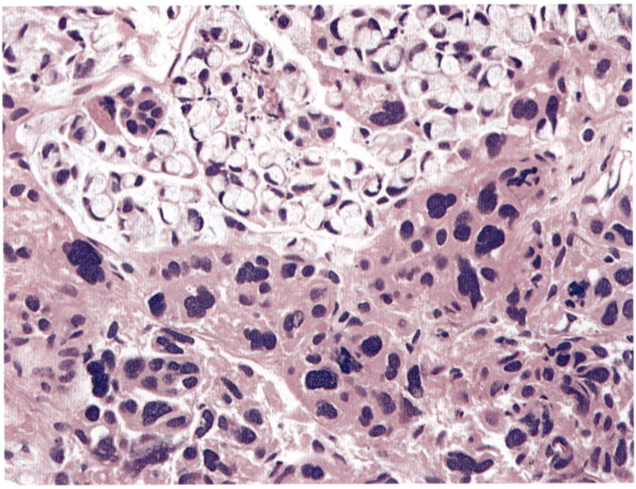

FIGURE 8.35 Urothelial carcinoma signet-ring cell adenocarcinoma differentiation.

seen together with usual urothelial carcinoma, the pathologist should use the terminology of "*urothelial carcinoma with ____ differentiation*," inserting the type of differentiation observed. Divergent differentiation is usually present in a setting of high-grade disease. Wherein it is commonly encountered in invasive disease, its presence does not appear to affect prognosis, once corrected for stage,[29,30,32] although this issue remains somewhat controversial.

CLEAR CELL ADENOCARCINOMA

Clear cell adenocarcinoma may arise in the bladder. Morphologically, these neoplasms have one or more of the three typical features seen in clear cell carcinomas of the female genital tract, including tubulocystic, papillary, and diffuse patterns (Figs. 8.36 and 8.37, eFigs. 8.81-8.84). These tumors initially were thought to arise from mesonephric rests in the trigone area, but we now believe that they may arise through a process of neometaplasia of the surface urothelium or from müllerian rests located within the bladder wall or perivesical soft tissue.[72-76] In a series of 13 cases, Oliva et al. found that 4 were likely of müllerian origin, whereas the remaining 9 could have arisen from the urothelium. Interestingly, their series included 11 females and 2 males. This strong female predominance is rare for urothelial tumors and suggests that müllerian origin may account for an even larger percent of these cases, although certainly most are likely to arise from the overlying urothelium as an expression of divergent differentiation.[74] Immunohistochemical studies are not useful in establishing histogenesis.

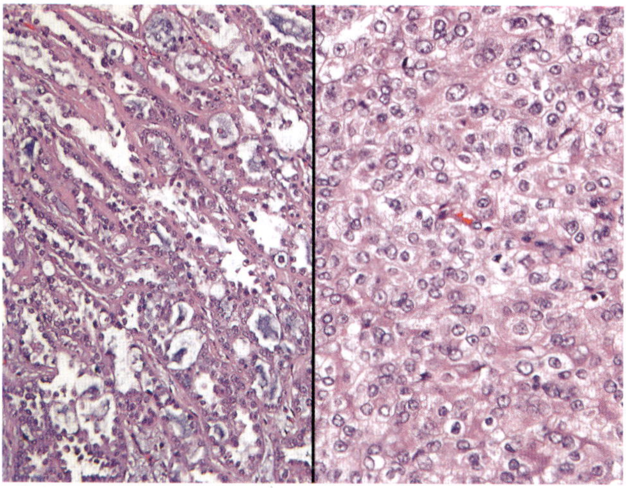

FIGURE 8.36 Clear cell adenocarcinoma with tubular (left) and solid (right) patterns.

The morphologic features are quite characteristic but vary between tumors as multiple patterns may be seen. Tubules and papillae are generally lined by flat, cuboidal, or rarely columnar cells. Sheetlike growth and cystic architecture may also be present. Clear cells are abundant in most tumors, although virtually all tumors also have cells with abundant eosinophilic cytoplasm as well. Hobnail cells are present in most tumors but are conspicuous in the minority. Nuclear atypia is moderate to severe, although rare cases with bland cytology have been described. Mitotic activity is present but may be quite variable. Necrosis may be evident.

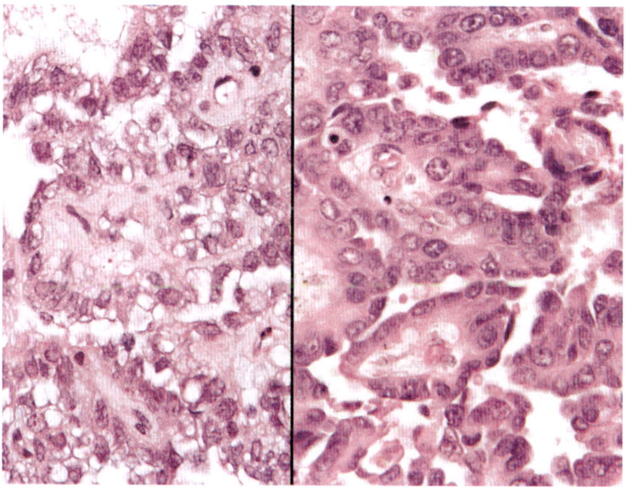

FIGURE 8.37 Clear cell adenocarcinoma with papillary fronds lined by cells with (left) and without (right) clear cytoplasm.

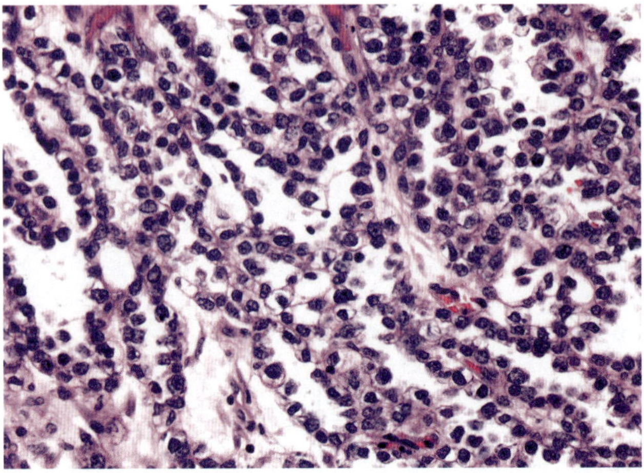

FIGURE 8.38 Area of clear cell adenocarcinoma composed of tubules, which on a small biopsy could be difficult to distinguish from nephrogenic adenoma.

Clear cell adenocarcinomas are high-grade, infiltrating carcinomas with frequent mitoses, nuclear pleomorphism, and areas of solid growth, all of which is absent in nephrogenic adenoma (metaplasia). However, in a limited biopsy, it may be very difficult to distinguish the two lesions (Figs. 8.38 and 8.39). Direct extension from an adjacent pelvic organ must also be ruled out clinically. In contrast to usual adenocarcinoma of the bladder but identical to its counterpart in the female genital system, clear cell adenocarcinoma of the bladder is positive for PAX8 and HNF-1 by immunohistochemistry, as is loss of ARID-1A. Other reported markers include AMACR, napsin, CK20 (focal), CEA, CK7, and CA125.

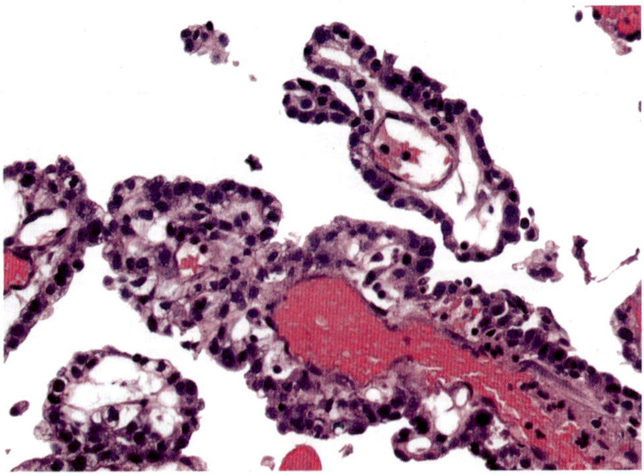

FIGURE 8.39 Area of papillary clear cell adenocarcinoma, which on a small biopsy could be difficult to distinguish from nephrogenic adenoma.

MESONEPHRIC ADENOCARCINOMA AND MESONEPHRICLIKE ADENOCARCINOMA

Rarely, true mesonephric adenocarcinomas can arise in the urothelial tract associated with mesonephric remnants and show morphological features similar to those of mesonephric adenocarcinomas of the uterine cervix.[77] Even more rare are mesonephriclike adenocarcinomas arising in the urothelial tract analogous to those seen in the ovary and endometrium, which are thought to arise from müllerian origin and shows no association with mesonephric remnants. Morphologically, these tumors are identical and heterogeneous with tubular and glandular/pseudoendometrioid/ductal features and variably solid, papillary, villoglandular, and glomeruloid features. Distinctive luminal eosinophilic colloidlike material/secretions are seen in all cases, most commonly with the tubular pattern. Cytological features are typified by cuboidal or columnar cells with minimal cytoplasm and overlapping/crowded nuclei often with grooves. Cases are diffusely positive for Pax8 and display a luminal pattern of CD10 staining. Gata3 and TTF-1 are variably positive. Urinary tract mesonephric adenocarcinomas and mesonephriclike adenocarcinomas share similar histopathogenesis, morphology, and immunophenotype to their counterparts in the female genital tract and differ from clear cell adenocarcinoma of the bladder, which historically in some cases was incorrectly labeled as *mesonephric* or *mesonephroid* or *mesonephriclike adenocarcinoma*. In contrast, clear cell adenocarcinoma commonly displays tubulocystic, papillary, and solid patterns with much more cytological atypia with hobnail morphology and areas with clear cytoplasm. Clear cell adenocarcinoma has no association with mesonephric remnants/hyperplasia and usually lack Gata3, TTF-1, and CD10 expression.

ENDOMETRIOSIS, ENDOCERVICOSIS, AND MÜLLERIANOSIS

While most glandular lesions involving the urinary bladder arise through a process of metaplasia of the surface urothelium, that is not the case with these types of lesions. Genitourinary involvement by endometriosis occurs in 1%-2% of cases. More than 200 cases of vesical endometriosis have been described, making the urinary bladder the most common site of involvement within the urinary tract.[78-80] Classically, it affects women between the second and fifth decade of life but may rarely be seen in postmenopausal women receiving exogenous estrogen.[81] Interestingly, rare cases of vesical endometriosis have been described in males with prostate carcinoma who were receiving exogenous estrogen therapy.[82,83] The occurrence in males is intriguing, and most likely, it represents activation of müllerian rests by exogenous estrogens. Clinically, patients present with urgency, frequency, suprapubic pain, and rarely hematuria. A mass is frequently apparent by either palpation or cystoscopic examination.[83,84] The lesion may reside in

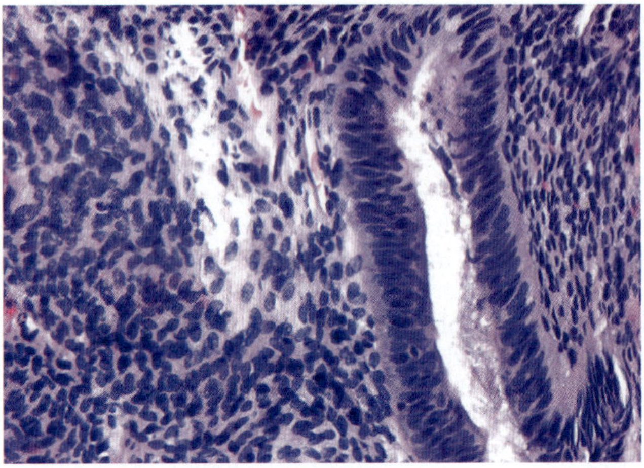

FIGURE 8.40 Endometriosis.

the superficial or deep layers of the vesical wall or in the adjacent perivesical soft tissue so that a simple transurethral biopsy may not always provide diagnostic tissue. Microscopically, the lesion resembles endometriosis elsewhere; endometriumlike glandular epithelium is present in association with endometrial stromal cells and recent or old hemorrhage (Fig. 8.40, eFig. 8.85). Rarely, one finds only glands or stroma. In the former case, the differential diagnosis must include infiltrating adenocarcinoma from which it is distinguished by their recognizable growth pattern characteristics and by the uniform and orderly glands of endometriosis. Endometriosis may involve the lower third of the ureter where it may produce obstructive symptoms. Endometriosis involving the urethra is extremely rare.

Endocervicosis of the urinary bladder is a rare condition first described as a distinct entity by Clement and Young[85] in 1992. It is seen in women of childbearing age who present with a mass in the posterior wall or posterior dome, usually associated with suprapubic pain, frequency, and dysuria. It is thought to arise from müllerian rests and is characterized by extensive involvement of the bladder wall by benign or mildly atypical, columnar, mucin-secreting endocervical-like glands (eFigs. 8.86-8.92). Extravasation of mucin may be present in cases secondary to gland rupture. Since endocervicosis of the bladder is commonly located deep within the viscus and associated with a mass, it must be distinguished from an invasive carcinoma clinically and from adenocarcinoma morphologically.[86] In contrast to adenocarcinoma, there is no–or at most–minimal atypia, no mitotic figures, and no tissue reaction.

In 1996, Clement and Young described müllerianosis of the urinary bladder.[85] These rare lesions occur in the same clinical setting as endocervicosis, differing only in that the lesion may contain other benign

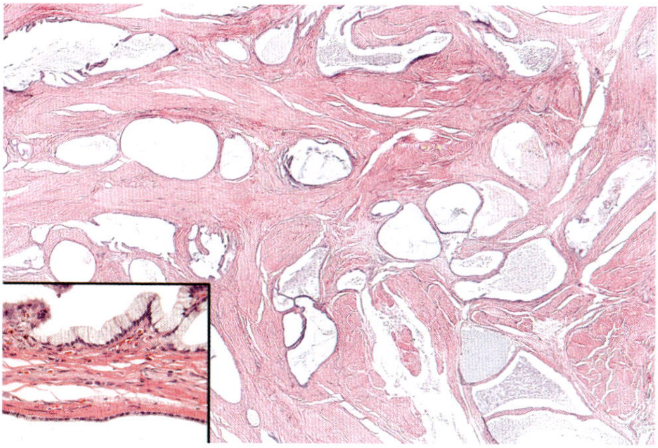

FIGURE 8.41 Endocervicosis (higher magnification [inset]).

müllerian-type components including endometrial and/or tubal epithelium (Figs. 8.41-8.44). Once again, care must be taken not to confuse such lesions with adenocarcinoma.[87-89]

NEPHROGENIC ADENOMA

The other lesion that may mimic adenocarcinoma is nephrogenic adenoma (eFigs. 8.93-8.97). They usually arise in the setting of prior urothelial injury, such as past surgery (60%), calculi (14%), or trauma (9%).[90] Eight percent have a history of renal transplantation. Approximately two-thirds of individuals affected with nephrogenic adenoma are male, and in one-third, the lesion is found in patients <30 years of age. Nephrogenic adenomas appear as papillary, polypoid, hyperplastic, fungating, friable, or velvety lesions.

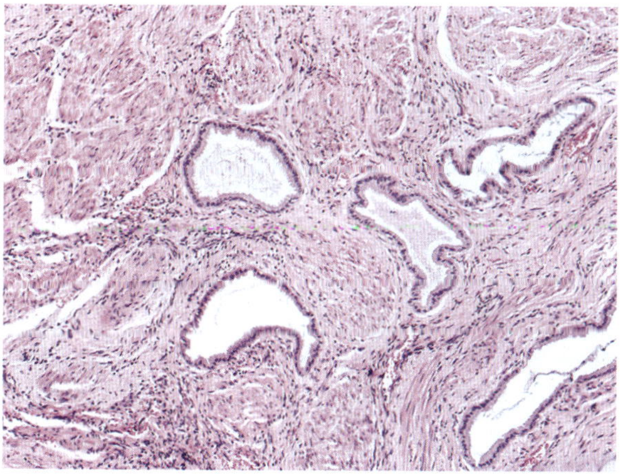

FIGURE 8.42 Müllerianosis.

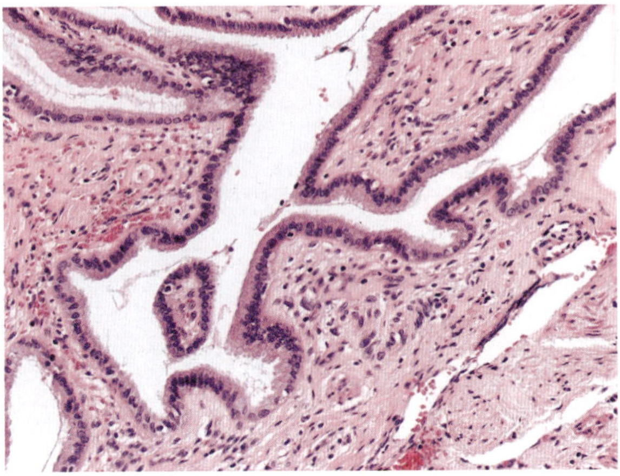

FIGURE 8.43 Müllerianosis.

They are located throughout the bladder, though rarely found on the anterior wall. Eighty percent are localized to the bladder, with 12% seen in the urethra and 8% in the ureter. Most measure <1 cm, although they may attain dimensions as large as 7 cm. In 18% of cases, multiple lesions are identified.

Nephrogenic adenomas have a broad histologic spectrum.[90-92] A common pattern consists of tubules lined by low columnar to cuboidal epithelium (Fig. 8.45). Nuclear atypia is virtually absent with mitoses either absent or rare, although prominent nucleoli may be visualized. Nuclear atypia, when present, appears degenerative. Nuclei are enlarged and hyperchromatic, yet have a smudged indistinct chromatin pattern. These atypical nuclei often reside in cells with an endothelial or hobnail appearance

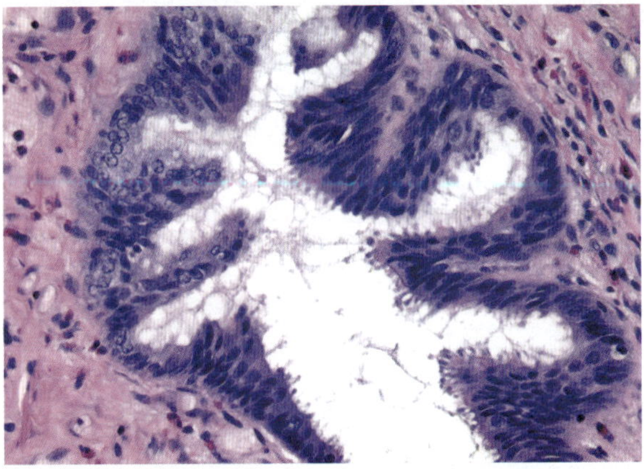

FIGURE 8.44 Endocervicosis with reactive atypia.

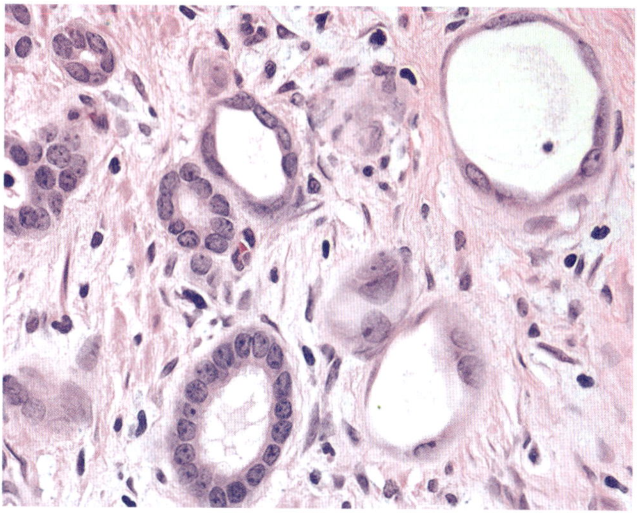

FIGURE 8.45 Nephrogenic adenoma with tubules (note some with nucleoli).

lining vascularlike dilated tubules (Fig. 8.46). Cystic tubules may contain colloidlike eosinophilic or basophilic secretions (Fig. 8.47). Uncommonly, tubules are lined by either more columnar cells with pale cytoplasm or signet-appearing cells; clear cells are rare, and glycogen is usually absent (Figs. 8.48 and 8.49). Nephrogenic adenomas may also be papillary, usually lined by low cuboidal cells with scant cytoplasm or on occasion by

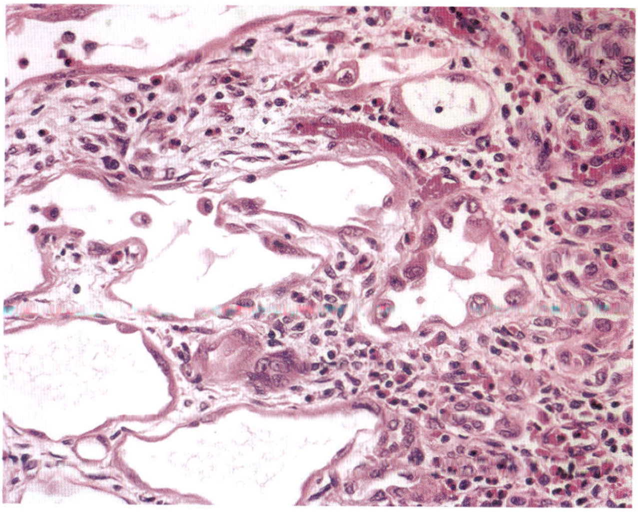

FIGURE 8.46 Nephrogenic adenoma with structures resembling vessels and hobnail atypia.

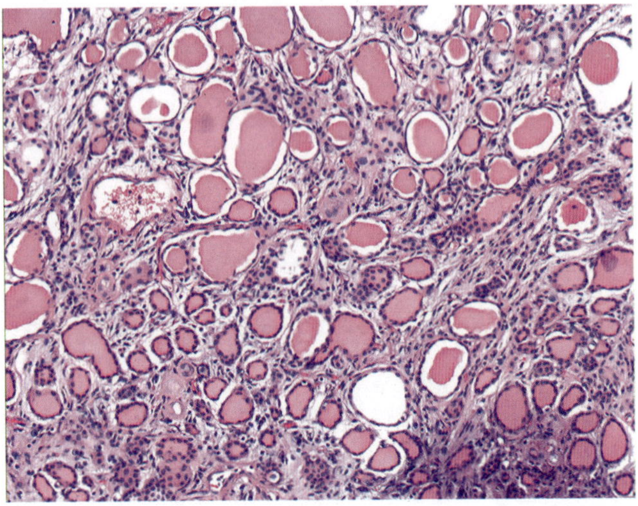

FIGURE 8.47 Nephrogenic adenoma with thyroidlike secretions.

oxyphilic cells (Figs. 8.50-8.52). Tubules in nephrogenic adenoma are often surrounded by a thickened and hyalinized basement membrane and do not incite a stromal response; the stroma may be edematous (Fig. 8.53). A focal solid growth pattern may be present though it is frequently associated with other patterns. A variant of nephrogenic adenoma is one with a fibromyxoid pattern, consisting of compressed spindled cells within a fibromyxoid background, with only rare tubular and cordlike structures,

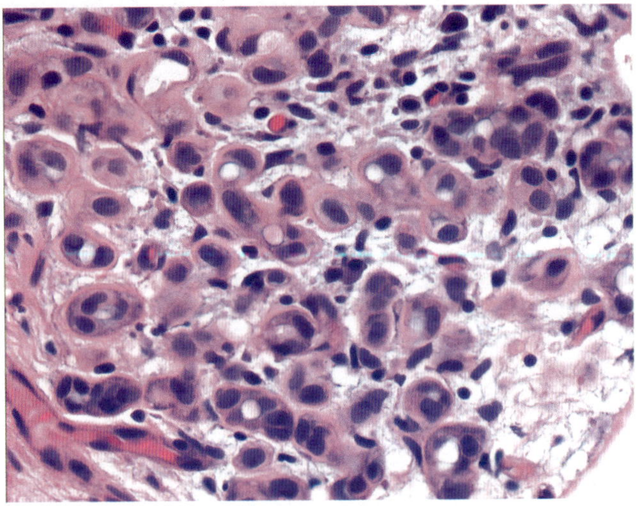

FIGURE 8.48 Nephrogenic adenoma with signet-ring cell–like small tubules.

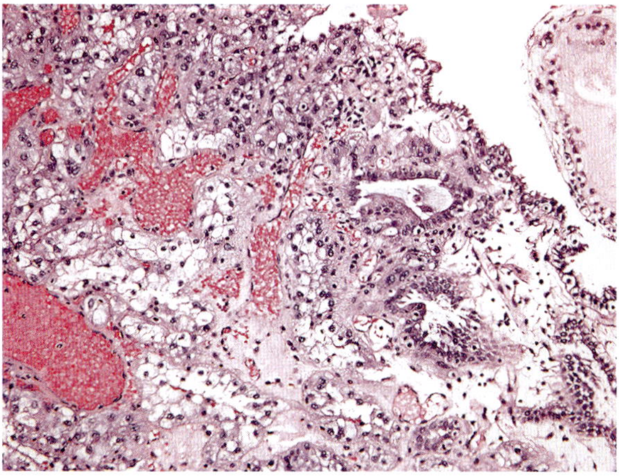

FIGURE 8.49 Nephrogenic adenoma with areas of clear cell change.

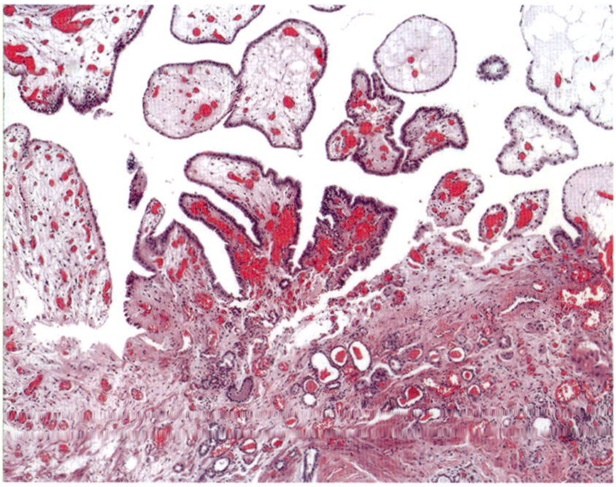

FIGURE 8.50 Nephrogenic adenoma with papillary formation and glandular architecture with thyroidlike secretions.

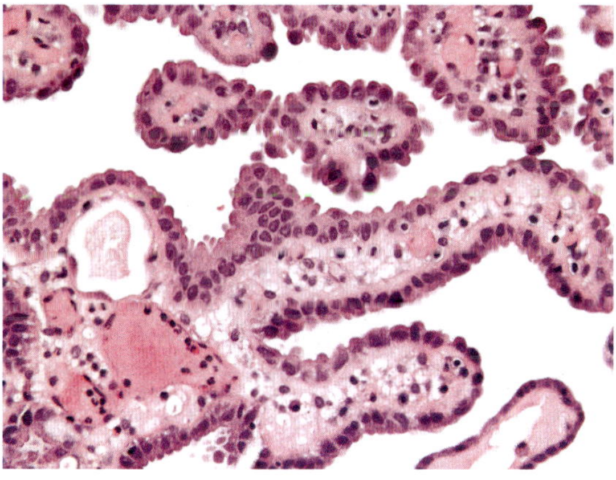

FIGURE 8.51 Nephrogenic adenoma with papillary formation.

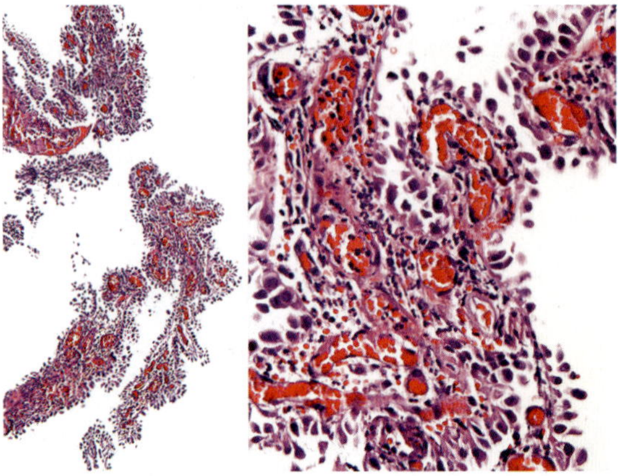

FIGURE 8.52 **Nephrogenic adenoma with papillary formation.** Note there is a slightly greater degree of cytologic atypia in this case (higher magnification **[right]**).

closely mimicking infiltrating carcinoma (Fig. 8.54).[93,94] Variable numbers of acute and chronic inflammatory cells are commonplace within the bladder wall. A flat pattern of nephrogenic adenoma has been described, characterized by urothelial surface involvement by a single cell or two to three cell layers of hobnailed cells mimicking flat urothelial atypia but representing surface involvement by cells from the nephrogenic adenoma.[95] This pattern is invariably associated with more classic components and can be easily highlighted by immunohistochemistry. The differential diagnosis of nephrogenic adenoma includes urothelial carcinoma with tubular and microcystic patterns and adenocarcinoma. In contrast to carcinomas, nephrogenic adenomas lack conspicuous solid growth patterns, mitotic activity, prominent cytological atypia, and are not typically large, deeply

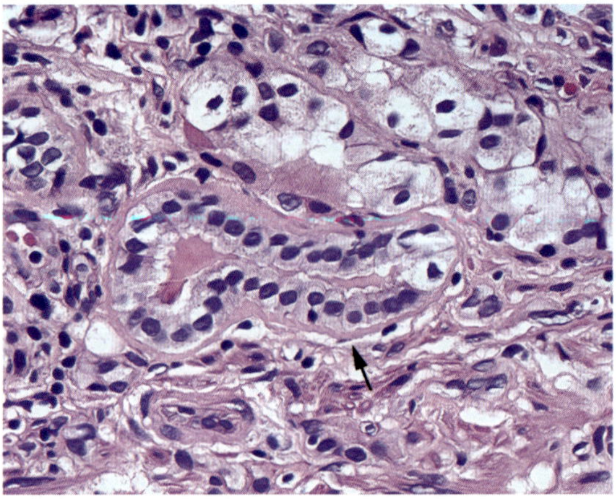

FIGURE 8.53 **Nephrogenic adenoma.** Note hyaline basement membrane–like material (***arrow***).

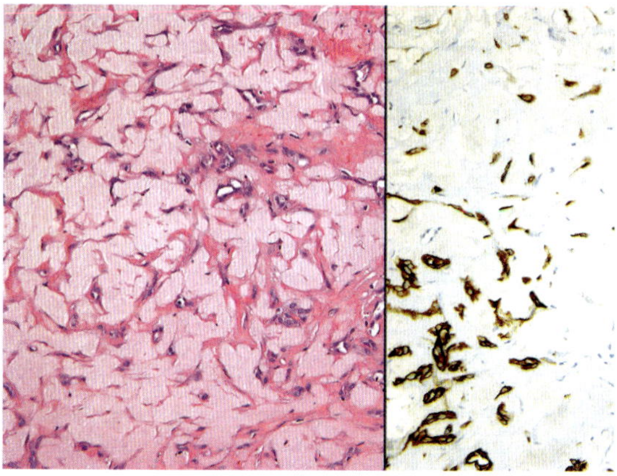

FIGURE 8.54 Fibromyxoid variant of nephrogenic adenoma, highlighted by keratin (right).

invasive lesions. We have seen rare cases of nephrogenic adenomas focally involve the superficial aspects of the muscularis propria. Nephrogenic adenoma may be weakly immunoreactive for PSA or PSAP, can be negative for 34βE12/p63, and positive for racemase as a further pitfall in the differential diagnosis with adenocarcinoma of the prostate. PAX-8 and GATA3 are not able to distinguish nephrogenic adenoma from urothelial carcinoma, given significant overlap in staining.[96] Positive napsin staining may occasionally be helpful.

The histogenesis of nephrogenic adenoma remains controversial. One theory is that it is a metaplastic phenomenon due to an inflammatory insult or local injury and thus belongs in the spectrum of proliferative cystitis.[97-100] Another hypothesis has been proposed by Mazal et al.[101] who studied cases of nephrogenic adenoma in kidney transplant recipients. Based on FISH and lectin studies, they concluded that these lesions were derived from shed tubular cells originating from the transplanted kidney rather than a metaplastic process. Other recent studies have supported this opinion based on the fact that nephrogenic adenomas are immunoreactive for PAX-8 similar to renal tubules.[93-95] The theory would be that areas of irritation or ulceration along the lower urinary tract are receptive to seeding and implantation or renal tubules shed from the kidney. Given the fact that antigen expression alone is insufficient evidence to establish site of origin and the fact that nephrogenic adenoma expresses other markers not associated with renal tubular epithelium, such as GATA3 and CA 125, it is likely that both mechanisms play a role in the histogenesis of this lesion.

REFERENCES

1. Mostofi FK. Potentialities of bladder epithelium. *J Urol*. 1954;71:705-714.
2. Davies G, Castro JE. Cystitis glandularis. *Urology*. 1977;10:128-129.

3. Young RH, Bostwick DG. Florid cystitis glandularis of intestinal type with mucin extravasation: a mimic of adenocarcinoma. *Am J Surg Pathol.* 1996;20:1462-1468.
4. Jacobs LB, Brooks JD, Epstein JI. Differentiation of colonic metaplasia from adenocarcinoma of urinary bladder. *Hum Pathol.* 1997;28:1152-1157.
5. Corica FA, Husmann DA, Churchill BM, et al. Intestinal metaplasia is not a strong risk factor for bladder cancer: study of 53 cases with long-term follow-up. *Urology.* 1997;50:427-431.
6. Gordetsky J, Epstein JI. Intestinal metaplasia of the bladder with dysplasia: a risk factor for carcinoma? *Histopathology.* 2015;67:325-330.
7. Engel RM, Wilkinson HA. Bladder exstrophy. *J Urol.* 1970;104:699-704.
8. Nielsen K, Nielsen KK. Adenocarcinoma in exstrophy of the bladder–the last case in scandinavia? A case report and review of literature. *J Urol.* 1983;130:1180-1182.
9. Newman J, Antonakopoulos GN. Widespread mucous metaplasia of the urinary bladder with nephrogenic adenoma. *Arch Pathol Lab Med.* 1985;109:560-563.
10. Assor D. A villous tumor of the bladder. *J Urol.* 1978;119:287-288.
11. Miller DC, Gang DL, Gavris V, et al. Villous adenoma of the urinary bladder: a morphologic or biologic entity? *Am J Clin Pathol.* 1983;79:728-731.
12. Cheng L, Montironi R, Bostwick DG. Villous adenoma of the urinary tract: a report of 23 cases, including 8 with coexistent adenocarcinoma. *Am J Surg Pathol.* 1999;23:764-771.
13. Seibel JL, Prasad S, Weiss RE, et al. Villous adenoma of the urinary tract: a lesion frequently associated with malignancy. *Hum Pathol.* 2002;33:236-241.
14. Almassi N, Whiting K, Toubaji A, et al. Clinical and genomic characterization of bladder carcinomas with glandular phenotype. *JCO Precis Oncol.* 2022;6:e2100392.
15. Chan TY, Epstein JI. In situ adenocarcinoma of the bladder. *Am J Surg Pathol.* 2001;25:892-899.
16. Miller J, Epstein J. Noninvasive urothelial carcinoma of the bladder with glandular differentiation: report of 24 cases. *Am J Surg Pathol.* 2009;33:1241-1248.
17. Wheeler JD, Hill WT. Adenocarcinoma involving the urinary bladder. *Arch Pathol Lab Med.* 1954;7:119-135.
18. Mostofi FK, Thomson RV, Dean AL. Mucous adenocarcinoma of the urinary bladder. *Cancer.* 1955;8:741-758.
19. Nocks BN, Heney NM, Daly JJ. Primary adenocarcinoma of urinary bladder. *Urology.* 1983;21:26-29.
20. Anderstrom C, Johansson SL, von Schultz L. Primary adenocarcinoma of the urinary bladder. *A clinicopathologic and prognostic study. Cancer.* 1983;52:1273-1280.
21. Grignon DJ, Ro JY, Ayala AG, et al. Primary adenocarcinoma of the urinary bladder. A clinicopathologic analysis of 72 cases. *Cancer.* 1991;67:2165-2172.
22. Jones WA, Gibbons RP, Correa RJ Jr, et al. Primary adenocarcinoma of bladder. *Urology.* 1980;15:119-122.
23. Malek RS, Rosen JS, O'Dea MJ. Adenocarcinoma of bladder. *Urology.* 1983;21:357-359.
24. Compérat E, Amin MB, Epstein JI, et al. The Genitourinary Pathology Society update on classification of variant histologies, T1 substaging, molecular taxonomy, and immunotherapy and PD-L1 testing implications of urothelial cancers. *Adv Anat Pathol.* 2021;28(4):196-208.
25. Shaaban AA, Elbaz MA, Tribukait B. Primary nonurachal adenocarcinoma in the bilharzial urinary bladder: deoxyribonucleic acid flow cytometric and morphologic characterization in 93 cases. *Urology.* 1998;51:469-476.
26. el-Mekresh MM, el-Baz MA, Abol-Enein H, et al. Primary adenocarcinoma of the urinary bladder: a report of 185 cases. *Br J Urol.* 1998;82:206-212.
27. Dean AL, Mostofi FK, Thompson RV. A restudy of the first fourteen hundred tumors in the bladder tumor registry. *J Urol.* 1954;74:571-590.

28. Melicow MM. Tumors of the urinary bladder: a clinicopathological analysis of over 2,500 specimens and autopsies. *J Urol*. 1955;74:498-521.
29. Rogers CG, Palapattu GS, Shariat SF, et al. Clinical outcomes following radical cystectomy for primary nontransitional cell carcinoma of the bladder compared to transitional cell carcinoma of the bladder. *J Urol*. 2006;175:2048-2053. discussion 2053.
30. Dalbagni G, Genega E, Hashibe M, et al. Cystectomy for bladder cancer: a contemporary series. *J Urol*. 2001;165:1111-1116.
31. Kim SP, Frank I, Cheville JC, et al. The impact of squamous and glandular differentiation on survival after radical cystectomy for urothelial carcinoma. *J Urol*. 2012;188:405-409.
32. Linder BJ, Boorjian SA, Cheville JC, et al. The impact of histological reclassification during pathology re-review–evidence of a will rogers effect in bladder cancer? *J Urol*. 2013;190:1692-1696.
33. Bischoff W, Bohm N. Adenocarcinoma of the appendix penetrating the bladder. *J Urol*. 1980;123:123.
34. Tavora F, Epstein JI. Urothelial carcinoma with abundant myxoid stroma. *Hum Pathol*. 2009;40:1391-1398.
35. McKenney JK, Amin MB. The role of immunohistochemistry in the diagnosis of urinary bladder neoplasms. *Semin Diagn Pathol*. 2005;22:69-87.
36. Amin MB, Trpkov K, Lopez-Beltran A, et al. Best practices recommendations in the application of immunohistochemistry in the bladder lesions: report from the International Society of Urologic Pathology consensus conference. *Am J Surg Pathol*. 2014;38:e20-e34.
37. Higgins JP, Kaygusuz G, Wang L, et al. Placental s100 (s100p) and gata3: markers for transitional epithelium and urothelial carcinoma discovered by complementary DNA microarray. *Am J Surg Pathol*. 2007;31:673-680.
38. Miettinen M, McCue PA, Sarlomo-Rikala M, et al. Gata3: a multispecific but potentially useful marker in surgical pathology: a systematic analysis of 2500 epithelial and nonepithelial tumors. *Am J Surg Pathol*. 2014;38:13-22.
39. Ordonez NG. Value of gata3 immunostaining in tumor diagnosis: a review. *Adv Anat Pathol*. 2013;20:352-360.
40. Broede A, Oll M, Maurer A, et al. Differential diagnosis of bladder versus colorectal adenocarcinoma: keratin 7 and GATA3 positivity in nuclear β-catenin-negative glandular tumours defines adenocarcinoma of the bladder. *J Clin Pathol*. 2016;69:307-312.
41. Smith SC, Mohanty SK, Kunju LP, et al. Uroplakin ii outperforms uroplakin iii in diagnostically challenging settings. *Histopathology*. 2014;65:132-138.
42. Li W, Liang Y, Deavers MT, et al. Uroplakin II is a more sensitive immunohistochemical marker than uroplakin III in urothelial carcinoma and its variants. *Am J Clin Pathol*. 2014;142:864-871.
43. Bernstein SA, Reuter VE, Carroll PR, et al. Primary signet-ring cell carcinoma of urinary bladder. *Urology*. 1988;31:432-436.
44. Braun EV, Ali M, Fayemi AO, et al. Primary signet-ring cell carcinoma of the urinary bladder: review of the literature and report of a case. *Cancer*. 1981;47:1430-1435.
45. Poore TE, Egbert B, Jahnke R, et al. Signet ring cell adenocarcinoma of the bladder: linitis plastica variant. *Arch Pathol Lab Med*. 1981;105:203-204.
46. Choi H, Lamb S, Pintar K, et al. Primary signet-ring cell carcinoma of the urinary bladder. *Cancer*. 1984;53:1985-1990.
47. Grignon DJ, Ro JY, Ayala AG, et al. Primary signet-ring cell carcinoma of the urinary bladder. *Am J Clin Pathol*. 1991;95:13-20.
48. Al-Ahmadie H, Iyer G, Mehra R, et al. E-cadherin (CDH1) is frequently mutated in urothelial carcinoma with signet-ring cell and plasmacytoid morphology. *Mod Pathol*. 2013;26:191A.

49. Ro JY, Shen SS, Lee HI, et al. Plasmacytoid transitional cell carcinoma of urinary bladder: a clinicopathologic study of 9 cases. *Am J Surg Pathol.* 2008;32:752-757.
50. Zukerberg LR, Harris NL, Young RH. Carcinomas of the urinary bladder simulating malignant lymphoma. A report of five cases. *Am J Surg Pathol.* 1991;15:569-576.
51. Nigwekar P, Tamboli P, Amin MB, et al. Plasmacytoid urothelial carcinoma: detailed analysis of morphology with clinicopathologic correlation in 17 cases. *Am J Surg Pathol.* 2009;33:417-424.
52. Lim MG, Adsay NV, Grignon DJ, et al. E-cadherin expression in plasmacytoid, signet ring cell and micropapillary variants of urothelial carcinoma: comparison with usual-type high-grade urothelial carcinoma. *Mod Pathol.* 2011;24:241-247.
53. Dayyani F, Czerniak BA, Sircar K, et al. Plasmacytoid urothelial carcinoma, a chemosensitive cancer with poor prognosis, and peritoneal carcinomatosis. *J Urol.* 2013;189:1656-1661.
54. Pontes JE, Oldford JR. Metastatic breast carcinoma to the bladder. *J Urol.* 1970;104:839-842.
55. Epstein JI, Lieberman PH. Mucinous adenocarcinoma of the prostate gland. *Am J Surg Pathol.* 1985;9:299-308.
56. Epstein JI, Kuhajda FP, Lieberman PH. Prostate-specific acid phosphatase immunoreactivity in adenocarcinomas of the urinary bladder. *Hum Pathol.* 1986;17:939-942.
57. Schubert GE, Pavkovic MB, Bethke-Bedurftig BA. Tubular urachal remnants in adult bladders. *J Urol.* 1982;127:40-42.
58. Johnson DE, Hodge GB, Abdul-Karim FW, et al. Urachal carcinoma. *Urology.* 1985;26:218-221.
59. Jakse G, Schneider HM, Jacobi GH. Urachal signet-ring cell carcinoma, a rare variant of vesical adenocarcinoma: incidence and pathological criteria. *J Urol.* 1978;120:764-766.
60. Alonso-Gorrea M, Mompo-Sanchis JA, Jorda-Cuevas M, et al. Signet ring cell adenocarcinoma of the urachus. *Eur Urol.* 1985;11:282-284.
61. Gopalan A, Sharp D, Fine SW, et al. Urachal carcinoma: a clinicopathologic analysis of 24 cases with outcome correlation. *Am J Surg Pathol.* 2009;33:659-668.
62. Ghazizadeh M, Yamamoto S, Kurokawa K. Clinical features of urachal carcinoma in Japan: review of 157 patients. *Urol Res.* 1983;11:235-238.
63. Eble JN, Hull MT, Rowland RG, et al. Villous adenoma of the urachus with mucusuria: a light and electron microscopic study. *J Urol.* 1986;135:1240-1244.
64. Hayman J. Carcinoma of the urachus. *Pathology.* 1984;16:167-171.
65. Herr HW, Bochner BH, Sharp D, et al. Urachal carcinoma: contemporary surgical outcomes. *J Urol.* 2007;178:74-78; discussion 78.
66. Sheldon CA, Clayman RV, Gonzalez R, et al. Malignant urachal lesions. *J Urol.* 1984;131:1-8.
67. Ashley RA, Inman BA, Sebo TJ, et al. Urachal carcinoma: clinicopathologic features and long-term outcomes of an aggressive malignancy. *Cancer.* 2006;107:712-720.
68. Ashley RA, Inman BA, Sebo TJ, et al. Urachal carcinoma: clinicopathologic features and long-term outcomes of an aggressive malignancy. *Cancer.* 2006;107(4):712-720.
69. Zaleski MP, Chen H, Roy-Chowdhuri S, et al. Distinct gene mutations are associated with clinicopathologic features in urachal carcinoma. *Am J Clin Pathol.* 2022;158(2):263-269.
70. Paner GP, Lopez-Beltran A, Sirohi D, et al. Updates in the pathologic diagnosis and classification of epithelial neoplasms of urachal origin. *Adv Anat Pathol.* 2016;23(2):71-83.
71. Amin MB, Smith SC, Eble JN, et al. Glandular neoplasms of the urachus: a report of 55 cases emphasizing mucinous cystic tumors with proposed classification. *Am J Surg Pathol.* 2014;38:1033-1045.

72. Skor AB, Warren MM. Mesonephric adenocarcinoma of bladder. *Urology*. 1977;10: 64-65.

73. Schultz RE, Bloch MJ, Tomaszewski JE, et al. Mesonephric adenocarcinoma of the bladder. *J Urol*. 1984;132:263-265.

74. Young RH, Scully RE. Clear cell adenocarcinoma of the bladder and urethra. A report of three cases and review of the literature. *Am J Surg Pathol*. 1985;9:816-826.

75. Oliva E, Amin MB, Jimenez R, et al. Clear cell carcinoma of the urinary bladder: a report and comparison of four tumors of mullerian origin and nine of probable urothelial origin with discussion of histogenesis and diagnostic problems. *Am J Surg Pathol*. 2002;26:190-197.

76. Sung MT, Zhang S, MacLennan GT, et al. Histogenesis of clear cell adenocarcinoma in the urinary tract: evidence of urothelial origin. *Clin Cancer Res*. 2008;14: 1947-1955.

77. Xing D, Liang SX, Gao FF, et al. Mesonephric adenocarcinoma and mesonephric adenocarcinoma-like adenocarcinoma of the urinary tract. *Mod Pathol*. 2023;36(1):100031.

78. Nixon WCW. Endometriosis of the bladder. *Lancet*. 1940;1:405-406.

79. Fein RL, Horton BF. Vesical endometriosis: a case report and review of the literature. *J Urol*. 1966;95:45-50.

80. Lichtenfeld FR, McCauley RT, Staples PP. Endometriosis involving the urinary tract: a collective review. *Obstet Gynecol Surv*. 1961;17:762-768.

81. Stewart WW, Ireland GW. Vesical endometriosis in a postmenopausal woman: a case report. *J Urol*. 1977;118:480-481.

82. Pinkert TC, Catlow CE, Straus R. Endometriosis of the urinary bladder in a man with prostatic carcinoma. *Cancer*. 1979;43:1562-1567.

83. Schrodt GR, Alcorn MO, Ibanez J. Endometriosis of the male urinary system: a case report. *J Urol*. 1980;124:722-723.

84. Comiter CV. Endometriosis of the urinary tract. *Urol Clin North Am*. 2002;29:625-635.

85. Clement PB, Young RH. Endocervicosis of the urinary bladder. A report of six cases of a benign mullerian lesion that may mimic adenocarcinoma. *Am J Surg Pathol*. 1992;16:533-542.

86. Julie C, Boye K, Desgrippes A, et al. Endocervicosis of the urinary bladder. Immunohistochemical comparative study between a new case and normal uterine endocervices. *Pathol Res Pract*. 2002;198:115-120.

87. Young RH, Clement PB. Mullerianosis of the urinary bladder. *Mod Pathol*. 1996;9: 731-737.

88. Kim HJ, Lee TJ, Kim MK, et al. Muellerianosis of the urinary bladder, endocervicosis type: a case report. *J Korean Med Sci*. 2001;16:123-126.

89. Donne C, Vidal M, Buttin X, et al. Mullerianosis of the urinary bladder: clinical and immunohistochemical findings. *Histopathology*. 1998;33:290-292.

90. Bhagavan BS, Tiamson EM, Wenk RE, et al. Nephrogenic adenoma of the urinary bladder and urethra. *Hum Pathol*. 1981;12:907-916.

91. Allan CH, Epstein JI. Nephrogenic adenoma of the prostatic urethra: a mimicker of prostate adenocarcinoma. *Am J Surg Pathol*. 2001;25:802-808.

92. Rahemtullah A, Oliva E. Nephrogenic adenoma: an update on an innocuous but troublesome entity. *Adv Anat Pathol*. 2006;13:247-255.

93. Hansel DE, Nadasdy T, Epstein JI. Fibromyxoid nephrogenic adenoma: a newly recognized variant mimicking mucinous adenocarcinoma. *Am J Surg Pathol*. 2007;31: 1231-1237.

94. Li L, Williamson SR, Castillo RP, et al. Fibromyxoid nephrogenic adenoma: A series of 43 cases reassessing predisposing conditions, clinical presentation, and morphology. *Am J Surg Pathol*. 2023;47(1):37-46.

95. Pina-Oviedo S, Shen SS, Truong LD, et al. Flat pattern of nephrogenic adenoma: previously unrecognized pattern unveiled using pax2 and pax8 immunohistochemistry. *Mod Pathol.* 2013;26:792-798.
96. McDaniel AS, Chinnaiyan AM, Siddiqui J, et al. Immunohistochemical staining characteristics of nephrogenic adenoma using the pin-4 cocktail (p63, amacr, and ck903) and gata-3. *Am J Surg Pathol.* 2014;38:1664-1671.
97. Stilmant MM, Siroky MB. Nephrogenic adenoma associated with intravesical bacillus calmette-guerin treatment: a report of 2 cases. *J Urol.* 1986;135:359-361.
98. Navarre RJ Jr, Loening SA, Platz C, et al. Nephrogenic adenoma: a report of 9 cases and review of the literature. *J Urol.* 1982;127:775-779.
99. Molland EA, Trott PA, Paris AM, et al. Nephrogenic adenoma: a form of adenomatous metaplasia of the bladder. A clinical and electron microscopical study. *Br J Urol.* 1976;48:453-462.
100. Ford TF, Watson GM, Cameron KM. Adenomatous metaplasia (nephrogenic adenoma) of urothelium. An analysis of 70 cases. *Br J Urol.* 1985;57:427-433.
101. Mazal PR, Schaufler R, Altenhuber-Muller R, et al. Derivation of nephrogenic adenomas from renal tubular cells in kidney-transplant recipients. *N Engl J Med.* 2002;347:653-659.

9

SQUAMOUS LESIONS

SQUAMOUS METAPLASIA

Squamous epithelium, particularly in the area of the trigone, is a common finding in women (Fig. 9.1) (also see Chapter 1). Trigonal squamous epithelium in women represents a normal histologic variation occurring under hormonal influence unassociated with local injury. Chronic irritation, such as with recurrent urinary tract infections, long-term catheterization, urinary lithiasis, chronic urinary tract obstruction, fistulae, bladder exstrophy, neurogenic bladder, prior bladder surgery or radiation, parasite infection, and vitamin A deficiency, can result in keratinizing squamous metaplasia.[1] In this condition, the squamous epithelium exhibits parakeratosis and hyperkeratosis and may even acquire a granular layer (Fig. 9.2). This metaplastic epithelium is not preneoplastic *per se*, but under some circumstances, especially when extensive, chronic and involving large regions of the bladder, it may lead to squamous carcinoma.[2] This is the sequence of events, for example, in patients with long-standing schistosomiasis of the urinary bladder or, in the case of squamous carcinoma, arising in bladder diverticula.[3-5] In these cases, it may be possible to observe keratinizing squamous metaplasia and dysplastic changes adjacent to *in situ* and invasive squamous carcinoma. The pathologist is obligated to mention the presence and extent of keratinizing squamous metaplasia in a transurethral biopsy specimen. Khan and colleagues[6] described their experience with 34 patients with keratinizing squamous metaplasia. Although the extent of involvement correlated with subsequent risk of carcinoma, any degree of keratinizing squamous metaplasia is a significant risk factor for the development of subsequent carcinoma as well as other complications such as bladder contracture and obstruction.[6] Lesions are treated by transurethral resection and close follow-up to rule out progression to carcinoma. In some cases, the metaplasia can resolve, especially if the inciting cause of injury has been removed.[1] If extensive squamous metaplasia is present, a comment that sampling of all lesional tissue is recommended because of the association with dysplastic, *in situ* or invasive squamous, or rarely urothelial lesions.

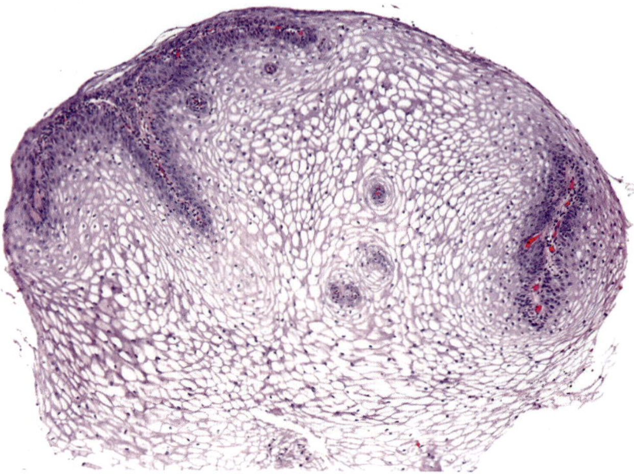

FIGURE 9.1 Glycogenated squamous metaplasia.

VERRUCOUS SQUAMOUS HYPERPLASIA

Verrucous squamous hyperplasia consists of a spiking or church spire-like squamous hyperplasia (Fig. 9.3). Marked hyperkeratosis, parakeratosis, and elongation of the rete pegs are also present, but the lesions lack the broad invasive tongues seen with verrucous carcinoma. Although this lesion has only been relatively recently reported in the urinary bladder, verrucous squamous hyperplasia is well recognized in the oral cavity and upper respiratory tract. In these sites, verrucous squamous hyperplasia is an irreversible lesion with a considerable risk for evolving into verrucous or other forms of squamous cell carcinoma. The entire lesion should be excised before this diagnosis is rendered, so as to not miss a verrucous

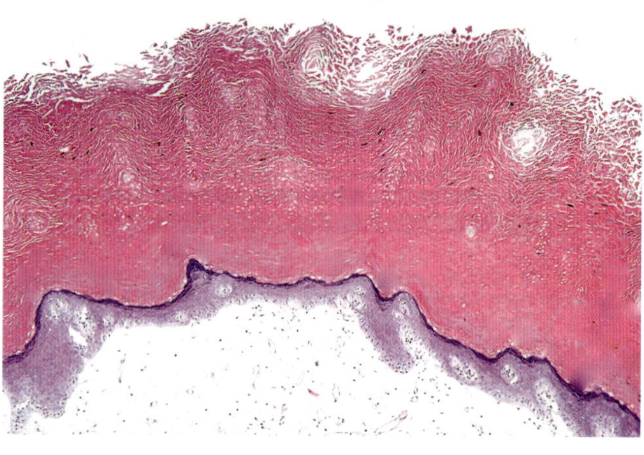

FIGURE 9.2 Keratinizing squamous metaplasia.

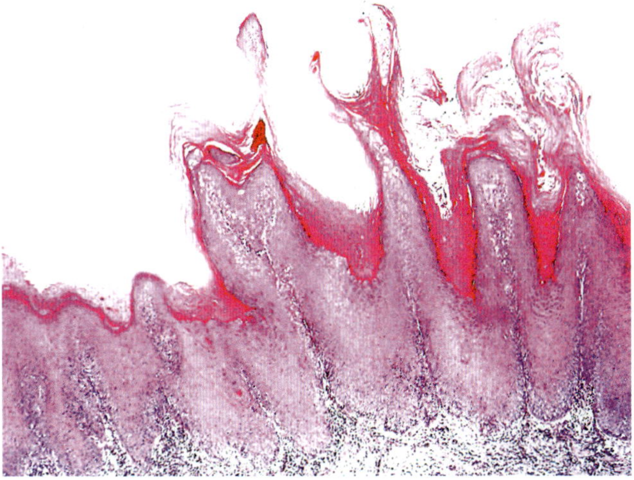

FIGURE 9.3 Verrucous squamous hyperplasia.

carcinoma. Flat squamous hyperplasia (normal cytology/with or without reactive changes) may be associated with verrucous lesions.

In the largest series to date on this entity, a total of 23 cases of verrucous squamous hyperplasia of the urinary bladder were identified.[7] Of these, 11 (47.8%) had concurrent *in situ* or invasive carcinoma. Of the 12 cases (52.2%) without concurrent carcinoma, clinical follow-up was too limited for meaningful assessment. Of 11 patients with concurrent carcinoma, 4 (36.4%) had extensive verrucous squamous hyperplasia with at least squamous cell CIS/cannot rule out superficial invasion. Two (18.2%) had mixed sarcomatoid urothelial carcinoma with squamous cell carcinoma in separately submitted parts. Two (18.2%) had invasive, well-differentiated squamous cell carcinoma, 1 (9.1%) of whom had long-standing schistosomiasis. One (9.1%) had invasive poorly differentiated squamous cell carcinoma. One (9.1%) had invasive high-grade squamous cell carcinoma with a prominent associated lymphocytic infiltrate. In another biopsy from a separate location, this patient also had concurrent invasive high-grade urothelial carcinoma with squamous differentiation. One (9.1%) had urothelial CIS, cannot exclude invasion.

In 4 patients (36.4%) with available clinical follow-up, 3 (75%) were dead from disease (6-24 months). HPV was negative in all cases tested. In summary, verrucous squamous hyperplasia of the bladder is unrelated to HPV infection and frequently associated with invasive carcinoma, most frequently squamous cell carcinoma. In cases unassociated with carcinoma, progression risk is unclear given the limited number of cases with adequate follow-up. Until more is known about the entity and in light of its strong association with carcinoma, close clinical follow-up is recommended in patients with a diagnosis of verrucous squamous hyperplasia.

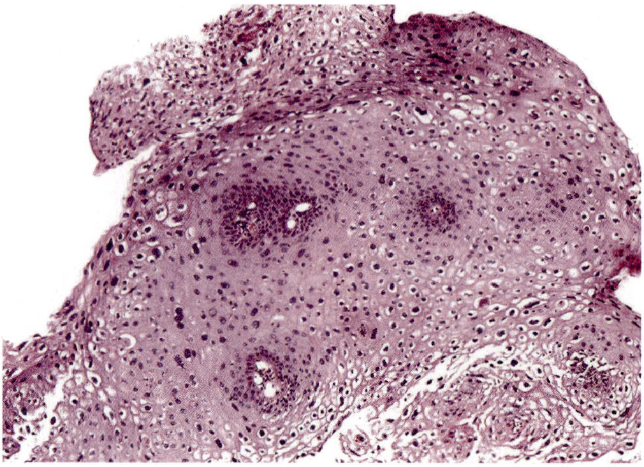

FIGURE 9.4 Condyloma acuminatum.

CONDYLOMA ACUMINATA

Condyloma acuminata are common sexually transmitted benign tumors caused by human papillomavirus (HPV) (Figs. 9.4 and 9.5, eFigs. 9.1-9.7). Condylomas are composed of thickened nonkeratinizing squamous epithelium arranged in verrucous folds with thin fibrovascular cores, typically lacking "free-floating" papillary fronds. There is cytoplasmic clearing around nuclei (koilocytosis) and with atypia restricted to crinkly mostly small nuclei, lacking hyperchromasia or mitoses unless accompanied by moderate to severe dysplasia. They occur most frequently on mucocutaneous surfaces of the external genitalia, perineum, and anus, but extension into the urethra is not uncommon, occurring in up to 20% of cases.

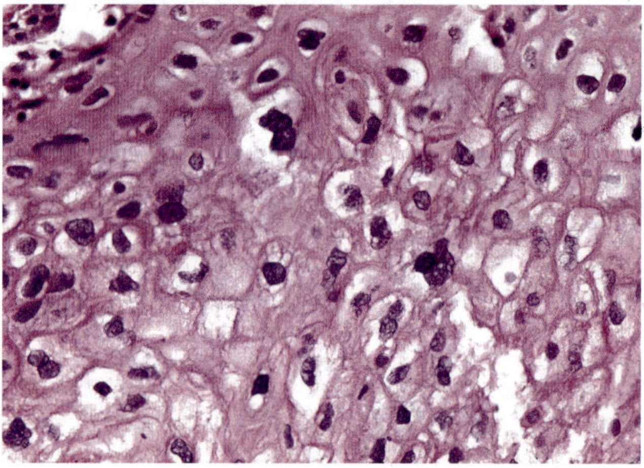

FIGURE 9.5 Condyloma acuminatum (higher magnification of Figure 9.4).

Samarska and Epstein published the largest study on this entity consisting of 51 cases of condyloma acuminatum of the urinary bladder from transurethral resections of the urinary bladder of 38 patients.[8] This study showed a strong association of condyloma acuminatum of the urinary bladder with squamous cell carcinoma of the bladder; 44.7% of patients were diagnosed with squamous cell carcinoma (either *in situ* or invasive) at the time of presentation with condyloma or within 1 year of follow-up. Condyloma acuminata was related to squamous cell carcinoma independently from squamous metaplasia. Overall, 50% of the patients in this study had condylomas that were negative for both LR-HPV and HR-HPV. HPV-negative condylomas have been described previously, with possible explanations related due to the presence of other nontested HPV subtypes or low viral loads. The results of ISH were also often different between multiple lesions removed at different times originating from the same patients. Thus, negative RNA ISH for HPV is still consistent with a diagnosis of condyloma acuminatum if the histology is classic. Although it is known that LR-HPV (HPV types 6/11) is associated with a low risk for neoplastic transformation, in this study, there was an association of squamous cell carcinoma and condylomas with positivity for LR-HPV and HR-HPV.

Although in the prior literature, anogenital condylomas acuminatum have been considered to be a predisposing factor for subsequent bladder involvement. In the study by Samarska and Epstein, only 1 male patient had a history of anogenital condylomas and anal intraepithelial neoplasia *in situ*. Three female patients had a history of HPV-related lesions of cervix and vagina, which were present before their first bladder condyloma acuminatum. Although prior HPV-related lesions of the anogenital region appear to be associated with condyloma acuminatum of the urinary bladder, they only occur in a minority of cases.

Immunodeficiency has also been suggested as a risk factor for developing condyloma acuminatum of the bladder. In the above study, 8 patients had a history of immunosuppression with 7 of 8 patients from this group having multiple and/or recurrent condylomas. However, 7 patients without any relevant history of predisposing factors had condyloma acuminatum and synchronous squamous cell carcinoma, either invasive. This study reinforced the relation of condyloma acuminatum in the bladder with squamous cell carcinoma of the bladder. The diagnosis of squamous cell carcinoma is commonly made within 1 year after the diagnosis of the bladder condyloma acuminatum. The short interval between the diagnosis of condyloma and squamous cell carcinoma and the high frequency of squamous cell carcinoma (~50%) associated with condyloma of the bladder suggests a close relationship between the two entities. Patients with bladder condylomas need close follow-up and sampling of the bladder for concurrent or subsequent *in situ* or invasive squamous cell carcinoma.

SQUAMOUS PAPILLOMA

In 2000, Cheng and colleagues[9] described a series of seven cases of squamous papilloma of the bladder, five occurring in the urinary bladder and

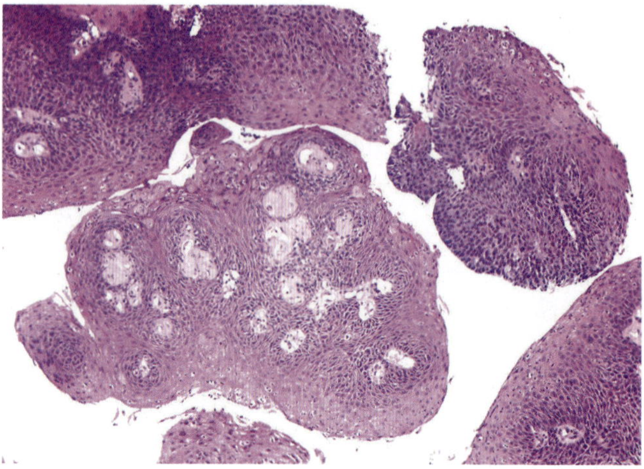

FIGURE 9.6 Squamous papilloma.

the others in the urethra (Figs. 9.6 and 9.7). These lesions were characterized by a proliferation of mature and benign-appearing squamous epithelium surrounding a central fibrovascular core. Koilocytes were not present, and *in situ* hybridization for HPV was negative in all cases. Most of the patients were women, and none had history of genital, perianal, or perineal condyloma. In the five cases without prior urothelial carcinoma, subsequent biopsies showed repeated squamous papilloma in one case and no evidence of disease in the other four cases. In a later study by Guo et al.,[10] among four patients with bladder squamous papillomas who had follow-up, only one patient developed a low-grade urothelial carcinoma and the other three patients had no evidence of disease. The case with low-grade urothelial carcinoma on follow-up had a history of low-grade urothelial

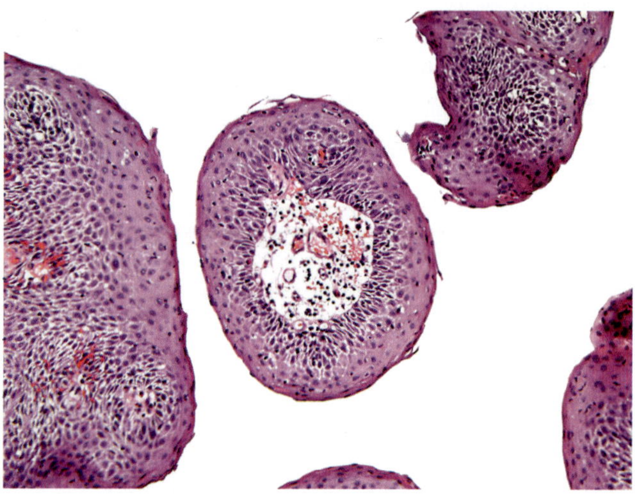

FIGURE 9.7 Squamous papilloma.

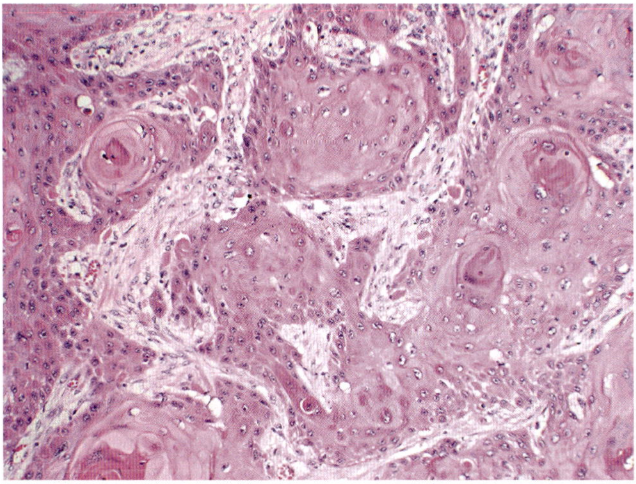

FIGURE 9.8 Infiltrating squamous cell carcinoma.

carcinoma that preceded the diagnosis of squamous papilloma, such that the recurrence of urothelial carcinoma in this patient is most likely unrelated to the squamous papilloma. Squamous papilloma appears to be a benign proliferative, non–HPV-associated squamous lesion without an appreciable risk factor for bladder cancer.

SQUAMOUS CELL CARCINOMA

The diagnosis of squamous cell carcinoma should be reserved for those tumors that are purely or almost entirely keratin forming and exhibiting intercellular bridges (Figs. 9.8 and 9.9, eFigs. 9.8-9.10). For urothelial

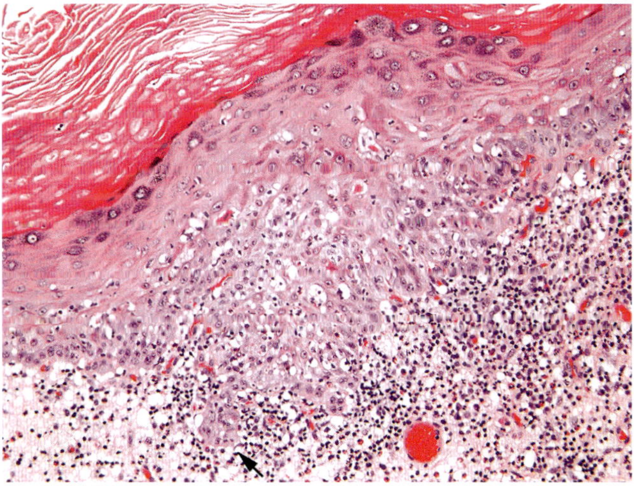

FIGURE 9.9 ***In situ*** and superficially invasive (*arrow*) squamous cell carcinoma.

tumors with variable amounts of squamous differentiation, the term *urothelial carcinoma with squamous differentiation* should be used (see Chapter 8 for general concepts regarding divergent differentiation). Squamous cell carcinoma occurs in two settings, one related to and the other not associated with schistosomal infections.

Schistosomal-Associated Squamous Cell Carcinoma

Between 60% and 90% of carcinomas associated with urinary schistosomiasis are squamous cell carcinomas, with 5%-15% being adenocarcinomas and the rest urothelial carcinomas.[11] Nitrates in the urine, particularly present in individuals living in agricultural areas where nitrate fertilizers are used liberally, may be reduced to carcinogenic nitrosamines as a result of secondary bacterial infection. Other contributing factors include mechanical irritation of the bladder by the parasitic eggs, smoking, and pesticides. Squamous carcinoma used to be the most common form of bladder cancer in Egypt as a result of the association with schistosomiasis, yet other countries share a high incidence of schistosomal-associated squamous cell carcinoma including Iraq, parts of Saudi Arabia, Yemen, and Sudan. Although bladder cancer is still the most common cancer in males in Egypt, urothelial carcinoma is currently more common than squamous carcinoma corresponding to a decrease in schistosomal infections[12-15] (see Chapter 10).

The male to female ratio of squamous cell carcinomas associated with schistosomiasis is 4-5:1, most likely related to the schistosomal exposure of men working in the fields. Patients affected by squamous cell carcinoma in endemic areas are 10-20 years younger than those in nonendemic areas with a long interval between initial exposure to the organisms and the development of squamous carcinoma. Symptoms associated with squamous carcinoma of the bladder are the same as those seen with chronic schistosomal infections of the bladder, which along with poverty, ignorance, and the lack of well-developed screening programs contribute to delays in diagnosis and late stage at presentation.

The tumors typically are nodular fungating masses most commonly involving the posterior and lateral walls. Tumors tend to be large at presentation, reflecting their late stage. Between 10% and 20% of tumors are multifocal. More than half of the squamous cell carcinomas associated with urinary schistosomiasis are well-moderately differentiated. Squamous metaplasia and squamous CIS are seen in the surrounding mucosa in ~80% and 50% of the cases, respectively.[16]

Compared to earlier dismal outcomes, the 5-year survival for schistosomal-associated squamous cell carcinoma is about 50%. Factors accounting for the better prognosis include lower pathological stage with increased screening, improved surgical skill, and less perioperative mortality. Survival is influenced by tumor stage, grade, and lymph node involvement, with <25% survival of tumors associated with nodal involvement. Treatment is radical cystoprostatectomy or radical cystectomy with little added benefit from radiation or chemotherapy.

Nonschistosomal-Associated Squamous Cell Carcinoma

Squamous carcinomas constitute 2%-7% of bladder cancers in Western countries.[17] Focal squamous differentiation in bladder tumors is not uncommon, seen in up to 20% of bladder tumors with an increase in higher-grade and higher-stage cancers.[18] It is the most common form of divergent differentiation in urothelial carcinoma.[19-21] The pathogenesis of nonendemic squamous carcinoma of the bladder relates to long-standing bladder irritation. Inciting agents include prolonged (>10 years) indwelling catheters as seen in patients with spinal cord injury, chronic infections, calculi, foreign bodies, and chronic bladder neck obstruction. Cigarette smoking is also a risk factor.[22] With rare exception, most large studies have shown that squamous cell carcinoma of the bladder is not associated with HPV infection.[23-25] There are rare cases of well-documented primary bladder invasive basaloid squamous cell carcinoma associated with neurogenic bladder and frequent catheterization that have been reported to be high-risk HPV positive.[26] While the *in situ* component is generally basaloid in appearance, the invasive component may lack basaloid features. With rare exception, the presence of an HPV-positive basaloid squamous cell carcinoma in a bladder TURP from a female typically represents spread from the uterine cervix (See Chapter 13). Immunohistochemistry for p16 cannot be used as a surrogate marker for HPV in the bladder as typical urothelial carcinoma is often diffusely positive.

The male to female ratio for squamous cell carcinoma is <2:1, lower than for urothelial carcinoma. The mean age is in the seventh decade with African Americans almost twice as likely to be affected.[27] The presenting symptoms of squamous carcinoma of the bladder are similar to those of urothelial carcinoma.

Squamous carcinomas in general tend to be sessile, ulcerated, infiltrative, and unifocal at the time of diagnosis. The histologic hallmarks of keratin pearl formation, intercellular bridges, and keratotic cellular debris are those of squamous carcinoma at any site. Most squamous cell carcinomas not associated with schistosomiasis are moderately poorly differentiated and more deeply invasive at the time of diagnosis than are the majority of urothelial carcinomas. In a large study of squamous cell carcinoma from the Cleveland Clinic, other findings in the surrounding mucosa included the following: keratinizing squamous metaplasia (62%), nonkeratinizing squamous metaplasia (44%), squamous cell CIS (36%), squamous metaplasia with dysplasia (9%), verrucous squamous hyperplasia (7%), and a single case with extensive condyloma accuminata (2%).[28] The differential diagnosis includes local extension from anal, penile, uterine cervical carcinomas (see Chapter 13), and pseudocarcinomatous urothelial hyperplasia with squamous differentiation. Immunohistochemically, most cases of squamous cell carcinoma of the bladder are positive for GATA3, thrombomodulin, CK7, p63, CK14, desmoglein, and high molecular weight cytokeratin and negative for uroplakins 2 and 3.[29] CK20 is usually negative.

The 5-year disease-free survival after radical cystectomy is 43%-57%.[19,28] Their generally poor prognosis can be attributed to the typically advanced stage at diagnosis, but stage for stage and even overall, the prognosis is similar for squamous and usual type of urothelial carcinoma.[19-21,30-35] There is also no difference in prognosis between pure squamous cell carcinoma of the bladder compared to urothelial carcinoma with squamous differentiation when other adverse factors such as stage are taken into consideration.[35] Prognostic factors for squamous cell carcinoma treated by radical cystectomy include pathological stage, age at diagnosis, tumor size, margin status, lymphovascular invasion, and perineural invasion.[36,37] Treatment for squamous cell carcinoma of the bladder is not different for urothelial carcinoma[38] although neoadjuvant chemotherapy is less standardized.

Whereas invasive squamous cell carcinoma may be associated with an *in situ* squamous cell carcinoma component, it is very rare to find isolated squamous cell CIS on bladder transurethral biopsy or resection specimens (Figs. 9.10-9.12, eFigs. 9.11-9.15). In the largest series of squamous cell CIS found on bladder biopsy, 3/7 patients with follow-up information were found to have invasive squamous cell carcinoma, 1/7 invasive urothelial carcinoma with squamous features, and 1/7 high-grade urothelial carcinoma.[10] Squamous cell CIS is associated with a significant risk of invasive squamous cell carcinoma. If squamous cell CIS is found on biopsy of the bladder, the need for rebiopsy and/or very close clinical follow-up of the patient for unsampled or subsequent development of invasive squamous carcinoma, respectively, should be communicated and recommended to the treating urologist.

There has also been one report of a poorly differentiated carcinoma with squamous differentiation arising in the bladder, characterized by rearrangement of the nuclear protein in testis (*NUT*) gene on chromosome 15q14. NUT carcinoma is a rare, highly lethal cancer that occurs in the

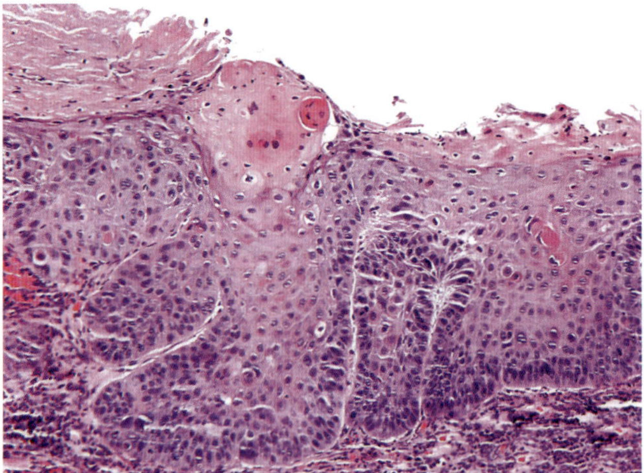

FIGURE 9.10 ***In situ*** squamous cell carcinoma.

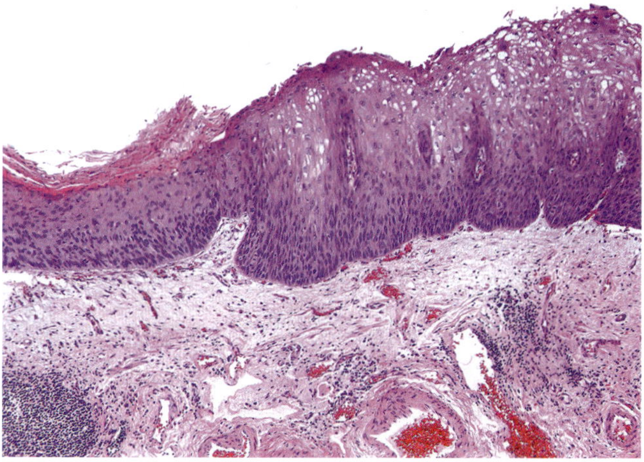

FIGURE 9.11 ***In situ*** squamous cell carcinoma.

midline, most commonly in the head, neck, or mediastinum, in children and adults of all ages.[39]

VERRUCOUS CARCINOMA

Verrucous carcinoma is a rare variant of infiltrating squamous carcinoma more commonly seen in the oral cavity, anus, or genital areas (Figs. 9.13 and 9.14, eFigs. 9.16-9.18). It is a very low-grade, orderly carcinoma (lacking atypia or disorganization) that is clinically indolent, characterized by local invasion by broad-pushing bulbous tongues of well-differentiated squamous epithelium. Pure verrucous carcinomas do not metastasize, yet

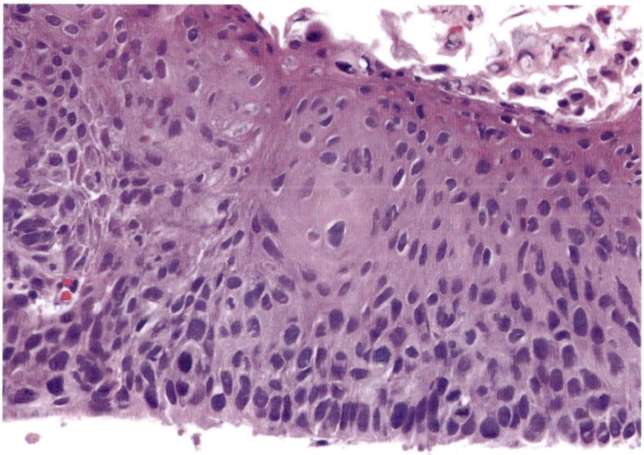

FIGURE 9.12 Higher magnification of Figure 9.11 showing ***In situ*** squamous cell carcinoma.

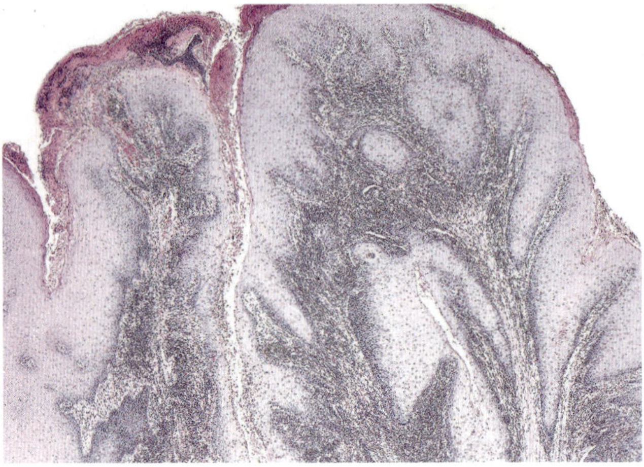

FIGURE 9.13 Verrucous carcinoma.

some verrucous carcinomas have a conventional squamous cell carcinoma component with destructive invasion, where the potential for metastatic behavior exists. The diagnosis of cancer is based on the finding that the squamous downgrowth of epithelium is too deep to represent an artifact of sectioning, verrucous hyperplasia, or pseudoepitheliomatous hyperplasia and hence must represent invasion. Few cases involving the bladder have been reported, usually in association with schistosomiasis.[40-47] Because transurethral resection specimens are rarely well oriented, it may be difficult to diagnose verrucous carcinoma on transurethral resection specimens, unless there is ample characteristic tumor or tumor is seen extending deep up to the muscularis propria. If pure verrucous carcinoma is seen in

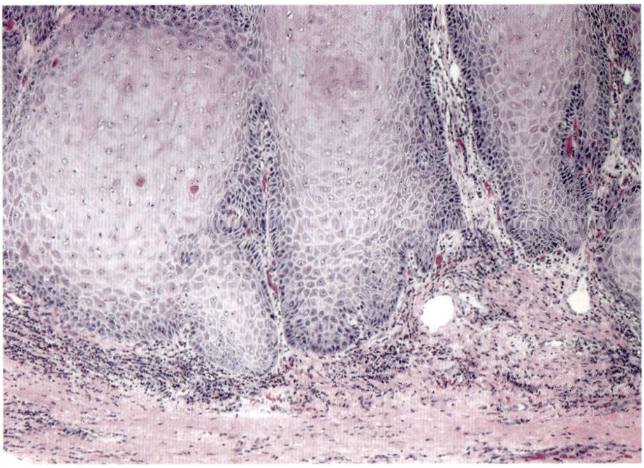

FIGURE 9.14 Base of verrucous carcinoma with pushing invasive border (same case as Figure 9.13).

a TUR specimen and if it is known or uncertain whether the entire tumor is resected, the diagnosis of "squamous cell carcinoma, well-differentiated, verrucous carcinoma histology" may be used with a comment that if pure verrucous histology is seen in the entire resected specimen, the diagnosis would be verrucous carcinoma.

REFERENCES

1. Ahmad I, Barnetson RJ, Krishna NS. Keratinizing squamous metaplasia of the bladder: a review. *Urol Int.* 2008;81:247-251.
2. Tannenbaum M. Inflammatory proliferative lesion of urinary bladder: squamous metaplasia. *Urology.* 1976;7:428-429.
3. Melekos MD, Asbach HW, Barbalias GA. Vesical diverticula: etiology, diagnosis, tumorigenesis, and treatment. Analysis of 74 cases. *Urology.* 1987;30:453-457.
4. Godwin JT, Hanash K. Pathology of bilharzial bladder cancer. *Prog Clin Biol Res.* 1984;162A:95-143.
5. Zahran MM, Kamel M, Mooro H, et al. Bilharziasis of urinary bladder and ureter: comparative histopathologic study. *Urology.* 1976;8:73-79.
6. Khan MS, Thornhill JA, Gaffney E, et al. Keratinising squamous metaplasia of the bladder: natural history and rationalization of management based on review of 54 years experience. *Eur Urol.* 2002;42:469-474.
7. Russell DH, Vang R, Epstein JI. Verrucous squamous hyperplasia of the urinary bladder: a series of 23 cases. *Arch Pathol Lab Med.* 2022;146(12):1508-1513.
8. Samarska IV, Epstein JI. Condyloma acuminatum of urinary bladder: Relation to squamous cell carcinoma. *Am J Surg Pathol.* 2019;43(11):1547-1553.
9. Cheng L, Leibovich BC, Cheville JC, et al. Squamous papilloma of the urinary tract is unrelated to condyloma acuminata. *Cancer.* 2000;88(7):1679-1686.
10. Guo CC, Fine SW, Epstein JI. Noninvasive squamous lesions in the urinary bladder: a clinicopathologic analysis of 29 cases. *Am J Surg Pathol.* 2006;30(7):883-891.
11. Abol Enein H, Kava BR, Carmack AJ. Nonurothelial cancer of the bladder. *Urology.* 2007;69:93-104.
12. Salem HK, Mahfouz S. Changing patterns (age, incidence, and pathologic types) of schistosoma-associated bladder cancer in Egypt in the past decade. *Urology.* 2012;79:379-383.
13. Salem S, Mitchell RE, El-Alim El-Dorey A, et al. Successful control of schistosomiasis and the changing epidemiology of bladder cancer in Egypt. *BJU Int.* 2011;107:206-211.
14. El-Sebaie M, Zaghloul MS, Howard G, et al. Squamous cell carcinoma of the bilharzial and non-bilharzial urinary bladder: a review of etiological features, natural history, and management. *Int J Clin Oncol.* 2005;10:20-25.
15. Felix AS, Soliman AS, Khaled H, et al. The changing patterns of bladder cancer in Egypt over the past 26 years. *Cancer Causes Control.* 2008;19:421-429.
16. Khafagy MM, el-Bolkainy MN, Mansour MA. Carcinoma of the bilharzial urinary bladder. A study of the associated mucosal lesions in 86 cases. *Cancer.* 1972;30:150-159.
17. Rausch S, Lotan Y, Youssef RF. Squamous cell carcinogenesis and squamous cell carcinoma of the urinary bladder: a contemporary review with focus on nonbilharzial squamous cell carcinoma. *Urol Oncol.* 2014;32:32.e11-32.e16.
18. Lopez-Beltran A, Requena MJ, Alvarez-Kindelan J, et al. Squamous differentiation in primary urothelial carcinoma of the urinary tract as seen by MAC387 immunohistochemistry. *J Clin Pathol.* 2007;60:332-335.
19. Monn MF, Kaimakliotis HZ, Pedrosa JA, et al. Contemporary bladder cancer: variant histology may be a significant driver of disease. *Urol Oncol.* 2015;33:18.e15-18.e20.

20. Soave A, Schmidt S, Dahlem R, et al. Does the extent of variant histology affect oncological outcomes in patients with urothelial carcinoma of the bladder treated with radical cystectomy? *Urol Oncol*. 2015;33:21.e1-21.e9.
21. Xylinas E, Rink M, Robinson BD, et al. Impact of histological variants on oncological outcomes of patients with urothelial carcinoma of the bladder treated with radical cystectomy. *Eur J Cancer*. 2013;49:1889-1897.
22. Kantor AF, Hartge P, Hoover RN, et al. Epidemiological characteristics of squamous cell carcinoma and adenocarcinoma of the bladder. *Cancer Res*. 1988;48(13):3853-3855.
23. Gordetsky J, Spieker AJ, Pena MDCR, et al. Squamous cell carcinoma of the bladder is not associated with high-risk HPV. *Urology*. 2020;144:158-163.
24. Collins K, Hwang M, Hamza A, et al. Prevalence of high-risk human papillomavirus in primary squamous cell carcinoma of urinary bladder. *Pathol Res Pract*. 2020;216(9):153084.
25. Schwartz LE, Khani F, Bishop JA, et al. Carcinoma of the uterine cervix involving the genitourinary tract: a potential diagnostic dilemma. *Am J Surg Pathol*. 2016;40(1):27-35.
26. Blochin EB, Park KJ, Tickoo SK, et al. Urothelial carcinoma with prominent squamous differentiation in the setting of neurogenic bladder: role of human papillomavirus infection. *Mod Pathol*. 2012;25(11):1534-1542.
27. Porter MP, Voigt LF, Penson DF, et al. Racial variation in the incidence of squamous cell carcinoma of the bladder in the United States. *J Urol*. 2002;168:1960-1963.
28. Lagwinski N, Thomas A, Stephenson AJ, et al. Squamous cell carcinoma of the bladder: a clinicopathologic analysis of 45 cases. *Am J Surg Pathol*. 2007;31:1777-1787.
29. Paner GP, Annaiah C, Gulmann C, et al. Immunohistochemical evaluation of novel and traditional markers associated with urothelial differentiation in a spectrum of variants of urothelial carcinoma of the urinary bladder. *Hum Pathol*. 2014;45:1473-1482.
30. Rogers CG, Palapattu GS, Shariat SF, et al. Clinical outcomes following radical cystectomy for primary nontransitional cell carcinoma of the bladder compared to transitional cell carcinoma of the bladder. *J Urol*. 2006;175:2048-2053.
31. Newman DM, Brown JR, Jay AC, et al. Squamous cell carcinoma of the bladder. *J Urol*. 1968;100:470-473.
32. Mitra AP, Bartsch CC, Bartsch G Jr, et al. Does presence of squamous and glandular differentiation in urothelial carcinoma of the bladder at cystectomy portend poor prognosis? An intensive case–control analysis. *Urol Oncol*. 2014;32:117-127.
33. Izard JP, Siemens DR, Mackillop WJ, et al. Outcomes of squamous histology in bladder cancer: a population-based study. *Urol Oncol*. 2015;33(10):425.e7-425.e13.
34. Ghoneim MA, Abdel-Latif M, el-Mekresh M, et al. Radical cystectomy for carcinoma of the bladder: 2,720 consecutive cases 5 years later. *J Urol*. 2008;180(1):121-127.
35. Ehdaie B, Maschino A, Shariat SF, et al. Comparative outcomes of pure squamous cell carcinoma and urothelial carcinoma with squamous differentiation in patients treated with radical cystectomy. *J Urol*. 2012;187:74-79.
36. Abdel-Rahman O. Squamous cell carcinoma of the bladder: a SEER database analysis. *Clin Genitourin Cancer*. 2017;15(3):e463-e468. doi:10.1016/j.clgc.2016.10.007
37. Zhang G, Li Z, Song D, Fang Z. Nomograms to predict individual prognosis of patients with squamous cell carcinoma of the urinary bladder. *BMC Cancer*. 2019;19(1):1200. doi:10.1186/s12885-019-6430-6
38. Rosiello G, Pecoraro A, Palumbo C, et al. Radical cystectomy plus chemotherapy in patients with pure squamous cell bladder carcinoma: a population-based study. *World J Urol*. 2021;39(3):813-822.
39. French CA, Kutok JL, Faquin WC, et al. Midline carcinoma of children and young adults with NUT rearrangement. *J Clin Oncol*. 2004;22:4135-4139.
40. el-Sebai I, Sherif M, el-Bolkainy MN, et al. Verrucous squamous carcinoma of bladder. *Urology*. 1974;4:407-410.

41. Faysal MH. Squamous cell carcinoma of the bladder. *J Urol.* 1981;126:598-599.
42. Holck S, Jorgensen L. Verrucous carcinoma of urinary bladder. *Urology.* 1983;22: 435-437.
43. Wyatt JK, Craig I. Verrucous carcinoma of urinary bladder. *Urology.* 1980;16:97-99.
44. el-Boulkany MN, Ghoneim MA, Mansour MA. Carcinoma of the bilharzial bladder in Egypt. Clinical and pathological features. *Br J Urol.* 1972;44(5):561-570.
45. Park S, Reuter VE, Hansel DE. Non-urothelial carcinomas of the bladder. *Histopathology.* 2019;74(1):97-111.
46. Ellsworth PI, Schned AR, Heaney JA, et al. Surgical treatment of verrucous carcinoma of the bladder unassociated with bilharzial cystitis: case report and literature review. *J Urol.* 1995;153(2):411-414.
47. Mahran MR, el-Baz M. Verrucous carcinoma of the bilharzial bladder. Impact of invasiveness on survival. *Scand J Urol Nephrol.* 1993;27(2):189-192.

10

CYSTITIS

INFECTIOUS

Encrusted Cystitis

Encrusted cystitis refers to inorganic salts being deposited in injured urothelial mucosa as a consequence of urea-splitting bacteria, alkalinizing urine.[1] This lesion is most common in women. Cystoscopically, the surface of the bladder is gritty. Histologically, deposits of calcium are present in the lamina propria, and the mucosal surface of the bladder is covered with fibrin mixed with calcific, necrotic debris associated with inflammatory cells. Rarely, carcinoma of the bladder may have overlying calcification and necrosis, and correlation with cystoscopy (mass lesion) is important.

Emphysematous Cystitis

This lesion, also known as pneumatosis of the bladder, refers to the presence of gas-filled blebs, predominantly within the lamina propria, which can be seen both at cystoscopy and on the gross examination.[2] This lesion is more typically found in women, often diabetic, and associated with bacterial infections. Predisposing conditions include trauma, fistula, instrumentation, and urinary stasis. In children, it may be a complication of necrotizing enterocolitis. Microscopically, the blebs consist of empty cavities lined by flattened cells surrounded by thin septa; frequently, there is an associated foreign body giant cell reaction focally lining the empty spaces (Figs. 10.1 and 10.2). Microbiologic studies are critical for patient management.

Fungal Cystitis

Fungal cystitis is uncommon and most often caused by *Candida albicans.*[3] Cases of cystitis caused by *Aspergillus* species and other fungi have also been rarely reported. Women are predominantly affected. Most patients are debilitated or immunocompromised or are on antibiotic therapy, with diabetic patients being another commonly affected group.

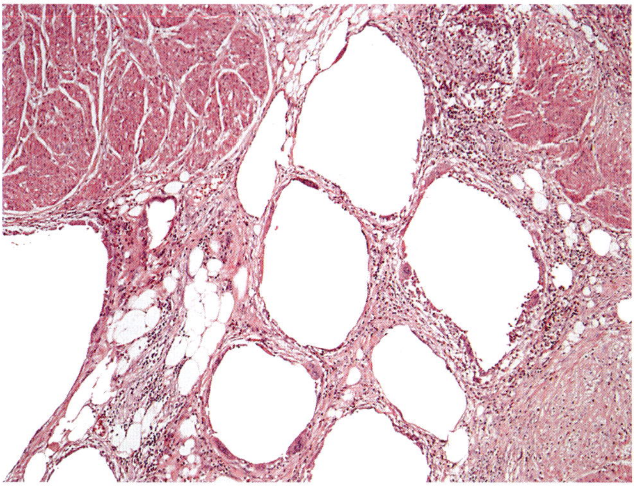

FIGURE 10.1 Emphysematous cystitis.

Tuberculosis (Including Bacillus Calmette-Guérin)

Most bladder lesions involved by *Mycobacterium* tuberculosis are secondary to renal involvement.[4] Typically, the infection begins around ureteral orifices with superficial ulceration, with acute and chronic inflammation, and initially noncaseating granulomas. Larger caseating granulomas may follow. Late complications include ulcers with fibrosis that can result in ureteral strictures and fibrosis of the bladder wall. The histology of tuberculosis more typically seen in current practice is that associated with intravesical bacillus Calmette-Guérin (BCG) immunotherapy for superficial

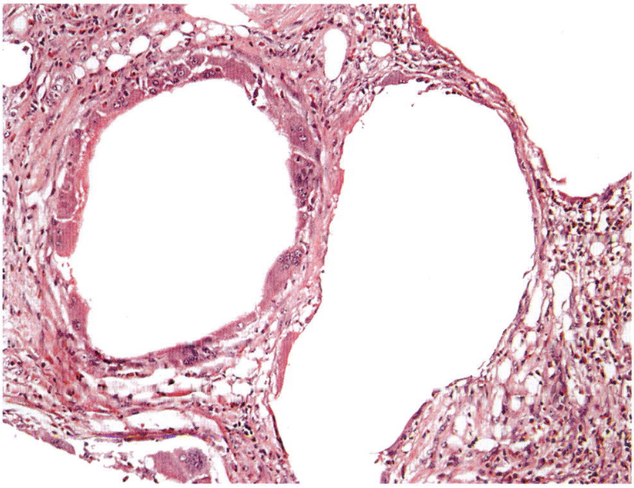

FIGURE 10.2 Higher magnification of Figure 10.1 showing empty spaces of air surrounded by giant cell reaction.

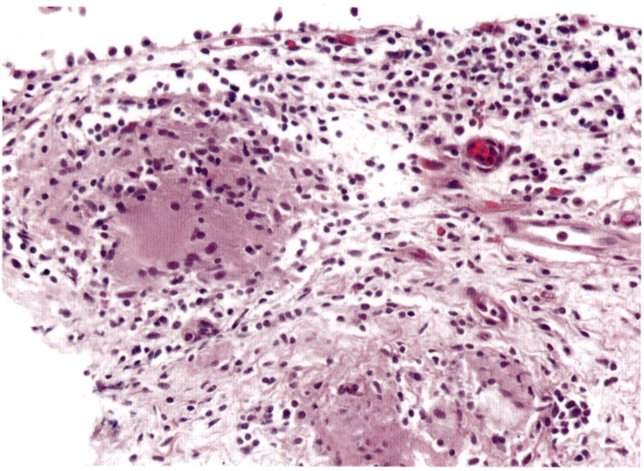

FIGURE 10.3 Small submucosal noncaseating granulomas following BCG immunotherapy.

bladder cancer and consists of small, noncaseating granulomas (Fig. 10.3) (see section "Treatment Related"). In patients with a known history of BCG immunotherapy and granulomas on bladder biopsy, we do not perform special stains for organisms. Postprocedural granulomas (usually with fibrinoid necrosis) are in the differential diagnosis.

Schistosomiasis

Schistosomiasis is a chronic disease involving the bladder caused by larvae of *Schistosoma haematobium*[5,6] (Figs. 10.4-10.6, eFigs. 10.1-10.5). Coupled adult male and female worms migrate to the veins of the vesical and pelvic

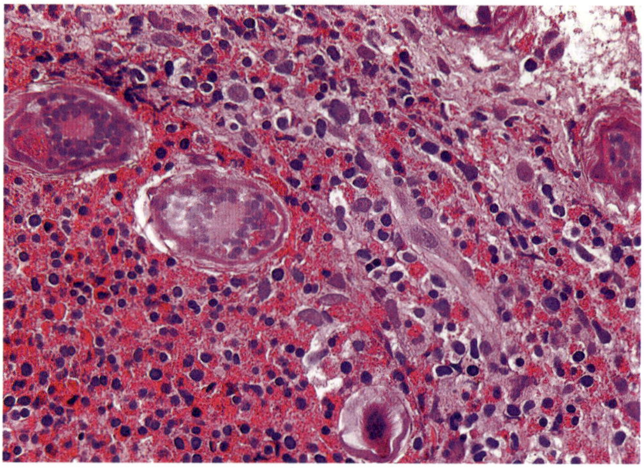

FIGURE 10.4 Eggs of schistosomiasis with associated prominent eosinophil infiltrate.

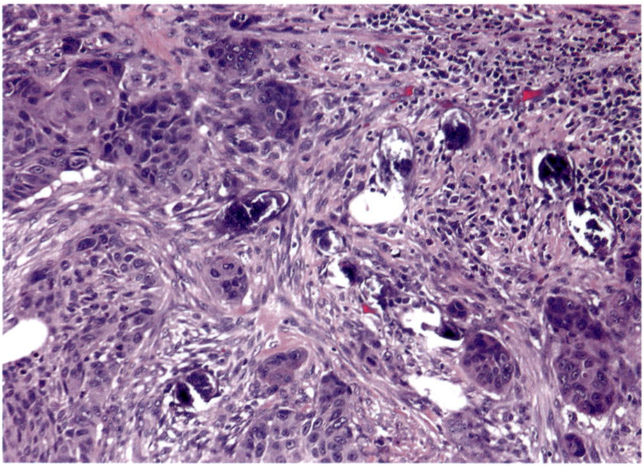

FIGURE 10.5 Calcified eggs of schistosomiasis associated with infiltrating squamous cell carcinoma.

plexuses, where they mate and females begin to lay eggs. Involvement of various urogenital organs correlates with the extent of the venous circulation, such that the urinary bladder with a rich venous supply is most heavily infected. Schistosomiasis most commonly occurs in the Middle East and in most of the African continent. The highest incidence is where irrigation agriculture is prevalent, such as in the Nile Valley and Delta. The initial response to *S haematobium* infection is a reaction of the host against the deposition of eggs. This lesion manifests as a granulomatous reaction to the eggs surrounded by numerous eosinophils. *S haematobium* eggs have terminal spines that differentiate them from other schistosomes, but this is difficult to appreciate in histologic sections. Another differentiating feature

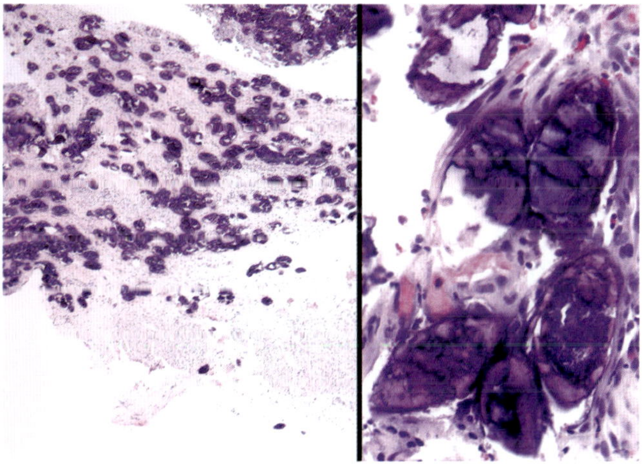

FIGURE 10.6 Numerous calcified eggs of schistosomiasis.

is that *S haematobium* eggshells are not acid-fast, whereas *Schistosoma mansoni* and *Schistosoma japonicum* eggs are. There are several histologic stages of schistosomiasis within the bladder. The background inflammatory pattern correlates with acuteness or chronicity of the disease including keratinizing metaplasia and dysplasia or intestinal metaplasia. Recent oviposition gives rise to perioval granulomatous inflammation, which can result in hyperemic polypoid masses. With greater chronicity and less ova position, eggs are destroyed or calcified and inflammation subsides. This gives rise to more fibrous tissue and "sandy patches," in which there is atrophy of the surface epithelium over the schistosomal lesion; old calcified schistosomal eggs buried immediately beneath the mucosa resemble sand seen through shallow water. One may also see schistosomal tubercles that are a manifestation of early active disease, appearing as seedlike, yellowish specks just beneath the urothelium. Each speck reflects a granuloma surrounded by a circle of hyperemia.

Patients with schistosomiasis of the lower urinary tract typically present with painful micturition, frequency, pyuria, and hematuria. Anemia and eosinophilia are common. With greater chronicity, individuals acquire "contracted bladder" syndrome, in which there is intense ova position involving all levels of the muscularis propria with dense fibrosis. Patients present with intractable frequency, painful urination, urgency, and incontinence. Surgery may be indicated when the bladder capacity is significantly reduced, requiring augmentation cystoplasty, using either the ileum or the colon. Another complication of schistosomiasis within the bladder is ulceration that is attributed to local ischemia caused by schistosomal obliteration of deeper vessels or onset of secondary bacterial infection. Although ulcers may respond to antischistosomal therapy, often total excision by partial cystectomy or endoscopic resection is required. Other nonneoplastic complications include bladder neck obstruction and ureteral strictures. Males are affected more than females in a 4:1 ratio. Carcinogenesis resulting from schistosomal infections is the result of chronic injury, often accompanying bacterial infection, foreign bodies, and urinary concentration of nitrosamines (see Chapter 9).

Malakoplakia

Malakoplakia may affect multiple organs, although the bladder is most commonly involved.[7] The lesion may manifest as a fibroinflammatory process with a mixed infiltrate including numerous plasma cells, histiocytes, and lymphocytes, or they may be rich with histiocytes (foamy or eosinophilic cytoplasm). The pathognomonic cells are large histiocytes, known as *von Hansemann cells*, containing small basophilic extracytoplasmic or intracytoplasmic calculopherules, called *Michaelis-Gutmann bodies* (Fig. 10.7, eFigs. 10.6-10.11). The bodies are found within the interstitium as well as within histiocytes. Bacteria or bacterial fragments (*Escherichia coli* and other Gram-negative bacilli) form a nidus for the calcium phosphate crystals that laminate the Michaelis-Gutmann bodies. A defect

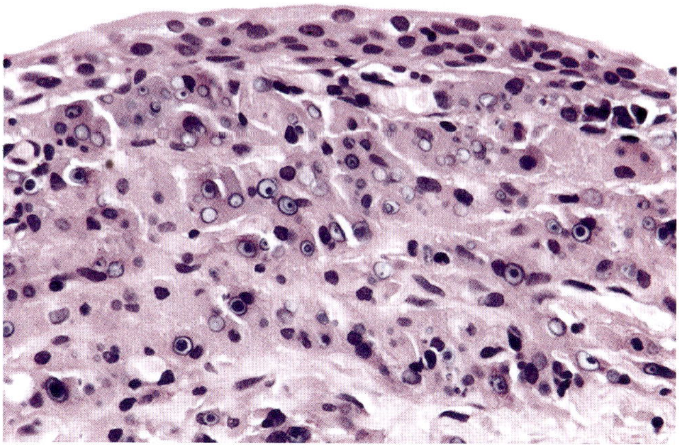

FIGURE 10.7 Malakoplakia with Michaelis-Gutmann bodies.

in intraphagosomal digestion, which accounts for the unusual immune response, gives rise to malakoplakia.[8-13] Electron microscopy reveals intact coliform bacteria and bacterial fragments within phagolysosomes within the foamy histiocytes. The overlying urothelium may be ulcerated, hyperplastic, or metaplastic. Some cases present primarily with sheets of histiocytes, while other have mixed inflammatory infiltrate. In long-standing lesions, the characteristic infiltrate is replaced by fibrosis and scarring. The characteristic Michaelis-Gutmann bodies may be hard to find, and one must have a high index of suspicion for malakoplakia in a chronic histiocytic inflammatory background. Most patients are middle aged with a female predominance of 4:1. Patients may be debilitated or immunosuppressed or have other chronic diseases. Cystoscopy reveals mucosal plaques and nodules that (malkos–soft; plakia–plaques), on occasion, become larger masses. There can be significant morbidity, including ureteral strictural stenosis, giving rise to renal obstruction or nonfunction. Management of malakoplakia is primarily based on controlling the urinary tract infections, which stabilizes the disease. Adding bethanechol, a cholinergic agent thought to increase intracellular cyclic guanosine monophosphate levels considered to be the defect causing macrophage dysfunction, may also be useful. Surgery may be necessary as the disease progresses, despite antimicrobial treatment. Malakoplakia may also result in death if it involves both kidneys. PAS with diastase, iron and calcium stains can highlight Michaelis-Gutmann bodies. The differential diagnosis includes extranodal Rosai-Dorfman disease, xanthogranulomatous inflammation, IgG4-related sclerosing disease, and atypical mycobacterial infection.

Viral Cystitis

Both adenovirus and herpes simplex type 2 virus have been associated with hemorrhagic cystitis in a few patients (Figs. 10.8 and 10.9).[14,15] Herpes

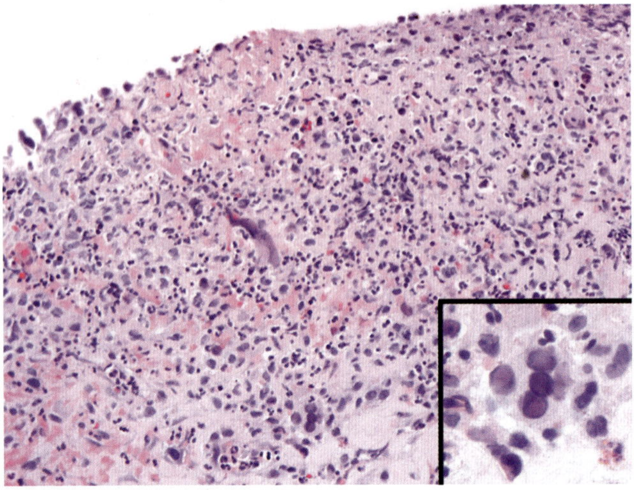

FIGURE 10.8 Denuded bladder tissue with extensive karyorrhexis and herpes viral inclusions (***inset***).

zoster and cytomegalovirus have also been rarely implicated in bladder infections.[16,17] HPV-associated lesions are covered in Chapter 9.

Patients with polyoma viruses and bladder involvement are usually immunosuppressed renal or bone marrow allograft recipients with hemorrhagic cystitis.[18,19] Despite the frequency of viruria and intranuclear inclusions seen in urinary cytology specimens in these patients, the identification of inclusions in histologic tissue sections is rare[20] (Figs. 10.10 and 10.11, eFigs. 10.12 and 10.13). The cytohistologic discordance might be due to the following reasons: (1) polyoma (BK) virus–infected cells are

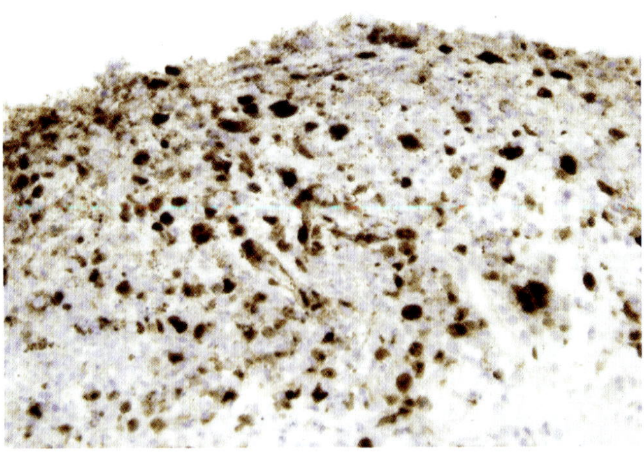

FIGURE 10.9 Immunohistochemistry for herpes virus demonstrates more virus than appreciable on H&E-stained section.

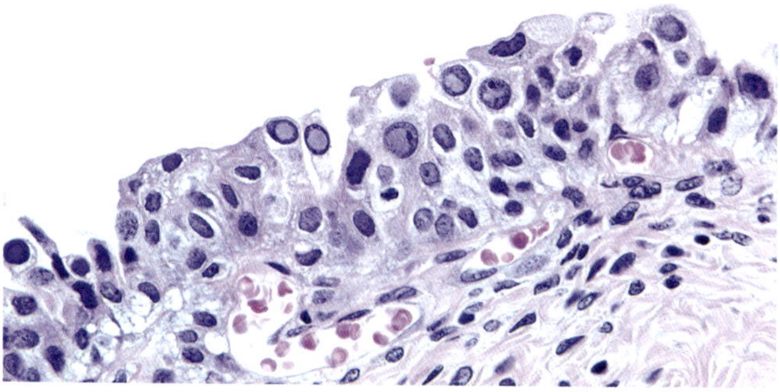

FIGURE 10.10 Polyoma virus infection.

shed from the tissue and collected in the urine; (2) polyoma virus changes may be focal and not sampled in directed tissue biopsies; and (3) polyoma virus changes may originate from sites in the genitourinary tract other than the bladder. Immunohistochemistry may be used to confirm the virus.

NONINFECTIOUS

Polypoid Cystitis

Polypoid cystitis may arise as a reaction to any inflammatory insult to the urinary mucosa[21-23] (eFigs. 10.14-10.46). The presence of indwelling catheters is a well-recognized etiology for polypoid cystitis.

However, any factor that irritates the bladder mucosa can result in polypoid cystitis, such as colovesical fistulas, calculi, urinary tract obstruction, and prior radiation therapy. It occurs equally in males and females, with an age range of 20 months to 79 years. Cystoscopically, it appears as

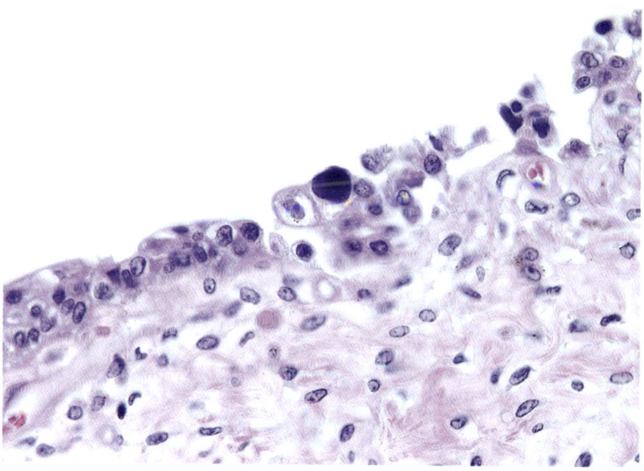

FIGURE 10.11 Polyoma virus infection.

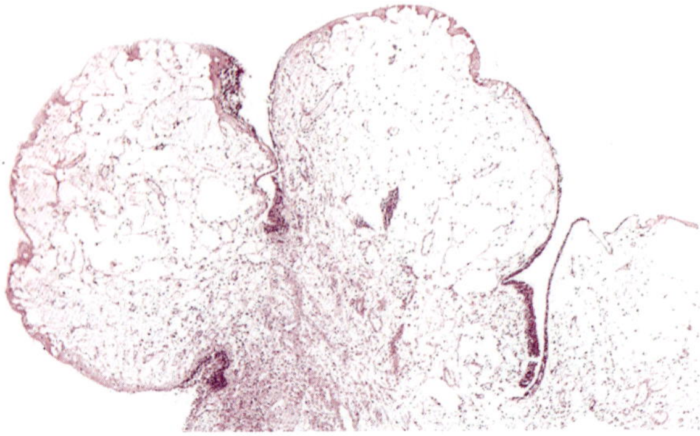

FIGURE 10.12 Polypoid cystitis (bullous cystitis).

either an area of friable mucosal irregularity or edematous broad papillae. Lesions may be multifocal and can range up to 5 mm in size.

In its most pronounced form, polypoid cystitis shows extensive submucosal edema with broad bulbous projections termed *bullous cystitis* (Fig. 10.12). Other cases of polypoid cystitis may be more difficult to distinguish from papillary urothelial neoplasm of low malignant potential and papillary urothelial carcinoma, especially in some areas of the biopsy. However, these examples of polypoid cystitis still show edematous fibrovascular cores that are broad based in contrast to narrow-necked, thin, and delicate fibrovascular cores of papillary urothelial neoplasm of low malignant potential and papillary urothelial carcinoma (Fig. 10.13). The fronds in polypoid cystitis do not branch into smaller papillae as can be seen in papillary urothelial carcinoma. While these are the classic features of polypoid cystitis, in a minority of cases, there may be narrow-based fronds, typically associated with broad-based fronds elsewhere in the lesion but occasionally as the sole finding (Fig. 10.14; Table 10.1).[21] Other overlapping

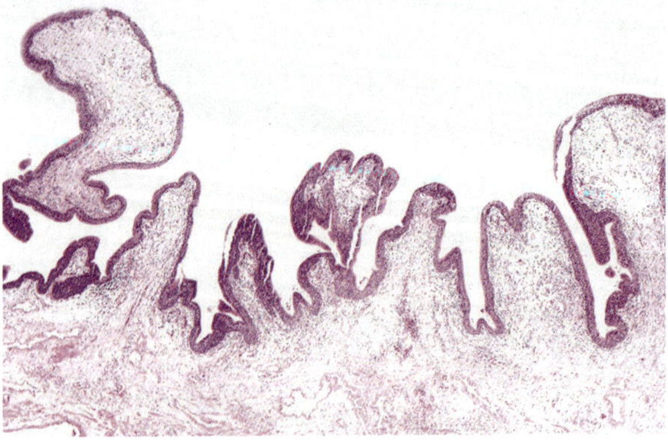

FIGURE 10.13 Polypoid cystitis.

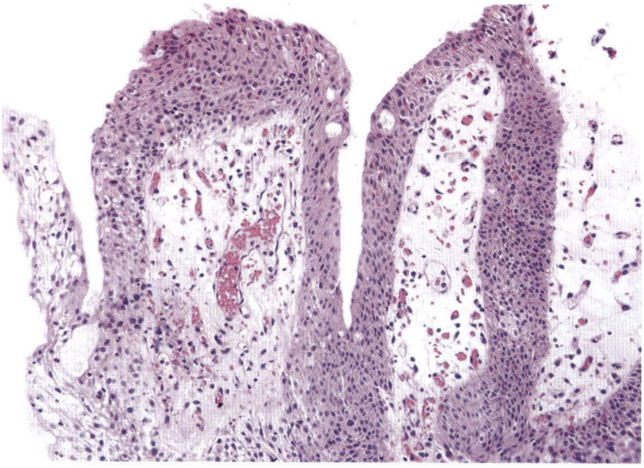

FIGURE 10.14 Polypoid cystitis with reactive cytologic atypia.

features can also lead to a misdiagnosis. Isolated papillary fronds within otherwise classic polypoid cystitis may lack edema and out of context can closely resemble a papillary neoplasm. Conversely, occasional fronds of papillary urothelial neoplasia may be edematous and have some inflammation. Similarly, in a minority of polypoid cystitis cases, the urothelium may

TABLE 10.1 Histology of Polypoid Cystitis

Architecture of Fronds	
Isolated fronds	76%
Branching	2%
Broad and narrow base	58%
Broad-only base	22%
Narrow-only base	7%
Stroma within Fronds	
Edematous	78%
Fibrosis	39%
Urothelium	
Diffusely thickened	19%
Focally thickened	12%
Umbrella cells	8%
Reactive urothelial atypia	63%
Mitotic figures	54%
Inflammation	
Acute and chronic	68%
Chronic	24%

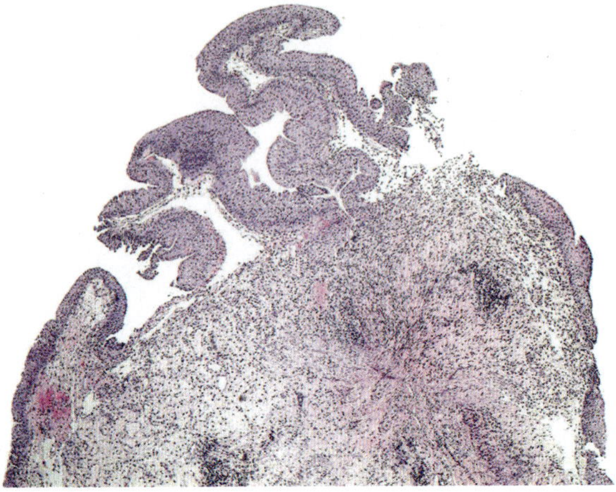

FIGURE 10.15 Polypoid cystitis (papillary cystitis) with inflamed fibrous tissue in stalk.

be focally or even diffusely thickened, although not typically to the extent seen in some papillary urothelial neoplasms.

With time, fronds of polypoid cystitis lesions become less edematous and are replaced by dense fibrosis often associated with chronic inflammation. These lesions may be referred to as *papillary cystitis*[21] (Figs. 10.15-10.17). The fibrous tissue in papillary cystitis differs from the delicate loose connective tissue within the fronds of papillary urothelial neoplasms. Out of context, several papillary fronds within polypoid cystitis may closely resemble papillary urothelial carcinoma (Figs. 10.18-10.23). However, one must assess the lesion in its entirety, and, if overall the lesion is that of polypoid cystitis, one should not overdiagnose isolated papillary fronds as carcinoma.

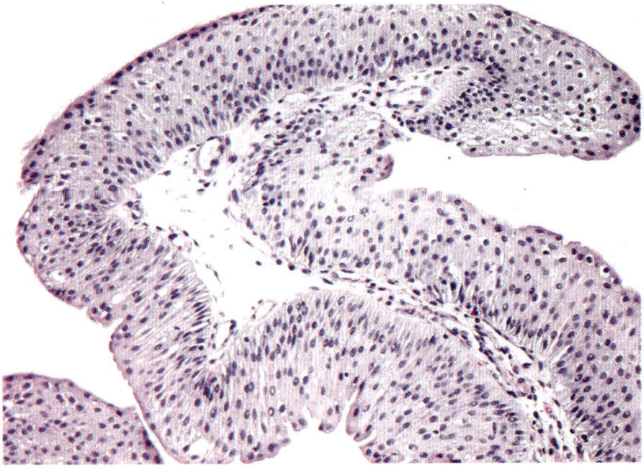

FIGURE 10.16 Papillary cystitis fronds that out of context may mimic papillary urothelial neoplasia.

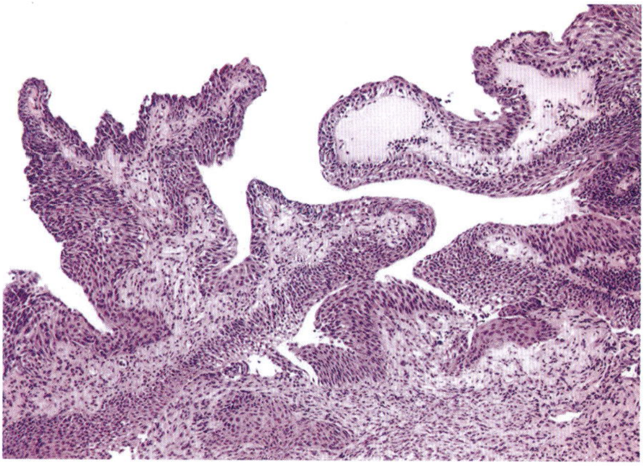

FIGURE 10.17 Papillary cystitis with branching frond containing fibrotic and chronically inflamed stroma (*left*). Note edematous frond (*upper right*).

The urothelial mucosa overlying the edematous stalks may be normal or show reactive urothelial atypia or squamous metaplasia with occasional mitotic figures that in some cases may be frequent (Figs. 10.20-10.25). The key to correctly diagnosing polypoid/papillary cystitis is to recognize at low magnification the reactive nature of the process with an inflamed background that is edematous or densely fibrous with predominantly simple, nonbranching, broad-based fronds of relatively normal thickness urothelium and not focus at higher power on the exceptional frond that may more closely resemble a urothelial neoplasm either architecturally or cytologically. In cases where the diagnosis of papillary neoplasia is not straightforward and there is a question of polypoid cystitis, pathologists should seek clinical history that might suggest a reactive process. Because the urologist can more often better recognize the inflammatory nature of the lesion than can the

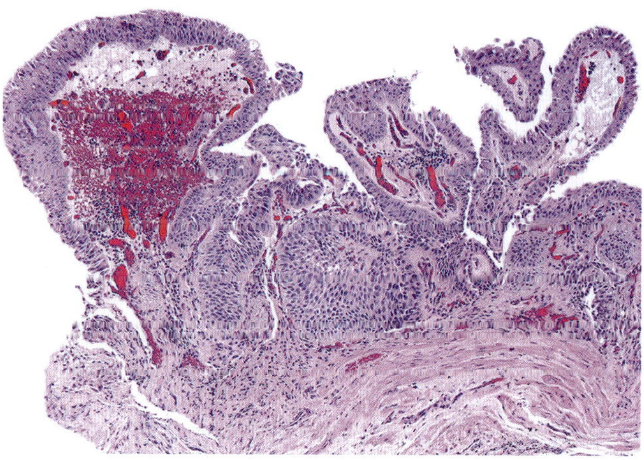

FIGURE 10.18 Polypoid cystitis with narrow-based simple fronds.

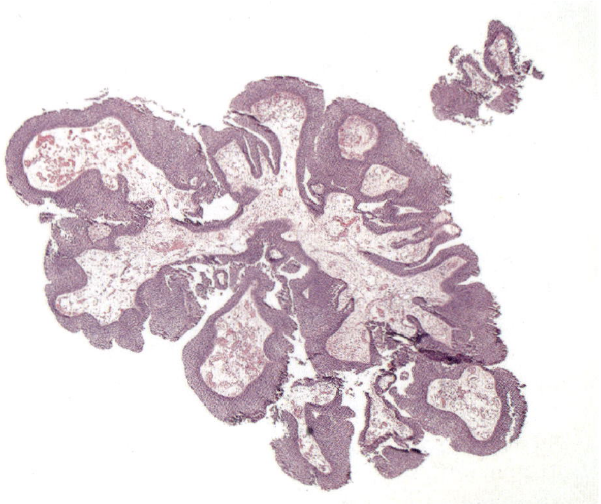

FIGURE 10.19 **Papillary/polypoid cystitis.** Fronds with edema and chronic inflammation are lined by bland hyperplastic cytologically unremarkable urothelium.

pathologist, the pathologist should hesitate diagnosing urothelial neoplasia when the cystoscopic impression is that of an inflammatory lesion. Polypoid cystitis is a benign lesion without any risk of evolving into carcinoma.

Eosinophilic Cystitis

Eosinophilic cystitis may be seen at all ages and is characterized by dense infiltrate of eosinophils within the lamina propria, submucosa, and, often,

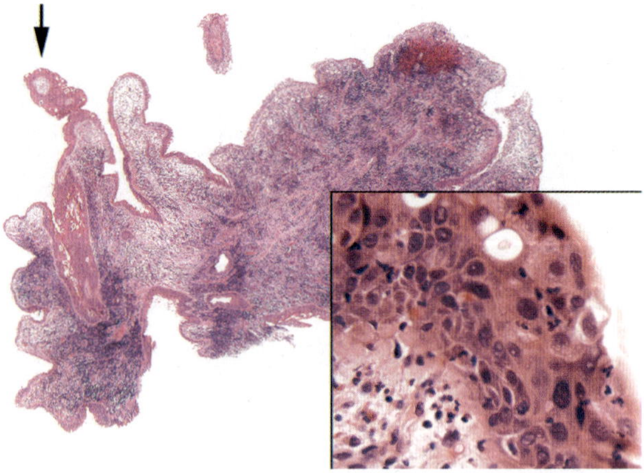

FIGURE 10.20 **Polypoid cystitis with marked inflammation with rare fronds that out of context can be misinterpreted as papillary urothelial neoplasia (*arrow*). *Inset* with reactive cytologic atypia.**

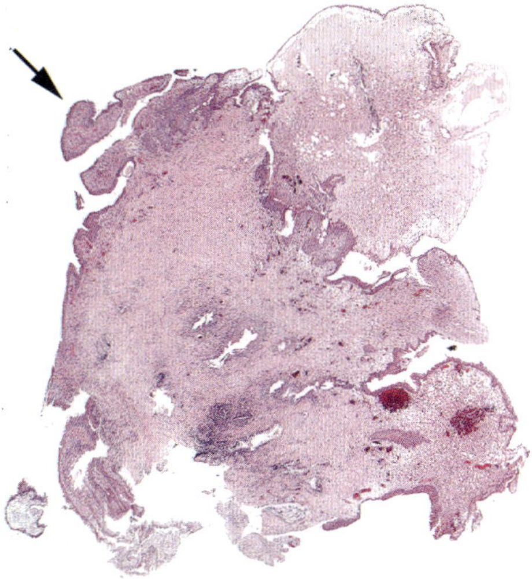

FIGURE 10.21 **Polypoid cystitis with broad-based edematous fronds (*right*).** Isolated fronds (*arrow*) with less edema mimics papillary neoplasia.

muscularis propria[24] (Figs. 10.26 and 10.27, eFigs. 10.47 and 10.48). There are two broad settings in which eosinophilic cystitis is found. The most common is that of a subacute, nonspecific inflammatory reaction caused by some other injury. Numerous eosinophils may be seen accompanying carcinomas, areas of prior surgery, various drugs, and as a response to

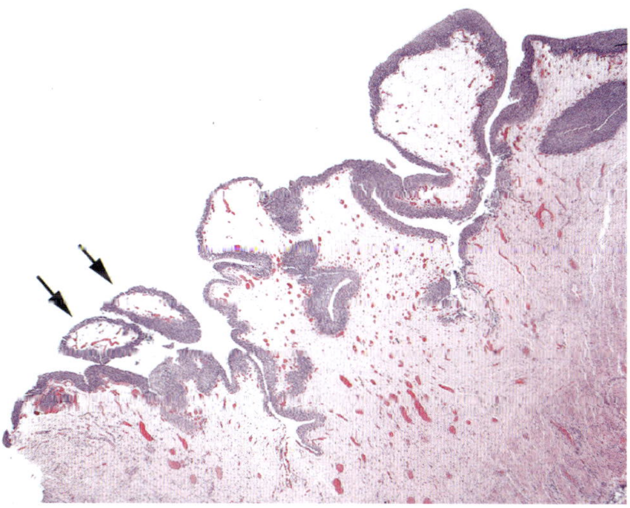

FIGURE 10.22 **Polypoid cystitis with broad-based edematous fronds (*center*) and several isolated fronds (*arrows*) mimicking papillary urothelial neoplasia.**

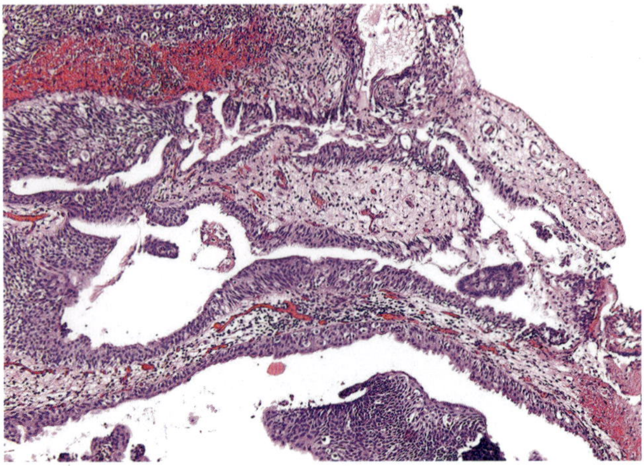

FIGURE 10.23 Thin stalks of polypoid cystitis with inflammation and minimal edema lined by normal-appearing urothelium.

catheterization. In most of these settings, the eosinophilic infiltrate is not symptomatic and is self-limited. More rarely, eosinophilic cystitis may be seen as a true allergic reaction, such as a reaction to a particular food or drug. Some of these patients may have associated peripheral eosinophilia or associated collagen vascular disease. Associated parasitic infection and chronic granulomatous disease of childhood may also be associated with an eosinophilic infiltrate in the lamina propria. Treatment in this setting

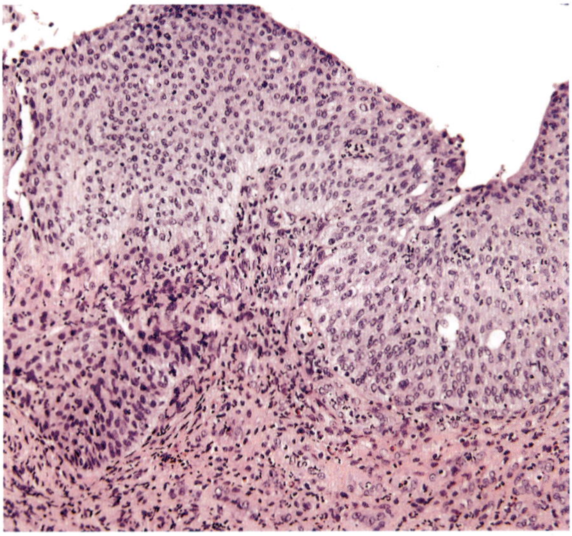

FIGURE 10.24 Polypoid cystitis with thickened acutely inflamed urothelium with reactive atypia.

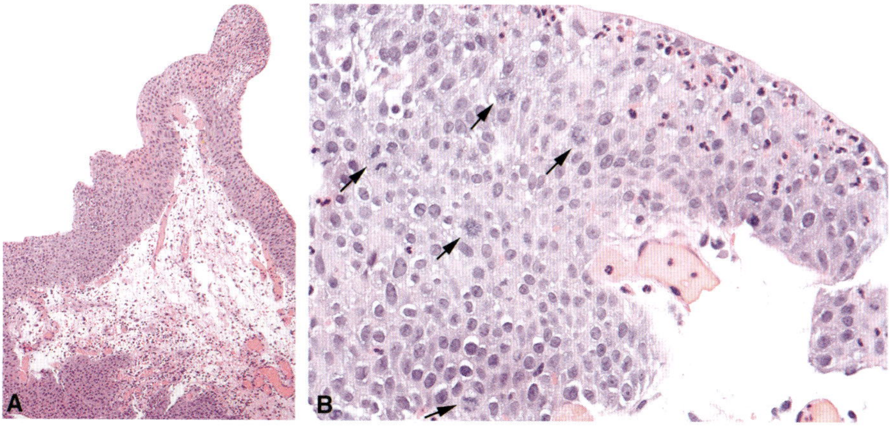

FIGURE 10.25 **A:** Polypoid cystitis in patient with indwelling catheter with simple edematous inflamed broad-based fold. **B:** Higher magnification with uniformly enlarged nuclei with single central nucleoli and lack of hyperchromasia, typical of reactive changes, associated with prominent acute inflammation. Note numerous mitotic figures (***arrows***).

consists of removing the suspected allergen and, in some cases, corticosteroids, anticholinergic drugs, and antiallergic drugs.

Follicular Cystitis

Follicular cystitis, which is more prevalent in children, consists of lymphoid follicles within the lamina propria[25] (Fig. 10.28, eFigs. 10.49-10.51). This lesion may be seen grossly as pinpoint white lesions. It is believed to be caused by the presence of bacteria in the bladder and can resolve following antibiotic therapy. Another association is with BCG immunotherapy and instrumentation. Only rarely, and when florid, the differential with a low-grade follicular lymphoma must be entertained.

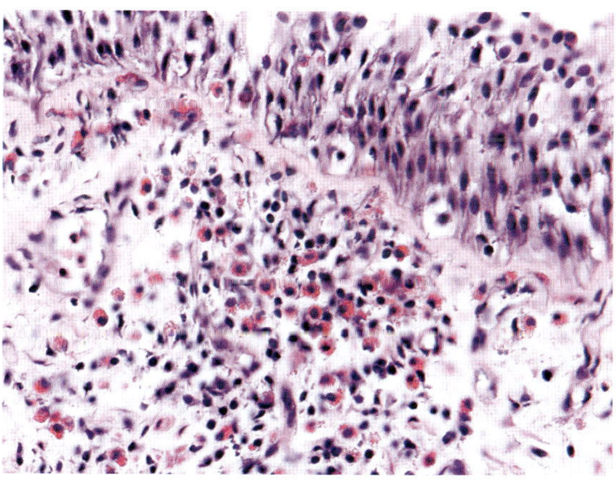

FIGURE 10.26 Eosinophilic cystitis.

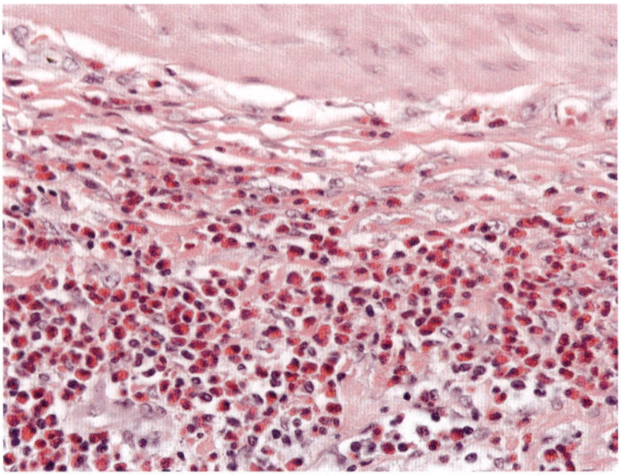

FIGURE 10.27 Eosinophilic cystitis with numerous eosinophils.

Giant Cell Cystitis

It is not uncommon to find with the lamina propria reactive-appearing stromal cells that are indistinguishable from the fibroblasts associated with radiation and/or chemotherapy. In contrast to sarcomas, the cells are sparse, have degenerative-appearing nuclear atypia, and no mitotic activity and do not form a mass lesion (Fig. 10.29, eFigs. 10.52 and 10.53).[26] In other cases, stromal cells that appear atypical at low magnification are merely multinucleated. It is unlikely that this lesion represents an inflammatory lesion.

TREATMENT RELATED

Granulomatous Cystitis Secondary to BCG Therapy or Transurethral Biopsy

Urothelial carcinoma *in situ* (CIS) and high-grade papillary carcinomas are commonly treated with intravesical installations of BCG, which usually

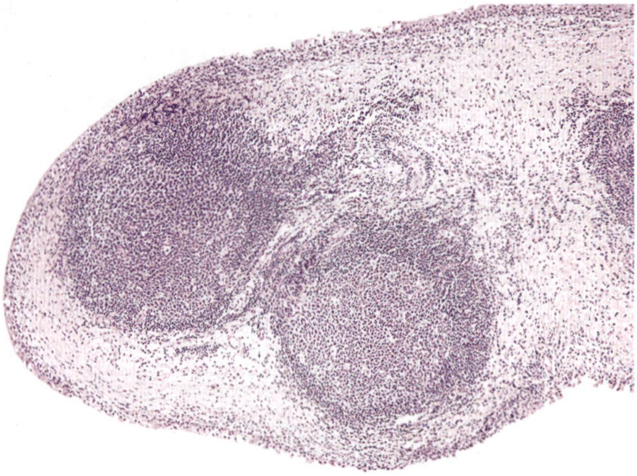

FIGURE 10.28 Follicular cystitis.

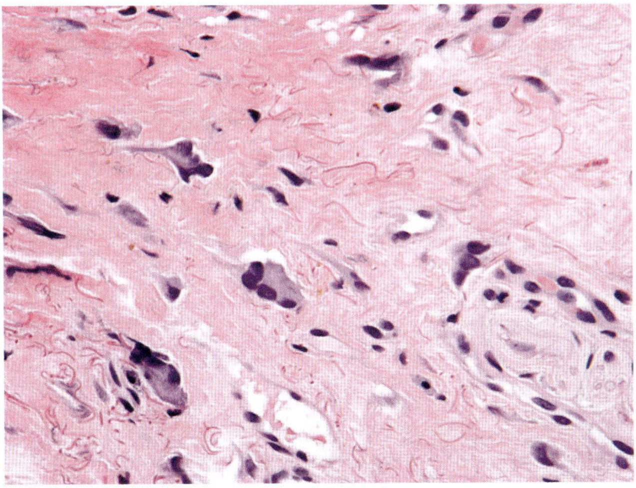

FIGURE 10.29 Giant cell cystitis.

induces an intense inflammatory reaction (BCG cystitis).[27-29] It is characterized by the presence of discrete noncaseating granulomas containing epithelioid histiocytes and multinucleated giant cells (Fig. 10.3). The granulomas are usually situated in the superficial third of the lamina propria and are associated with an intense lymphocytic infiltrate. The overlying urothelium may show nonspecific reactive atypia or may be partially or entirely denuded. Urine cytology commonly reveals inflammatory cells, including epithelioid histiocytes and occasional giant cells. Many patients undergoing this type of therapy become symptomatic, developing dysuria and occasionally hematuria. It is not necessary to perform special for acid-fast organisms; in some cases, stains will be positive, yet this is of no clinical significance. Only if a patient develops systemic signs of infection along with disseminated BCG to organs other than the bladder and prostate (ie, liver, lung, bones) is antibiotic therapy initiated.

Radiation Cystitis

Radiation cystitis may be acute or chronic and can occur any time the bladder is included in the treatment field. The clinical severity and histologic features of radiation cystitis are both time and dose dependent. Clinically, the acute symptoms of radiation cystitis may appear as early as 4-6 weeks after initiation of therapy, whereas late symptoms appear as late as 10 years later.[30] The toxic effects of irradiation are enhanced if administered in conjunction with cyclophosphamide.[31]

Microscopically, the early changes are characterized by marked edema and hyperemia. The edema produces thickened mucosal folds, resulting in a characteristic gross appearance termed *radiation cystitis*. These changes may be accompanied by desquamation and superficial ulceration of the bladder epithelium.[32] At this stage, the urothelium can take on atypical

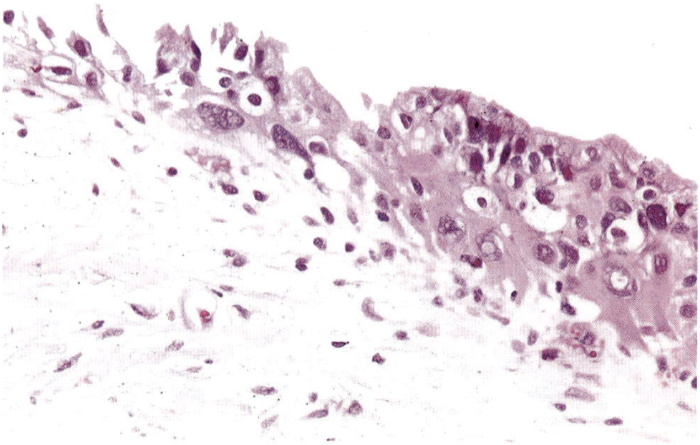

FIGURE 10.30 **Radiation atypia within urothelium.** Atypical cells have degenerative-appearing nuclei with vacuolization accompanied by abundant cytoplasm.

cytologic features mimicking and sometimes indistinguishable from CIS, although mitotic activity is rare, with variable karyorrhexis. The cells may become enlarged with prominent, hyperchromatic nuclei. However, the altered epithelial cells are typically more bizarre than cells of CIS, with giant cells and multinucleated cells that lack the crisp nuclear detail of nonirradiated cells and have abundant cytoplasm, which may be vacuolated[30] (Figs. 10.30-10.33, eFigs. 10.54-10.57). There are virtually no data on how long radiation atypia of the urothelium lasts after radiotherapy. In general, damaged urothelial cells are shed and replaced by normal urothelium, such that if the bladder last received radiation (most commonly for prostate cancer) over 1 year ago and surface urothelial severe atypia is still seen, strong consideration should be given to the diagnosis of CIS. This

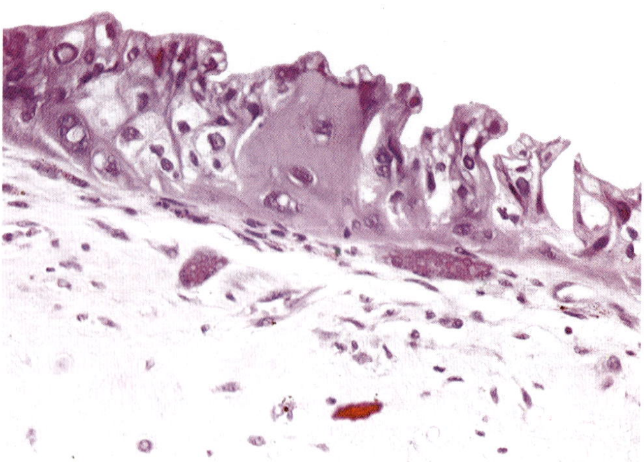

FIGURE 10.31 **Radiation atypia within urothelium characterized by multinucleated, vacuolated, degenerative-appearing nuclei.**

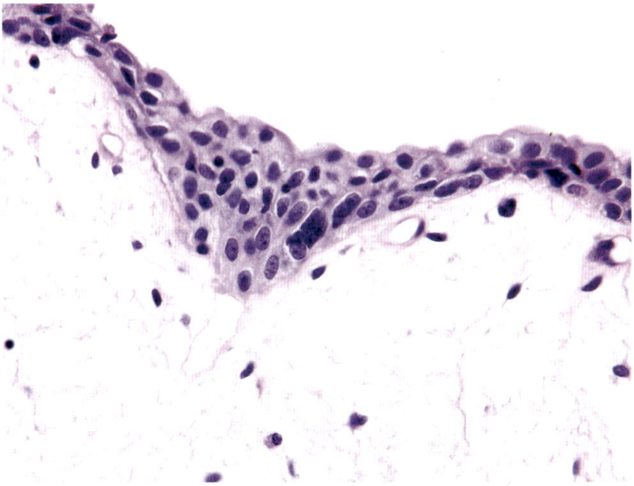

FIGURE 10.32 Radiation atypia within urothelium.

sequence of events would not be unexpected, as radiation is a risk factor for the development of CIS. A caveat is that radiation change may persist for longer intervals in von Brunn nests, where cells are not shed into the urine. With shorter intervals, it may not be possible to distinguish radiation atypia from CIS, and close follow-up is warranted.

Late radiation-induced changes include collagenization of the lamina propria and muscular fibers, myointimal proliferation or hyalinization of the media of arterioles, and, often, ulceration with abundant fibrinous exudate (Fig. 10.34, eFigs. 10.58 and 10.59). Atypical fibroblasts are invariably present in the scarred lamina propria (eFig. 10.60). The surface mucosa may mimic preneoplastic flat urothelial disease. Immunohistochemistry

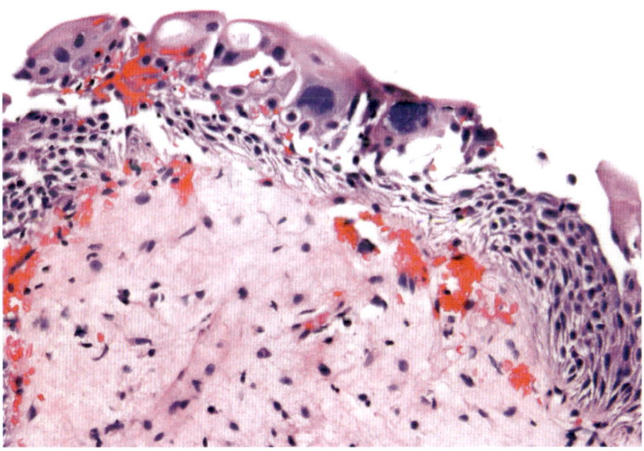

FIGURE 10.33 Radiation atypia within urothelium.

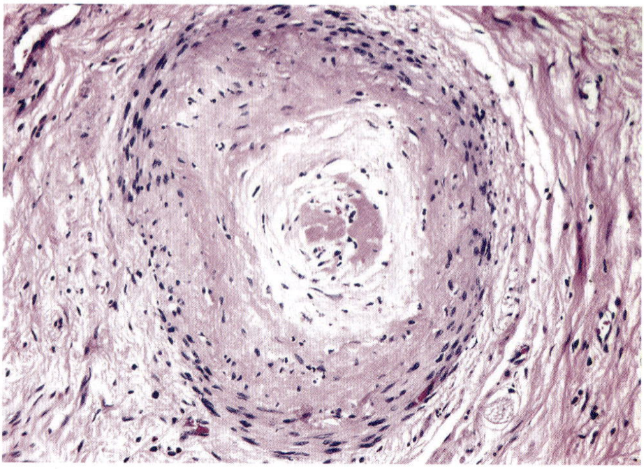

FIGURE 10.34 Radiation change within vessels.

for CK20, p53, and CD44 may be helpful, although p53 is least reliable in a posttreatment setting.[33] Most helpful is to require a high threshold and unmistakable changes to diagnose CIS in the setting of radiation.

In some cases, radiation injury to the bladder manifests as pseudocarcinomatous hyperplasia with epithelial cords and nests that extend into the lamina propria (Figs. 10.35-10.38, eFigs. 10.61-10.71).[34-37] In addition to architectural features typically associated with invasive urothelial carcinoma, pseudocarcinomatous lesions may have prominent nucleoli, mild-moderate nuclear pleomorphism, and mitotic activity. The eosinophilic cytoplasm seen with pseudocarcinomatous epithelial proliferation also mimics urothelial carcinoma with squamous differentiation or paradoxical differentiation seen with early invasive urothelial carcinoma. The key

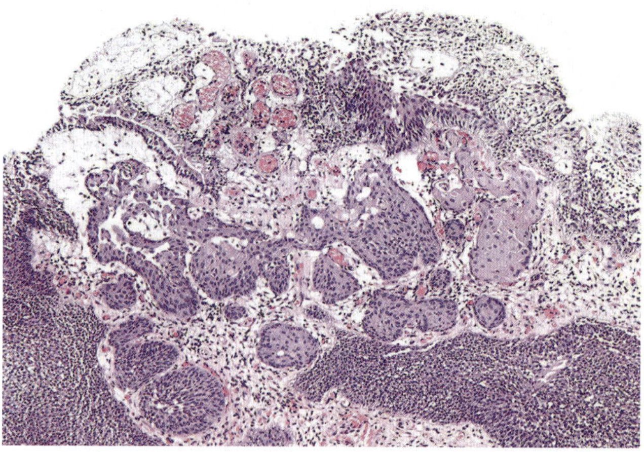

FIGURE 10.35 Pseudocarcinomatous hyperplasia resulting from radiotherapy.

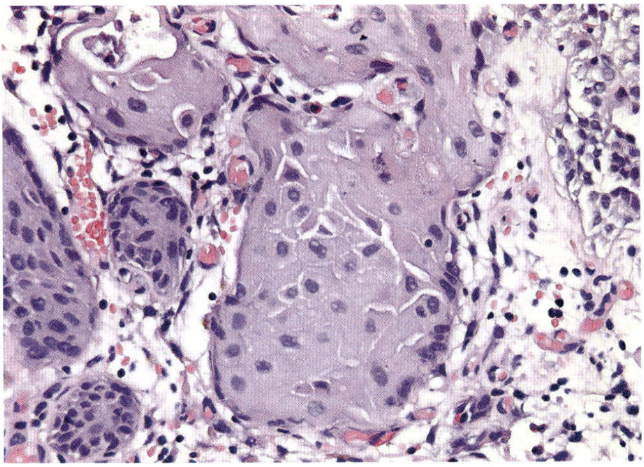

FIGURE 10.36 Pseudocarcinomatous hyperplasia resulting from radiotherapy (higher magnification of Fig. 10.35).

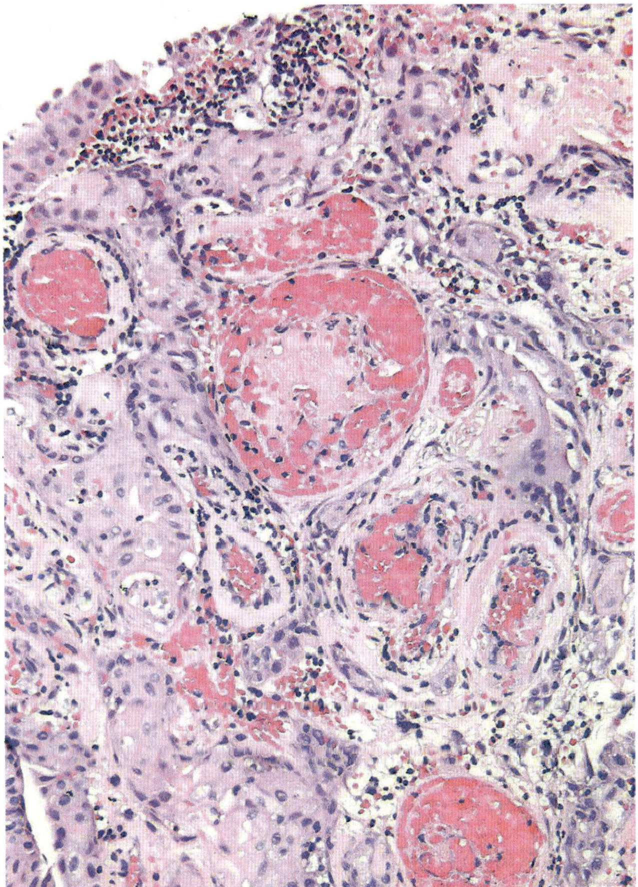

FIGURE 10.37 Pseudocarcinomatous hyperplasia resulting from radiotherapy.

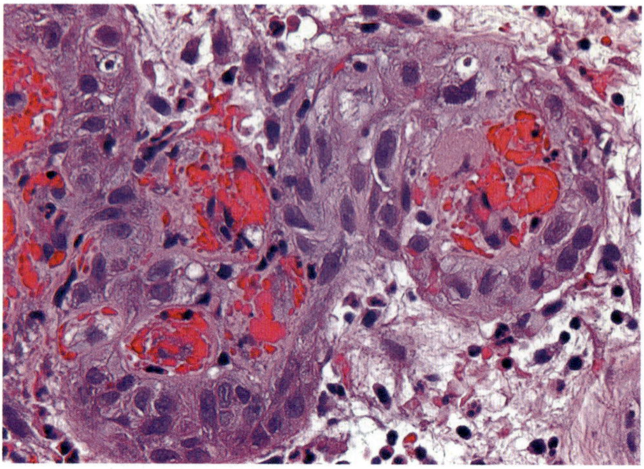

FIGURE 10.38 **Higher magnification of Figure 10.37.** Note epithelial islands wrapping around congested blood vessels and fibrin deposits.

to accurately recognizing pseudocarcinomatous hyperplasia is by paying attention to the background tissue in between the urothelial nests. The characteristic features of stromal hemorrhage, vascular fibrin thrombi, hemosiderin deposition, inflammation, edema, and ectatic vessels are not typically seen with invasive urothelial cancer. The close relationship (wrapping around) of urothelial nests around blood vessels is also a helpful feature. Pseudocarcinomatous epithelial hyperplasia can in a minority of cases be quite extensive in the lamina propria, but this entity does not involve the muscularis propria. It is unclear whether this pseudocarcinomatous epithelial hyperplasia results from preexisting florid von Brunn nests, with superimposed hemorrhage and vascular abnormalities or a *de novo* reactive proliferation. Most of the cases occur in men following irradiation for prostate cancer with a few other cases occurring subsequent to pelvic irradiation for endometrial or colon cancer. A few individuals with a history of systemic chemotherapy develop identical lesions. Less common conditions associated with this entity include chronic bladder irritation, generalized ischemia, long-standing urinary obstruction, and sickle cell trait.[35] The interval between radiation and discovery of the bladder lesion is on average 55 months with a range from 9 months to 13 years. Pseudocarcinomatous urothelial proliferation appears to reflect a general response of the bladder mucosa to long-standing ischemia. It is important to note that while one must be cautious in making a diagnosis of carcinoma in the background of radiation to the bladder field, there are rare instances of invasive urothelial carcinoma occurring in patients who have radiation to the pelvis.

Hemorrhagic Cystitis: Chemotherapy

In the late 1950s, systemic administration of cyclophosphamide was found to cause hemorrhagic cystitis (Fig. 10.39, eFigs. 10.72 and 10.73). At times,

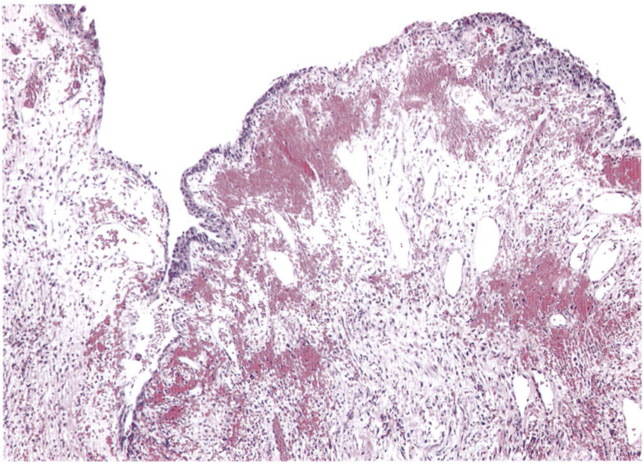

FIGURE 10.39 Hemorrhagic cystitis.

hematuria could be massive and uncontrollable, sometimes requiring cystectomy. Philips and colleagues[38] showed that the tissue damage that led to hemorrhagic cystitis was due to a topical effect of the metabolic by-products of cyclophosphamide, which were excreted through the kidney. The occurrence of hemorrhagic cystitis appears to be unrelated to dose and was reported in roughly 8% of patients receiving the drug.[39,40] Currently, patients are treated with forced fluids, and the incidence of hemorrhagic cystitis has been sharply reduced. More recently, another alkylating agent, busulfan, has been implicated as a rare cause of hemorrhagic cystitis.[41] Adenovirus infection in children may also result in hemorrhagic cystitis.

Microscopically, the bladder is characterized by marked edema and hemorrhage throughout the lamina propria, with extensive ulceration and an associated fibrinopurulent exudate. Where not ulcerated, the epithelium may be thinned and atypical. During the regenerative stage, macrophages and fibroblasts populate the lamina propria, while the overlying epithelium exhibits an increased mitotic rate, increased thickness, and marked atypia.[38,40] Intravesical installation of chemotherapeutic agents such as thiotepa and mitomycin C is also able to induce cytologic atypia, which can be confused with CIS, including cytomegaly, pleomorphism, and hyperchromasia (Fig. 10.40, eFig. 10.74).[42] Despite these changes, mitotic activity is not evident and superficial (umbrella) cells are preferentially affected.

Posttransurethral Resection

Following transurethral resections (TUR), either a nonspecific granulomatous inflammation with foreign body giant cells or necrotizing (fibrinoid necrosis) palisading granulomas, resembling rheumatoid nodules, may be

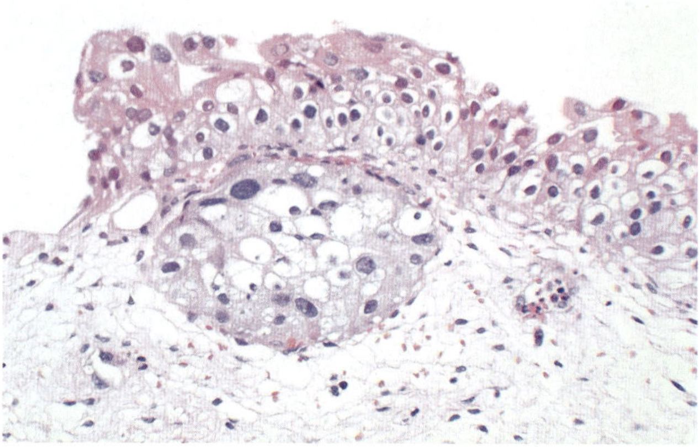

FIGURE 10.40 Chemotherapy atypia in von Brunn nest.

seen (Figs. 10.41 and 10.42, eFigs. 10.75-10.81).[43,44] There is coagulative/fibrinoid necrosis in the center surrounded by epithelioid histiocytes with occasional foreign body–type giant cells. In cases where the prior TUR is recent, the surrounding inflammatory infiltrate is often rich in eosinophils, which over time get replaced by lymphocytes and plasma cells and fibrosis.

In prior biopsy sites, aberrant keratin expression can be seen in myofibroblastic and smooth muscle cells (Figs. 10.43-10.45).[45] In contrast, residual keratin-positive tumor cells have a more epithelioid morphology. When interpreting cytokeratin stains for the detection of residual tumor cells, one should pay attention to the nature of the cells and not assume all cytokeratin staining cells are residual tumor cells. Florid epithelioid granulomatous reaction can also be confused with infiltrating urothelial

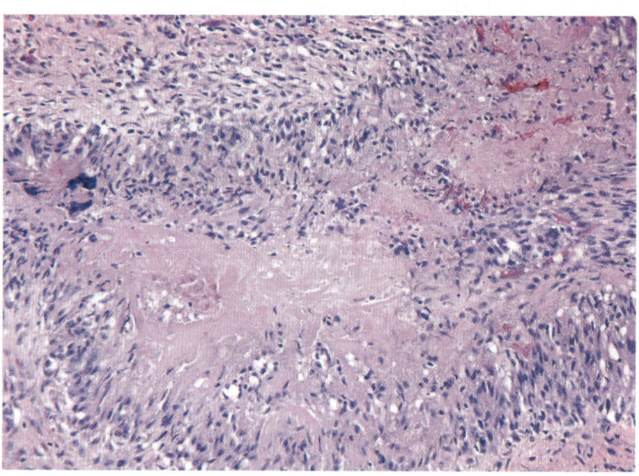

FIGURE 10.41 Posttransurethral resection granuloma.

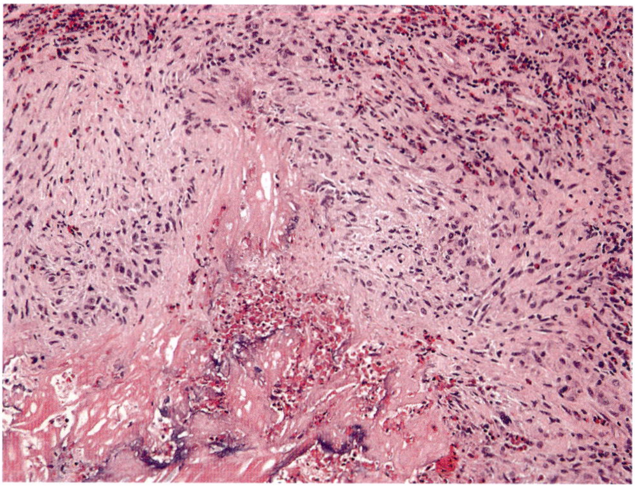

FIGURE 10.42 Posttransurethral resection granulomas associated with numerous eosinophils.

carcinoma, with immunohistochemistry for pancytokeratin and CD68 capable of resolving the issue (Fig. 10.46). Rarely, one can see bizarre reactive stromal cells in the areas of a biopsy site, analogous to what has been described in the gastrointestinal tract in areas of granulation tissue, resulting from hypoxia, inflammation, regeneration/repair, and cell turnover as a response to injury (Fig. 10.47).[46] The degenerative nature of the atypia, the setting of a prior biopsy site, along with the recognition of the spectrum of atypia that can occur in this reactive condition should prevent a misdiagnosis of malignancy.

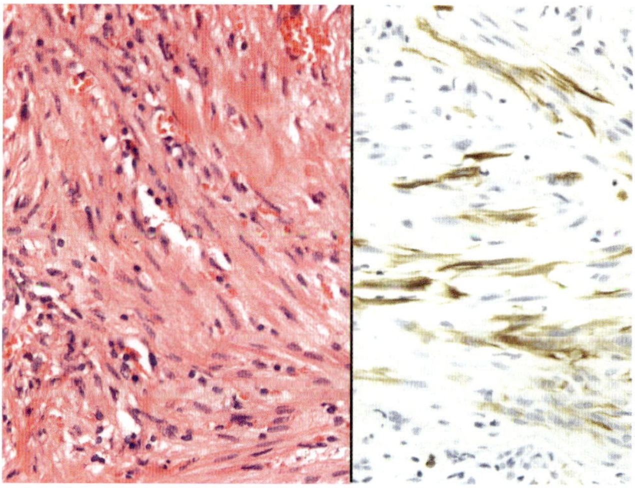

FIGURE 10.43 Prior biopsy site with myofibroblasts labeling with keratin AE1/AE3 (***right***).

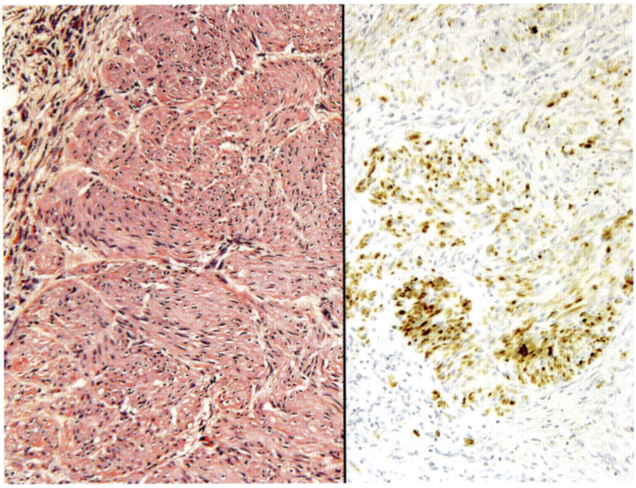

FIGURE 10.44 Prior biopsy site with bundles of smooth muscle labeling with keratin AE1/AE3 (*right*).

INTERSTITIAL CYSTITIS/BLADDER PAIN SYNDROME

The definition of interstitial cystitis/bladder pain syndrome (IC/BPS) agreed upon by the Society of Urodynamics, Female Pelvic Medicine & Urogenital Reconstruction: "An unpleasant sensation (pain, pressure, discomfort) perceived to be related to the urinary bladder, associated with lower urinary tract symptoms of more than 6-week duration, in the absence of infection or other identifiable causes."[47] However, different organizations have different definitions mainly relating to the duration of symptoms

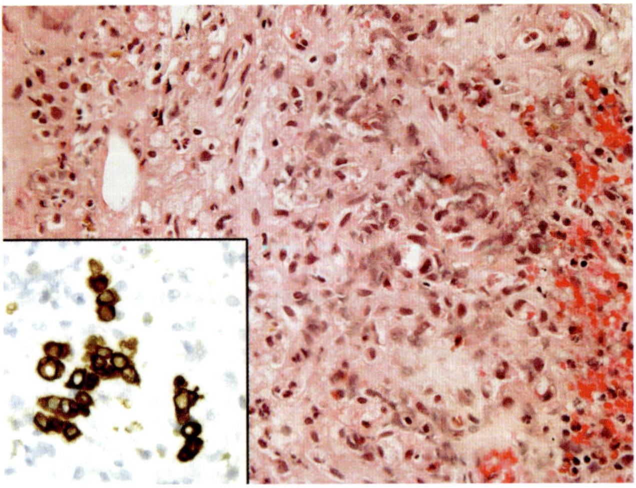

FIGURE 10.45 Prior biopsy site with residual carcinoma highlighted by clusters of epithelioid cells labeling with keratin AE1/AE3 (*inset*).

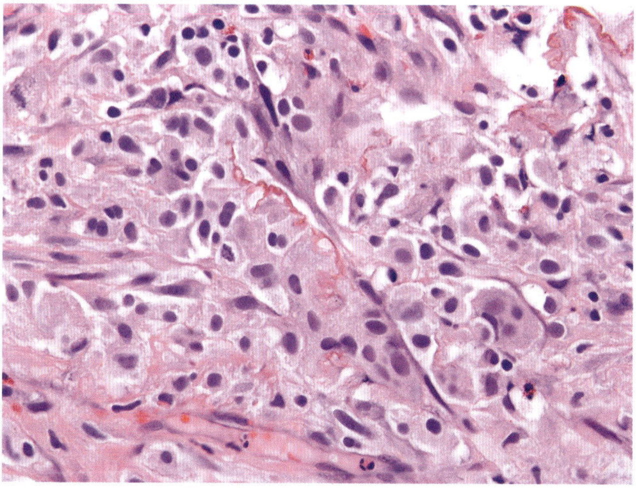

FIGURE 10.46 Prior biopsy site with florid granulomatous reaction mimicking urothelial carcinoma.

needed before establishing the diagnosis.[47-50] There is typically increased frequency, nocturnal frequency, and lower voiding volume with the pain typically improved after voiding. IC/PBS is very difficult to diagnose and is based on a combination of history, physical examination, postvoid residual, urinalysis and culture, symptom questionnaire, and pain evaluation. First-line treatments consist of stress and pain management patient education, and behavior modification with multiple sequential lines of various treatments if earlier attempts fail. The last resort in some patients may include cystectomy. IC/BPS is more common in women, but recently, it

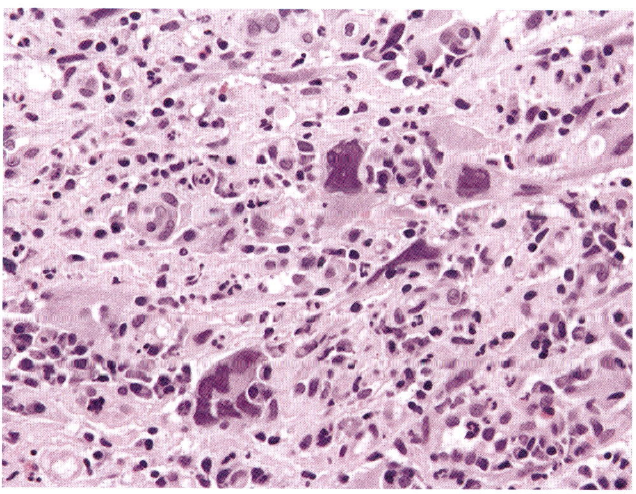

FIGURE 10.47 Prior biopsy site with marked degenerative atypia in stromal cells.

has been suggested that in men, the disease is often underdiagnosed. It is also common for IC/BPS to coexist with other unexplained medical conditions, such as fibromyalgia, irritable bowel syndrome, chronic fatigue syndrome, Sjögren syndrome, chronic headaches, and other gynecological pain syndromes. It is not known whether IC/BPS is a primary bladder disorder or whether the bladder symptoms of IC/BPS are secondary phenomena. An autoimmune etiology is postulated. Other possible etiologies include urothelial dysfunction, abnormal Tamm-Horsfall protein, mast cell activation, infection, production of antiproliferative factor, genetics, central sensitization of the spinal cord, and sensory processing.

The most critical tasks for the pathologist are to (1) accurately rule out other forms of cystitis and CIS, lesions that clinically and cystoscopically may mimic IC/BPS, and (2) in a documented case, provide correlations of histology with cystoscopic findings and clinical features. The ultimate diagnosis of IC/BPS is made after clinical and pathologic correlation.

There are two patterns of disease, one designated as nonclassic (nonulcerative, early) and the other as classic (ulcerative, late). The more common nonclassic disease exhibits multiple microhemorrhages within the lamina propria that are referred to as *glomerulations.* In the classic phase, the bladder on cystoscopy displays single or multiple patches of reddened mucosa with small blood vessels radiating from a central scar. Under hydrodistention, the mucosa ruptures, resulting in oozing of blood from the mucosal margins on the bottom of the ulcer; this is referred to as *glomerulations. In the late phase of the disease, classic ulcer formation (Hunner ulcer) may be seen.* The presence at cystoscopy of glomerulations or even Hunner ulcers is by itself not specific for IC/BPS but needs to be considered in conjunction with the clinical symptoms.

There are also no characteristic histologic features for IC/BPS.[51] In routine cystoscopic biopsies, suburothelial edema and telangiectasia are constantly observed regardless of whether the disease is the nonclassic or classic form. The findings in nonulcer patients are usually meager and limited to mucosal ruptures or tears and suburothelial hemorrhages that correspond to the cystoscopically observed glomerulations (Figs. 10.48 and 10.49, eFigs. 10.82-10.86). The mucosal ruptures may be single or multiple.

Some studies have shown significant differences in demographics, clinical presentation, urinary marker profiles, and treatment responses between patients with and without Hunner lesions, suggesting that they may represent two distinct diseases.[52-54]

In patients with Hunner ulcer, the mucosal ulcers are often covered by debris, fibrin, inflammatory cells, and red blood cells (Figs. 10.50-10.52, eFigs. 10.87-10.94). The ulcers vary in thickness but usually involve the upper half of the lamina propria. The ulcer base is composed of granulation tissue.

The inflammation is generally chronic and nonspecific in nature with a variable density and distribution of lymphocytes, macrophages, and

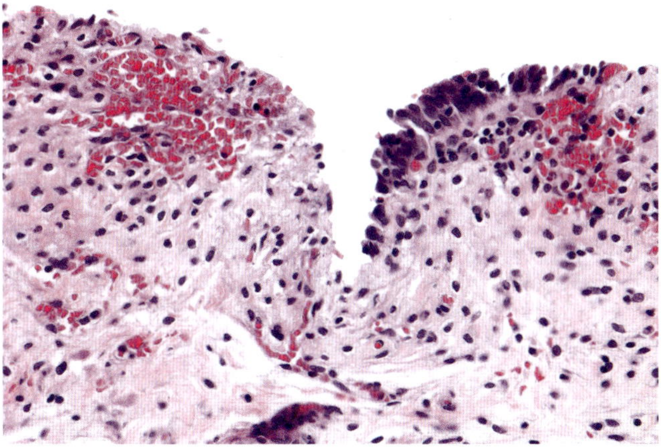

FIGURE 10.48 IC/BPS, nonulcerative type with foci of hemorrhage in lamina propria.

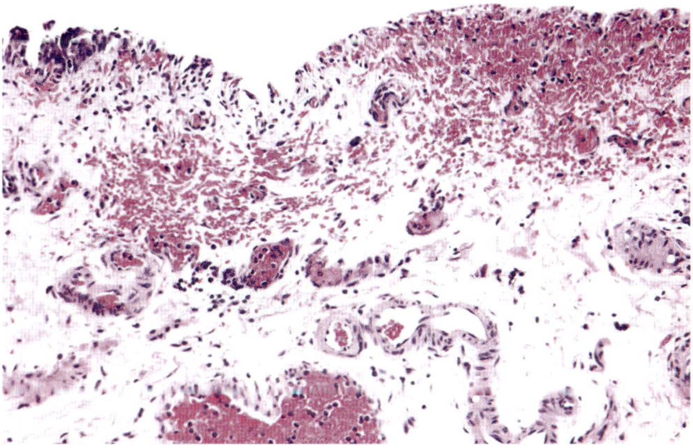

FIGURE 10.49 IC/BPS, nonulcerative type with more extensive hemorrhage in lamina propria.

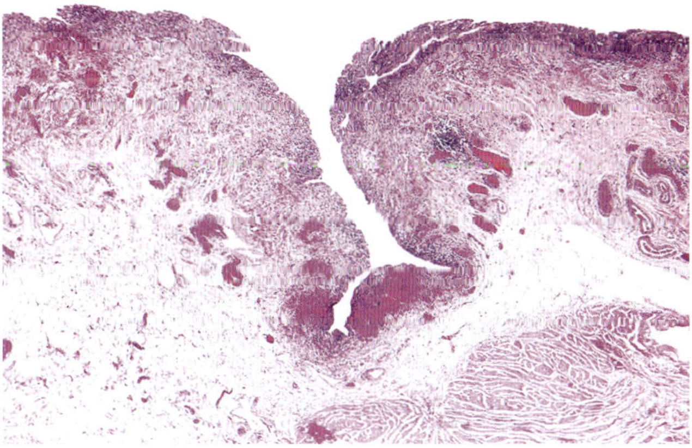

FIGURE 10.50 IC/BPS, ulcerative type.

plasma cells. Acute inflammation and eosinophils may be seen on rare occasions, but this is invariably seen in patients with ulcers. Fibrosis and inflammation may be seen in the muscularis propria, a finding that correlates with the decreased bladder capacity seen in advanced stages of the disease. The perivesical fat usually lacks significant inflammation. A high mast cell count in the muscularis propria of the bladder (detrusor muscle) was initially touted as a diagnostic histopathologic feature for IC/BPS. The significance of mast cells is controversial, in that mast cell counts in patients with IC/BPS overlap with counts in patients with bladder inflammation of other causes. Also, most mast cell counts do not correlate with clinical symptoms, cystoscopic findings, or response to therapy. We do not routinely comment on mast cells in specimens performed to diagnose IC/BPS. Rather, we add the following note to these cases: "The histologic findings of IC/BPS are nonspecific. Quantifying mast cells with mast cell stains are not diagnostic, as there are conflicting studies in the literature as to its specificity. Furthermore, the results of mast cell counts vary depending on the type of stain used, the staining technique used with a given stain, and where (mucosa, submucosa, muscularis propria) the mast cells are counted."

The most critical differential diagnosis in biopsies performed to IC/BPS is CIS. Although 25% of patients with CIS may be asymptomatic, most patients, especially those with *de novo* CIS, present with frequency, dysuria, nocturia, and suprapubic fullness. Cystoscopically, the involved areas of CIS exhibit erythema or granularity, which can also mimic IC/BPS. The extensive mucosal denudation that frequently occurs with CIS may result in a biopsy appearance of ulceration, vascular congestion, and inflammation further resembling IC/BPS. When the urothelium is absent

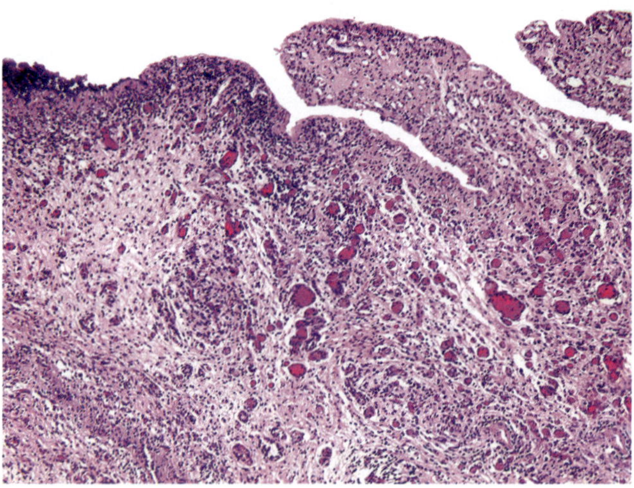

FIGURE 10.52 **IC/BPS, ulcerative type with granulation tissue at base of Hunner ulcer.**

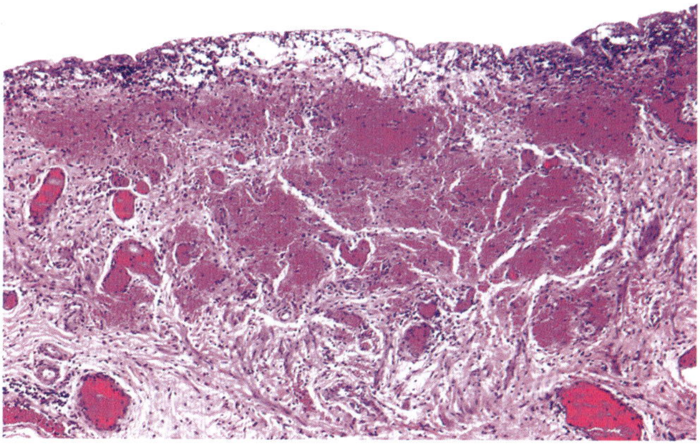

FIGURE 10.51 IC/BPS, ulcerative type with surface granulation tissue.

or scant, multiple levels should be obtained to look for atypical cells and to rule out the possibility of CIS. As a result of the overlap of symptoms of IC/BPS, urine cytology is recommended in patients who smoke and are at higher risk of developing urothelial carcinoma.

REFERENCES

1. Meria P, Desgrippes A, Arfi C, Le Duc A. Encrusted cystitis and pyelitis. *J Urol.* 1998;160:3-9.
2. Patel NP, Lavengood RW, Fernandes M, et al. Gas-forming infections in genitourinary tract. *Urology.* 1992;39:341-345.
3. Wise GJ, Talluri GS, Marella VK. Fungal infections of the genitourinary system: manifestations, diagnosis, and treatment. *Urol Clin North Am.* 1999;26:701-718. vii.
4. Christensen WI. Genitourinary tuberculosis: review of 102 cases. *Medicine (Baltimore).* 1974;53:377-390.
5. Ghoneim MA. Bilharziasis of the genitourinary tract. *BJU Int.* 2002;89(suppl 1):22-30.
6. Zahran MM, Kamel M, Mooro H, et al. Bilharziasis of urinary bladder and ureter: comparative histopathologic study. *Urology.* 1976;8:73-79.
7. Smith BH. Malacoplakia of the urinary tract: a study of twenty-four cases. *Am J Clin Pathol.* 1965;43:409-417.
8. Lewin KJ, Fair WR, Steigbigel RT, et al. Clinical and laboratory studies into the pathogenesis of malacoplakia. *J Clin Pathol.* 1976;29:354-363.
9. Lou TY, Teplitz C. Malakoplakia: pathogenesis and ultrastructural morphogenesis. A problem of altered macrophage (phagolysosomal) response. *Hum Pathol.* 1974;5:191-207.
10. Abdou NI, NaPombejara C, Sagawa A, et al. Malakoplakia: evidence for monocyte lysosomal abnormality correctable by cholinergic agonist in vitro and in vivo. *N Engl J Med.* 1977;297:1413-1419.
11. Qualman SJ, Gupta PK, Mendelsohn G. Intracellular *Escherichia coli* in urinary malakoplakia: a reservoir of infection and its therapeutic implications. *Am J Clin Pathol.* 1984;81:35-42.
12. Stanton MJ, Maxted W. Malacoplakia: a study of the literature and current concepts of pathogenesis, diagnosis and treatment. *J Urol.* 1981;125:139-146.

13. Stevens S, McClure J. The histochemical features of the Michaelis-Gutmann body and a consideration of the pathophysiological mechanisms of its formation. *J Pathol.* 1982;137:119-127.
14. Mufson MA, Belshe RB. A review of adenoviruses in the etiology of acute hemorrhagic cystitis. *J Urol.* 1976;115:191-194.
15. DeHertogh DA, Brettman LR. Hemorrhagic cystitis due to herpes simplex virus as a marker of disseminated herpes infection. *Am J Med.* 1988;84:632-635.
16. Richmond W. The genito-urinary manifestations of herpes zoster. Three case reports and a review of the literature. *Br J Urol.* 1974;46:193-200.
17. Wong TW, Warner NE. Cytomegalic inclusion disease in adults. Report of 14 cases with review of literature. *Arch Pathol.* 1962;74:403-422.
18. Vogeli TA, Peinemann F, Burdach S, et al. Urological treatment and clinical course of BK polyomavirus-associated hemorrhagic cystitis in children after bone marrow transplantation. *Eur Urol.* 1999;36:252-257.
19. Apperley JF, Rice SJ, Bishop JA, et al. Late-onset hemorrhagic cystitis associated with urinary excretion of polyomaviruses after bone marrow transplantation. *Transplantation.* 1987;43:108-112.
20. Herawi M, Parwani AV, Chan T, et al. Polyoma virus-associated cellular changes in the urine and bladder biopsy samples: a cytohistologic correlation. *Am J Surg Pathol.* 2006;30:345-350.
21. Lane Z, Epstein JI. Polypoid/papillary cystitis: a series of 41 cases misdiagnosed as papillary urothelial neoplasia. *Am J Surg Pathol.* 2008;32:758-764.
22. Ekelund P, Johansson S. Polypoid cystitis: a catheter associated lesion of the human bladder. *Acta Pathol Microbiol Scand A.* 1979;87A:179-184.
23. Young RH. Papillary and polypoid cystitis. A report of eight cases. *Am J Surg Pathol.* 1988;12:542-546.
24. Verhagen PC, Nikkels PG, de Jong TP. Eosinophilic cystitis. *Arch Dis Child.* 2001;84:344-346.
25. Hansson S, Hanson E, Hjalmas K, et al. Follicular cystitis in girls with untreated asymptomatic or covert bacteriuria. *J Urol.* 1990;143:330-332.
26. Wells HG. Giant cells in cystitis. *Arch Pathol Lab Med.* 1938;26:32-43.
27. Pagano F, Bassi P, Milani C, et al. Pathologic and structural changes in the bladder after BCG intravesical therapy in men. *Prog Clin Biol Res.* 1989;310:81-91.
28. Lage JM, Bauer WC, Kelley DR, et al. Histological parameters and pitfalls in the interpretation of bladder biopsies in bacillus Calmette-Guerin treatment of superficial bladder cancer. *J Urol.* 1986;135:916-919.
29. Betz SA, See WA, Cohen MB. Granulomatous inflammation in bladder wash specimens after intravesical bacillus Calmette-Guerin therapy for transitional cell carcinoma of the bladder. *Am J Clin Pathol.* 1993;99:244-248.
30. Fajardo LF, Berthrong M. Radiation injury in surgical pathology. Part I. *Am J Surg Pathol.* 1978;2:159-199.
31. Jayalakshmamma B, Pinkel D. Urinary-bladder toxicity following pelvic irradiation and simultaneous cyclophosphamide therapy. *Cancer.* 1976;38:701-707.
32. Warren S. Effects of radiation on normal tissues: effects of radiation on the urinary system. *Arch Pathol.* 1942;34: 079-1084.
33. Oliva E, Pinheiro NF, Heney NM, et al. Immunohistochemistry as an adjunct in the differential diagnosis of radiation-induced atypia versus urothelial carcinoma in situ of the bladder: a study of 45 cases. *Hum Pathol.* 2013;44:860-866.
34. Baker PM, Young RH. Radiation-induced pseudocarcinomatous proliferations of the urinary bladder: a report of 4 cases. *Hum Pathol.* 2000;31:678-683.

35. Lane Z, Epstein JI. Pseudocarcinomatous epithelial hyperplasia in the bladder unassociated with prior irradiation or chemotherapy. *Am J Surg Pathol.* 2008;32:92-97.
36. Chan TY, Epstein JI. Radiation or chemotherapy cystitis with "pseudocarcinomatous" features. *Am J Surg Pathol.* 2004;28:909-913.
37. Kryvenko ON, Epstein JI. Pseudocarcinomatous urothelial hyperplasia of the bladder: clinical findings and followup of 70 patients. *J Urol.* 2013,189:2083-2086.
38. Philips FS, Sternberg SS, Cronin AP, et al. Cyclophosphamide and urinary bladder toxicity. *Cancer Res.* 1961;21:1577-1589.
39. Lawrence HJ, Simone J, Aur RJ. Cyclophosphamide-induced hemorrhagic cystitis in children with leukemia. *Cancer.* 1975;36:1572-1576.
40. Beyer-Boon ME, de Voogt HJ, Schaberg A. The effects of cyclophosphamide treatment on the epithelium and stroma of the urinary bladder. *Eur J Cancer.* 1978;14:1029-1035.
41. Pode D, Perlberg S, Steiner D. Busulfan-induced hemorrhagic cystitis. *J Urol.* 1983;130:347-348.
42. Murphy WM, Soloway MS, Lin CJ. Morphologic effects of thio-TEPA on mammalian urothelium. Changes in abnormal cells. *Acta Cytol.* 1978;22:550-554.
43. Spagnolo DV, Waring PM. Bladder granulomata after bladder surgery. *Am J Clin Pathol.* 1986;86:430-437.
44. Eble JN, Banks ER. Post-surgical necrobiotic granulomas of urinary bladder. *Urology.* 1990;35:454-457.
45. Tamas EF, Epstein JI. Detection of residual tumor cells in bladder biopsy specimens: pitfalls in the interpretation of cytokeratin stains. *Am J Surg Pathol.* 2007;31:390-397.
46. Serra S, Chetty R. Bizarre stromal cells in ischemic bowel disease. *Ann Diagn Pathol.* 2005;9:193-196.
47. Hanno PM, Erickson D, Moldwin R, et al.; American Urological Association. Diagnosis and treatment of interstitial cystitis/bladder pain syndrome: AUA guideline amendment. *J Urol.* 2015;193:1545-1553.
48. Barr S. Diagnosis and management of interstitial cystitis. *Obstet Gynecol Clin North Am.* 2014;41:397-407.
49. Hanno PM. Painful bladder syndrome/interstitial cystitis and related disorders. In: Wein AJ, Kavoussi LR, Novick AC, et al., eds. *Campbell-Walsh Urology.* 9th ed. Saunders; 2007:330-370.
50. McLennan MT. Interstitial cystitis: epidemiology, pathophysiology, and clinical presentation. *Obstet Gynecol Clin North Am.* 2014;41:385-395.
51. Johansson SL, Fall M. Pathology of interstitial cystitis. *Urol Clin North Am.* 1994;21: 55-62.
52. Lai HH, Pickersgill NA, Vetter JM. Hunner lesion phenotype in interstitial cystitis/bladder pain syndrome: a systematic review and meta-analysis. *J Urol.* 2020;204(3):518-523.
53. Fall M, Nordling J, Cervigni M, et al. Hunner lesion disease differs in diagnosis, treatment and outcome from bladder pain syndrome: an ESSIC working group report. *Scand J Urol.* 2020;54(2):91-98.
54. Whitmore KE, Fall M, Sengiku A. Hunner lesion versus non-Hunner lesion interstitial cystitis/bladder pain syndrome. *Int J Urol.* 2019;26(suppl 1):26-34.

11

MESENCHYMAL TUMORS AND TUMORLIKE LESIONS

Benign mesenchymal neoplasms may arise within the urinary tract, although it is notable that they are less common than their malignant counterparts. Primary sarcomas of the urinary bladder are rare, more common in males than in females, and comprise <0.5% of malignant tumors arising at this site.[1-4] The majority are of muscle origin, and while myosarcomas may occur in any age group, rhabdomyosarcomas (RMS) predominate in children, while leiomyosarcomas (LMS) predominate in adults.

LEIOMYOMA

Leiomyoma is the most common benign mesenchymal neoplasm of the urinary bladder, exhibiting the same morphologic features seen at other sites[5-7] (Figs. 11.1 and 11.2, eFig. 11.1). While some are asymptomatic and discovered at the time of pelvic imaging, others can present with obstructive symptoms or dysuria. Most tumors are typically small and <2 cm in size and lack gross or microscopic infiltrative features. On transurethral resection (TUR), there is a tendency to overlook the neoplastic smooth muscle as fragments of muscularis propria, as the presence of circumscribed nodules cannot typically be appreciated. However, in contrast to the well-formed bundles of muscularis propria, leiomyomas in the context of a clinical/cystoscopic mass lesion are composed of large compact sheets of intersecting smooth muscle fascicles (Fig. 11.3). Typically, they exhibit low cellularity and minimal or no cytological atypia or mitoses, although may have coagulative necrosis. We have anecdotally seen leiomyomas of the bladder with degenerative atypia (symplastic leiomyoma), although there is no reported information on their clinical or biologic potential (see "Leiomyosarcoma" section). Leiomyomas express smooth muscle actin and desmin.

LEIOMYOSARCOMA

LMS are the most common sarcoma encountered in the urinary bladder in adults, although there have been cases reported in children.[1,3,5,8] Although most present *de novo*, isolated cases have been reported subsequent to

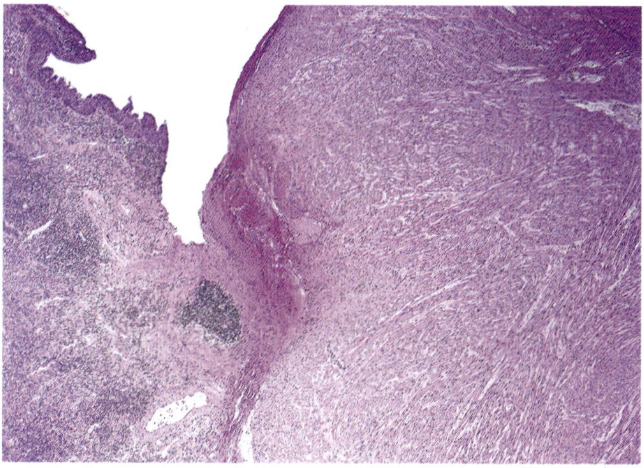

FIGURE 11.1 Leiomyoma.

chemotherapy with cyclophosphamide.[9-12] The tumors are usually well circumscribed, may protrude into the lumen, and ulcerate the overlying urothelium. Size is variable (mean 5 cm), although some may measure up to 20 cm. They occur more frequently in males than in females in a ratio of 2:1. Morphologic features are identical to those seen in other sites, including the presence of interlacing fascicles of spindle cells with variable amounts of eosinophilic cytoplasm with mild to marked nuclear atypia (Fig. 11.4, eFigs. 11.2-11.7). Some tumors may have prominent myxoid change, and others may have a prominent epithelioid morphology. The majority of cases will demonstrate tumor necrosis and mitotic activity of 10 per 10 high-power fields or more. Although the rarity of these tumors makes

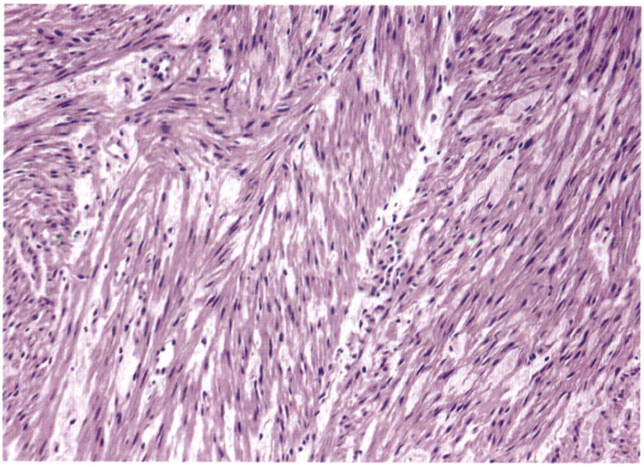

FIGURE 11.2 Leiomyoma (higher magnification of Fig. 11.1).

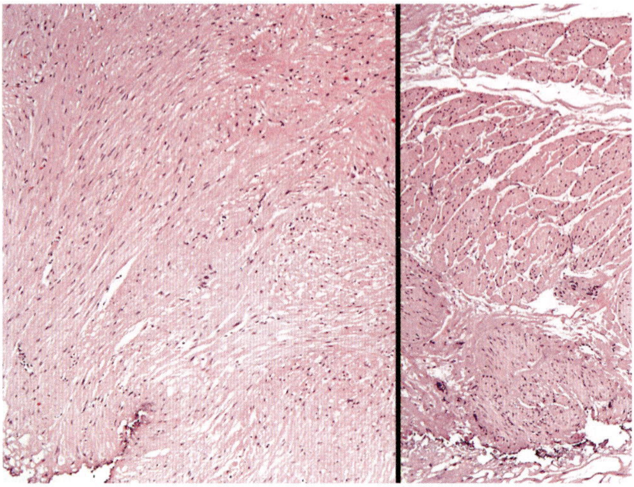

FIGURE 11.3 Leiomyoma composed of irregular sheets of smooth muscle (*left*) as opposed to well-formed discrete smooth muscle bundles of normal muscular propria (*right*).

it difficult to establish risk factors for progression, a recent study by Coiner et al. based on SEER data suggests that tumors >5 cm have an increased incidence of disease progression.[13] The data suggest that established grading schemes, particularly that defined by Fédération Nationale des Centres de Lutte Contre le Cancer (FNCLCC), may provide useful prognostic information.[14] Although most smooth muscle tumors of the bladder are overtly either benign or malignant, there are some tumors with low cellularity yet with atypia or rare mitotic activity. In the uterus, these lesions would be classified as benign, even if accompanied by a few readily identifiable

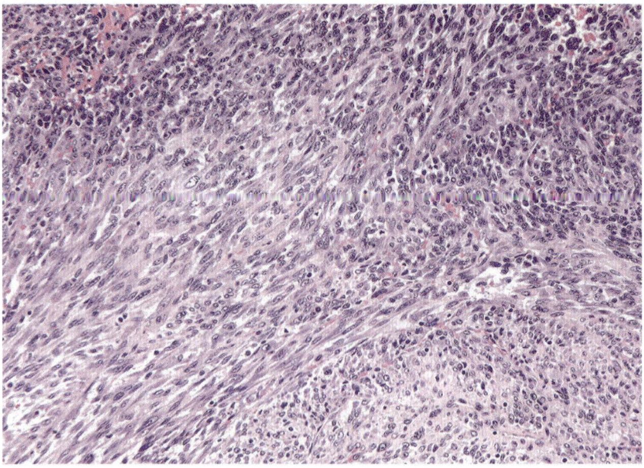

FIGURE 11.4 Leiomyosarcoma.

mitotic figures. Large tumors may show a prominent myxoid morphology, and occasionally, an epithelioid appearance may be striking. As there are no follow-up data in the literature for comparable lesions in the bladder, it may be more prudent to designate these lesions as "atypical smooth muscle tumors" describing their findings and stating that their biological behavior is unknown. For those lesions without mitotic figures, it can be added that it is likely that they will behave in an indolent fashion.

Sarcomatoid carcinoma may mimic LMS and must be excluded by adequate sampling of the specimen (to identify a carcinomatous or *in situ* component) and appropriate immunohistochemical studies. LMS of the bladder are so rare that this diagnosis should be made only after excluding all other possibilities, particularly sarcomatoid carcinoma but also secondary involvement from an adjacent organ. LMS (~50%) may express a minimal or occasionally a moderate degree of cytokeratin[15,16] but typically are composed of regular intersecting fascicles as opposed to the more haphazard growth pattern of sarcomatoid carcinoma. One must also rule out reactive spindle cell lesions, which may occur after local surgery or trauma. These reactive lesions are composed of spindle cells that may also consistently express smooth muscle markers by immunohistochemistry but are of myofibroblastic origin (see below). Other differential diagnostic considerations include perivascular epithelioid cell neoplasms (less dense pink and more filamentous cytoplasm, spindle cells radiating off of vessels, variable epithelioid morphology, and coexpression of HMB45 with smooth muscle markers), solitary fibrous tumor (distinctive collagenous stroma, staghorn blood vessels, and expression of CD34 and STAT 6), and gastrointestinal stromal tumor (c-kit and DOG 1 expression). Over two-thirds of LMS will demonstrate immunoreactivity of both smooth muscle actin (1A4) and muscle-specific actin (HHF-35). Desmin will be positive in some of the cases, whereas epithelial membrane antigen is usually negative. It has been suggested that caldesmon will be positive in LMS but negative in myofibroblastic lesions[17] (Table 11.1). A review of the Surveillance, Epidemiology, and End Results (SEER) database found that grade, advanced disease at diagnosis, and failure to undergo surgical excision correlated with poor outcome.[18]

RHABDOMYOSARCOMA

In children, 20%-27% of RMS arise in the genitourinary tract. The bladder, prostate, and paratesticular region are the most common primary sites in males and the bladder and vagina in females[16,19-22] (Figs. 11.5 and 11.6, eFigs. 11.8 and 11.9). The mean age at diagnosis for vesical RMS is 4 years. Most are embryonal rhabdomyosarcoma and exophytic (polypoid), with or without a "botryoid" component. Microscopically, the botryoid variant of RMS has a superficial condensation of tumor cells (so-called cambium layer), including strap cells and rhabdomyoblasts, located immediately beneath the

TABLE 11.1 Spindle Cell Neoplasms of the Bladder: Immunoreactivity

Antibody	RMS	LMS	SFT	IMT/PMP	SC[a]
Vim	+	+	+	+	+
SMA (1A4)	−/+	+	−/+	+/−	−
MCA (HHF-35)	+	+	−/+	+	−
Desmin	+	+/−	−	−/+	−
Myogenin	+	−	−	−	−
CD34	−	−	+	−	−
Bcl-2	−	−/+	+	−/+	−/+
EMA	−	−	−	−	+/−
CAM 5.2/ AE1/AE3	−	−/+	−	−/+	+/−
34BE12	−	−	−	−	+/−
ALK (IHC)	−	−	−	+/−	−
ALK (FISH)	−	−	−	+/−	−

[a]Sarcomatoid carcinomas with mesenchymal differentiation may express muscle markers.

RMS, rhabdomyosarcoma; LMS, leiomyosarcoma; SFT, solitary fibrous tumor; IMT, inflammatory myofibroblastic tumor; PMP, pseudosarcomatous myofibroblastic proliferation; SC, sarcomatoid carcinoma; Vim, vimentin; SMA, smooth muscle actin (clone 1A4); MCA, muscle common actin (clone HHF-35); EMA, epithelial membrane antigen (clone MC5); ALK, anaplastic lymphoma kinase; +, positive in >75% of cases; +/−, positive in >50% of cases; −/+, positive in <50% of cases; −, negative in <5% of cases.

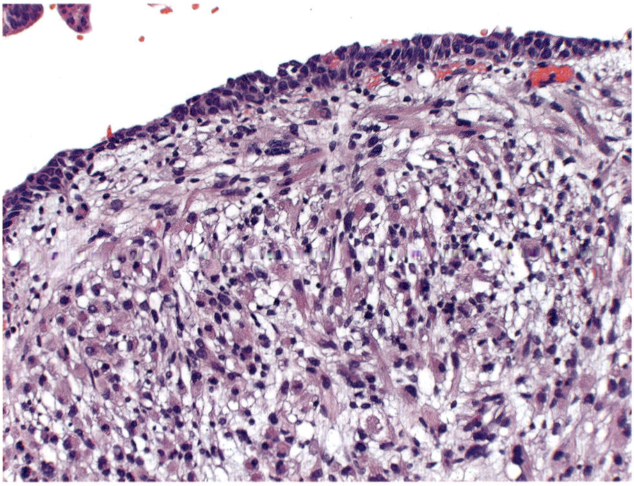

FIGURE 11.5 Rhabdomyosarcoma.

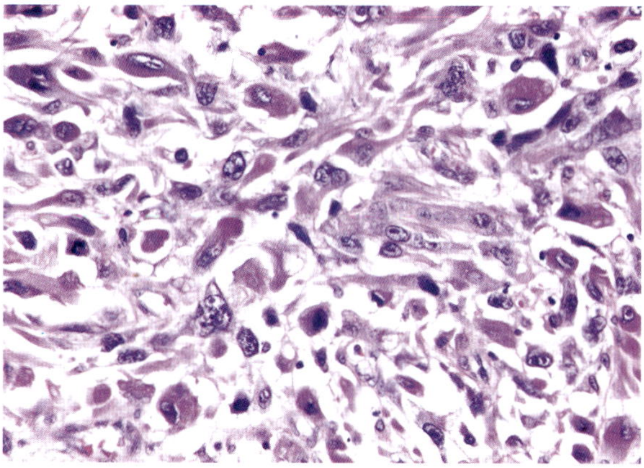

FIGURE 11.6 Rhabdomyosarcoma.

urothelium (Figs. 11.7 and 11.8). The underlying stroma is hypocellular and myxoid, and here, the tumor cells may have a more bland appearance. In other polypoid tumors, the neoplastic cells are diffusely distributed throughout. A significant percentage of vesical RMS does not have an exophytic component, and in these, the tumor cells infiltrate the bladder wall diffusely.[22] The spindle cell and alveolar variants of RMS may be rarely encountered. Typical rhabdomyoblasts and cross striations are seen frequently in exophytic RMS but rarely seen in the spindle cell and alveolar types (defined by translocations involving FOXO1). Rare cases of vesical rhabdomyosarcoma have been described in adults, and these may have embryonal, pleomorphic, or alveolar patterns.[19] Rhabdomyosarcoma should enter in the differential diagnosis of all spindle, round cell, and myxoid lesions of the genitourinary tract in the pediatric age group. Tumor cells will be at least focally immunoreactive for desmin and myogenin, or myoD1, the latter two markers in a nuclear distribution.[14] Immunoreactivity for myoglobin is also diagnostic, although it is positive in a minority of cases (Table 11.1).

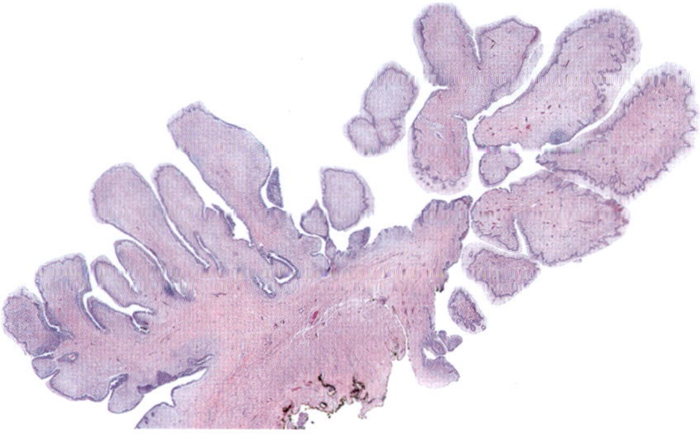

FIGURE 11.7 Botryoid variant of rhabdomyosarcoma.

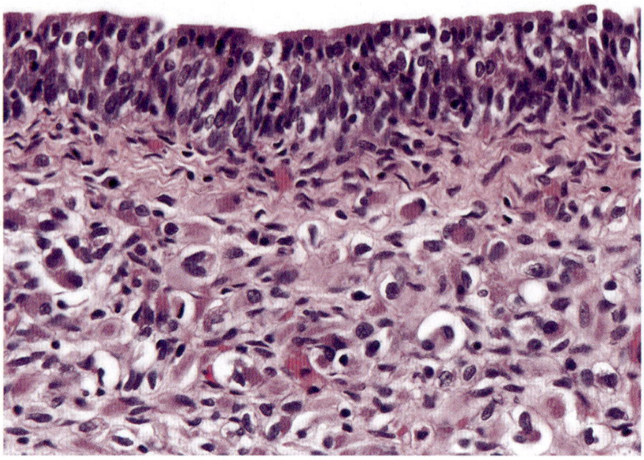

FIGURE 11.8 Cambium layer of botryoid variant of rhabdomyosarcoma (higher magnification of Fig. 11.7).

A subset of these tumors may have remarkable overlap in morphology with small cell carcinoma, as the typical alveolar morphology may not be obvious and there may be greater degree of anaplasia (Fig. 11.9). Synaptophysin immunoreactivity, which can be seen in these tumors, further complicates this differential diagnosis, although myoD1, myogenin, and desmin should help confirm the diagnosis.[23] Gupta et al. found that ASCL1 protein expression was present only in high-grade neuroendocrine carcinoma, while both a pure alveolar rhabdomyosarcoma and sarcomatoid rhabdomyosarcoma of the urinary bladder demonstrated a fusion involving PPP1R12A.[24]

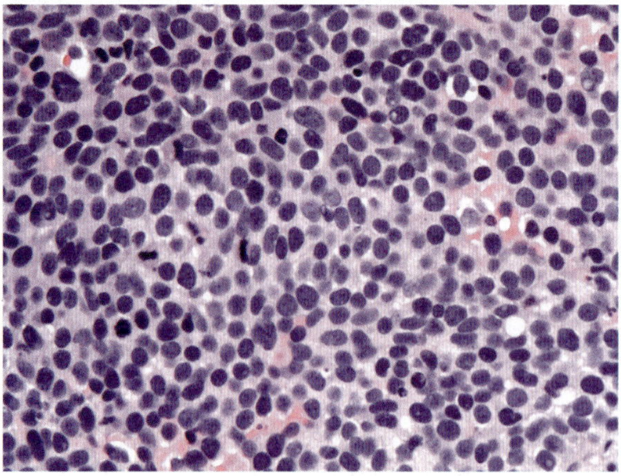

FIGURE 11.9 Rhabdomyosarcoma resembling small cell carcinoma.

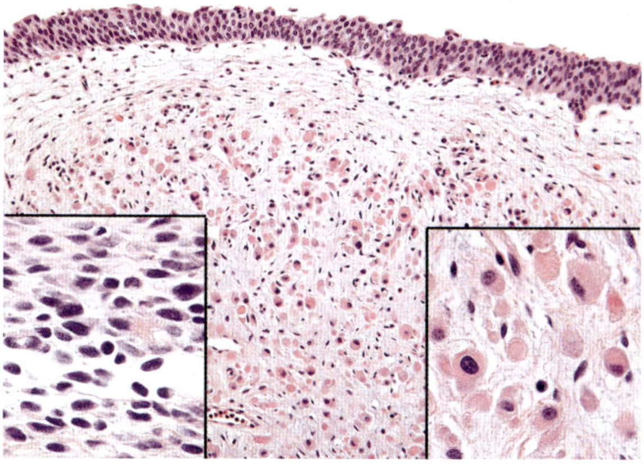

FIGURE 11.10 **Rhabdomyosarcoma postchemotherapy.** Areas of the tumor showed mature rhabdomyoblasts (***right inset***), while others demonstrated cellular, more poorly differentiated sarcoma (***left inset***).

Presently, there is no specific translocation associated with embryonal rhabdomyosarcoma, although they exhibit a significant amount of genomic instability in the form of copy number abnormalities. Fusion of *FOXO1* on chromosome 13 with either *PAX3* on chromosome 2 or *PAX7* on chromosome 1 is present in up to 75% of alveolar RMS and preferentially in advanced or clinically aggressive tumors. The rare spindle cell or sclerosing variants, more commonly seen in adults, exhibit somatic mutations of *MYOD1* and/or *PIK3CA*.

In general, RMS have a poor prognosis in adults. Combination therapy with surgery and chemotherapy has greatly improved survival in the pediatric age group. Studies have suggested that exophytic RMS have a better prognosis than those that infiltrate the bladder wall diffusely.[22] Patterns of embryonal RMS with a better prognosis include the spindle cell, botryoid, and tumors lacking diffuse anaplasia (criteria similar to Wilms tumors). Alveolar and pleomorphic variants are associated with a relatively poor outcome. Interestingly, treated tumors commonly exhibit morphologic evidence of "maturation" as evidenced by a greater number of myoblasts and cross striations (Fig. 11.10).

MYOFIBROBLASTIC PROLIFERATIONS OF THE BLADDER: INFLAMMATORY MYOFIBROBLASTIC TUMOR AND REACTIVE PSEUDOSARCOMATOUS MYOFIBROBLASTIC PROLIFERATION

Lesions of myofibroblastic origin that involve the urinary bladder mimic sarcoma or sarcomatoid carcinoma. They have been described under a variety of names including inflammatory pseudotumor, pseudosarcomatous myofibroblastic tumor, pseudosarcomatous myofibroblastic proliferation (PMP), pseudosarcomatous fibromyxoid tumor, nodular fasciitis, postoperative spindle cell nodule, and most recently inflammatory myofibroblastic tumor (IMT). It is evident that myofibroblasts can give rise to two types of lesions, one reactive (PMP) and the other neoplastic (IMT). Importantly, both have significant overlapping histologic features (eFigs. 11.10-11.49). In 1984, Proppe et al.[25] reported on nine cases of spindle cell tumors, two of which involved the bladder and three the prostatic urethra, all appearing within months of a TUR. They named the lesions "postoperative spindle cell nodules of the genitourinary tract." These apparently benign proliferative lesions are characterized histologically by plump, stellate, or elongated spindle cells, which infiltrate the bladder wall and focally can destroy muscle. Marked cytologic atypia is not present. The lesion can be quite cellular. A prominent feature of these tumors is a delicate network of small blood vessels in an edematous or myxoid stroma with little to moderate collagen deposition. Mitotic figures may be present and even frequent, but they are not atypical. The surface urothelium is usually ulcerated with an acute inflammatory cell infiltrate superficially and chronic inflammatory infiltrate scattered throughout the remainder of the lesion. Pseudosarcomatous reaction, often prominent, may be seen associated with invasive urothelial carcinoma and iatrogenic soft tissue filters used for stress incontinence.

Histologically, similar lesions were described by other authors and called "inflammatory pseudotumor,"[26,27] "pseudosarcomatous fibromyxoid tumor,"[28] and "pseudosarcomatous myofibroblastic proliferation."[29] A similar pseudosarcomatous lesion was reported by Roth.[30] The lesions were either pedunculated or polypoid, with a low mitotic rate. They appeared either spontaneously or in a background of chronic cystitis and differed from the cases reported by Proppe in that they were not necessarily related to a recent operative procedure.

Studies have suggested that some myofibroblastic proliferations arise unassociated with prior instrumentation or local trauma and are clonal, confirming that they are neoplastic rather than reactive in nature.[31-33] This fact is further supported by studies that demonstrate immunoreactivity for anaplastic lymphoma kinase (ALK) in up to 60% of cases and ALK rearrangement confirmed by fluorescent *in situ* hybridization (FISH). These neoplasms fall under the category of IMT. Some experts, including some of the authors of this book, consider that regardless of whether there is prior instrumentation or the lesions arise *de novo*, they are the same entity as (1) ALK gene rearrangements have been described in some postoperative lesions; (2) lesions have identical morphology, prognosis, and treatment whether they arise with or without the setting of prior instrumentation; and (3) it is conceivable that instrumentation could be the initiating event leading to a clonal neoplasm as opposed to a reactive process. This point of view is certainly not universal, with other experts highlighting the fact that myofibroblastic response to local injury of the bladder, particularly posttransurethral resection, is very frequent and usually localized to this area and yet the development of a true neoplasm is fleetingly rare.

IMTs have a wide age distribution but are preferentially seen in children and young adults, with the urinary bladder being one of the most commonly involved viscera. As previously mentioned, the morphology may overlap significantly with reactive myofibroblastic proliferations. The appearance is identical to that seen in nodular fasciitis lesions seen in soft tissue. Classically, one encounters stellate cells in a myxoid and mixed inflammatory background, while other cases are characterized by spindle cells arranged in fascicles. Less commonly, the spindle cells are embedded in a sparsely cellular collagenized stroma, where the delicate network of small blood vessels is less apparent. These patterns may coexist within the same tumor and result in "zonation" with hypocellular areas toward the surface and hypocellular areas at the advancing edge.

The differential diagnosis usually is with LMS and sarcomatoid carcinoma.[34,35] Large size of some of the lesions, necrosis, cellularity, and muscle infiltration compound the differential with a malignant process. Sarcomatoid carcinoma is likely to exhibit a greater degree of cytologic atypia, at least focally, and close examination may reveal subtle transitions to a more obvious epithelial neoplasm. Mitotic activity may be brisk, but atypical mitoses, which are encountered in sarcomas and sarcomatoid carcinoma, are not seen myofibroblastic lesions, either reactive or neoplastic. Caution must be observed since invasive or metastatic urothelial carcinoma may also incite a pseudosarcomatous stromal reaction, which may be confused with a myofibroblastic proliferation or with sarcoma.[31,32,36] Although sarcomatoid carcinomas are likely to invade deeply into the muscularis propria, IMTs are similarly locally invasive. A reactive myofibroblastic proliferation should always be suspected when a spindle cell lesion is encountered shortly after instrumentation or in a setting of local injury. The best clues to its diagnosis are a delicate but abundant vascular network, absence of atypical mitotic figures, absence of nuclear hyperchromasia, edematous or myxoid stroma, and a sprinkling of chronic inflammatory cells deep within the lesion (Figs. 11.11-11.19). Tumor cells will usually have the features of

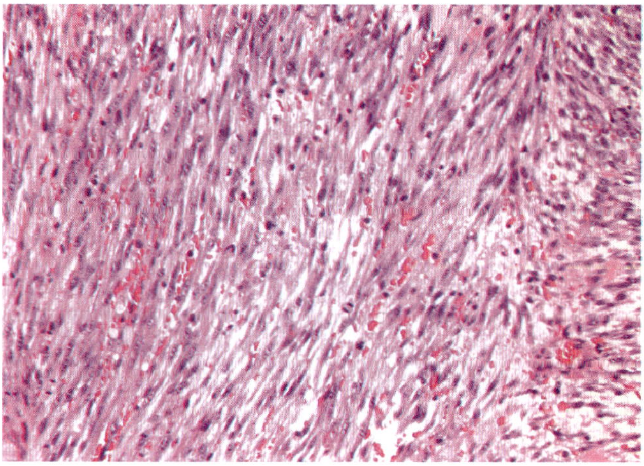

FIGURE 11.11 Inflammatory myofibroblastic tumor/pseudosarcomatous myofibroblastic proliferation (IMT/PMP).

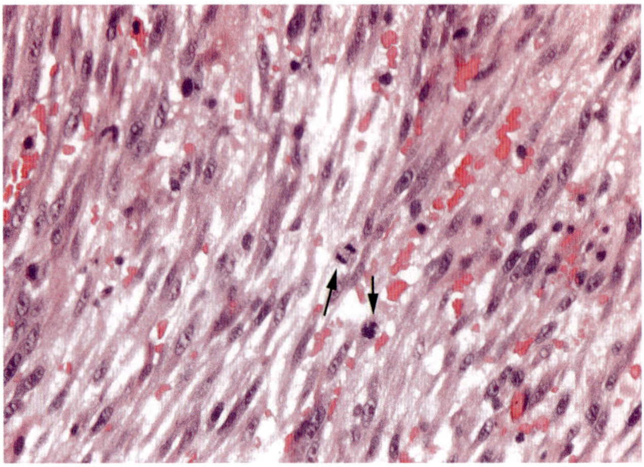

FIGURE 11.12 **IMT/PMP.** Note mitotic figures (*arrows*).

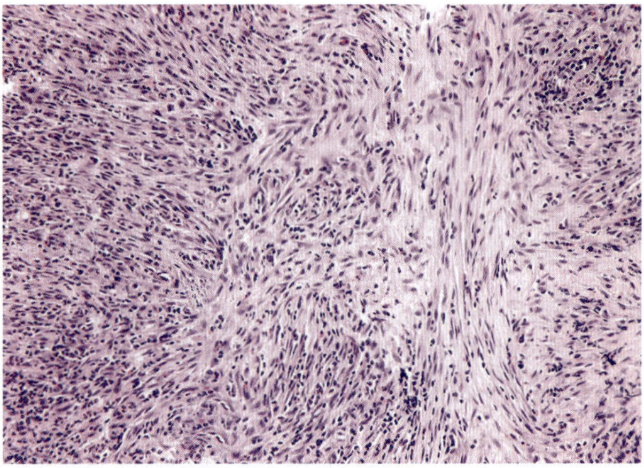

FIGURE 11.13 **IMT/PMP with interspersed inflammatory cells.**

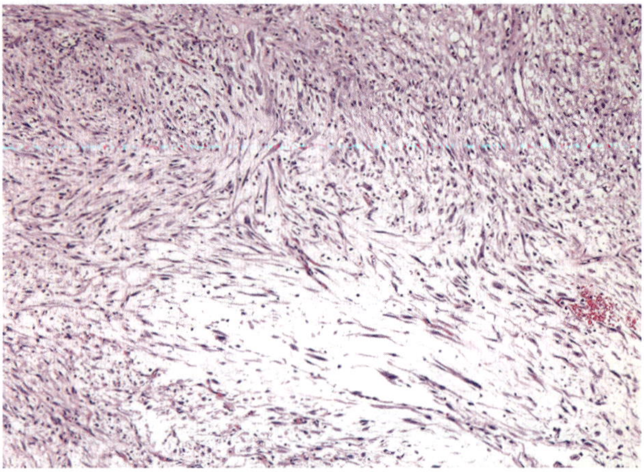

FIGURE 11.14 **IMT/PMP with myxoid areas.**

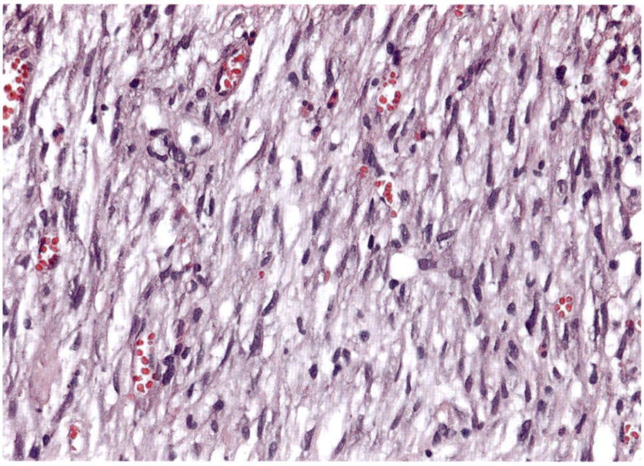

FIGURE 11.15 Inflammatory myofibroblastic tumor/pseudosarcomatous myofibroblastic proliferation (IMT/PMP).

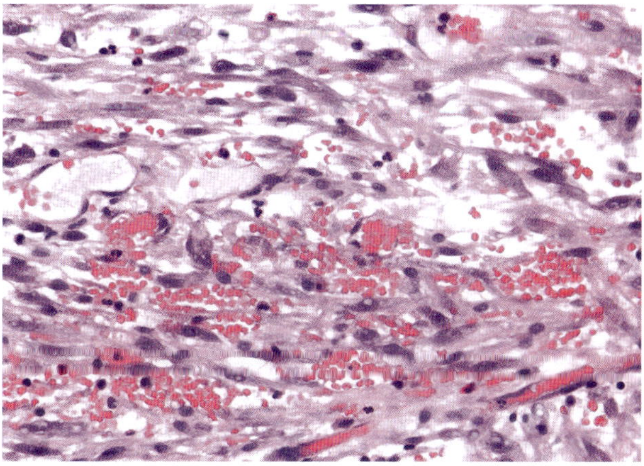

FIGURE 11.16 IMT/PMP with extravasated red blood cells.

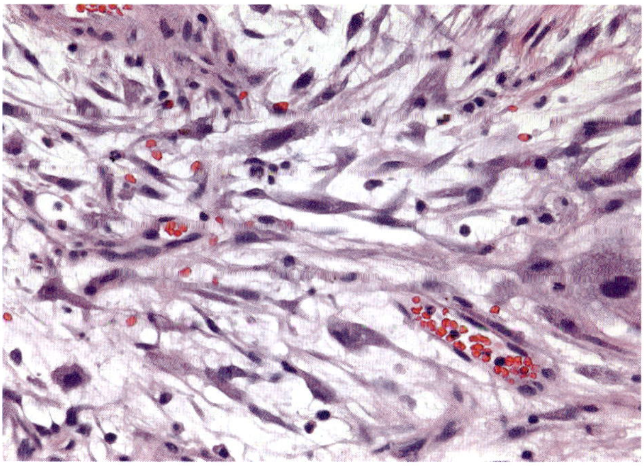

FIGURE 11.17 IMT/PMP with tissue culture–like cells.

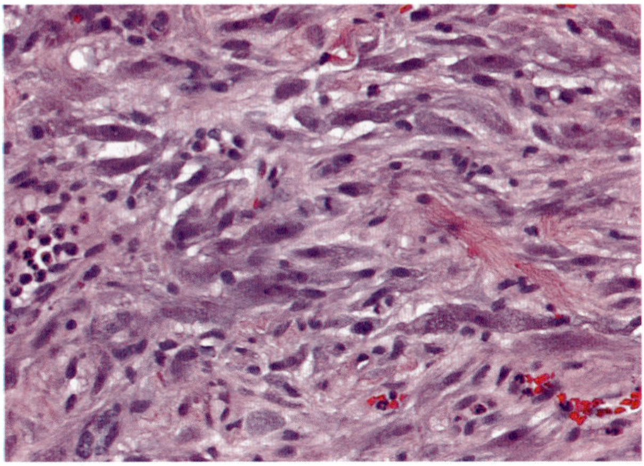

FIGURE 11.18 IMT/PMP (note mitotic figure).

myofibroblasts with large, plump, stellate, or elongated spindle cells with abundant eosinophilic cytoplasm; occasionally, ganglionlike cells with prominent nucleoli are present. Often, IMT/PMP have zonation-more myxoid toward the surface and more cellular toward the base. Immunohistochemical studies will help to prove the myofibroblastic nature of the cells.[15,32,34,35,37,38] Nevertheless, extreme caution is warranted in the interpretation of the immunohistochemical stains since proliferating myofibroblasts may be positive for cytokeratins and actin,[39] although not caldesmon or rarely epithelial membrane antigen (Table 11.1). Given the marked immunohistochemical overlap between IMT, LMS, and sarcomatoid carcinoma, a panel composed of GATA3, cytokeratin (AE1/3), desmin, smooth muscle actin, ALK, high molecular weight cytokeratin, p63, and CK5/6 expression should be interpreted in the context of the clinical scenario, morphology, and overall staining pattern. The expression of GATA3 as

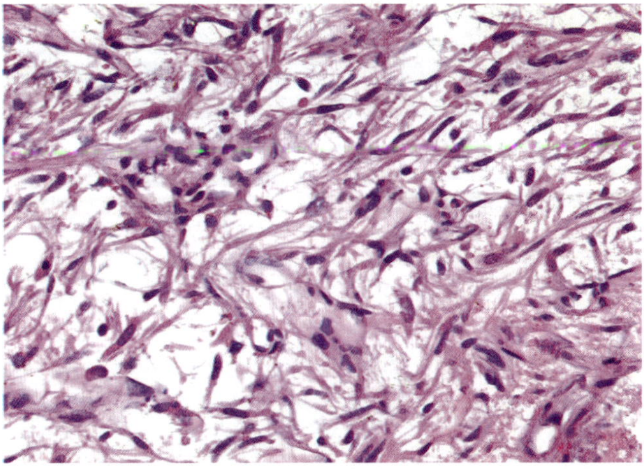

FIGURE 11.19 IMT/PMP with tissue culture–like cells.

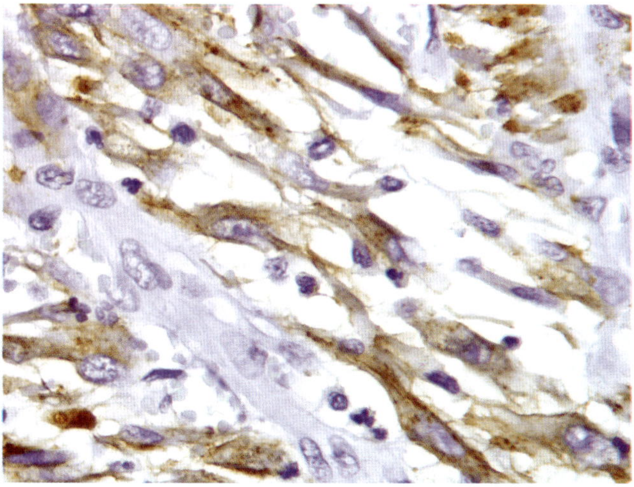

FIGURE 11.20 **IMT/PMP with positivity for ALK-1 protein.**

well as several cytokeratins, especially high molecular weight cytokeratin, CK5/6, and p63, favors sarcomatoid carcinoma, while immunoreactivity for smooth muscle actin and desmin with overall absence of other markers favors LMS.[13,14] Approximately two-thirds of IMTs express ALK by immunohistochemistry.[40] This ALK overexpression goes along with the finding of a recurrent translocation involving chromosome band 2p23, site of the ALK gene, in these tumors up to 70% of cases (Figs. 11.20 and 11.21).

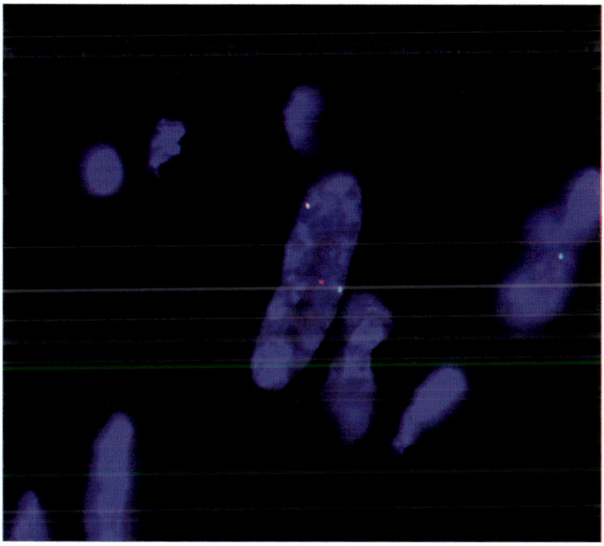

FIGURE 11.21 **IMT with 2p23 break point on chromosome 2 (rearranged as a result of a translocation).** The *orange* and *green* signals are separated and are visualized as distinct signals more than one signal width apart. The abnormal specimen thus has one fusion for the normal chromosome 2 and one *orange* and one *green* signal for the rearranged chromosome 2.

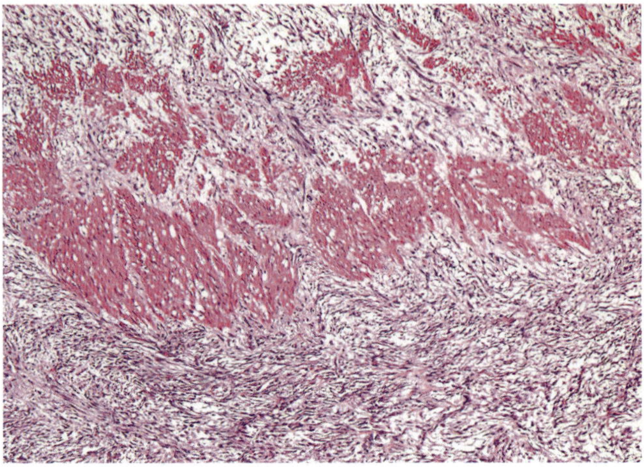

FIGURE 11.22 IMT/PMP involving muscularis propria.

Consideration should be given to confirmation by FISH, if this assay is available. USP6, ETV6, or ROS1 rearrangements are not typical of IMT/myofibroblastic lesions of the bladder.

IMT can invade deeply into the muscularis propria and even into the perivesical adipose tissue (Fig. 11.22). However, typically, these tumors once resected, even incompletely, tend to regress or stay stable. However, occasionally, these tumors may recur, causing local morbidity and potentially even necessitating radical surgery. Close follow-up is recommended.

We have noted increasing cellularity and atypia in some cases of recurrences and have observed exceptionally rare sarcomatous transformation in recurrences, such that at least complete conservative excision of all lesional tissue and maintained follow-up is required for all IMT of the bladder. A unique case has been described with many morphological features of IMT/PMP and an ALK rearrangement, yet overtly sarcomatous. This tumor led to death from intra-abdominal metastatic disease at 9 months (Fig. 11.23).[31] Comparison of histology of primary tumors with recurrent tumors is strongly advised to assess for increasing cellularity, atypia, or mitotic activity.

MISCELLANEOUS BENIGN MESENCHYMAL TUMORS

A wide spectrum of benign and borderline malignant vascular lesions occurs in the bladder including hemangioma, hemangiopericytoma, arteriovenous malformations, intravascular papillary endothelial hyperplasia, and epithelioid hemangioendothelioma[41] (Figs. 11.24-11.27). In a series of schwannomas and neurofibromas of the bladder, it was emphasized that the importance of accurately diagnosing plexiform neurofibromas of the bladder is that a subset harbors neurofibromatosis.[42] If the lesion is focal,

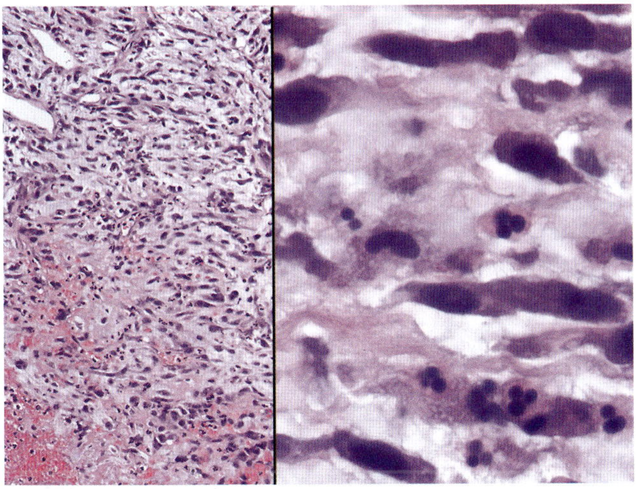

FIGURE 11.23 Malignant IMT with hyperchromatic nuclei (higher magnification [*right*]).

conservative excision is the choice of treatment with a low risk of recurrence. Diffuse neurofibromas can be difficult to diagnose leading to delay of treatment and potentially the need for a more extensive excision. The diagnosis of diffuse neurofibroma in the bladder may be problematic as the lamina propria and submucosa are replaced by a homogenous delicate eosinophilic matrix that is easily overlooked as normal (Figs. 11.28-11.30, eFigs. 11.50 and 11.51). The key to its recognition is that the tissue in the lamina propria and submucosa appears denser and Wagner-Meissner bodies may be found. Other benign mesenchymal tumors arising at this site

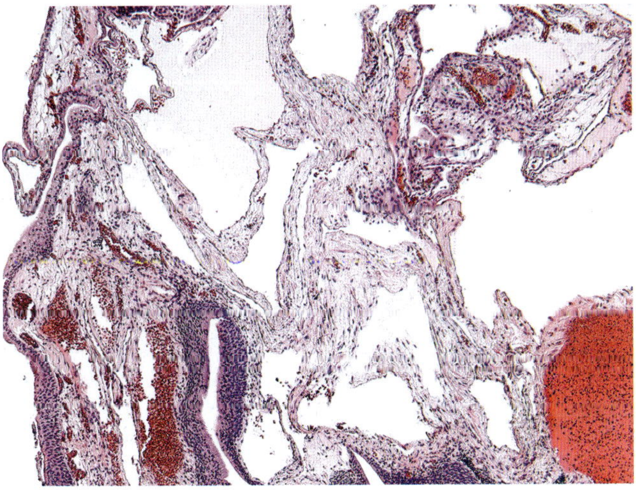

FIGURE 11.24 Cavernous hemangioma.

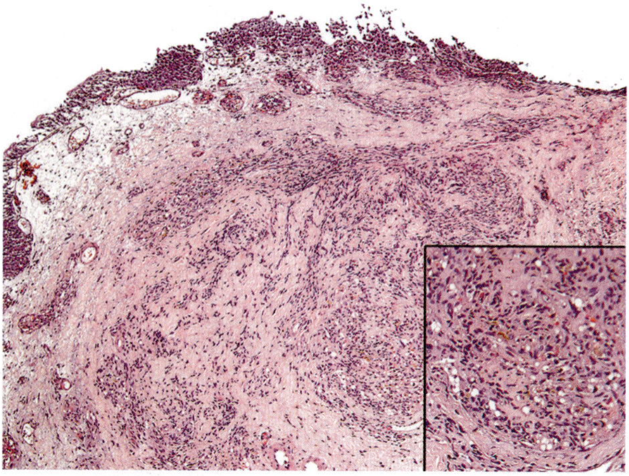

FIGURE 11.25 Capillary hemangioma (higher magnification [*inset*]).

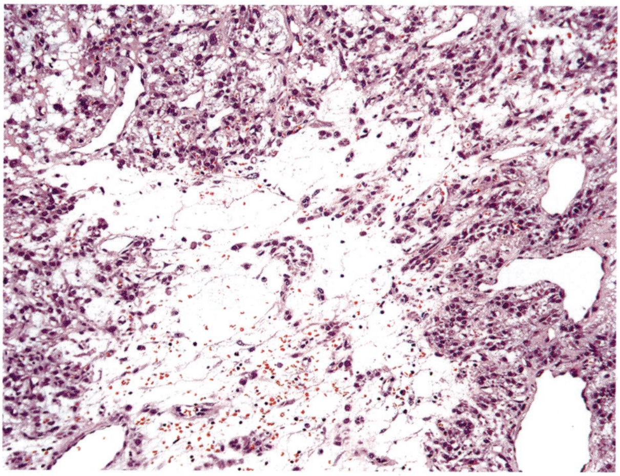

FIGURE 11.26 Epithelioid hemangioendothelioma.

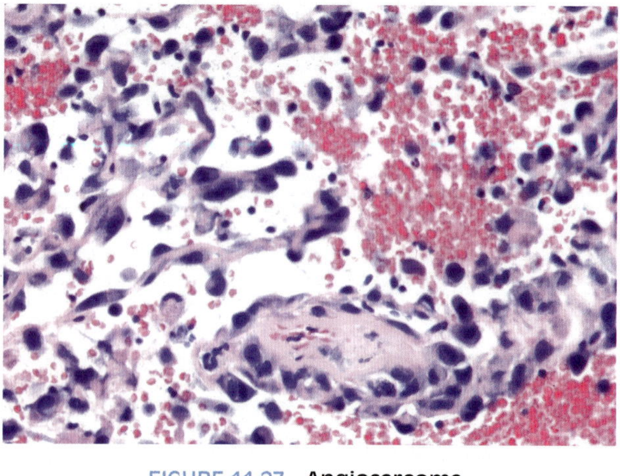

FIGURE 11.27 Angiosarcoma.

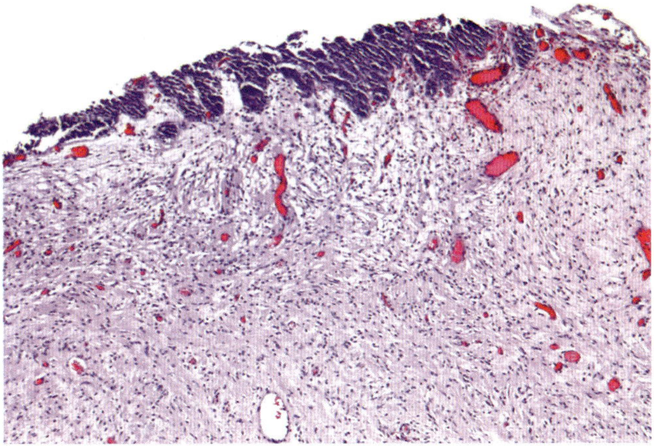

FIGURE 11.28 Neurofibroma within lamina propria.

include fibroma,[43,44] granular cell tumors,[45-47] and glomus tumor. Granular cell tumors are composed of large polygonal cells with voluminous granular eosinophilic cytoplasm. The morphology is identical to what has been described at other sites. They may occur at any age but are preferentially seen in adults. Although mostly benign, at least one case with locally advanced disease developed metastases.[47] They are thought to be of Schwann cell origin and are immunoreactive for S100 protein. Rare cases of perivascular epithelioid cell tumor (PEComa) and (extra) gastrointestinal stromal tumors have been described in the bladder[48,49] (Fig. 11.31). The vesical PEComas described in the literatures have not been associated with tuberous sclerosis complex. As in other sites, the tumor cells may be either epithelioid or spindled and are arranged in either nests or fascicles. The

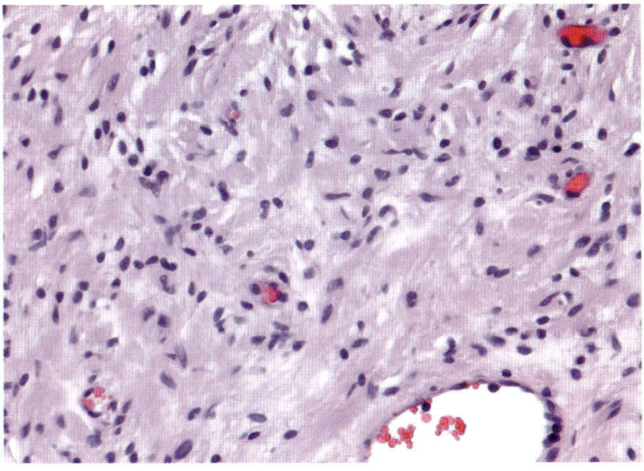

FIGURE 11.29 Neurofibroma (higher magnification of Fig. 11.28).

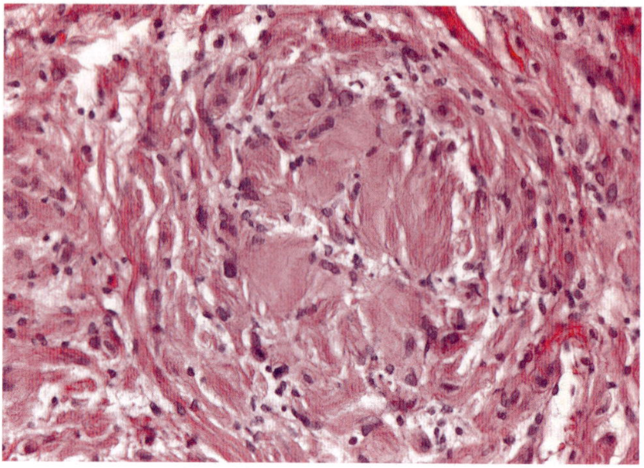

FIGURE 11.30 Neurofibroma with Wagner-Meissner body.

cytoplasm is either clear or granular eosinophilic. Vascularity is prominent with areas of perivascular sclerosis. While the majority of tumors described in the bladder have followed an indolent clinical course, criteria associated with malignant behavior include size >5 cm, necrosis, high nuclear grade, increase cellularity, and infiltrative margins.[50,51] These tumors are immunoreactive actin as well as melanocytic-related markers, including HMB45, melan A, tyrosinase, microphthalmia transcription factor (MiTF), and cathepsin K.[52,53] TFE3 is expressed in a subset of tumors, but this marker is difficult to perform in a CLIA environment.[53] Assessing TFE3 rearrangement by FISH or targeted RNA sequencing is more sensitive and specific.

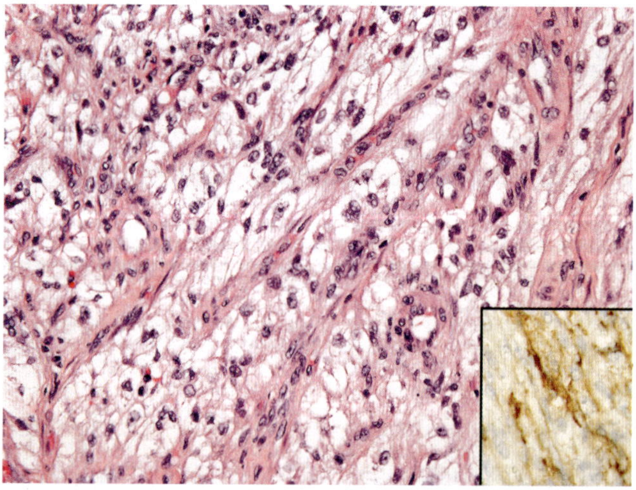

FIGURE 11.31 PEComa. (***Inset*** shows HMB45 positivity).

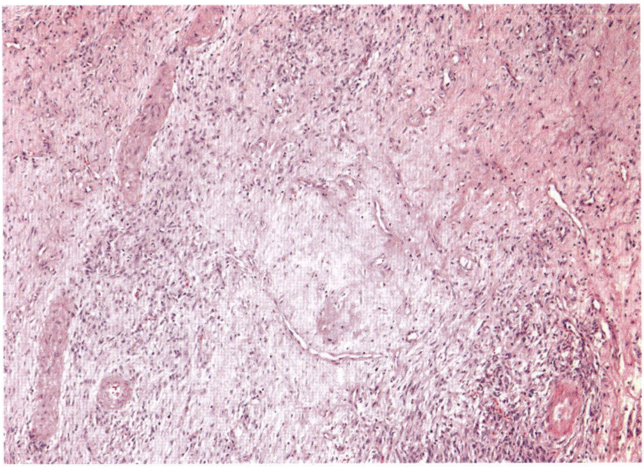

FIGURE 11.32 Solitary fibrous tumor.

SOLITARY FIBROUS TUMOR

Solitary fibrous tumors (SFT) may originate within the pelvis, including the bladder and prostate[54-56] (Figs. 11.32-11.35, eFigs. 11.52-11.60). They can be asymptomatic or associated with hematuria, obstruction, or pelvic pain. SFT of the bladder presents as a submucosal mass, which may be ulcerated. Microscopic features are identical to those seen at other sites, including spindle cells arranged in a haphazard or storiform pattern, zones of hypocellularity and hypercellularity, deposition of intercellular dense collagen, and staghorn vasculature. Classic examples behave in a benign fashion if completely excised, although incompletely resected and unresectable cases will recur locally. Malignant examples with cellular

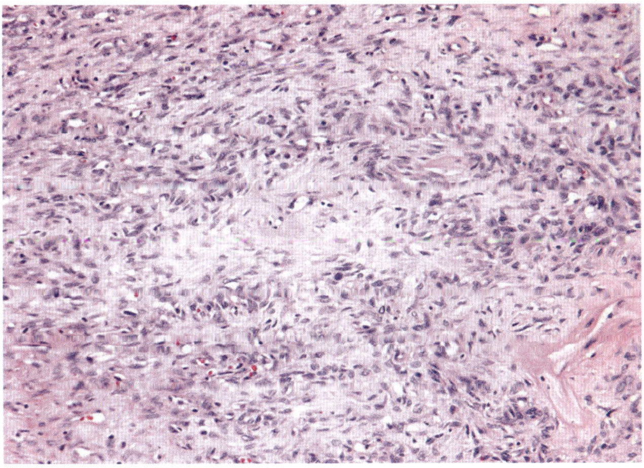

FIGURE 11.33 Solitary fibrous tumor.

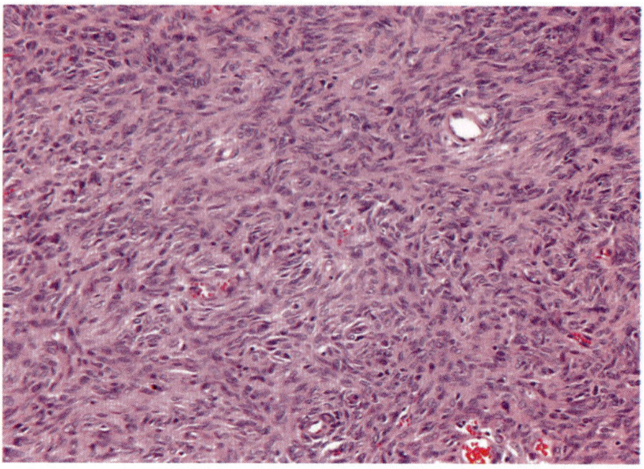

FIGURE 11.34 Solitary fibrous tumor with cellular areas.

pleomorphism and high mitotic rate (>4 per high-power field) have been described (eFigs. 11.61-11.65).

Despite classic cytologic and growth pattern characteristics seen in most cases, even in TUR specimens, these tumors are commonly misdiagnosed as sarcoma or sarcomatoid carcinoma. Immunohistochemistry for CD34 and bcl-2 are positive in SFT, aiding in their classification[56,57] (Table 11.1). Cytokeratins, epithelial membrane antigen, and smooth muscle markers will be negative. Spindle cell tumors of dedicated prostatic stroma may secondarily involve the bladder and may also express these markers as well as progesterone receptors, the latter being negative in SFT. Since these tumors are associated with an NAB2-STAT6 gene fusion, STAT6 immunohistochemistry has become the most reliable marker in establishing the diagnosis.

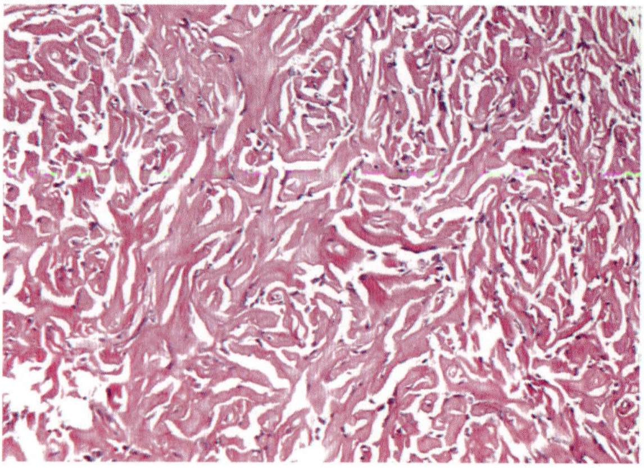

FIGURE 11.35 Solitary fibrous tumor with collagenized basket weave pattern.

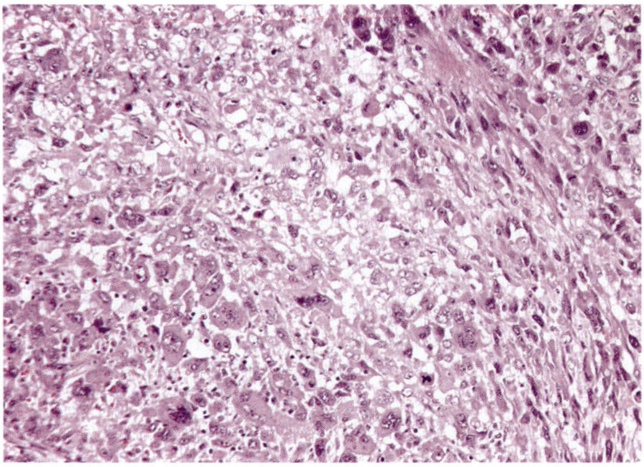

FIGURE 11.36 Undifferentiated pleomorphic sarcoma.

MISCELLANEOUS MALIGNANT MESENCHYMAL TUMORS

Other sarcomas that have been described in the bladder include angiosarcoma,[41] malignant "fibrous histiocytoma",[57,58] osteosarcoma,[59] fibrosarcoma,[60] alveolar soft part sarcoma,[61] and liposarcoma[62] (Fig. 11.36, eFigs. 11.66-11.72). Epithelioid angiosarcoma of the bladder is a rare malignancy that is frequently misdiagnosed as high-grade carcinoma, especially due to positive immunostaining for cytokeratins.[63] This tumor is more frequent in older men with a history of radiotherapy to the pelvis. Morphologic features that should suggest the vascular origin of the tumor include highly atypical nuclei with interspersed erythrocytes, hemorrhagic background, and occasional intracytoplasmic lumens (Fig. 11.37). Patients usually present with muscle-invasive disease, and the prognosis is dismal.

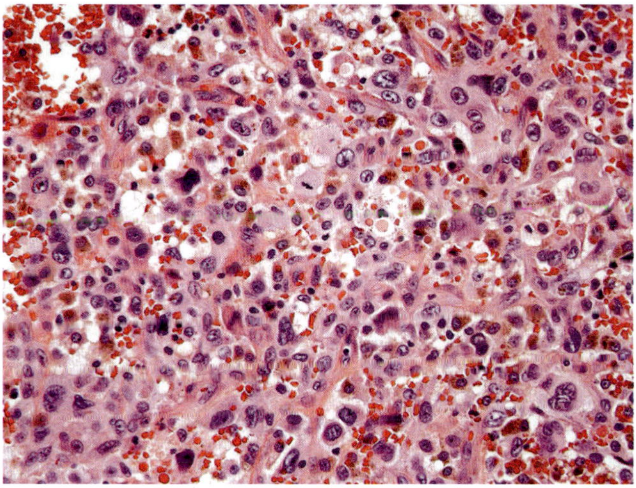

FIGURE 11.37 **Epithelioid angiosarcoma of the bladder with extravasated red blood cells.** Tumor was positive for CD31 and keratin.

While it is possible for these tumors to arise in the bladder, it is more likely that they originate in other sites and involve the bladder secondarily. The possibility that these represent elements of heterologous differentiation in a sarcomatoid carcinoma should be ruled out by liberal sampling to rule out an epithelial component either in the *in situ* or invasive component. We would consider tumors in patients with a prior history of treated high-grade urothelial carcinoma with a predominant sarcoma histology as likely to be sarcomatoid carcinoma. The only exception is a patient treated with radiation therapy who develops a tumor 8 years or more after completing treatment. In this setting, the tumor may represent a postradiation sarcoma.

REFERENCES

1. Mackenzie AR, Whitmore WF Jr, Melamed MR. Myosarcomas of the bladder and prostate. *Cancer*. 1968;22:833-844.
2. Russo P, Brady MS, Conlon K, et al. Adult urological sarcoma. *J Urol*. 1992;147:1032-1036. discussion 1036-1037.
3. Weitzner S. Leiomyosarcoma of urinary bladder in children. *Urology*. 1978;12:450-452.
4. Dotan ZA, Tal R, Golijanin D, et al. Adult genitourinary sarcoma: the 25-year Memorial Sloan-Kettering experience. *J Urol*. 2006;176:2033-2038. discussion 2038-2039.
5. Martin SA, Sears DL, Sebo TJ, et al. Smooth muscle neoplasms of the urinary bladder: a clinicopathologic comparison of leiomyoma and leiomyosarcoma. *Am J Surg Pathol*. 2002;26:292-300.
6. Lake MH, Kossow AS, Bokinsky G. Leiomyoma of the bladder and urethra. *J Urol*. 1981;125:742-743.
7. Yusim IE, Neulander EZ, Eidelberg I, et al. Leiomyoma of the genitourinary tract. *Scand J Urol Nephrol*. 2001;35:295-299.
8. Swartz DA, Johnson DE, Ayala AG, et al. Bladder leiomyosarcoma: a review of 10 cases with 5-year followup. *J Urol*. 1985;133:200-202.
9. Tanguay C, Harvey I, Houde M, et al. Leiomyosarcoma of urinary bladder following cyclophosphamide therapy: report of two cases. *Mod Pathol*. 2003;16:512-514.
10. Pedersen-Bjergaard J, Jonsson V, Pedersen M, et al. Leiomyosarcoma of the urinary bladder after cyclophosphamide. *J Clin Oncol*. 1995;13:532-533.
11. Motta L, Porcaro AB, Ficarra V, et al. Leiomyosarcoma of the bladder fourteen years after cyclophosphamide therapy for retinoblastoma. *Scand J Urol Nephrol*. 2001;35:248-249.
12. Rowland RG, Eble JN. Bladder leiomyosarcoma and pelvic fibroblastic tumor following cyclophosphamide therapy. *J Urol*. 1983;130:344-346.
13. Coiner BL, Cates J, Kamanda S, et al. Leiomyosarcoma of the urinary bladder: A SEER database study and comparison to leiomyosarcomas of the uterus and extremities/trunk. *Ann Diagn Pathol*. 2021;53:151743.
14. Lindberg MR, Fisher C, Thway K, et al. Leiomyosarcoma of the urinary bladder: a clinicopathological study of 34 cases. *J Clin Pathol*. 2010;63(8):708-713.
15. Westfall DE, Folpe AL, Paner GP, et al. Utility of a comprehensive immunohistochemical panel in the differential diagnosis of spindle cell lesions of the urinary bladder. *Am J Surg Pathol*. 2009;33:99-105.

16. Amin MB, Trpkov K, Lopez-Beltran A, et al. Best practices recommendations in the application of immunohistochemistry in the bladder lesions: report from the international society of urologic pathology consensus conference. *Am J Surg Pathol.* 2014;38: e20-e34.

17. Watanabe K, Baba K, Saito A, et al. Pseudosarcomatous myofibroblastic tumor and myosarcoma of the urogenital tract. *Arch Pathol Lab Med.* 2001;125:1070-1073.

18. Rodriguez D, Preston MA, Barrisford GW, et al. Clinical features of leiomyosarcoma of the urinary bladder: analysis of 183 cases. *Urol Oncol.* 2014;32:958-965.

19. Maurer HM, Moon T, Donaldson M, et al. The intergroup rhabdomyosarcoma study: a preliminary report. *Cancer.* 1977;40:2015-2026.

20. Scholtmeijer RJ, Tromp CG, Hazebroek FW. Embryonal rhabdomyosarcoma of the urogenital tract in childhood. *Eur Urol.* 1983;9:69-74.

21. Henriksson C, Zetterlund CG, Boiesen P, et al. Large rhabdomyosarcoma of the urinary bladder in an adult. Case report. *Scand J Urol Nephrol.* 1985;19:237-239.

22. Leuschner I, Harms D, Mattke A, et al. Rhabdomyosarcoma of the urinary bladder and vagina: a clinicopathologic study with emphasis on recurrent disease: a report from the Kiel Pediatric Tumor Registry and the German CWS study. *Am J Surg Pathol.* 2001;25:856-864.

23. Paner GP, McKenney JK, Epstein JI, et al. Rhabdomyosarcoma of the urinary bladder in adults: predilection for alveolar morphology with anaplasia and significant morphologic overlap with small cell carcinoma. *Am J Surg Pathol.* 2008;32:1022-1028.

24. Gupta S, Sosa CP, Kosari F, et al. A comparison of adult rhabdomyosarcoma and high-grade neuroendocrine carcinoma of the urinary bladder reveals novel PPP1R12A fusions in rhabdomyosarcoma. *Hum Pathol.* 2019;88:48-59.

25. Proppe KH, Scully RE, Rosai J. Postoperative spindle cell nodules of genitourinary tract resembling sarcomas. A report of eight cases. *Am J Surg Pathol.* 1984;8:101-108.

26. Nochomovitz LE, Orenstein JM. Inflammatory pseudotumor of the urinary bladder is—possible relationship to nodular fasciitis. Two case reports, cytologic observations, and ultrastructural observations. *Am J Surg Pathol.* 1985;9:366-373.

27. Jones EC, Clement PB, Young RH. Inflammatory pseudotumor of the urinary bladder. A clinicopathological, immunohistochemical, ultrastructural, and flow cytometric study of 13 cases. *Am J Surg Pathol.* 1993;17:264-274.

28. Ro JY, Ayala AG, Ordonez NG, et al. Pseudosarcomatous fibromyxoid tumor of the urinary bladder. *Am J Clin Pathol.* 1986;86:583-590.

29. Albores-Saavedra J, Manivel JC, Essenfeld H, et al. Pseudosarcomatous myofibroblastic proliferations in the urinary bladder of children. *Cancer.* 1990;66:1234-1241.

30. Roth JA. Reactive pseudosarcomatous response in urinary bladder. *Urology.* 1980; 16:635-637.

31. Montgomery EA, Shuster DD, Burkart AL, et al. Inflammatory myofibroblastic tumors of the urinary tract: a clinicopathologic study of 46 cases, including a malignant example inflammatory fibrosarcoma and a subset associated with high-grade urothelial carcinoma. *Am J Surg Pathol.* 2006;30:1502-1512.

32. Harik LR, Merino C, Coindre JM, et al. Pseudosarcomatous myofibroblastic proliferations of the bladder: a clinicopathologic study of 42 cases. *Am J Surg Pathol.* 2006;30: 787-794.

33. Hirsch MS, Dal Cin P, Fletcher CD. ALK expression in pseudosarcomatous myofibroblastic proliferations of the genitourinary tract. *Histopathology.* 2006;48:569-578.

34. Young RH. Spindle cell lesions of the urinary bladder. *Histol Histopathol.* 1990;5: 505-512.

35. McKenney JK. An approach to the classification of spindle cell proliferations in the urinary bladder. *Adv Anat Pathol.* 2005;12:312-323.

36. Mahadevia PS, Alexander JE, Rojas-Corona R, et al. Pseudosarcomatous stromal reaction in primary and metastatic urothelial carcinoma. A source of diagnostic difficulty. *Am J Surg Pathol.* 1989;13:782-790.
37. Reuter VE. Sarcomatoid lesions of the urogenital tract. *Semin Diagn Pathol.* 1993;10: 188-201.
38. Iczkowski KA, Shanks JH, Gadaleanu V, et al. Inflammatory pseudotumor and sarcoma of urinary bladder: differential diagnosis and outcome in thirty-eight spindle cell neoplasms. *Mod Pathol.* 2001;14:1043-1051.
39. Wick MR, Brown BA, Young RH, et al. Spindle-cell proliferations of the urinary tract. An immunohistochemical study. *Am J Surg Pathol.* 1988;12:379-389.
40. Cook JR, Dehner LP, Collins MH, et al. Anaplastic lymphoma kinase (ALK) expression in the inflammatory myofibroblastic tumor: a comparative immunohistochemical study. *Am J Surg Pathol.* 2001;25:1364-1371.
41. Tavora F, Montgomery E, Epstein JI. A series of vascular tumors and tumorlike lesions of the bladder. *Am J Surg Pathol.* 2008;32:1213-1219.
42. Wang W, Montgomery E, Epstein JI. Benign nerve sheath tumors on urinary bladder biopsy. *Am J Surg Pathol.* 2008;32:907-912.
43. Murao T, Kamoi M, Asano K. Fibroma of the urinary bladder: a light and ultrastructural study of a case with review of the literature in Japan. *Acta Med Okayama.* 1979;33: 113-120.
44. Winfield HN, Catalona WJ. An isolated plexiform neurofibroma of the bladder. *J Urol.* 1985;134:542-543.
45. Fletcher MS, Aker M, Hill JT, et al. Granular cell myoblastoma of the bladder. *Br J Urol.* 1985;57:109-110.
46. Mouradian JA, Coleman JW, McGovern JH, et al. Granular cell tumor (myoblastoma) of the bladder. *J Urol.* 1974;112:343-345.
47. Sun Y, Reuter VE, Magi-Galluzzi C, et al. Granular cell tumor of the bladder: a report of six cases. *Urology.* 2018;121:203e1-203e5.
48. Neumann NM, Haffner MC, Argani P, et al. Histopathologic characterization of bladder perivascular epithelioid cell neoplasms (PEComa): a series of 11 cases with a subset having TFE3 rearrangements. *Am J Surg Pathol.* 2021;45(2):169-177.
49. Weinreb I, Howarth D, Latta E, et al. Perivascular epithelioid cell neoplasms (PEComas): four malignant cases expanding the histopathological spectrum and a description of a unique finding. *Virchows Arch.* 2007;450:463-470.
50. Hamza A, Guo CC. Perivascular epithelioid cell tumor of the urinary bladder: a systematic review. *Int J Surg Pathol.* 2020;28(4):393-400.
51. Wu YL, Lang L, Ma Q, et al. Perivascular epithelioid cell tumor of urinary bladder. *Am J Clin Pathol.* 2021;156(1):56-71.
52. Williamson SR, Bunde PJ, Montironi R, et al. Malignant perivascular epithelioid cell neoplasm (PEComa) of the urinary bladder with TFE3 gene rearrangement: clinicopathologic, immunohistochemical, and molecular features. *Am J Surg Pathol.* 2013;37: 1619-1626.
53. Martignoni G, Pea M, Zampini C, et al. PEComas of the kidney and of the genitourinary tract. *Semin Diagn Pathol.* 2015;32:140-159.
54. Mentzel T, Bainbridge TC, Katenkamp D. Solitary fibrous tumour: clinicopathological, immunohistochemical, and ultrastructural analysis of 12 cases arising in soft tissues, nasal cavity and nasopharynx, urinary bladder and prostate. *Virchows Arch.* 1997;430:445-453.
55. Westra WH, Grenko RT, Epstein J. Solitary fibrous tumor of the lower urogenital tract: a report of five cases involving the seminal vesicles, urinary bladder, and prostate. *Hum Pathol.* 2000;31:63-68.

56. Corti B, Carella R, Gabusi E, et al. Solitary fibrous tumour of the urinary bladder with expression of bcl-2, cd34, and insulin-like growth factor type ii. *Eur Urol.* 2001;39: 484-488.
57. Henriksen OB, Mogensen P, Engelholm AJ. Inflammatory fibrous histiocytoma of the urinary bladder: clinicopathological report of a case. *Acta Pathol Microbiol Immunol Scand A.* 1982;90:333-337.
58. Turner AG. Malignant fibrous histiocytoma involving the bladder. *Br J Urol.* 1985; 57:237-238.
59. Berenson RJ, Flynn S, Freiha FS, et al. Primary osteogenic sarcoma of the bladder. Case report and review of the literature. *Cancer.* 1986;57:350-355.
60. Foote JW, Seemayer TA, Duignan JP. Desmoid tumor involving the bladder: case report. *J Urol.* 1975;114:147-149.
61. Amin MB, Patel RM, Oliveira P, et al. Alveolar soft-part sarcoma of the urinary bladder with urethral recurrence: a unique case with emphasis on differential diagnoses and diagnostic utility of an immunohistochemical panel including TFE3. *Am J Surg Pathol.* 2006;30:1322-1325.
62. Rosi P, Selli C, Carini M, Rosi MF. Myxoid liposarcoma of the bladder. *J Urol.* 1983;130:560-561.
63. Matoso A, Epstein JI. Epithelioid angiosarcoma of the bladder: a series of 9 cases. *Am J Surg Pathol.* 2015;39:1377-1382.

12

MISCELLANEOUS NONTUMORS AND TUMORS

NONTUMORS

Amyloidosis

The bladder may be involved in cases of systemic amyloidosis but rarely is the primary site of this disease.[1,2] The usual clinical presentation is that of hematuria. On cystoscopy, a localized amyloid tumor will be seen as an elevated mass that can be confused with an invasive neoplasm. Less frequently, the disease may diffusely involve the bladder wall. Microscopically, the amyloid protein is an eosinophilic, afibrillar material deposited preferentially in the lamina propria and extending into the connective tissue surrounding muscle fascicles[2] (Figs. 12.1 and 12.2, eFigs. 12.1-12.7). Less frequently, and usually in systemic amyloidosis, there are perivascular amyloid deposits. Congestion and hemorrhage are common, but inflammatory cells are scanty unless the overlying epithelium is ulcerated. A few fibroblastlike cells are usually interspersed within the eosinophilic material. An unusual association of bladder amyloidosis with urothelial carcinoma has been by one of us in half the cases of bladder amyloidosis seen in our practice.[3] However, it is unlikely that there is a causal relationship between these lesions. Special stains such as Congo red, crystal violet, or van Gieson will help establish the diagnosis. In a minority of cases, there may be a diffuse plasma cell infiltrate. In these cases, studies should be performed for light chain restriction to rule out associated plasma cell dyscrasia. Patients with localized lesions are usually successfully managed by transurethral resection (TUR), but patients with more diffuse involvement may require more radical surgery to control the bleeding.[4] In selected cases, treatment will require additional subtyping, which can be achieved by laser capture microdissection and mass spectrometry analysis.[5]

Diverticular Disease

Bladder diverticula are relatively common, yet their etiology remains controversial. Most investigators agree that they occur secondary to increased intravesical pressure as a result of obstruction distal to the diverticulum.[6-10] The obstruction brings about compensatory muscle hypertrophy and eventual mucosal herniation in areas of weakness. Others feel that at least

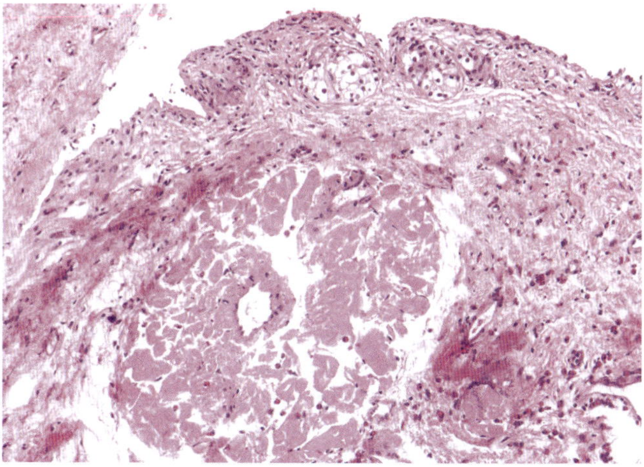

FIGURE 12.1 Amyloidosis surrounding a blood vessel.

some diverticula are a consequence of congenital defects in the bladder musculature, and they cite as evidence cases of diverticula in young patients with or without evidence of obstruction.[11,12] In the pediatric population, a significant number of cases are associated with other congenital defects, but this association has not been seen in adults. In addition, tumors associated with diverticula rarely occur in children.[13] The most common sites of diverticula are adjacent to the ureteral orifices, the bladder dome (probably related to an urachal remnant), and the region of the internal urethral orifice. Grossly one sees distortion of the external surface of the bladder. The diverticula may be widely patent but usually have a narrow os in symptomatic patients. The mucosa adjoining the diverticulum is usually hyperemic or ulcerated. At this site, the urothelium as well as the underlying bladder wall may exhibit reactive changes. Very commonly, there is inflammation

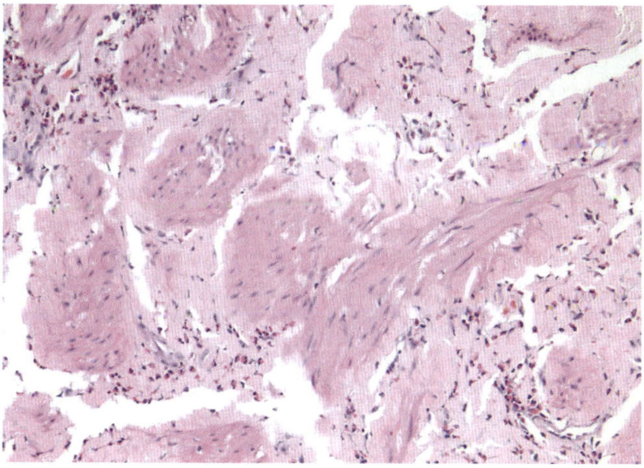

FIGURE 12.2 Amyloidosis infiltrating and destroying the muscularis propria.

involving the lamina propria and muscularis in the area of the diverticular os. The wall of the diverticulum itself consists of urothelium and underlying connective tissue, similar to the bladder mucosa with lamina propria. Fascicles of smooth muscle will be identified in the majority of cases of acquired diverticula but, when present, represent muscularis mucosae, which may be hyperplastic. In fact, in some cases, these hyperplastic muscularis mucosae may appear as a relatively thick, continuous layer of smooth muscle (Fig. 1.5). By definition, bladder diverticula in adults do not contain muscularis propria, an important fact that influences pathological staging of tumors (Fig. 12.3). The true "congenital" diverticula seen in the pediatric age group contain a thinned outer muscle layer. The urothelium lining the sac may undergo squamous or glandular metaplasia due to local irritation associated with urine stasis, irritation, or stone. In these cases, it is not unusual for the diverticular wall to become extensively fibrotic.

Major complications of bladder diverticula include infection, lithiasis with subsequent obstruction, and carcinoma.[14-16] It is believed that 2%-7% of patients with bladder diverticula will develop an associated urothelial neoplasm, presumed secondary to the chronic inflammatory stimuli mentioned above. The neoplasms may develop at the orifice or may occur within the diverticula, making endoscopic evaluation difficult. While "usual" urothelial carcinomas predominate, there is a relative increase in urothelial tumors with divergent differentiation in the form of squamous

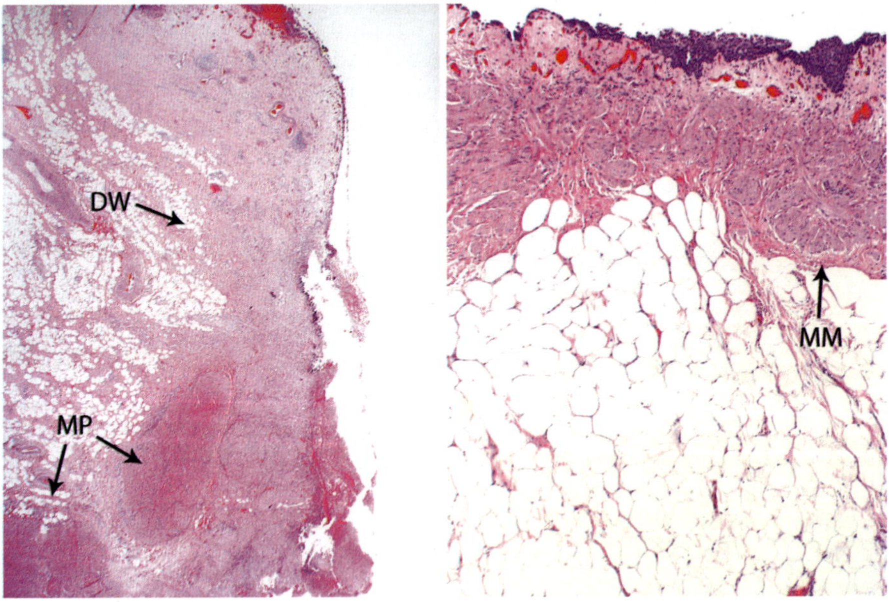

FIGURE 12.3 **Wall of the bladder diverticulum: image on the *left* shows the junction of the bladder wall, which contains muscularis propria (MP) and the wall of the diverticular wall (DW), devoid of muscularis propria.** On the ***right*** is the diverticular wall with a relatively thin lamina propria and thickened muscularis mucosae (MM) in direct contact with peridiverticular fat.

carcinoma, adenocarcinoma, at times associated with squamous or glandular metaplasia in the lining urothelium. Rare cases of small cell carcinoma have been described. Sarcomas also have been reported in association with bladder diverticula, but we feel that most, if not all, of these cases are likely to represent sarcomatoid transformation in high-grade urothelial carcinomas.[16] Survival is dependent on completeness of excision (negative margins) and stage at the time of resection with tumors invading the lamina propria (pT1) having a better disease-specific survival than tumors that extend into the peridiverticular soft tissue (pT3).[17,18]

Ectopic Prostatic Tissue

Ectopic prostatic polyps within the bladder are usually single, polypoid lesions usually around the trigone.[19,20] Etiology is not clear, but possibilities include seeding and persistence of embryonic remnants. These lesions typically present with gross and microscopic hematuria. They may occur over a wide age range but are more frequently detected in young men. Histologically, the submucosal component of the urethral polyps is composed of stroma and prostatic glands (Fig. 12.4). The glands may be closely packed, and in some areas, they may be cystically dilated at the periphery. The surface of urethral polyps is often papillary with broad papillae lined by urothelial cells, prostatic epithelial cells, or a combination of both. Rarely, these polyps have broad fingerlike villous projections lined by benign prostatic epithelium. The presence of corpora amylacea and double layered is a helpful clue to the prostatic origin of the lesions, and rarely prostate-specific immunohistochemistry may be required to rule out other benign mimics including cystitis glandularis.[20] These lesions are totally benign.

Fibroepithelial Polyp

Fibroepithelial polyp of the lower urinary tract is a relatively rare disease entity that is considered to be a nonneoplastic condition, some arising

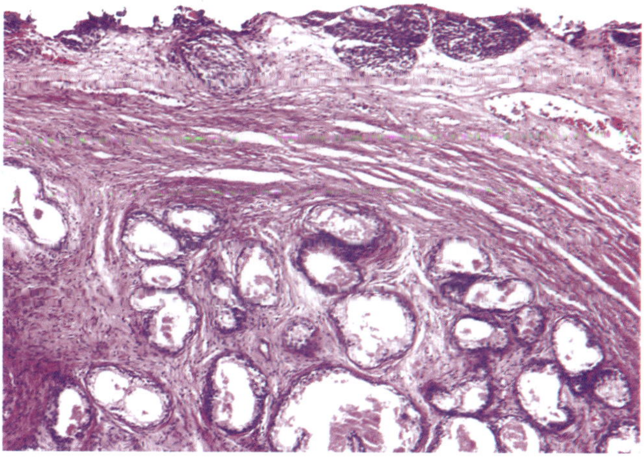

FIGURE 12.4 **Ectopic prostate tissue.**

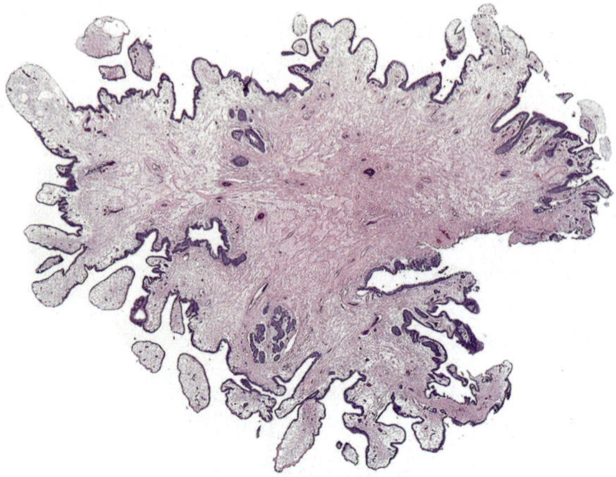

FIGURE 12.5 Fibroepithelial polyp lined by the urothelium.

from acquired conditions and others congenitally.[21] It has a marked male predominance. More than half of the reported cases occur in neonates or children, some of which are associated with urogenital malformations. However, cases have also been reported from the second to fourth decades and are unlikely to be congenital. Their main clinical manifestations are urinary obstruction, urinary hesitancy, dysuria, enuresis, hematuria, infection, and flank pain.[22,23] They are usually diagnosed by cystourethrography or cystoscopy and are treated by TUR, following which the lesion does not usually recur. Most cases are located near the verumontanum or the bladder neck. Histologically, fibroepithelial polyps with broad stalks predominantly composed of urothelial epithelium and fibrovascular stroma showing a fingerlike or polypoid growth pattern (Figs. 12.5-12.7,

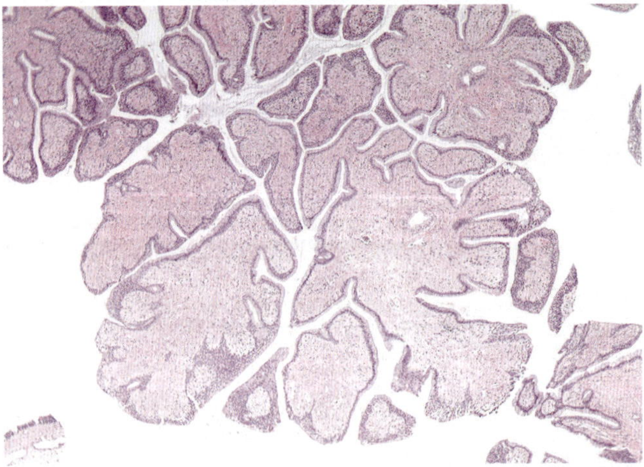

FIGURE 12.6 Fibroepithelial polyp lined by glandular epithelium.

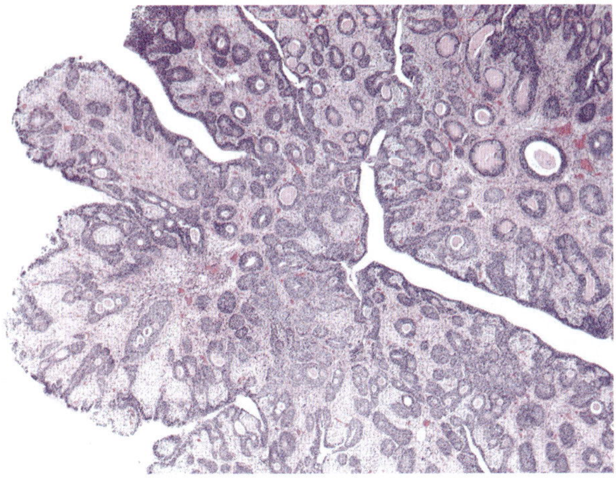

FIGURE 12.7 Fibroepithelial polyp resembling cystitis cystica.

eFigs. 12.8-12.11). Urothelium shows tubular or anastomosing structures with colloidlike secretions in some cases, resembling cystitis cystica. Although some of the urothelium shows focal squamous or mucinous metaplasia or becomes thin or denuded, none contain significant cytological atypia. The stroma of the polyps typically contains relatively frequent small vessels, some of which are dilated or congested. Stromal edema, either focal or extensive, is also a common finding. Although the stromal cells can show atypia with multinucleated cells and hyperchromasia, the atypia appears degenerative in nature, lacking prominent nucleoli and mitoses.

Urothelial papilloma may be difficult to differentiate because both lesions show a polypoid or fingerlike growth pattern and lack of cytological atypia of the urothelium. However, urothelial papilloma usually has thin fibrovascular cores in contrast to the relatively broad stroma of fibroepithelial polyp. Rarely, exstrophy of the bladder may present as a polyp.[24,25] While the age and the clinical setting are typical, deep penetrating nests of urothelium or metaplastic glandular epithelium with or without cystic change may result in diagnostic difficulty with a neoplasm. A unique cuff of periepithelial fibrosis also helps in the correct diagnosis.

Other Lesions

Other rare nonneoplastic lesions we have encountered in the urinary bladder but have been poorly described in the literature include Langerhans cell histiocytosis and crystal storing histiocytosis (Figs. 12.8 and 12.9). Mesonephric rests may be seen in the bladder although they are much more common in the prostate[22,26] (Fig. 12.10). As in the prostate, these rests should not be confused with adenocarcinoma, prostatic in origin or otherwise.

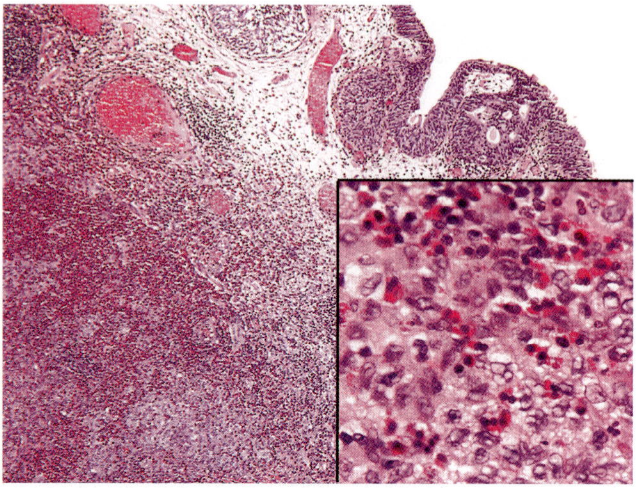

FIGURE 12.8 **Langerhans cell histiocytosis.** (***Inset*** shows histiocytes with longitudinal nuclear grooves in a background of eosinophils.)

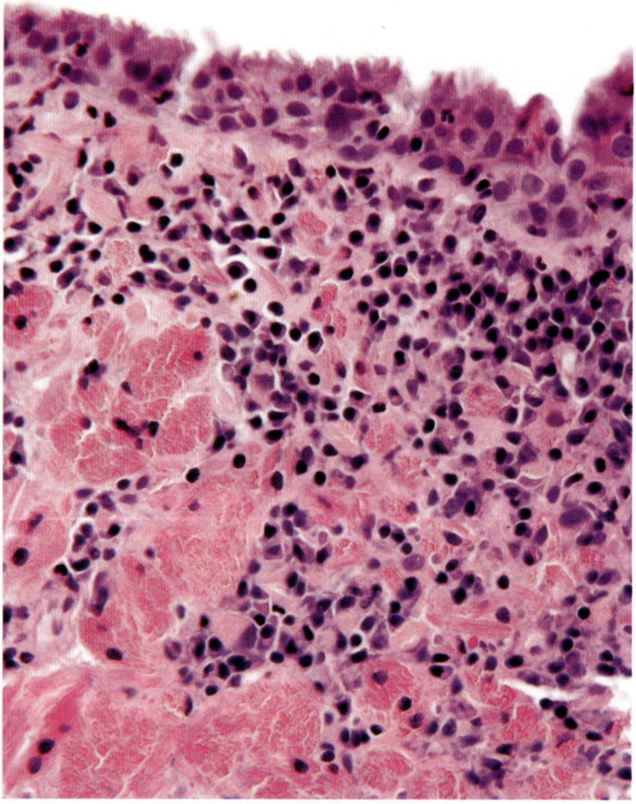

FIGURE 12.9 **Crystal storing histiocytosis.**

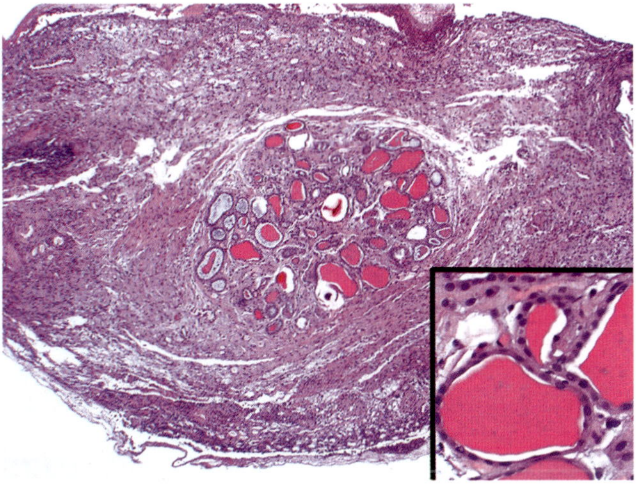

FIGURE 12.10 Hyperplasia of mesonephric remnants involving urinary bladder (higher magnification [*inset*]).

Caruncle

Caruncles usually occur in the urethra but may be encountered by pathologists examining bladder biopsies. These are pedunculated or sessile polypoid lesions that have a fleshy, pink-red appearance and bleed easily. Three clinically irrelevant histologic subgroups are described: papillomatous, angiomatous, and granulomatous, based on the most prominent feature of the lesion. The surface epithelium may be either "transitional" or squamous or rarely columnar and is invariably inflamed. The epithelium may become hyperplastic. The underlying stroma is richly vascular and inflamed, at times containing atypical degenerative-appearing reactive mesenchymal cells (Fig. 12.11).

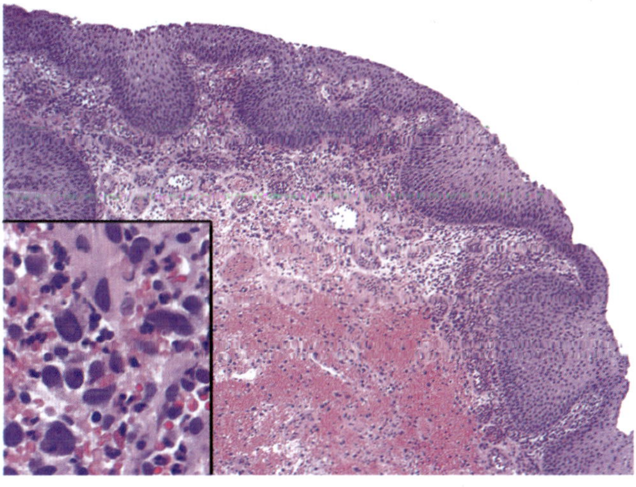

FIGURE 12.11 Urethral caruncle with degenerative stromal atypia (higher magnification of stromal atypia [*inset*]).

TUMORS

Paraganglioma

Of paragangliomas throughout the body, 10% occur in extra-adrenal sites, and of these extra-adrenal tumors, 10% are found in the bladder wall.[27,28] Paragangliomas of the urinary bladder account for <0.5% of bladder tumors. Primary paragangliomas of the bladder have a female to male ratio of 3-2 with an average age diagnosis of 41 years. Some case may occur in the setting of either germ line or somatic succinate dehydrogenase (*SDH*) mutations, which seen in 27%-52% of bladder paragangliomas,[29] suggesting some authors to advocate for potential role for SDHB immunohistochemistry in these tumors for appropriate triaging for genetic counseling (see below). There is a wide age distribution from childhood to the elderly. Most tumors are located on either the dome or the trigone. Although the majority of patients have exophytic lesions with an intact mucosa, in a minority of cases, there may be ulceration of the overlying mucosa. Lesions vary greatly in size from 2 mm to 10 cm. The majority of patients present with solitary lesions. It is not unusual for these cases to be misdiagnosed as invasive urothelial carcinomas with an inverted/nested growth pattern.

Paragangliomas can often be diagnosed on clinical grounds. Seventy-five percent of patients experience micturition attacks. When the bladder fills or upon urination, there ensues bursts of headaches, palpitations, hypertension, blurred vision, sweating, anxiety, tremulousness, and sometimes syncope. Hypertension can also be induced by intraoperative manipulation of the tumor. Hematuria is found in 60% of patients, whereas dysuria is uncommon. Increases in serum or urine catecholamines can provide laboratory confirmation of the diagnosis in 60%-80% of patients. Radiologically, bladder paragangliomas may be diagnosed using arteriography, selective venous sampling, CT or MRI, and scintigraphy with meta-I131 iodobenzylguanidine (I131-MIBG) or FDG-PET.

Paragangliomas typically are composed of nests (Zellballen) separated by either a thin delicate plexiform vascular network or more fibrous septa (Figs. 12.12-12.14, eFigs. 12.12-12.22). At higher magnification, polyhedric cells have acidophilic to amphophilic cytoplasm with central or eccentric nuclei and visible nucleoli (Fig. 12.15). As in many endocrine tumors, occasional bizarre nuclei may be seen (Figs. 12.16-12.19). Their chromatin appears smudged and hyperchromatic without mitoses, typical of degenerative atypia rather than the atypia of a high-grade malignant tumor. Mitoses in other tumor cells may be present yet are usually not numerous. Paragangliomas of the bladder can invade deeply into the muscle or show vascular invasion (Figs. 12.20 and 12.21). Focal hemorrhage and necrosis may also be present. Occasionally, one can discern neuroblastic or ganglioneuromatous differentiation. Cases of paraganglioma

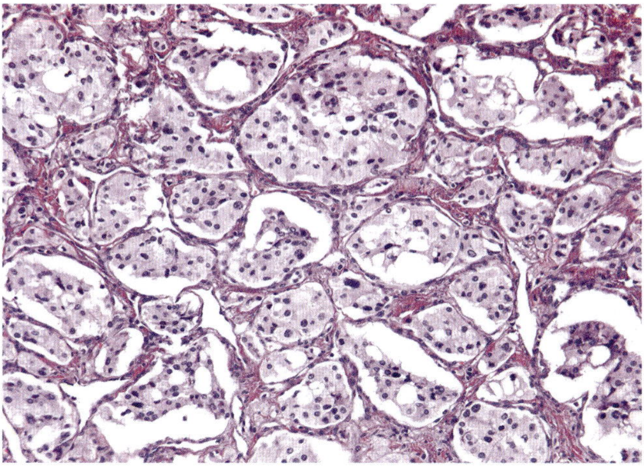

FIGURE 12.12 Paraganglioma with nested pattern.

of the urinary bladder have been described in patients with neurofibromatosis. Invasive urothelial carcinoma on occasion grows in a nesting pattern reminiscent of paraganglioma (Fig. 12.22).[30,31] They are likely to be associated with a malignant noninvasive component, while the urothelium overlying a paraganglioma is normal, reactive, or ulcerated. In contrast to paragangliomas, urothelial carcinomas exhibit cytologic atypia consisting of enlarged nuclei, prominent nucleoli, and numerous mitotic figures. Furthermore, the nesting and vascular pattern in urothelial carcinoma tends to be only focally present. In cases where the authors have seen paragangliomas misdiagnosed as urothelial carcinoma, the major histological features that led to the incorrect diagnosis included a diffuse growth pattern, focal clear cells, necrosis, and muscularis propria invasion, with significant cautery artifact compounding the diagnostic problems.[30] Distinction

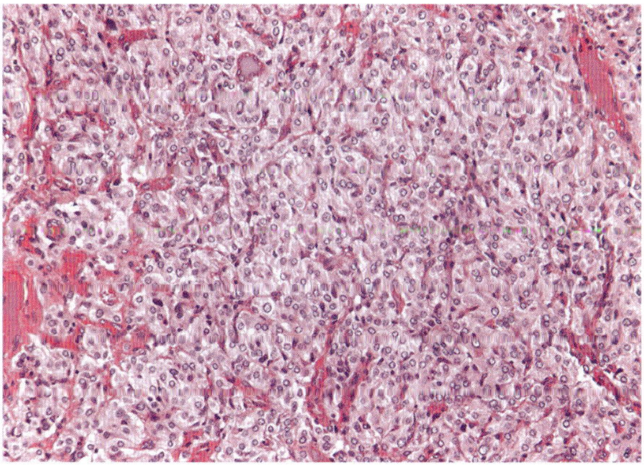

FIGURE 12.13 Paraganglioma with nested to solid growth pattern.

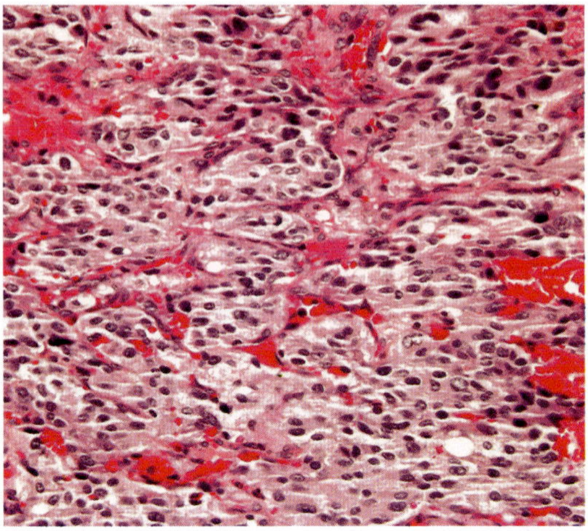

FIGURE 12.14 **Paraganglioma with nested pattern.**

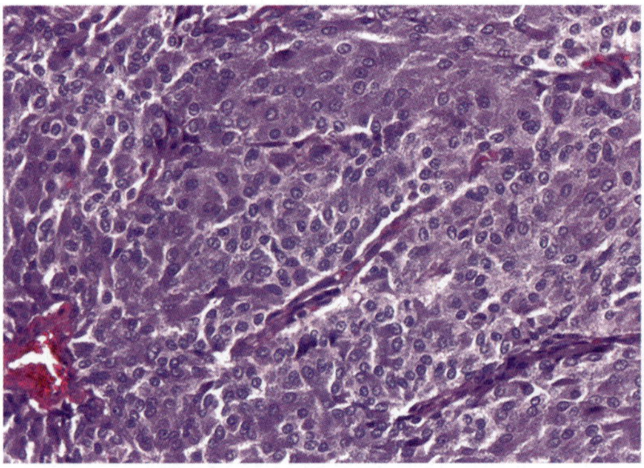

FIGURE 12.15 **Paraganglioma with amphophilic granular cytoplasm.**

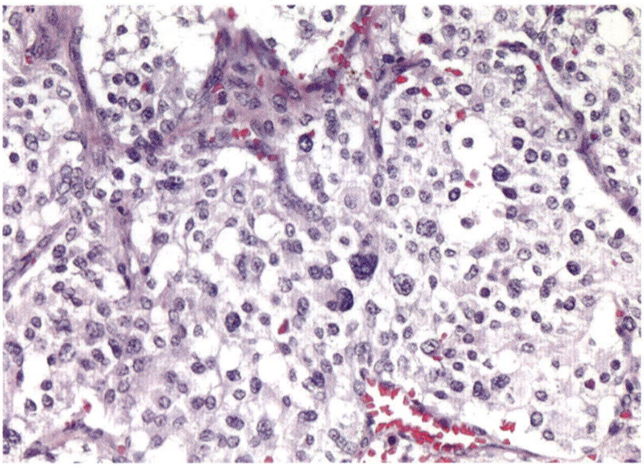

FIGURE 12.16 **Paraganglioma with degenerative atypia.** Note there is greater clearing of cytoplasm in this case.

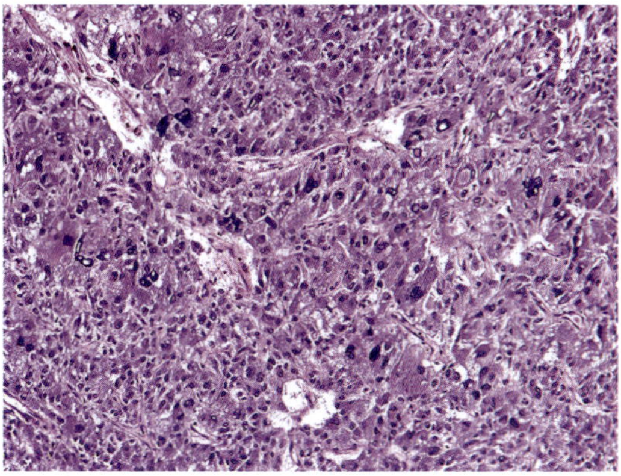

FIGURE 12.17 Paraganglioma with degenerative atypia.

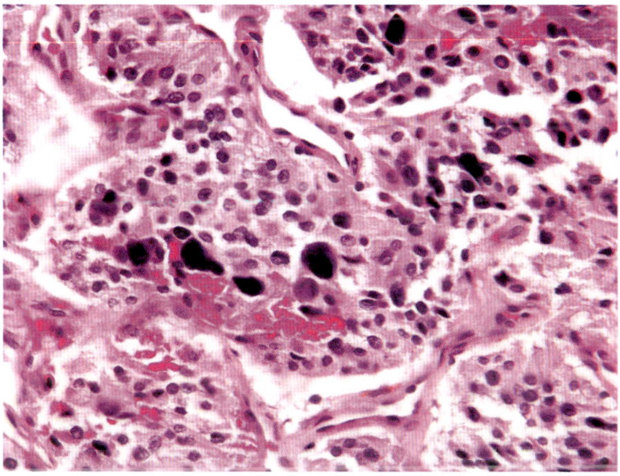

FIGURE 12.18 Paraganglioma with degenerative atypia.

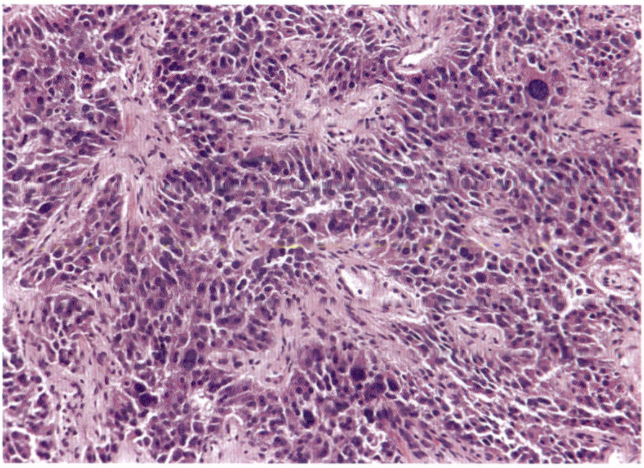

FIGURE 12.19 **Paraganglioma with eosinophilic cytoplasm and degenerative atypia.** Lesion mimics urothelial carcinoma.

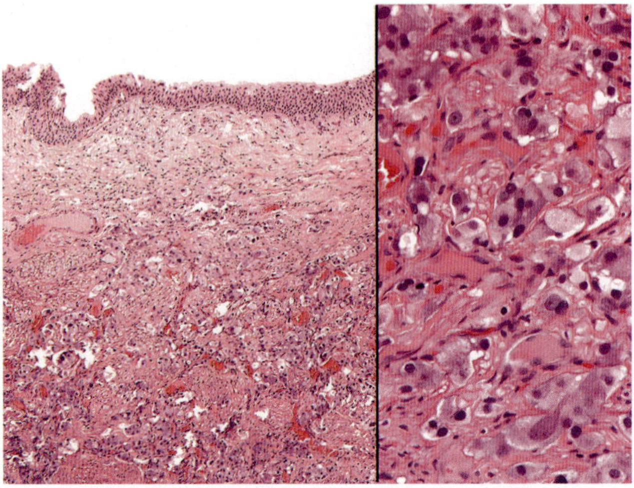

FIGURE 12.20 Paraganglioma invading beneath mucosa extending into muscularis propria (higher magnification [*right*]).

between paraganglioma and urothelial cancer is critical because of different therapeutic options and potential implications for assessment for syndromal associations.

Paragangliomas usually react with antisera to CD56, synaptophysin, and chromogranin and are negative for keratin (Fig. 12.23). Immunostains for S100 show sustentacular cells surrounding tumor nests. Cases associated with *SDH* mutations show loss of SDH protein expression.[29] Invasive urothelial carcinomas that are poorly differentiated can also show focal neuroendocrine differentiation, although striking positivity for cytokeratin will usually help resolve any diagnostic dilemma. Cases of pigmented paragangliomas within the bladder, containing melanin, have been reported.

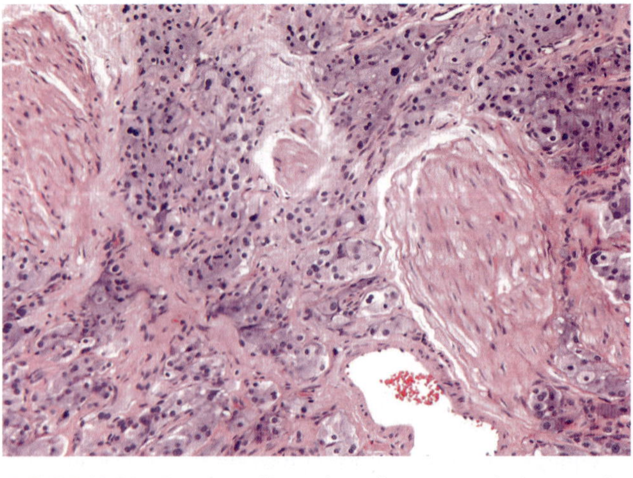

FIGURE 12.21 Paraganglioma invading muscularis propria.

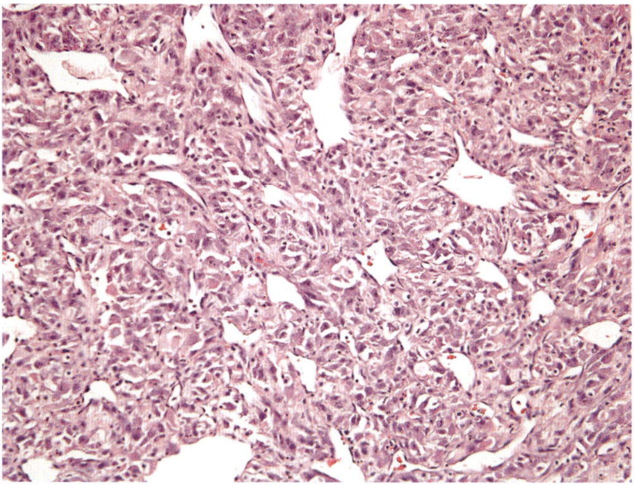

FIGURE 12.22 Invasive urothelial carcinoma with nested pattern resembling paraganglioma.

Approximately 10%-15% of paragangliomas of the bladder are malignant. There are no histologic criteria (ie, atypia, vascular invasion, size, etc.) predictive of which lesions are capable of distant spread. Only those tumors that have metastasized are diagnosed as malignant. Most local metastases are to the iliohypogastric lymph nodes with distant spread most commonly to the lung. Localized tumors are treated by TUR, wedge resection, or partial cystectomy. Treatment for malignant paraganglioma of the bladder is radical cystectomy with removal of metastases if possible. Radiation and chemotherapy appear to have limited effectiveness. Ancillary studies, such as DNA ploidy, p53 expression, and proliferation (MIB-1 labeling), do not appear predictive of clinical outcome. In one large series, a better prognosis was seen in patients with stage T1 or T2 tumors, which were able to be completely resected. Tumors with SDHB mutations have an increased association with malignancy and multiple tumors. It has been recommended that all bladder paragangliomas be tested with immunohistochemistry for SDHB to (1) identify patients at risk for additional paragangliomas in other sites; (2) identify associated syndromes, such as the Carney-Stratakis syndrome with gastric GISTs and paragangliomas; and (3) predict an increased risk of malignancy.

Paragangliomas of the bladder most likely arise from paraganglia that may uncommonly be found in the bladder neck smooth muscle[32] (eFigs. 12.23-12.26). Rarely, paraganglia may be seen on TURP or on needle biopsy where their distinction from carcinoma must be made. They consist of clusters of clear or amphophilic cells with fine cytoplasmic granules and a prominent vascular pattern, often intimately related to nerves. Nucleoli are not prominent, and if nuclear atypia is present, it is degenerative in appearance as seen in endocrine lesions. Verification of the diagnosis can be accomplished with positive immunostaining for neuroendocrine markers and for

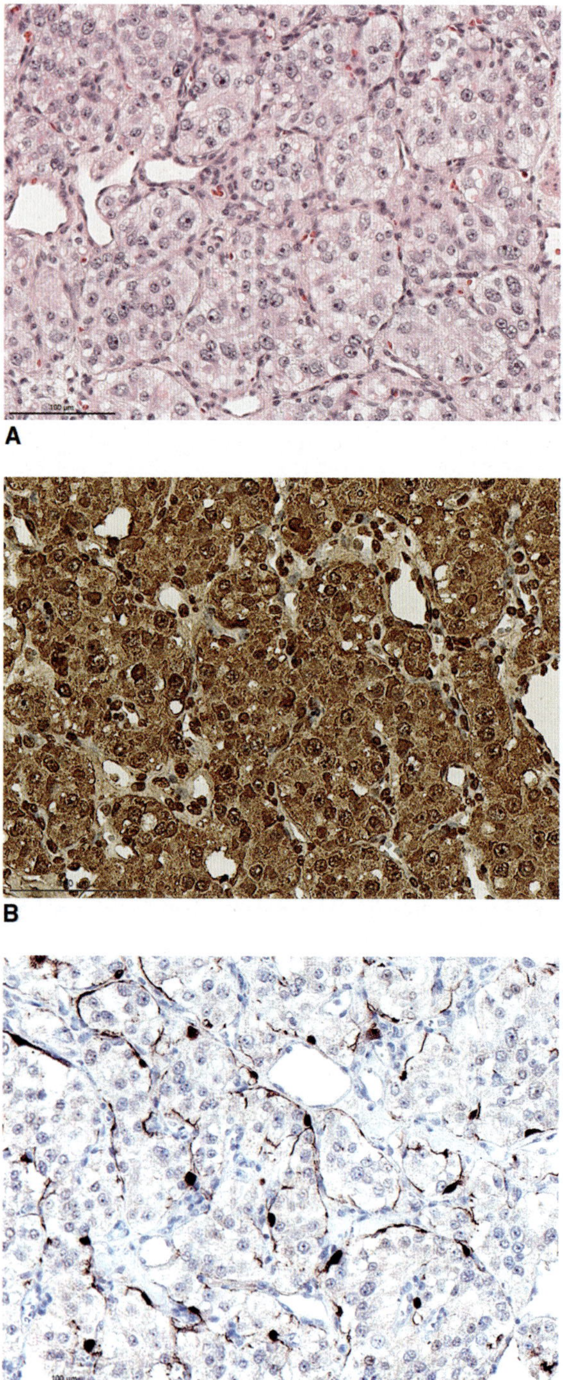

FIGURE 12.23 **Paraganglioma of the bladder mimicking urothelial carcinoma.** **A**: H&E. **B**: Diffuse and intense chromogranin immunoreactivity. **C**: S-100 highlighting sustentacular cells.

S100 in sustentacular cells. If paraganglial tissue is seen on a mucosal biopsy, the distinction between a paraganglioma and paraganglia must be made on clinical grounds, where the former are clinically apparent tumors and the latter are incidentally found lesions measuring a few millimeters.

Well-Differentiated Neuroendocrine Tumor (Carcinoid)

The term well-differentiated neuroendocrine tumor is preferred over carcinoid. Very few true cases have been described.[33-35] These tumors are thought to arise from isolated neuroendocrine cells located in the basal layer of the urothelium, which may become more numerous in reactive conditions. They do not arise or are a variant of urothelial carcinoma. They present as small polypoid masses in the bladder (neck or trigone) or in the urethra classically associated with hematuria. They exhibit the classic histologic features described at other sites, including uniform cells with basophilic cytoplasm arranged in glandular, acinar, cribriform, or trabecular arrangements. In the bladder, there is a tendency for well-differentiated neuroendocrine tumors to be small, have a prominent glandular appearance, and be associated with cystitis cystica et glandularis. In the differential diagnosis, it is important to remember that high-grade urothelial carcinomas may exhibit focal carcinoidlike or organoid growth, but in this case, one is likely to encounter an increased mitotic rate and apoptotic bodies as well as transitions to other overtly carcinomatous areas. Another important consideration in the differential diagnosis is the possibility of metastatic disease from more common sites such as the gastrointestinal tract; occasionally, an extension from a conventional acinar carcinoma of the prostate with "carcinoidlike appearance" may also enter in the differential diagnosis (Fig. 12.24).

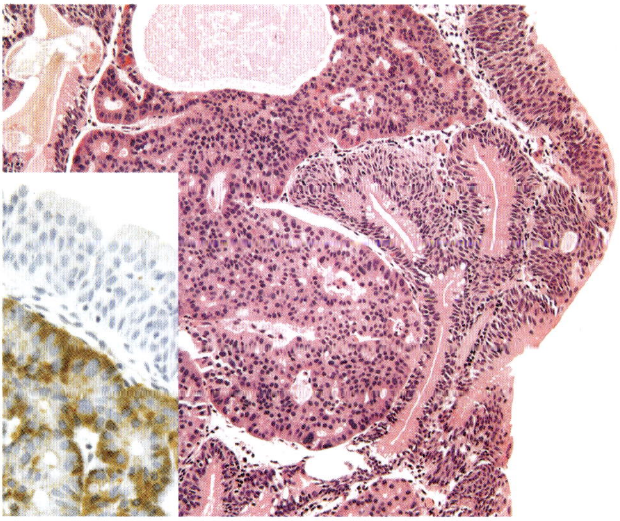

FIGURE 12.24 **Well-differentiated neuroendocrine tumor (carcinoid tumor).** (***Inset*** shows chromogranin positivity.)

Hematological Malignancies

Lymphomas involving the bladder have a female tendency with most reported cases in middle-aged women.[36-38] Tumors may be classified as (1) primary localized in the bladder, (2) presenting in the bladder as the first sign of systemic disease, and (3) recurrent in patients with a history of malignant lymphoma (secondary lymphoma). Primary lymphomas localized to the bladder are rare, accounting for only between 0.15% and 2% of all extranodal lymphomas. Most are B-cell non-Hodgkin lymphoma, with the most common subtype being MALT-type lymphoma. Lymphoepithelial lesions are found in only a minority of reported bladder MALT-type lymphomas. Lymphomas presenting in the bladder and secondary lymphomas are predominantly of large B-cell type. Other subtypes of lymphomas have been reported in the bladder, often as case reports, with follicular small cleaved being relatively more represented (Fig. 12.25, eFigs. 12.27-12.31). Patients typically present nonspecifically with hematuria and sometimes with frequency and dysuria. Urine cytology is typically not diagnostic and a tissue biopsy is required. Grossly, lymphomatous lesions of the bladder appear as solitary submucosal masses, although they may be multifocal. The urothelium is typically intact, although ulceration has been recorded. Treatment typically consists of TUR followed by chemotherapy and/or radiotherapy. Prognosis depends on the type of lymphoma present, with MALT-type lymphomas having a good prognosis with a tendency to remain localized to the bladder for a long time, with low risk of dissemination. On the other hand, diffuse large cell lymphomas have a more aggressive course. Patients with recurrent lymphoma have the worst prognosis, often measured in months, as it is a sign of widely disseminated disease resistant to therapy. When presented with an undifferentiated tumor within the bladder, the presumption may be that it is an undifferentiated carcinoma,

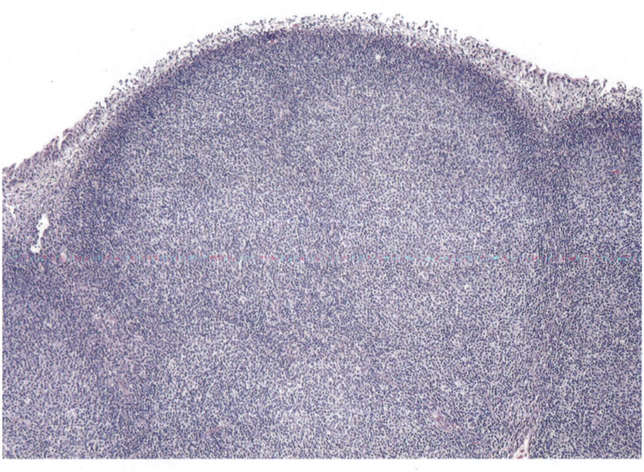

FIGURE 12.25 Malignant lymphoma, small cleaved type, follicular pattern (eFig. 12.31 shows higher magnification).

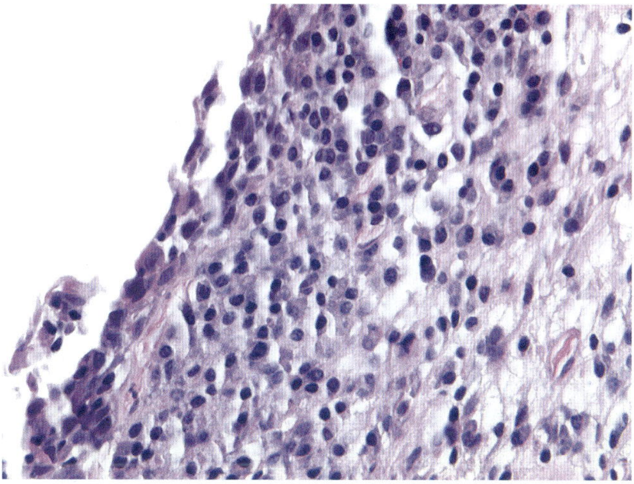

FIGURE 12.26 Plasmacytoma (eFigs. 12.32 and 12.33 show lambda light chain restriction).

given that is the overwhelming majority of bladder tumors. Immunohistochemical stains for epithelial and lymphoid markers should be performed in this setting.

The bladder is a rare site of primary plasmacytoma 39 (Fig. 12.26, eFigs. 12.32 and 12.33). Care must be taken to exclude urothelial carcinoma with plasmacytoid features (see Chapter 6). Immunohistochemical stains for keratin and kappa and lambda light chains can help resolve the differential diagnosis. CD 138 is not helpful as it stains urothelial carcinoma as well as plasma cells. The majority of patients with extramedullary plasmacytoma are adults with nonspecific symptoms of hematuria and dysuria. Although the lesions may be diffusely infiltrative, they tend to form intraluminal masses. Patients who have been treated with cystectomy have had excellent results, although typically, extramedullary plasmacytomas in other sites are treated with radiotherapy.

REFERENCES

1. Malek RS, Greene LF, Farrow GM. Amyloidosis of the urinary bladder. *Br J Urol.* 1971;43:189-200.
2. Al-Obaidy KI, Grignon DJ. Primary amyloidosis of the genitourinary tract. *Arch Pathol Lab Med.* 2021;145(6):699-703.
3. Sirohi D, Gandhi J, Amin MB, et al. Amyloidosis of the bladder and association with urothelial carcinoma: report of 29 cases. *Hum Pathol.* 2019;93:48-53.
4. Akhtar M, Valencia M, Thomas AM. Solitary primary amyloidosis of urinary bladder. Light and electron microscopic study. *Urology*. 1978;12:721-724.
5. Holub D, Flodrova P, Pika T, et al. Mass Spectrometry amyloid typing is reproducible across multiple organ sites. *Biomed Res Int.* 2019;2019:3689091.
6. Miller A. The aetiology and treatment of diverticulum of the bladder. *Br J Urol.* 1958;30:43-56.

7. Kertsschmer HL. Diverticula of the urinary bladder: a clinical study of 236 cases. *Surg Gynecol Obstet.* 1940;71:491-503.
8. Fox M, Power RF, Bruce AW. Diverticulum of the bladder: presentation and evaluation of treatment of 115 cases. *Br J Urol.* 1962;34:286-298.
9. Idrees MT, Alexander RE, Kum JB, et al. The spectrum of histopathologic findings in vesical diverticulum: implications for pathogenesis and staging. *Hum Pathol.* 2013;44:1223-1232.
10. Kong MX, Zhao X, Kheterpal E, et al. Histopathologic and clinical features of vesical diverticula. *Urology.* 2013;82:142-147.
11. Schiff M Jr, Lytton B. Congenital diverticulum of the bladder. *J Urol.* 1970;104:111-115.
12. Barrett DM, Malek RS, Kelalis PP. Observations on vesical diverticulum in childhood. *J Urol.* 1976;116:234-236.
13. Alexander RE, Kum JB, Idrees M. Bladder diverticulum: clinicopathologic spectrum in pediatric patients. *Pediatr Dev Pathol.* 2012;15:281-285.
14. Abeshouse BS. Primary carcinoma in a diverticulum of the bladder: a report of four cases and a review of the literature. *J Urol.* 1943;49:534-547.
15. Faysal MH, Freiha FS. Primary neoplasm in vesical diverticula. A report of 12 cases. *Br J Urol.* 1981;53:141-143.
16. Ward MP. Sarcoma of vesical diverticula. *Br J Urol.* 1958;30:57-59.
17. Golijanin D, Yossepowitch O, Beck SD, et al. Carcinoma in a bladder diverticulum: presentation and treatment outcome. *J Urol.* 2003;170:1761-1764.
18. Tamas EF, Stephenson AJ, Campbell SC, et al. Histopathologic features and clinical outcomes in 71 cases of bladder diverticula. *Arch Pathol Lab Med.* 2009;133:791-796.
19. Remick DG Jr, Kumar NB. Benign polyps with prostatic-type epithelium of the urethra and the urinary bladder. A suggestion of histogenesis based on histologic and immunohistochemical studies. *Am J Surg Pathol.* 1984;8:833-839.
20. Halat S, Eble JN, Grignon DJ, et al. Ectopic prostatic tissue: histogenesis and histopathological characteristics. *Histopathology.* 2011;58(5):750-758.
21. Young RH. Fibroepithelial polyp of the bladder with atypical stromal cells. *Arch Pathol Lab Med.* 1986;110:241-242.
22. Samaratunga H, Delahunt B, Yaxley J, et al. Tumour-like lesions of the urinary bladder. *Pathology.* 2021;53(1):44-55.
23. Tsuzuki T, Epstein JI. Fibroepithelial polyp of the lower urinary tract in adults. *Am J Surg Pathol.* 2005;29(4):460-466. doi:10.1097/01.pas.0000155153.64360.1a
24. Novak TE, Lakshmanan Y, Frimberger D, et al. Polyps in the exstrophic bladder. A cause for concern? *J Urol.* 2005;174:1522-1526. discussion 1526.
25. Fan R, Grignon DJ, Rhee A, et al. Exstrophy polyp is a unique pathology entity. *Pediatr Dev Pathol.* 2012;15:471-477.
26. Young RH. Tumor-like lesions of the urinary bladder. *Mod Pathol.* 2009;22(suppl 2):S37-S52. doi:10.1038/modpathol.2008.201
27. Cheng L, Leibovich BC, Cheville JC, et al. Paraganglioma of the urinary bladder: can biologic potential be predicted? *Cancer.* 2000;88:844-852.
28. Nakatani T, Hayama T, Uchida J, et al. Diagnostic localization of extra-adrenal pheochromocytoma: comparison of (123)I-MIBG imaging and (131)I-MIBG imaging. *Oncol Rep.* 2002;9:1225-1227.
29. Giubellino A, Lara K, Martucci V, et al. Urinary bladder paragangliomas: how immunohistochemistry can assist to identify patients with SDHB germline and somatic mutations. *Am J Surg Pathol.* 2015;39:1488-1492.
30. Zhou M, Epstein JI, Young RH. Paraganglioma of the urinary bladder: a lesion that may be misdiagnosed as urothelial carcinoma in transurethral resection specimens. *Am J Surg Pathol.* 2004;28:94-100.

31. Lopez-Beltran A, Cheng L. Histologic variants of urothelial carcinoma: differential diagnosis and clinical implications. *Hum Pathol.* 2006;37:1371-1388.
32. Ostrowski ML, Wheeler TM. Paraganglia of the prostate. Location, frequency, and differentiation from prostatic adenocarcinoma. *Am J Surg Pathol.* 1994;18:412-420.
33. Chen YB, Epstein JI. Primary carcinoid tumors of the urinary bladder and prostatic urethra: a clinicopathologic study of 6 cases. *Am J Surg Pathol.* 2011;35:442-446.
34. Murali R, Kneale K, Lalak N, et al. Carcinoid tumors of the urinary tract and prostate. *Arch Pathol Lab Med.* 2006;130:1693-1706.
35. Fine SW. Neuroendocrine lesions of the genitourinary tract. *Adv Anat Pathol.* 2007;14:286-296.
36. Wazait HD, Chahal R, Sundurum SK, et al. Malt-type primary lymphoma of the urinary bladder: clinicopathological study of 2 cases and review of the literature. *Urol Int.* 2001;66:220-224.
37. Kempton CL, Kurtin PJ, Inwards DJ, et al. Malignant lymphoma of the bladder: evidence from 36 cases that low-grade lymphoma of the malt-type is the most common primary bladder lymphoma. *Am J Surg Pathol.* 1997;21:1324-1333.
38. Ho DS, Patterson AL, Orozco RE, Murphy WM. Extramedullary plasmacytoma of the bladder: case report and review of the literature. *J Urol.* 1993;150:473-474.

13

SECONDARY TUMORS OF THE BLADDER

The bladder may be involved secondarily by tumors from adjacent sites such as the prostate, seminal vesicles, lower intestinal tract, and the female genital tract.[1-5] These tumors more commonly involve the bladder by direct extension and can also metastasize to the bladder. Malignant lymphoma or leukemia may also secondarily involve the bladder as part of a more disseminated or systemic manifestation (see Chapter 12). Less commonly, the bladder may be involved by metastatic tumor from distant sites (eg, melanoma, gastric, breast, ovary, and kidney). The diagnostic problems posed for the pathologist in cases of secondary involvement vary according to the morphology of the primary neoplasm.

TUMORS INVOLVING THE BLADDER PRIMARILY BY DIRECT EXTENSION

Carcinomas of the prostate, rectosigmoid, and uterine cervix account for the most common primary neoplasms involving the bladder by direct extension, although other cancers such as those from the endometrium, ovary, appendix, and other segments of the colon may rarely directly involve the bladder.[1,3,6,7]

Prostate

A common diagnostic problem is in differentiating on transurethral resection of the prostate (TURP) between a poorly differentiated urothelial carcinoma of the bladder and a poorly differentiated prostatic adenocarcinoma (Figs. 13.1-13.3, eFigs. 13.1-13.8). The therapy of these two diseases differs significantly, making the distinction between these two entities crucial. Most urothelial cancers grow in nests, whereas poorly differentiated prostate adenocarcinoma forms sheets of cells. The findings of infiltrating cords of cells or focal cribriform glandular differentiation are other features more typical of prostatic adenocarcinoma than urothelial carcinoma. Another useful differentiating feature in high-grade prostatic adenocarcinoma is a subtle attempt at cribriform gland formation. The tumor is so

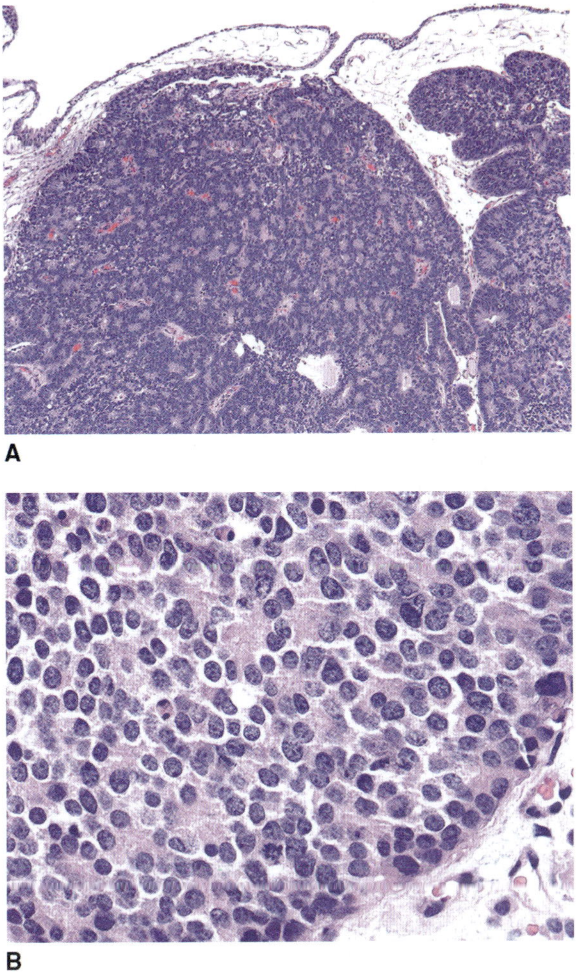

FIGURE 13.1 A: Metastatic prostate adenocarcinoma with poor cribriform glandular formation resembling rosettes undermining urothelium. B: Higher magnification of Figure 13.1A showing rosettelike structures.

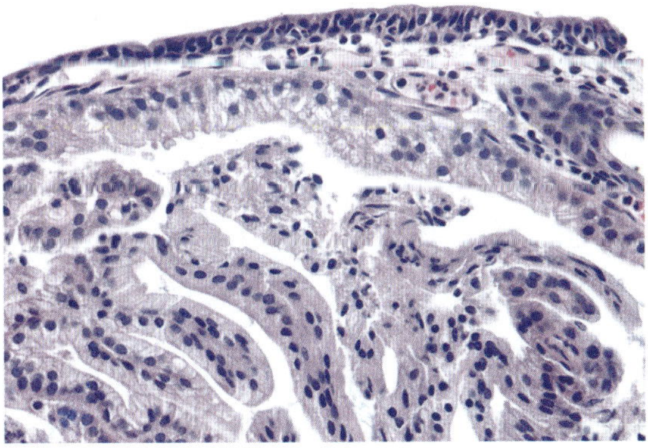

FIGURE 13.2 Metastatic prostate adenocarcinoma underneath the urothelial surface.

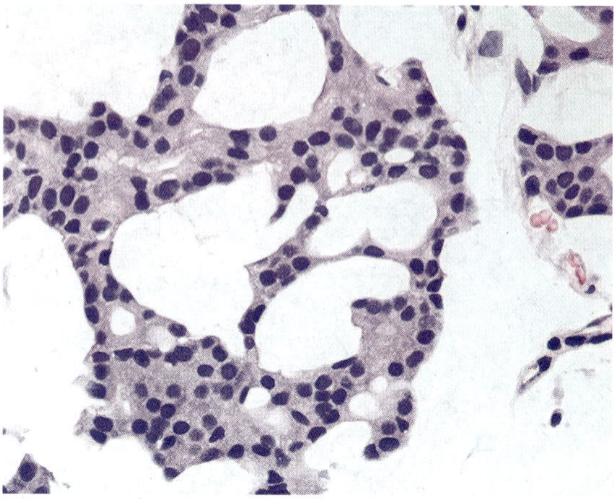

FIGURE 13.3 Metastatic prostate adenocarcinoma with mucinous features.

poorly differentiated that it cannot form true lumina, but there are rosette-like areas of cytoplasm in an attempt at glandular differentiation. Urothelial carcinoma lacks this morphology (Fig. 13.1). Cytologically, there are also several distinctions based on routine H&E-stained sections. Even in poorly differentiated prostatic adenocarcinomas, there is typically relatively little pleomorphism or mitotic activity compared to poorly differentiated urothelial carcinoma. Poorly differentiated prostate adenocarcinomas may have enlarged nuclei and prominent nucleoli; yet usually, there is little variability in nuclear shape or size from one nucleus to another (Fig. 13.4). High-grade urothelial carcinomas often reveal marked pleomorphism occasionally with tumor giant cells. A subtler finding is that the cytoplasm of prostatic adenocarcinoma is often very foamy and pale imparting a "soft" appearance. In contrast, urothelial carcinomas may demonstrate

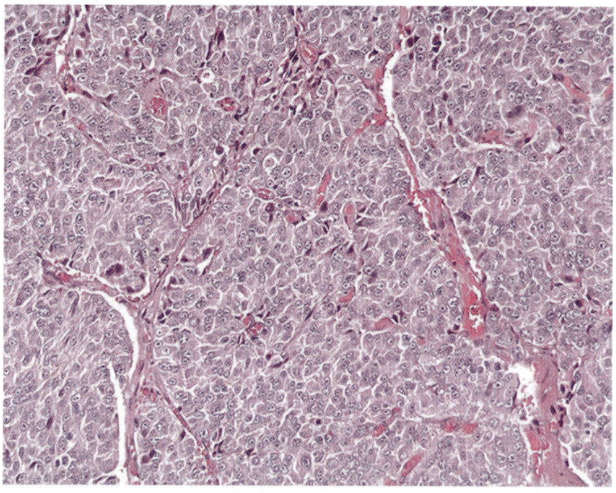

FIGURE 13.4 Poorly differentiated adenocarcinoma of the prostate lacking pleomorphism typically seen with urothelial carcinoma.

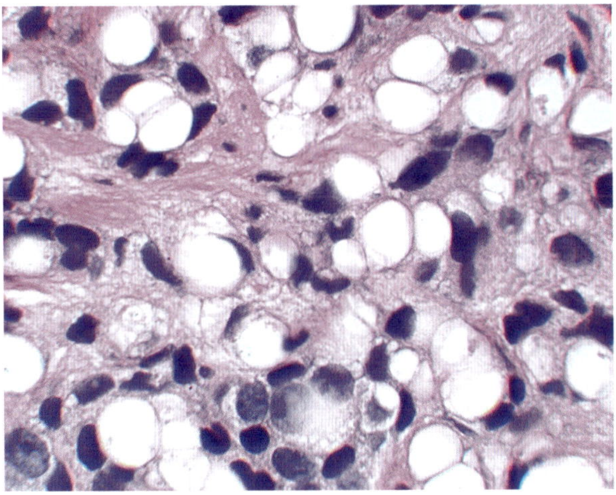

FIGURE 13.5 Metastatic prostate adenocarcinoma with signet-ring–like cell features.

hard glassy eosinophilic cytoplasm or more prominent squamous differentiation. In contrast to urothelial carcinoma with glandular differentiation, adenocarcinoma of the prostate rarely contains mucin-positive signet cells. Some carcinomas of the prostate will have a signet-ring cell appearance, yet the vacuoles appear empty and do not contain intracytoplasmic mucin (Fig. 13.5).[8] Only a few cases of prostate cancer have been reported with mucin-positive signet cells.[6,7] Despite the above distinctions, there are often cases that overlap in their morphology. Although most urothelial cancers tend to grow in nests, in some cases, there are sheets of tumor. Another pitfall is that poorly differentiated prostatic adenocarcinoma can fall apart away from its blood supply, giving rise to pseudopapillary structures closely mimicking papillary urothelial carcinoma (Fig. 13.6).[9]

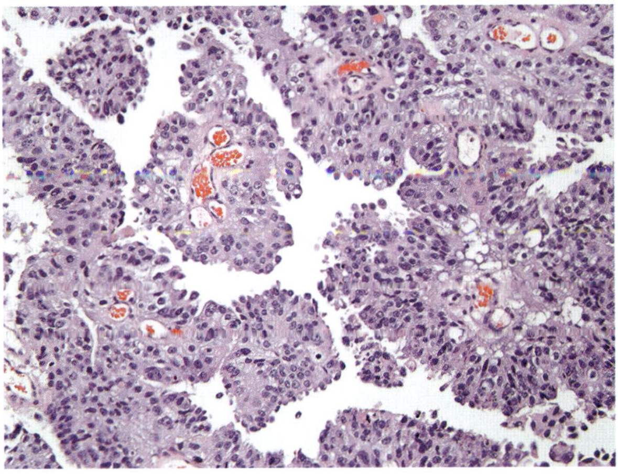

FIGURE 13.6 Pseudopapillary pattern in prostate adenocarcinoma mimicking urothelial carcinoma.

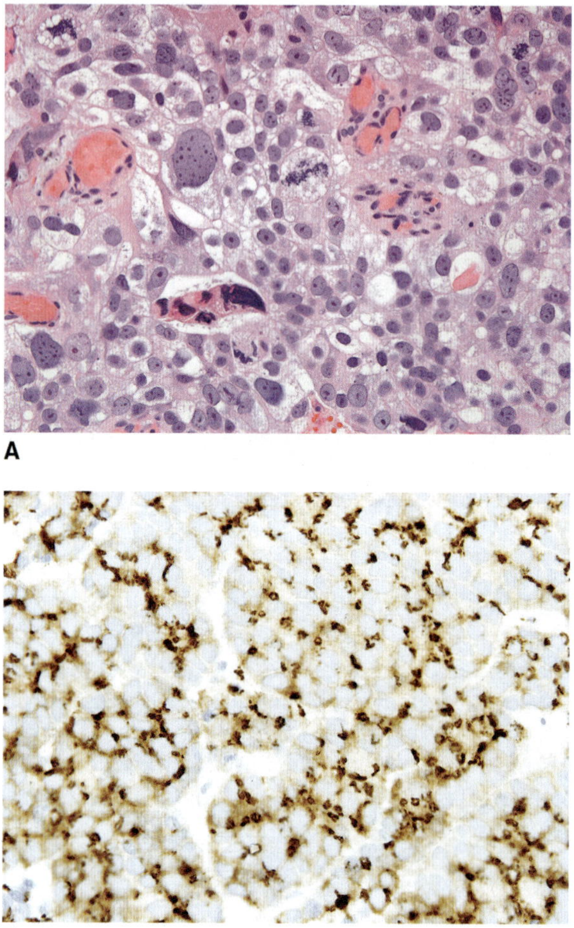

A

B

FIGURE 13.7 **A:** Poorly differentiated adenocarcinoma of the prostate with marked pleomorphism mimicking urothelial carcinoma. **B:** Tumor is positive for P501S verifying prostate origin.

Cytologically, rare cases of prostate adenocarcinoma have marked pleomorphism identical to urothelial carcinoma (Fig. 13.7).[10] Presence of concomitant urothelial carcinoma *in situ* (CIS) is helpful for proving an urothelial primary, although on very rare occasions, both urothelial and prostate cancers are seen in TURBT specimens. Almost 50% of cystoprostatectomy specimens performed for urothelial carcinoma also contain adenocarcinoma of the prostate.[11] Therefore, the finding in a TURP of a small focus of well-differentiated adenocarcinoma of the prostate should not necessarily influence whether a separate focus of poorly differentiated tumor is urothelial carcinoma or adenocarcinoma of the prostate.

Consequently, in a poorly differentiated tumor involving the bladder and prostate without any glandular differentiation typical of prostate adenocarcinoma, the case should be worked up immunohistochemically. Approximately 90% of poorly differentiated prostatic adenocarcinomas show PSA, although it may be focal, sometimes limited to isolated cells.[12-14] In the setting of a poorly differentiated carcinoma where the differential diagnosis is prostatic adenocarcinoma vs urothelial carcinoma where PSA is negative and urothelial markers (see below) are negative, then other prostate markers should be utilized. Prostate-specific membrane antigen (PSMA) and androgen receptor (AR) have high sensitivity but lower specificity and are not recommended.[15-19] The two prostate markers that are more sensitive than PSA and are just as specific are prostein (P501S) and NKX3.1.[15] P501S has the benefit of distinctive clumpy granular immunoreactivity, and NKX3.1 is a very sensitive and specific nuclear antibody.

Some of the most commonly currently used antibodies to label urothelial carcinoma are not recommended, and others lack specificity. Finally, CK7 and CK20 are of limited utility in this differential given that they may both be positive in a subset of prostatic adenocarcinoma.[20,21] High molecular weight cytokeratin and p63 are positive in approximately two-thirds of urothelial carcinoma but can be focally expressed in prostate adenocarcinoma, especially poorly differentiated prostate cancer where urothelial carcinoma is in the differential diagnosis.[15,22] Also, HMWCK labels squamous epithelia including areas of squamous differentiation in posttherapy recurrent prostate carcinoma lesions.[10] Although highly specific for urothelial differentiation, uroplakin III and the newer uroplakin II lack sensitivity in high-grade invasive urothelial carcinoma, and we have not found them to be useful in this differential diagnosis.[23,24] Thrombomodulin suffers from the same lack of sensitivity, although it is fairly specific in terms of not labeling prostate cancer.[15,25,26] The best current urothelial marker in the differential diagnosis of urothelial carcinoma vs prostate adenocarcinoma is GATA3. In the two largest studies by Liu et al.[26] and Miettinen et al.,[27] 86% and >90% of urothelial carcinomas were positive for GATA3, respectively. The nuclear staining is usually diffuse in >50% of cells. In rare cases, prostatic adenocarcinoma can be positive for GATA3.[27-29]

Finally, prostatic ductal carcinoma, prostatic carcinoma with neuroendocrine differentiation (particularly small cell carcinoma), and sarcomatoid carcinoma of prostate may also secondarily involve the prostate and raise differential diagnosis with primary enteric adenocarcinoma, small cell carcinoma, sarcomatoid urothelial carcinoma, and even sarcomas of the bladder. Identification of an acinar prostatic carcinoma component and history of prostate cancer are useful in differentiating from primary bladder malignancies.

Colorectal

Colorectal carcinoma most commonly involves the bladder by direct invasion but also by discontinuous metastases. Distinction of a colon vs a bladder primary adenocarcinoma is difficult to impossible, because colonic tumors can even involve the bladder mucosa and secondarily colonize it to

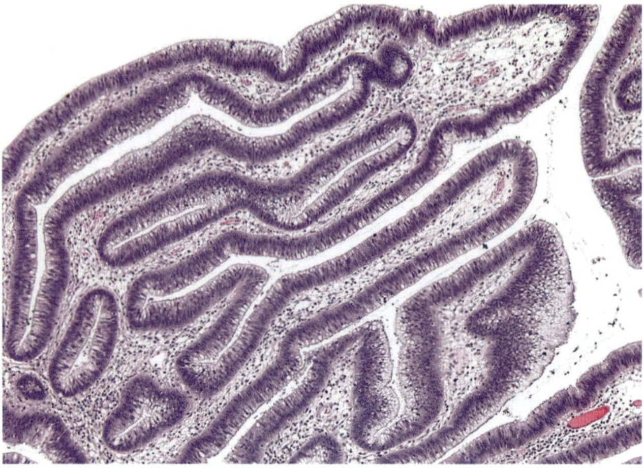

FIGURE 13.8 **Metastatic adenocarcinoma from the colon.** In areas, tumor mimics primary villous adenoma of the bladder.

create a villous architecture that would suggest a primary bladder tumor[30,31] (Figs. 13.8-13.11, eFigs. 13.9-13.19). Urothelial carcinoma with enteric differentiation may show obvious conventional urothelial carcinoma histology or urothelial CIS, which may help to establish a bladder primary. A history of high-grade, high-stage colon cancer is important, and, if present, an adenocarcinoma in the bladder with enteric histology should be considered as a metastasis. Immunohistochemical studies are not definitive as

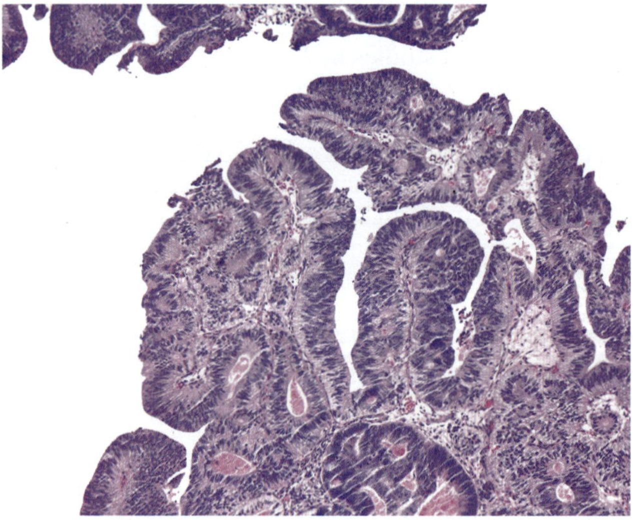

FIGURE 13.9 **Metastatic adenocarcinoma from the colon.** When tumor reaches the bladder luminal surface, it develops papillary fronds mimicking primary adenocarcinoma of the bladder.

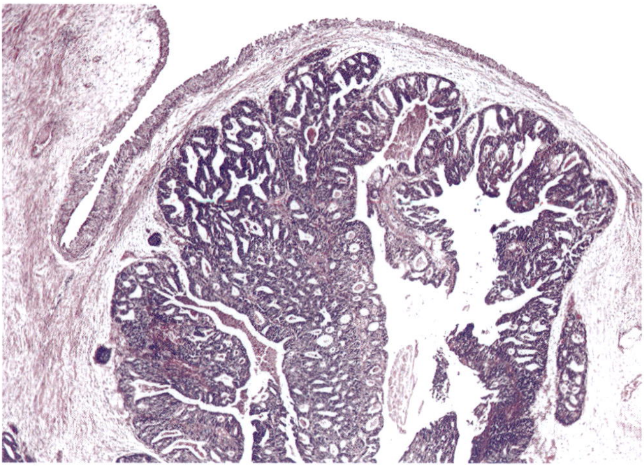

FIGURE 13.10 Metastatic adenocarcinoma from the colon undermining urothelium.

"intestinal" markers, such as CDX2, SATB2, villin, are variably expressed in adenocarcinoma of the bladder.[31-36] The one exception is that strong diffuse nuclear beta-catenin expression is highly suggestive of adenocarcinoma of the colon, as only rare cases of bladder adenocarcinoma express focal weak nuclear positivity. Most bladder adenocarcinomas express both CK7 and CK20, in contrast to typical adenocarcinoma of the colon, which is often negative for CK7.[31-33,36] GATA3 is typically not positive in enteric subtype of bladder adenocarcinoma such that it is not that useful in this differential diagnosis, and uroplakin can be positive in colorectal adenocarcinoma.[37-39] None of the immunohistochemical studies are sufficiently diagnostic to be definitive as to the source of the adenocarcinoma.

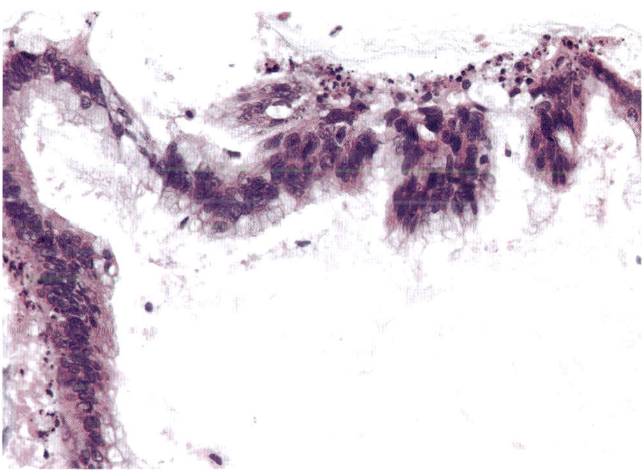

FIGURE 13.11 Metastatic adenocarcinoma from the colon (higher magnification of Fig. 13.10).

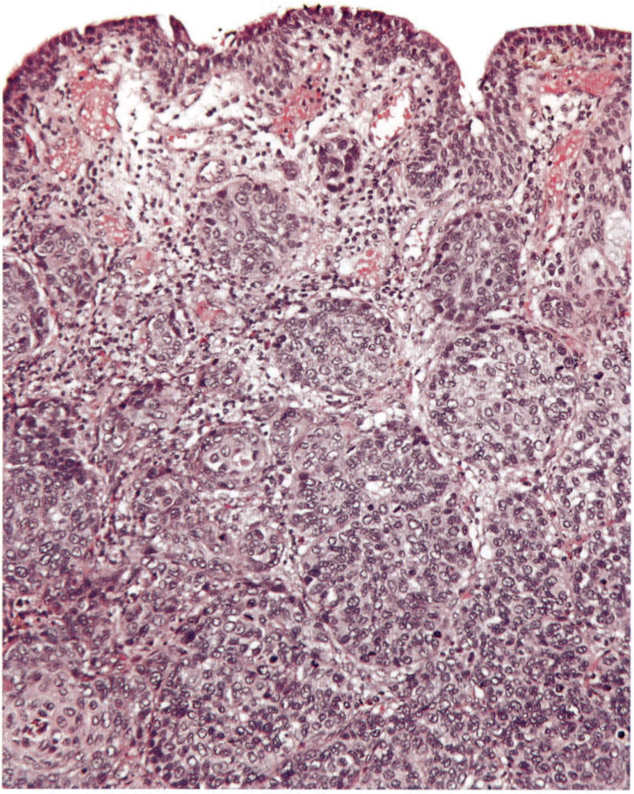

FIGURE 13.12 Uterine cervical squamous carcinoma invading the bladder.

Consequently, in the setting of an adenocarcinoma with enteric morphology involving the bladder, it is best to state: "Although this tumor may be primary in the bladder, an intestinal adenocarcinoma with spread to the bladder should be excluded on clinical grounds." The potential of subjecting a patient to radical cystectomy for colorectal cancer involving the bladder, erroneously thought to be a primary adenocarcinoma of the bladder, justifies a routine recommendation of imaging studies or colonoscopy to exclude an intestinal tumor in the setting of an adenocarcinoma with enteric morphology on bladder biopsy.

Uterine Cervix

The morphology of cervical carcinoma can mimic the often variable and nonspecific histologic appearance of urothelial carcinoma (Figs. 13.12 and 13.13). Urothelial carcinoma can appear similar to cervical squamous cell carcinoma as it can demonstrate a squamoid as well as a nested appearance. Further, cervical carcinoma involving the bladder can colonize

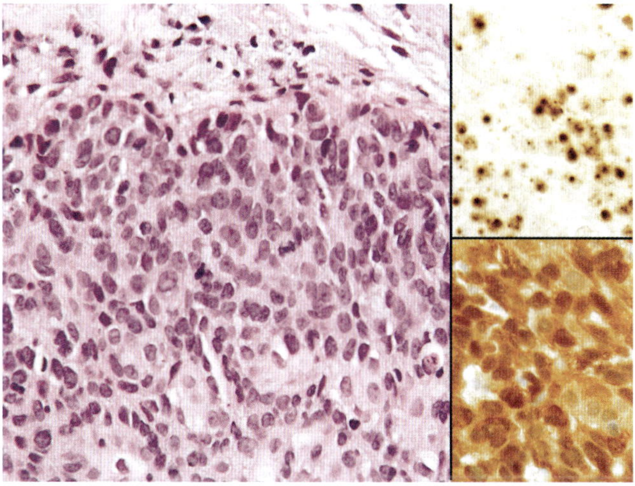

FIGURE 13.13 Uterine cervical squamous carcinoma invading the bladder. ***Upper right inset*** shows positive *in situ* hybridization for HPV16/18. ***Lower right inset*** demonstrates p16 immunoreactivity.

surface urothelium mimicking urothelial carcinoma. The lack of surface involvement and nests of tumor cells involving deep muscular tissue seen in some cervical cases invading the bladder can provide a clue that there is cervical tumor secondarily involving the bladder rather than a primary, although this histology can occasionally be seen in a primary urothelial carcinoma. Histologically, primary adenocarcinomas of the bladder typically resemble colonic (enteric-type) adenocarcinoma with larger glands containing markedly atypical elongated and stratified nuclei or show signet-ring cell differentiation. When adenocarcinomas within the bladder are composed of small glands with usually one cell layer of cuboidal cells often with relatively bland cytology, secondary involvement of the bladder by a pancreaticobiliary or endocervical primary should be excluded clinically. Gynecologic clinical history is critical to the evaluation of these specimens; however, this is often lacking, and patients may present solely with urinary symptoms.[13] Uterine cervical carcinoma is typically negative for GATA3, but a minority can show variable staining.[27,40,41] Furthermore, GATA3 is of limited diagnostic utility in bladder adenocarcinomas, as it only rarely shows nuclear positivity.[37] More recent studies specifically evaluating primary bladder squamous cell carcinoma and primary bladder adenocarcinoma for HPV are few but suggest that HPV plays no significant role in the development of these types of carcinoma in the bladder, with the exception of a few case reports (see Chapter 9). *In situ* hybridization for high-risk HPV is positive in the majority of cases of cervical carcinoma. However, a minority can be negative, highlighting the variable sensitivity reported with HPV ISH and illustrating that negative HPV ISH does not definitively rule out cervical origin of a tumor. p16 overexpression and

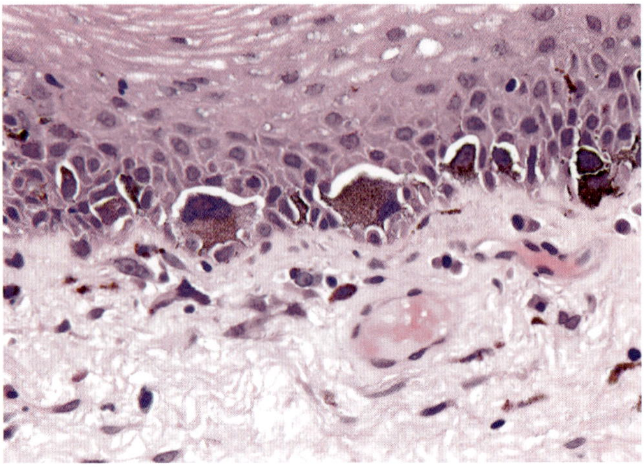

FIGURE 13.14 Melanoma involving urothelial trigonal mucosa extending from vaginal primary.

positive p16 immunohistochemical staining in primary bladder neoplasms, including urothelial carcinoma with squamous differentiation, primary bladder squamous cell carcinoma, and primary bladder adenocarcinoma, demonstrate that p16 in general does not act as a surrogate marker for HPV infection and does not rule out a bladder primary (reviewed in Ref.[40]). The critical nature of differentiating cervical carcinoma involving the genitourinary tract from primary neoplasms of the genitourinary tract cannot be emphasized enough as the treatment of these two clinical situations is extremely different.

METASTASES TO THE BLADDER

Of malignancies arising from distant sites, melanomas appear to be the most common (Fig. 13.14).[3] In particular, it could be difficult to distinguish urothelial carcinomas with plasmacytoid histology, rhabdoid or large cell undifferentiated carcinomas of the bladder from melanoma (eFigs. 13.20-13.23). Other relatively common sites include the breast (see below), stomach, lung, and kidney (Figs. 13.15-13.17),[1,3,42-48] Signet-ring cell adenocarcinomas of the bladder can be GATA3 positive, which may suggest a bladder primary.[37] Rare examples of other primary sites with tumors metastatic to the bladder are the pancreas, testis, gallbladder, liver, ovary, uterus including endometrial stromal sarcoma, skin, appendix, and tongue (Figs. 13.18 and 13.19).[1,3,4,49-53] In general, a metastasis should be suspected when there is an absence of a mucosal abnormality (urothelial or glandular CIS or a mucosal based mass), frequent vascular invasion, involvement of muscularis propria only, or a histology not conforming to the commonly encountered histologic patterns of bladder cancer. In these cases, it is important to determine the pattern of involvement (whether a tumor

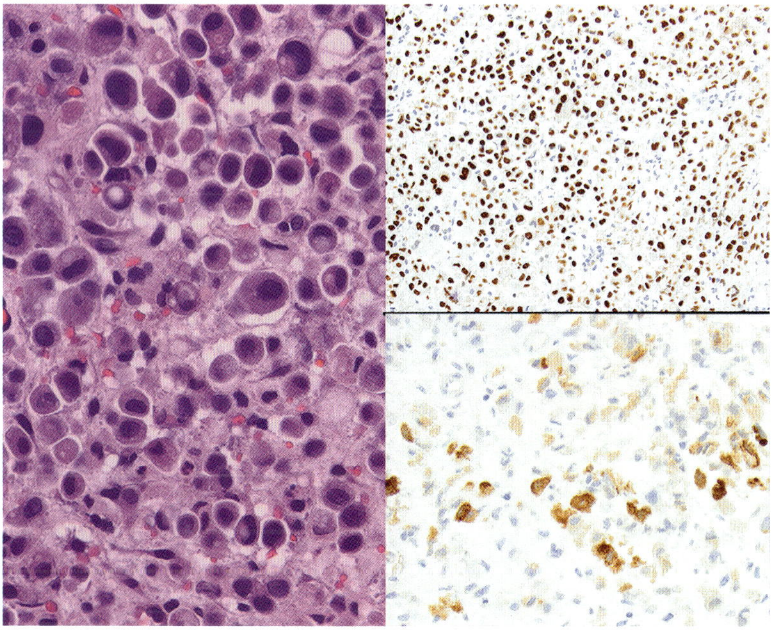

FIGURE 13.15 Metastatic adenocarcinoma from the breast (*upper right* inset shows positive ER staining; *lower right* inset shows positivity for GCDFP-15).

involves the bladder from "outside in") and correlate findings with imaging studies and clinicopathologic findings.

Breast

It is critical to recognize metastatic breast carcinoma to the bladder, given the implications for therapy.[42,54] Breast cancer should be a consideration for tumors with a signet-ring cell or plasmacytoid morphology, cases composed of individual tumor cells resembling lobular carcinoma, or micropapillary carcinoma (Fig. 13.15, eFigs. 13.24 and 13.25). There is significant histological and immunohistochemical overlap with plasmacytoid urothelial carci-

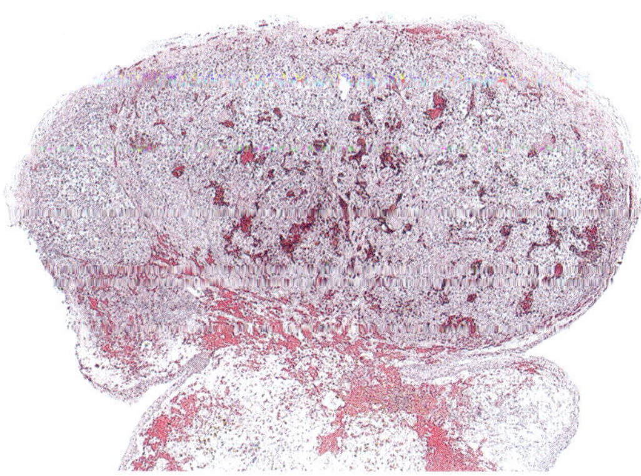

FIGURE 13.16 Metastatic clear cell renal cell carcinoma.

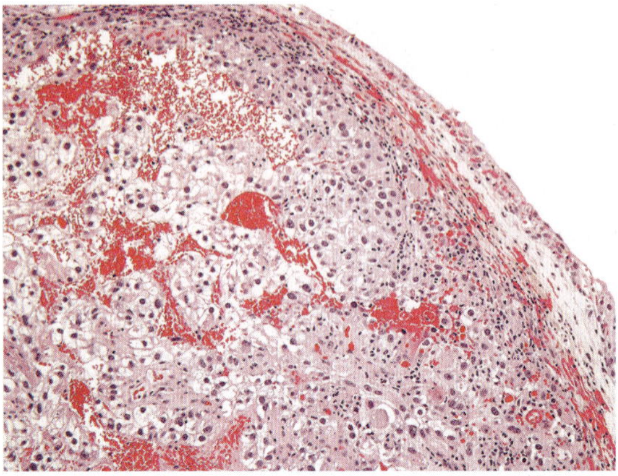

FIGURE 13.17 Metastatic clear cell renal cell carcinoma (higher magnification of Fig. 13.16).

noma and pleomorphic lobular carcinoma metastatic to bladder, including loss of e-cadherin expression. The history of breast cancer can be remote. ER, mammaglobin, and TRPS1 appear to be preferentially expressed in pleomorphic lobular carcinoma but not plasmacytoid urothelial cancer. GATA3, GCDFP-15, PR, HMWK, keratin 5/6, and AR have overlapping patterns of staining and cannot assist in differential diagnosis.

Carcinoma With Micropapillary Histology Involving the Bladder

Carcinomas with micropapillary morphology can occur in the bladder, breast, pancreas, ovary, salivary glands, and lung.[55] These tumors will commonly overexpress Her-2, limiting its clinical utility. The best markers to identify infiltrating micropapillary urothelial carcinoma are uroplakin 2

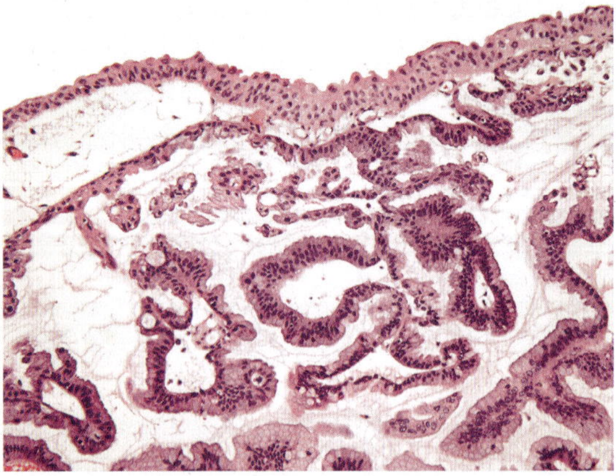

FIGURE 13.18 Metastatic pancreatic adenocarcinoma.

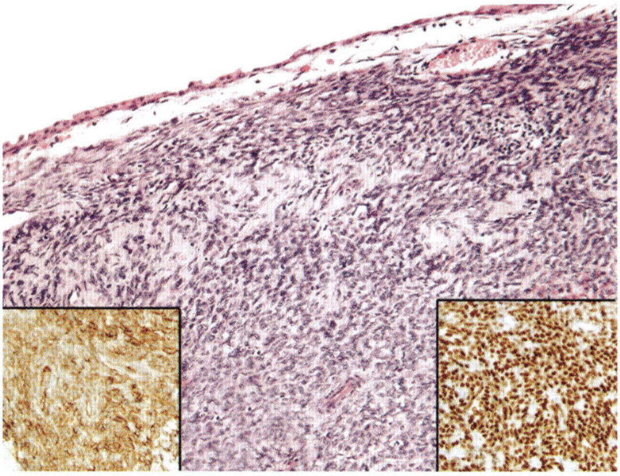

FIGURE 13.19 Metastatic endometrial stromal sarcoma positive for estrogen receptor (*lower right inset*) and CD10 (*lower left inset*).

and CK20, while p63 and thrombomodulin are less sensitive and specific (Table 13.1).[24,56] Breast infiltrating micropapillary carcinomas are ER, GATA3, and mammaglobin positive and PAX8/WT-1 negative, while ovarian micropapillary carcinomas are ER positive and PAX8/WT-1 positive. The vast majority of lung micropapillary carcinomas are uniformly TTF-1 positive. When invasive micropapillary carcinoma occurs in the bladder without an associated *in situ* or conventional urothelial carcinoma component, the above panel should be performed to establish the origin of the tumor. Clinicopathologic correlation is also critical.

Carcinomas With Clear Cell Morphology

It is critical to recognize that urothelial carcinoma can have strikingly clear cytoplasm (see Chapter 6). Metastatic clear cell renal cell carcinoma typically has a prominent vascular pattern and if necessary can be evaluated immunohistochemically with antibodies to RCC and PAX8 (Figs. 13.14 and 13.15).[45]

TABLE 13.1 Recommended Immunohistochemistry Panel for Micropapillary Carcinomas

	Uroplakins II and III	CK20	TTF-1	ER	WT-1	PAX8	Mammaglobin
Bladder	~80%	54%	0%	0%	0%	0%	0%
Breast	0%	0%	0%	88%	0%	0%	56%
Lung	0%	17%	100%	17%	0%	0%	0%
Ovary	0%	0%	0%	92%	91%	100%	0%

CK, cytokeratin; ER, estrogen receptor.

Clear cell adenocarcinoma of the bladder or urethra is histologically indistinguishable from the same tumor found in the ovary (see Chapter 8). In some cases, clear cell adenocarcinoma of the bladder is accompanied by urothelial carcinoma, which indicates a bladder primary.[57] Otherwise, clinical correlation is required. On occasion, prostate cancer may have a prominent clear to foamy appearance.

Small Cell Carcinoma Involving the Bladder

Small cell carcinoma of the bladder is identical to small cell carcinoma from other sites, such as the lung. In up to 40%-50% of bladder small cell carcinomas, identification of CIS or invasive urothelial carcinoma will help verify that the small cell cancer is primary to the bladder. If at the time of diagnosis of small cell carcinoma involving the bladder, tumor appears localized to the bladder, it unlikely represents spread from an occult pulmonary primary. Approximately 40% of primary bladder small cell carcinomas are positive for TTF-1.[58] Another differential diagnosis is with small cell carcinoma of the prostate secondarily involving the bladder. Clinical history of prostate cancer, presence of conventional prostate cancer, and ERG detection by FISH (and not immunohistochemistry) are very helpful in this differential.[59] However, systemic treatment for small cell carcinoma, whether arising in the bladder or prostate, is similar, although cystectomy would not be indicated if it is metastatic to the bladder.

REFERENCES

1. Klinger ME. Secondary tumors of the genito-urinary tract. *J Urol.* 1951;65:144-153.
2. Melicow MM. Tumors of the urinary bladder: a clinico-pathological analysis of over 2500 specimens and biopsies. *J Urol.* 1955;74:498-521.
3. Velcheti V, Govindan R. Metastatic cancer involving bladder: a review. *Can J Urol.* 2007;14:3443-3448.
4. Young RH, Johnston WH. Serous adenocarcinoma of the uterus metastatic to the urinary bladder mimicking primary bladder neoplasia. A report of a case. *Am J Surg Pathol.* 1990;14:877-880.
5. Xiao GQ, Chow J, Unger PD. Metastatic tumors to the urinary bladder: clinicopathologic study of 11 cases. *Int J Surg Pathol.* 2012;20:342-348.
6. Uchijima Y, Ito H, Takahashi M, et al. Prostate mucinous adenocarcinoma with signet ring cell. *Urology.* 1990;36:267-268.
7. Hejka AG, England DM. Signet ring cell carcinoma of prostate. Immunohistochemical and ultrastructural study of a case. *Urology.* 1989;34:155-158.
8. Ro JY, el-Naggar A, Ayala AG, et al. Signet-ring-cell carcinoma of the prostate. Electron-microscopic and immunohistochemical studies of eight cases. *Am J Surg Pathol.* 1988;12:453-460.
9. Gordetsky J, Epstein JI. Pseudopapillary features in prostatic adenocarcinoma mimicking urothelial carcinoma: a diagnostic pitfall. *Am J Surg Pathol.* 2014;38:941-945.
10. Parwani AV, Herawi M, Epstein JI. Pleomorphic giant cell adenocarcinoma of the prostate: report of 6 cases. *Am J Surg Pathol.* 2006;30:1254-1259.
11. Schellhammer PF, Bean MA, Whitmore WF Jr. Prostatic involvement by transitional cell carcinoma: pathogenesis, patterns and prognosis. *J Urol.* 1977;118:399-403.

12. Ellis DW, Leffers S, Davies JS, et al. Multiple immunoperoxidase markers in benign hyperplasia and adenocarcinoma of the prostate. *Am J Clin Pathol.* 1984;81:279-284.
13. Ford TF, Butcher DN, Masters JR, et al. Immunocytochemical localisation of prostate-specific antigen: specificity and application to clinical practice. *Br J Urol.* 1985;57:50-55.
14. Svanholm H. Evaluation of commercial immunoperoxidase kits for prostatic specific antigen and prostatic specific acid phosphatase. *Acta Pathol Microbiol Immunol Scand A.* 1986;94:7-12.
15. Chuang AY, DeMarzo AM, Veltri RW, et al. Immunohistochemical differentiation of high-grade prostate carcinoma from urothelial carcinoma. *Am J Surg Pathol.* 2007;31: 1246-1255.
16. Downes MR, Torlakovic EE, Aldaoud N, et al. Diagnostic utility of androgen receptor expression in discriminating poorly differentiated urothelial and prostate carcinoma. *J Clin Pathol.* 2013;66:779-786.
17. Miyamoto H, Yao JL, Chaux A, et al. Expression of androgen and oestrogen receptors and its prognostic significance in urothelial neoplasm of the urinary bladder. *BJU Int.* 2012;109:1716-1726.
18. Mohanty SK, Smith SC, Chang E, et al. Evaluation of contemporary prostate and urothelial lineage biomarkers in a consecutive cohort of poorly differentiated bladder neck carcinomas. *Am J Clin Pathol.* 2014;142:173-183.
19. Epstein JI, Egevad L, Humphrey PA; Members of the ISUP Immunohistochemistry in diagnostic urologic pathology group, et al. Best practices recommendations in the application of immunohistochemistry in the prostate: report from the International Society of Urologic Pathology consensus conference. *Am J Surg Pathol.* 2014;38:e6-e19.
20. Genega EM, Hutchinson B, Reuter VE, et al. Immunophenotype of high-grade prostatic adenocarcinoma and urothelial carcinoma. *Mod Pathol.* 2000;13:1186-1191.
21. Mhawech P, Uchida T, Pelte MF. Immunohistochemical profile of high-grade urothelial bladder carcinoma and prostate adenocarcinoma. *Hum Pathol.* 2002;33:1136-1140.
22. Varma M, Morgan M, Amin MB, et al. High molecular weight cytokeratin antibody (clone 34betaE12): a sensitive marker for differentiation of high-grade invasive urothelial carcinoma from prostate cancer. *Histopathology.* 2003;42:167-172.
23. Logani S, Oliva E, Amin MB, et al. Immunoprofile of ovarian tumors with putative transitional cell (urothelial) differentiation using novel urothelial markers: histogenetic and diagnostic implications. *Am J Surg Pathol.* 2003;27:1434-1441.
24. Smith SC, Mohanty SK, Kunju LP, et al. Uroplakin II outperforms uroplakin III in diagnostically challenging settings. *Histopathology.* 2014;65:132-138.
25. Parker DC, Folpe AL, Bell J, et al. Potential utility of uroplakin III, thrombomodulin, high molecular weight cytokeratin, and cytokeratin 20 in noninvasive, invasive, and metastatic urothelial (transitional cell) carcinomas. *Am J Surg Pathol.* 2003;27:1-10.
26. Liu H, Shi J, Wilkerson ML, Lin F. Immunohistochemical evaluation of GATA3 expression in tumors and normal tissues: a useful immunomarker for breast and urothelial carcinoma. *Am J Clin Pathol.* 2012;138:57-64.
27. Miettinen M, McCue PA, Sarlomo-Rikala M, et al. GATA3: a multispecific but potentially useful marker in surgical pathology: a systematic analysis of 2500 epithelial and nonepithelial tumors. *Am J Surg Pathol.* 2014;38(1):13-22.
28. McDonald TM, Epstein JI. Aberrant GATA3 Staining in prostatic adenocarcinoma: a potential diagnostic pitfall. *Am J Surg Pathol.* 2021;45(3):341-346
29. Chang A, Amin A, Gabrielson E, et al. Utility of GATA3 immunohistochemistry in differentiating urothelial carcinoma from prostate adenocarcinoma and squamous cell carcinomas of the uterine cervix, anus, and lung. *Am J Surg Pathol.* 2012;36:1472-1476.
30. Silver SA, Epstein JI. Adenocarcinoma of the colon simulating primary urinary bladder neoplasia. A report of nine cases. *Am J Surg Pathol.* 1993;17:171-178.

31. Tamboli P, Mohsin SK, Hailemariam S, et al. Colonic adenocarcinoma metastatic to the urinary tract versus primary tumors of the urinary tract with glandular differentiation: a report of 7 cases and investigation using a limited immunohistochemical panel. *Arch Pathol Lab Med.* 2002;126:1057-1063.
32. Thomas AA, Stephenson AJ, Campbell SC, et al. Clinicopathologic features and utility of immunohistochemical markers in signet-ring cell adenocarcinoma of the bladder. *Hum Pathol.* 2009;40(1):108-116.
33. Raspollini MR, Nesi G, Baroni G, et al. Immunohistochemistry in the differential diagnosis between primary and secondary intestinal adenocarcinoma of the urinary bladder. *Appl Immunohistochem Mol Morphol.* 2005;13:358-362.
34. Suh N, Yang XJ, Tretiakova MS, et al. Value of CDX2, villin, and alpha-methylacyl coenzyme A racemase immunostains in the distinction between primary adenocarcinoma of the bladder and secondary colorectal adenocarcinoma. *Mod Pathol.* 2005;18:1217-1222.
35. Werling RW, Yaziji H, Bacchi CE, et al. CDX2, a highly sensitive and specific marker of adenocarcinomas of intestinal origin: an immunohistochemical survey of 476 primary and metastatic carcinomas. *Am J Surg Pathol.* 2003;27:303-310.
36. Wang HL, Lu DW, Yerian LM, et al. Immunohistochemical distinction between primary adenocarcinoma of the bladder and secondary colorectal adenocarcinoma. *Am J Surg Pathol.* 2001;25:1380-1387.
37. Ellis CL, Chang AG, Cimino-Mathews A, et al. GATA-3 immunohistochemistry in the differential diagnosis of adenocarcinoma of the urinary bladder. *Am J Surg Pathol.* 2013;37:1756-1760.
38. Amin MB, Trpkov K, Lopez-Beltran A; Members of the ISUP Immunohistochemistry in Diagnostic Urologic Pathology Group, et al. Best practices recommendations in the application of immunohistochemistry in the bladder lesions: report from the International Society of Urologic Pathology consensus conference. *Am J Surg Pathol.* 2014;38:e20-e34.
39. Klopfer K, Delahunt B, Adamson M, et al. Value of uroplakin III in distinguishing variants of primary bladder urothelial carcinoma from malignancy metastatic to the urinary bladder. *Anticancer Res.* 2014;34:6779-6784.
40. Schwartz LE, Khani F, Bishop JA, et al. Carcinoma of the uterine cervix involving the genitourinary tract: a potential diagnostic dilemma. *Am J Surg Pathol.* 2016;40(1):27-35.
41. Zhao L, Antic T, Witten D, et al. Is GATA3 expression maintained in regional metastases?: a study of paired primary and metastatic urothelial carcinomas. *Am J Surg Pathol.* 2013;37:1876-1881.
42. Silverstein LI, Plaine L, Davis JE, et al. Breast carcinoma metastatic to bladder. *Urology.* 1987;29:544-547.
43. van Driel MF, Ypma AF, van Gelder B. Gastric carcinoma metastatic to the bladder. *Br J Urol.* 1987;59:193-194.
44. Coltart RS, Stewart S, Brown CH. Small cell carcinoma of the bronchus: a rare cause of haematuria from a metastasis in the urinary bladder. *J R Soc Med.* 1985;78:1053-1054.
45. Zhang M, Wah C, Epstein JI. Metastatic renal cell carcinoma to the urinary bladder: a report of 11 cases. *Am J Surg Pathol.* 2014;38:1516-1521.
46. Raymond KW, Hin TS, Fai KC, et al. Urinary bladder metastasis from lung adenocarcinoma: a rare cause of hematuria. *Urol Ann.* 2014;6:359-362.
47. Vigliar E, Marino G, Matano E, et al. Signet-ring-cell carcinoma of stomach metastatic to the bladder: a case report with cytological and histological correlation and literature review. *Int J Surg Pathol.* 2013;21:72-75.
48. Matsumoto K, Hayakawa N, Nakamura S, et al. Bladder metastasis from renal cell carcinoma: retrospective analysis of 65 reported cases. *Clin Exp Metastasis.* 2015;32:135-141.
49. Chalbaud RA, Johnson DE. Adenocarcinoma of tongue metastatic to bladder. *Urology.* 1974;4:454-455.

50. Chung SD, Ho CH, Hung SF, et al. Metastatic hepatocellular carcinoma in the urinary bladder with radiation-induced hemorrhagic cystitis. *J Formos Med Assoc.* 2007; 106:861-863.
51. Henry R, Bracken RB, Ayala A. Appendiceal carcinoma mimicking primary bladder cancer. *J Urol.* 1980;123:590-591.
52. Strasser H, Amann K, Schrott KM, et al. Solitary metastasis of a Merkel cell tumor to the urinary bladder. *Anticancer Res.* 2008;28:1361-1364.
53. Tian W, Latour M, Epstein JI. Endometrial stromal sarcoma involving the urinary bladder: a study of 6 cases. *Am J Surg Pathol.* 2014;38:982-989.
54. Zhang G, Susnik B, Paulsen EJ, et al. Metastatic pleomorphic lobular carcinoma of the breast to the urinary bladder: a report of 10 cases. *Am J Surg Pathol* (in press).
55. Ramalingam P, Middleton LP, Tamboli P, et al. Invasive micropapillary carcinoma of the breast metastatic to the urinary bladder and endometrium: diagnostic pitfalls and review of the literature of tumors with micropapillary features. *Ann Diagn Pathol.* 2003;7: 112-119.
56. Lotan TL, Ye H, Shih IM, et al. Immunohistochemical panel to distinguish micropapillary urothelial carcinoma from breast, lung and ovarian micropapillary carcinomas. *Am J Surg Pathol.* 2009;33:1037-1041.
57. Oliva E, Amin MB, Jimenez R, et al. Clear cell carcinoma of the urinary bladder: a report and comparison of four tumors of mullerian origin and nine of probable urothelial origin with discussion of histogenesis and diagnostic problems. *Am J Surg Pathol.* 2002;26:190-197.
58. Jones TD, Kernek KM, Yang XJ, et al. Thyroid transcription factor 1 expression in small cell carcinoma of the urinary bladder: an immunohistochemical profile of 44 cases. *Hum Pathol.* 2005;36:718-723.
59. Lotan TL, Gupta NS, Wang W, et al. ERG gene rearrangements are common in prostatic small cell carcinomas. *Mod Pathol.* 2011;24:820-828.

14

BIOPSY OF THE RENAL PELVIS AND URETER

Urothelial lesions of the renal pelvis and upper ureter are infrequent, accounting for ~5% of urothelial malignancies and 10% of renal tumors diagnosed every year in the United States.[1] The spectrum of urothelial pathology in the renal pelvis and ureter is similar to that seen in the bladder, and these lesions are often associated with bladder lesions of the same grade.[2] Tumors of the upper urothelial tract may present *de novo* or following a bladder primary. Up to 40% of upper tract urothelial tumors will recur along the lower urinary tract, particularly the bladder.

VARIANTS/SUBTYPES

In a large SEER registry study, of 11 809 upper urinary tract tumors, 97.3% were urothelial carcinoma, 1.3% squamous cell carcinoma, 0.7% adenocarcinoma, 0.3% neuroendocrine carcinoma, and 0.3% other variants of urothelial carcinoma, now called subtypes (previous histologic variants and urothelial carcinoma with divergent differentiation) in the latest edition of the WHO classification of tumors. A caveat is that the SEER data have no centralized pathology review.[3] In a more detailed pathological study of 39 patients with histological "variants" in the upper tract, squamous divergent differentiation was the most common morphology (20%) followed by sarcomatoid (18%), glandular (15%), clear cell (13%), lipid rich (10%), micropapillary (10%), inverted growth (10%), and diffuse plasmacytoid (8%) with some cases having more than one variant pattern.[4] Nested, giant cell, lymphoepitheliomalike, small cell, trophoblastic, rhabdoid, microcystic, lymphoid-rich stroma, or myxoid stroma/chordoid were other morphologies noted (Fig. 14.1, eFig. 14.1). Only 5/39 (13%) of the cases had pure variant/subtype histology (sarcomatoid [n = 1], inverted growth [n = 3]; lymphoid-rich stroma [n = 1]). Variant (subtype/divergent differentiation) histology was typically seen in patients with high pathological stage (pT2-pT4) (82%) with lower survival rate (median survival 31 months). Similar findings were reported in a systematic review and meta-analysis.[5] However, it is important to recognize that the overall poor prognosis of histologic subtypes is driven only by some of the variants that are more aggressive (ie, micropapillary, high-grade neuroendocrine, sarcomatoid,

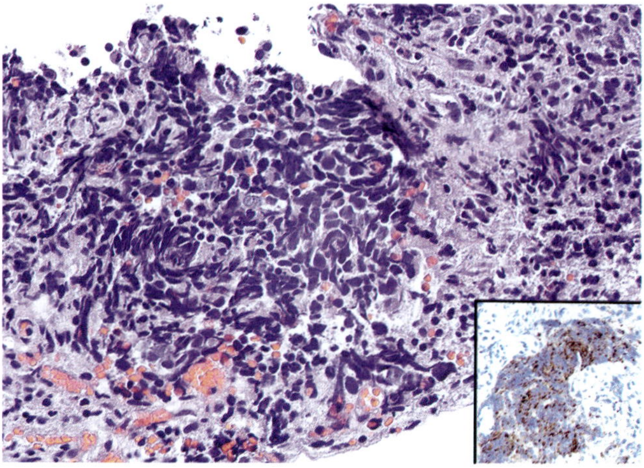

FIGURE 14.1 **Biopsy of small cell carcinoma from the renal pelvis.** *Inset* shows positive chromogranin. Immunostains for cytokeratin, CD56, and synaptophysin were also positive.

rhabdoid, and micropapillary), whereas the other variants do not impact prognosis. As expected, the aggressive subtypes tend to present with locally advanced disease. Whether decreased survival is due to advanced stage or histology remains controversial, but response to systemic therapy is similar for all subtypes. One of the variants with a predilection for the renal pelvis and proximal ureter is undifferentiated urothelial carcinoma with osteoclastic giant cells.[6]

A few separate larger studies on specific variants/subtypes have also been reported. In a large series of 18 cases of micropapillary urothelial carcinoma of the upper tract, the majority (72%) of patients had ≥pT3 disease at the time of resection.[7] Cancer-specific and recurrence-free survivals were 3.29 and 1.69 years, respectively. There was no survival difference between conventional upper tract urothelial carcinoma and micropapillary urothelial carcinoma when matched for age, stage, grade, lymphovascular invasion, and margins. None of the patients with micropapillary urothelial carcinoma receiving neoadjuvant and adjuvant chemotherapy had apparent pathologic downstaging, and of those receiving adjuvant chemotherapy, two-thirds died of disease within 2 years. In a separate study of 10 cases of lymphoepithelial-like urothelial carcinomas (LELC) of the upper tract, survival analysis showed no differences between LELC and conventional upper urinary tract urothelial carcinoma, with pathological stage being the only significant prognostic parameter.[8] Microscopically, all tumors contained pure ($n = 3$) or predominant ($n = 7$) LELC, which composed 60%–80% of the entire tumor. A series of 23 cases with squamous differentiation in upper tract urothelial carcinoma showed that the presence of squamous differentiation was significantly associated with a worse prognosis, but in multivariate analyses, squamous differentiation was not significantly associated with patient outcomes.[9]

NEPHROURETERECTOMY OR URETERECTOMY WITHOUT BIOPSY

Tumors in the upper tract may be treated by nephroureterectomy sometimes without a prior biopsy. In a study from University of Michigan, the results of upper tract biopsy and/or cytology specimens influenced the decision to proceed to radical nephroureterectomy or ureterectomy in 62% cases.[10] In the remaining cases, the decision to proceed with resection was made based on clinical features, including size (52%), multifocal disease (7%), hydronephrosis or other imaging findings (7%), presence in an area that is difficult to access endoscopically (5%), or presence of residual/recurrent tumor despite therapy (11%). In the remaining 18% of the cases, there was a combination of more than one of the previously listed clinical features that influenced the decision for resection. As a result, some benign urothelial tumors in the upper tract undergo resection where a prior biopsy is not done or not influential. These include inverted urothelial papillomas, which can occur in the renal pelvis or ureter.[11] Another benign urothelial neoplasm that exclusively occurs in the renal pelvis/proximal ureter is polypoid urothelial tumor with inverted growth pattern (PUTIP) (Fig. 14.2).[12] The masses range in size from 0.5 to 3.2 cm (mean, 1.6 cm). PUTIP is a polypoid, plaquelike lesion with features of the following: (1) inverted papillary urothelial neoplasm of low malignant potential, lacking an exophytic papillary component; (2) florid von Brunn nest proliferation within and radiating outward from the polypoid lesion; and (3) in some cases, an inverted papilloma with densely hyalinized collagenous stroma. PUTIP clinically forms a tumor and is typically treated by nephroureterectomy, despite the tumor having to date no malignant potential.

In some instances, as a result of sampling artifact and the scant tissue sent for pathologic examination, the diagnosis of a biopsy of the upper tract is benign, yet there is extensive cancer present on follow-up. Consequently, in selected cases despite a nondiagnostic or benign biopsy report, urologists may still elect to proceed with radical resection on the basis of ureteroscopic findings and radiographic studies, recognizing that repeat biopsy may not always be helpful.

DIFFICULTY IN OBTAINING DIAGNOSTIC TISSUE

Due to the technical difficulties involved in performing ureteral and renal pelvis biopsies, ureteroscopic biopsy specimens are generally smaller than cystoscopic samples. In a study by Vashistha et al., the median biopsy sample size was 0.3 cm (mean, 0.7 cm; range, 0.1-4.0 cm).[13] For this reason, specimens from the upper urinary tract are particularly challenging for pathologists when it comes to accurate tumor grading, staging, and diagnosis. Biopsies from the ureter and renal pelvis have a higher likelihood compared to those from the bladder of having nondiagnostic tissue. Some examples of the histology seen in these insufficient biopsies are scant

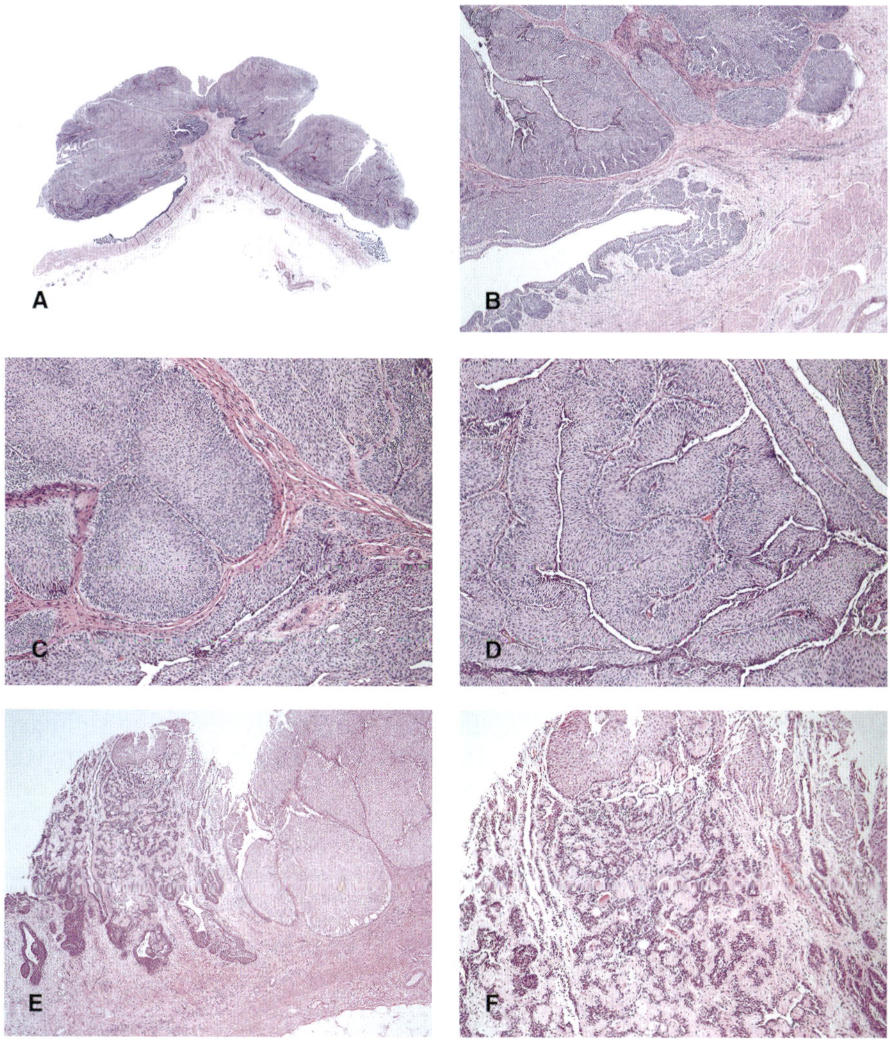

FIGURE 14.2 A: Low-power image of PUTIP with pedunculated appearance. B: Same case—base of stalk with the shoulder of areas resembling VBN proliferation and larger bland urothelial nests. C: Same case—medium-power image of large nests with bland cytology. D: Same case—medium-power image of nests with inverted papilloma–like features of anastomosing cords with bland cytology. E: Another case of PUTIP with inverted papilloma–like areas (*left*) and inverted PUNLMP-like areas (*right*). F: Same case with higher-power image of collagen within inverted papilloma–like areas.

fragments of benign urothelium, granulation tissue, tissue too small to survive processing, acellular debris, or stroma with crush artifact[10] (Fig. 14.3). A specimen can also be insufficient if it is minute and does not sample adequately the tumor (Fig. 14.4). The following data are from a systematic review and meta-analysis analyzing the diagnostic accuracy of biopsies in predicting stage and grade in the upper tract.[14]

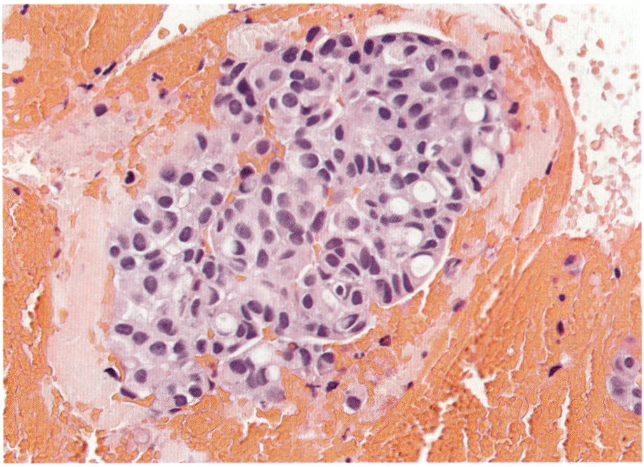

FIGURE 14.3 **Minute focus of atypical urothelial cells, insufficient for further diagnosis.** Was the only cluster from a biopsy of the renal pelvis.

NONDIAGNOSTIC SPECIMENS

The nondiagnostic biopsy rate is 8% and 3% for perbiopsy and perpatient analysis, respectively. This discrepancy is explained by the fact that whenever possible, the surgeon takes more than one biopsy over time per patient, which increases the likelihood of eventually obtaining sufficient samples to achieve the diagnosis. In the study by Vashistha et al., there was no statistical difference in size of the biopsies between true positives and true negatives vs false negatives.[13]

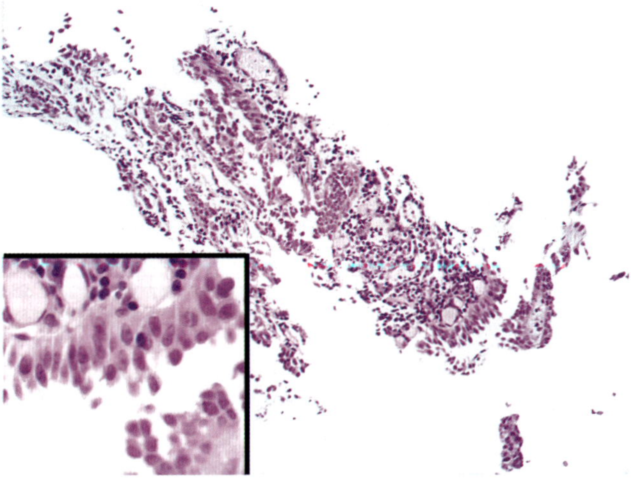

FIGURE 14.4 **Minute fragment of urothelium with prominent chronic inflammation and reactive-appearing urothelial cells (*inset*), which favors a reactive process.** Follow-up demonstrated a pT3-invasive high-grade papillary urothelial carcinoma.

CORRELATION OF GRADE BETWEEN BIOPSY AND RESECTION

The cumulative meta-analysis for grade-to-grade match between biopsy and the surgical specimen in the series using the current WHO/ISUP grading system, the grade-to-grade match is 66% and 95% for low-grade and high-grade tumors, respectively. Although undergrading of the biopsy relative to the resection specimen is more common due to sampling issues, overgrading of biopsies also exists. For example, in the study by Simon et al., of the 10 biopsies demonstrating a change in grade, 3 were from noninvasive low-grade to high-grade papillary urothelial carcinoma, 4 were from noninvasive low-grade papillary to invasive high-grade urothelial carcinoma, and 3 were downgraded from noninvasive high-grade to low-grade papillary urothelial carcinoma.[10] It is critical not to overgrade papillary urothelial carcinoma in the upper tract, since it could result in a nephroureterectomy or neoadjuvant systemic therapy that potentially could have been avoided. If the findings are not overtly high-grade but there are some features that are worrisome for a high-grade tumor (ie, increased mitotic figures in the absence of marked pleomorphism), then a designation of *noninvasive papillary urothelial carcinoma, borderline between low and high grade* is warranted and the decision to process to resection would not be solely based on the pathology but also factor in clinical and radiographic findings. Of note, if there is radiographic evidence of a mass, the patient may be eligible for neoadjuvant systemic therapy even if the biopsy is called low-grade carcinoma on biopsy.

CORRELATION OF BIOPSY GRADE AND STAGE AT RESECTION

The meta-analysis showed a significant association between high-grade tumor at biopsy and muscle-invasive disease at final pathology. When high-grade carcinoma was seen on biopsy, muscle-invasive disease at the final pathology was seen in 60% of cases. In contrast, when there was low-grade carcinoma on biopsy, there was non–muscle-invasive disease at the final pathology in 77% of cases.

CORRELATION OF STAGE BETWEEN BIOPSY AND RESECTION

The cumulative meta-analysis for stage to stage match showed that when biopsies showed invasion of the subepithelial connective tissue or muscularis propria invasion, in 94% of cases there was muscle-invasive disease at resection. In contrast, if on biopsy, there was carcinoma *in situ* (CIS) or noninvasive papillary urothelial carcinoma and there was non–muscle-invasive disease at resection in 60% of cases. Margolin et al. noted that the likelihood of missing invasion on biopsy in patients with muscle-invasive disease was increased when biopsy fragments were limited to 1 mm or less.[15]

SPECIAL HISTOLOGICAL CONSIDERATIONS

Equivocal Diagnoses

Upper tract biopsies are particularly challenging. In a study by one of the current authors, cases where a definitive diagnosis could not be made was in part due to inadequate tissue[16] (eFig. 14.2). The most commonly encountered problem was small sample size and lack of proper tissue orientation. Other cases where a definitive diagnosis cannot be made relates to cases with papillary formation, but where it was difficult to distinguish between artifactual papillary structures and true papillary neoplasms. A third scenario resulting in an equivocal diagnosis is when a papillary neoplasm is diagnosable, but a correct grade cannot be accurately assigned because of scant tissue often with mechanical distortion or because of the poor quality of the histologic slide or due to marked denudation (Fig. 14.5). If one applies data from the bladder of papillary tumors with denudation, most of these lesions represent noninvasive high-grade papillary urothelial carcinoma, but occasionally can be a low-grade papillary tumor with extensive denudation[17] (eFigs. 14.3 and 14.4). In the upper tract if a case has some features of low-grade papillary urothelial carcinoma (ie, preserved polarity and lack of marked pleomorphism) but has some features of high-grade papillary urothelial carcinoma (ie, increased mitotic activity), one should be careful not to overgrade the tumor, which could result in unnecessary systemic therapy and/or nephroureterectomy. In these cases, it is prudent to grade the tumor as *borderline between low and high grade* and have the urologists

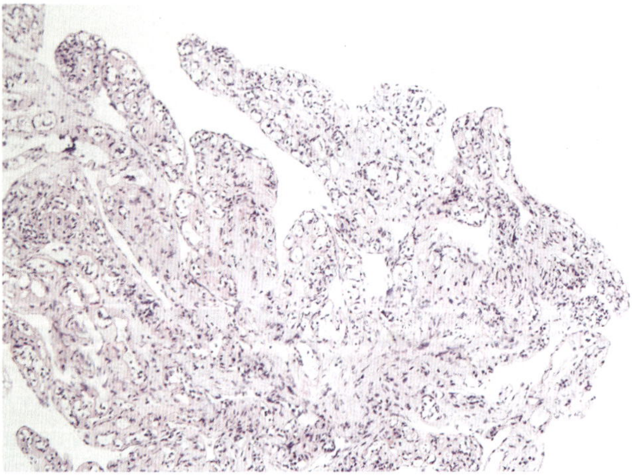

FIGURE 14.5 **Papillary urothelial neoplasm with marked denudation.** Due to extensive denudation, a grade cannot be assigned. Correlation with urine cytology and additional sampling should be considered. Most of these lesions represent noninvasive high-grade papillary urothelial carcinoma, although uncommonly low-grade lesions can show extensive denudation.

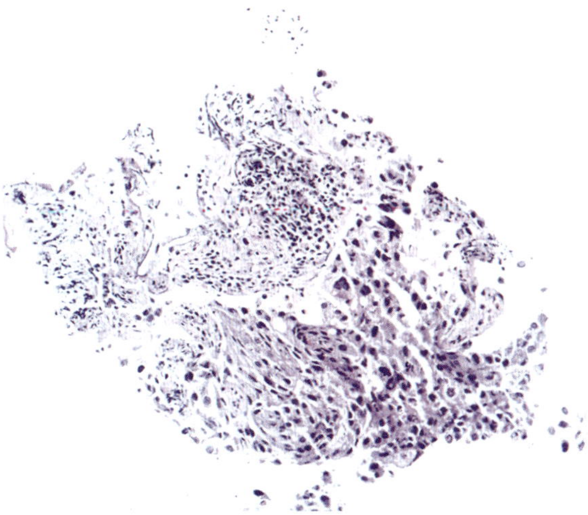

FIGURE 14.6 Scant specimen with high-grade urothelial carcinoma, invasion cannot be ruled out.

factor in other parameters such as the size of the lesion, multifocality, and sessile vs papillary growth to determine therapy (eFig. 14.5). An option remains to perform a repeat biopsy to try to arrive at a more definitive grade. El-Hakim et al. found that in ~80% of the cases, the grade of the tumor (low or high grade) was clinically correctly predicted.[18] Equivocal diagnoses can also result when there is definite high-grade carcinoma, yet invasion cannot be assessed because of the superficial nature of the biopsy (Fig. 14.6).

OVERDIAGNOSIS OF TUMOR

There is a significant likelihood of biopsies from the upper tract to be overdiagnosed as tumor, when on expert review they are benign.[16] Low-grade papillary urothelial neoplasm can be misdiagnosed as a papillary urothelial tumor when characterized by either: (1) detached pieces of urothelial tissue mimicking papillary formation or urothelium with pseudopapillary formation (Figs. 14.7-14.13, eFig. 14.6), (2) proliferations of von Brunn nests (Fig. 14.14), or (3) lamina propria edema (Figs. 14.15 and 14.16). The overdiagnosis of a neoplasm, even low-grade carcinoma, can have serious patient implications in this site, sometimes leading to unnecessary treatment.

Another situation resulting in overdiagnosis is in the setting of reactive urothelial cells associated with inflammation. In contrast to a low-grade papillary urothelial neoplasm, reactive cytological changes consist of urothelial cells with uniformly enlarged vesicular nuclei with central prominent nucleoli (Fig. 14.17). Extra care should be taken in cases where there is a history stent placement.

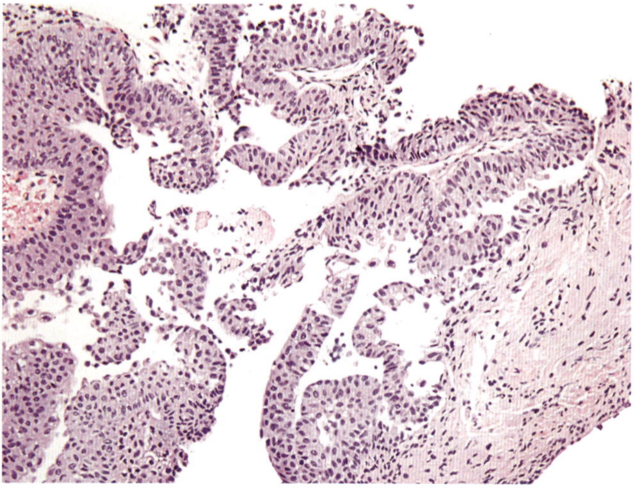

FIGURE 14.7 **Strips of benign urothelium mimicking a papillary urothelial neoplasm.**

Cases may also be misdiagnosed invasive nested urothelial carcinoma, given the predilection for florid proliferation of von Brunn nests to occur in the renal pelvis and ureter.[19] Upon resection, the benign nature of these proliferations is more evident, given the linear or lobular as opposed to infiltrative growth pattern. However, on a biopsy, one cannot appreciate whether the proliferation of small bland urothelial nests are infiltrative. Nested variant of urothelial carcinoma of the renal pelvis and ureter is extremely rare but does exist as a possible diagnosis at this site.[20] In contrast to nested variant of urothelial carcinoma in the bladder, where

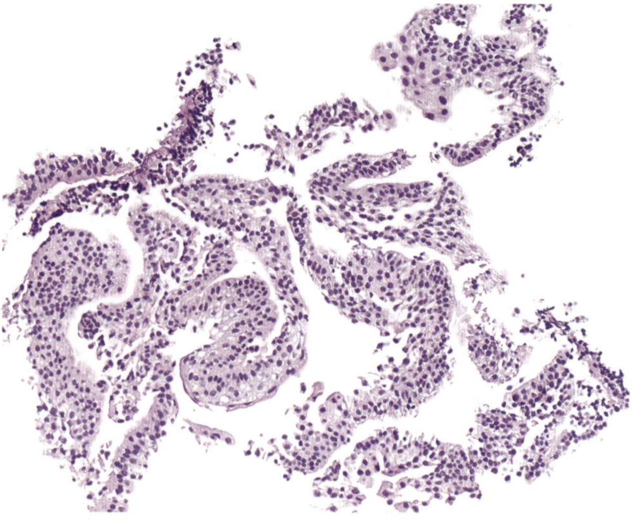

FIGURE 14.8 **Strips of benign urothelium mimicking a papillary urothelial neoplasm.**

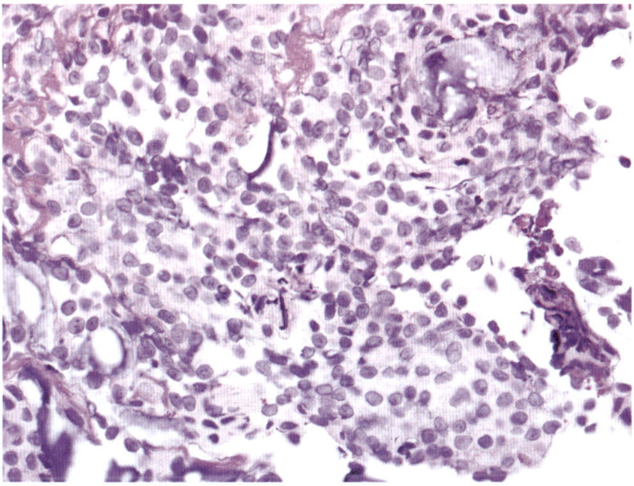

FIGURE 14.9 Compressed fragments of benign urothelium mimicking a papillary urothelial neoplasm.

there often is a lack of a surface precursor component, in the upper tract, nested urothelial carcinoma is often accompanied by papillary urothelial carcinoma, facilitating its diagnosis on biopsy. However, in the renal pelvis and ureter, some cases will need to be diagnosed as *atypical urothelial proliferation. The differential diagnosis is between florid proliferation of von Brunn nests and invasive nested urothelial carcinoma* (Fig. 14.18).

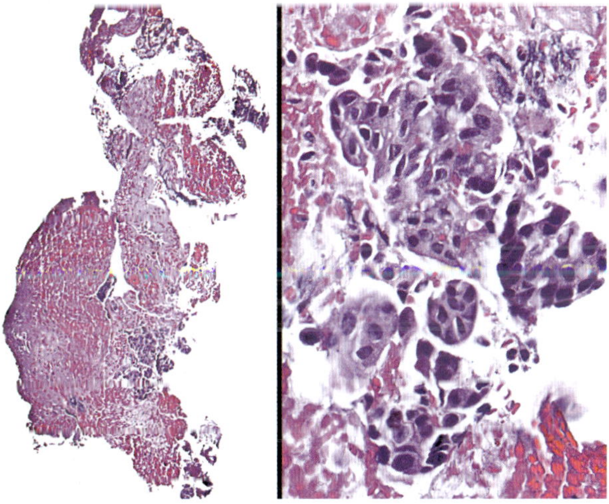

FIGURE 14.10 Scant specimen predominantly composed of blood and fibrin (*left*) with clusters of urothelium with uniformly enlarged nuclei (*right*) consistent with reactive urothelial changes.

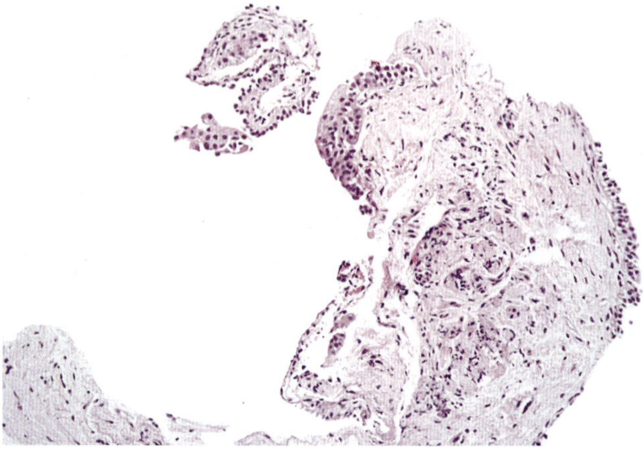

FIGURE 14.11 **Benign biopsy with artifactual papillary formation.** Note urothelium of normal thickness and cytology.

ESTABLISHING A DEFINITIVE TUMOR DIAGNOSIS

A definite diagnosis of papillary urothelial neoplasm can be established in the presence of papillary fronds with well-formed fibrovascular cores. These cases can be definitively diagnosed as low-grade (Figs. 14.19-14.22, eFigs. 14.7-14.12) or high-grade (Figs. 14.23 and 14.24, eFig. 14.13) noninvasive papillary urothelial carcinoma. In the renal pelvis and ureter, if there is a papillary urothelial tumor with thickened urothelium, but little or no

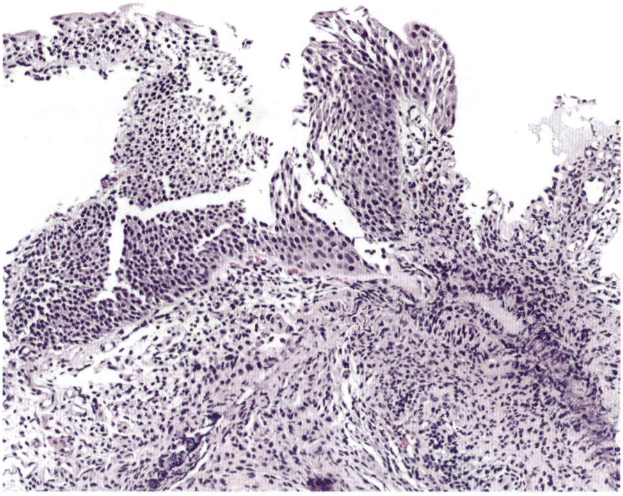

FIGURE 14.12 **Benign urothelial tissue with chronic inflammation in the stroma and focal protuberance mimicking a small papillae.** Follow-up showed no tumor.

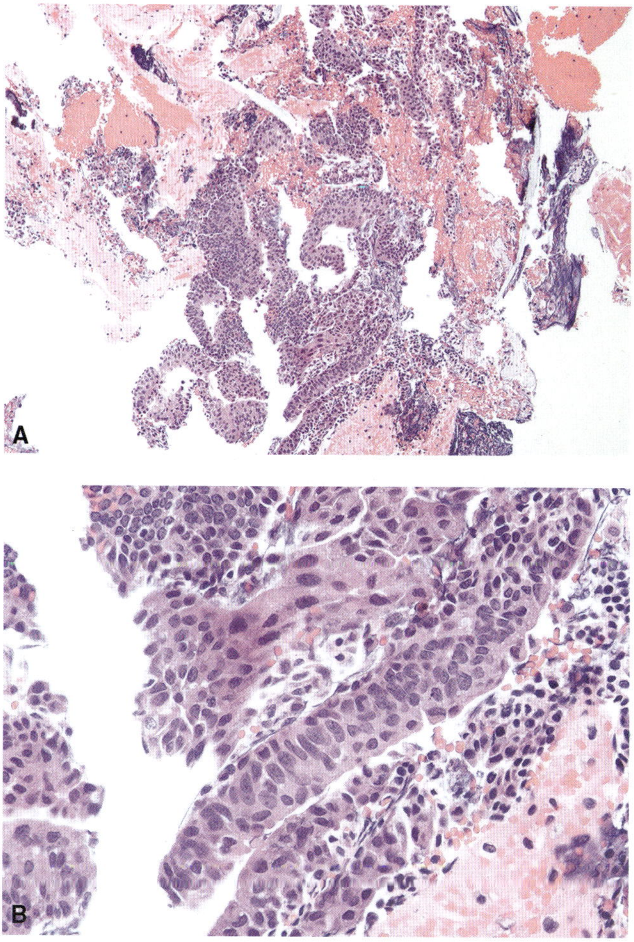

FIGURE 14.13 A: Biopsy from the renal pelvis with numerous strips of urothelium in blood and fibrin. B: Higher magnification with benign-appearing normal thickness urothelium and umbrella cells with more abundant eosinophilic cytoplasm.

cytologic atypia, a diagnosis can be made of low-grade papillary urothelial neoplasm where a grade could not be assigned (Fig. 14.25). The vast majority of these lesions upon resection will be noninvasive low-grade papillary urothelial carcinoma, given the likelihood of undersampling more definitive low-grade morphology, but uncommonly, the resected tumor will be a PUNLMP (eFig. 14.14). CIS (Fig. 14.26) and invasive urothelial carcinoma (Fig. 14.27, eFig. 14.15) can also be diagnosable on biopsies of the renal pelvis and ureter.

There are also rare cases of renal cell carcinoma where a major component of the tumor grows into the renal pelvic-calyceal system and can be first biopsied on ureteroscopic biopsy.[21] There is a significant chance in this scenario of misdiagnosing a minute fragments of renal cell carcinoma

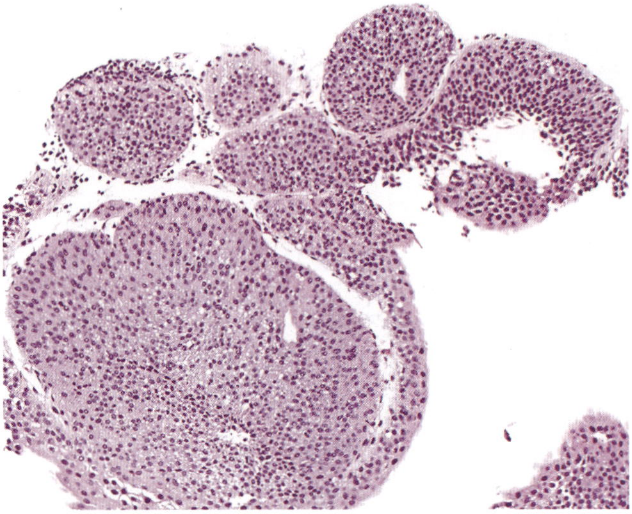

FIGURE 14.14 Benign urothelium with proliferation of von Brunn nests.

as urothelial carcinoma, since the diagnosis of renal cell carcinoma is not expected on ureteroscopic biopsy. These tumors can be associated with positive cytology, which can also lead to misdiagnosis.

CLINICOPATHOLOGICAL CORRELATION

There is a strong correlation between the presence of a mass noted radiographically or cystoscopically and the histologic diagnosis of a neoplasm.[16] However, the correlation is not perfect. In a minority of cases, despite the

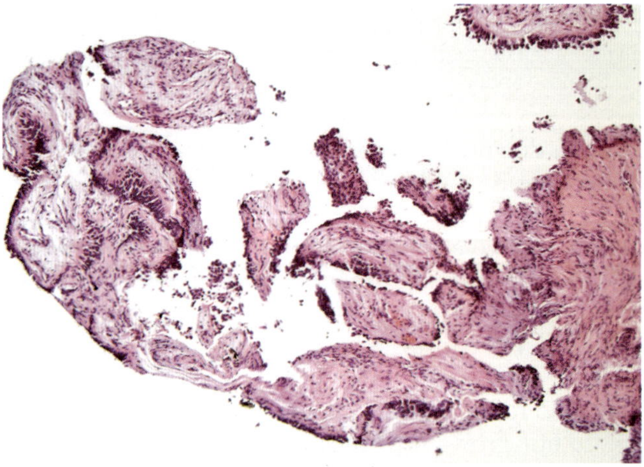

FIGURE 14.15 Benign urothelium and underlying stroma with lamina propria edema mimicking a papillary urothelial tumor.

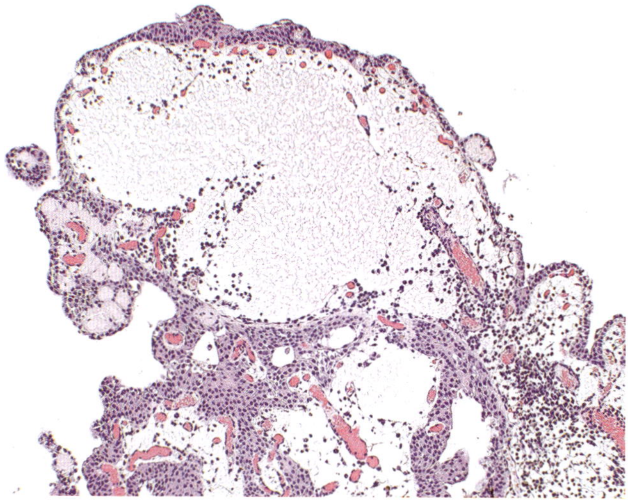

FIGURE 14.16 Polypoid pyelitis.

absence of a clinical mass, follow-up reveals a neoplasm. Explanations for this discrepancy may be explained by gross tumor that was subtle or tumor in a location in the pelvis or ureter that was difficult to image and/or visualize at ureteroscopy. Similarly, there is a minority of cases with a clinically suspected tumor present; yet both on histology and follow-up, there is no a neoplasm. It is well recognized that polypoid ureteritis/pyelitis, nephrogenic adenoma, fibroepithelial polyp, and proliferation of von Brunn nests can clinically mimic a neoplasm.

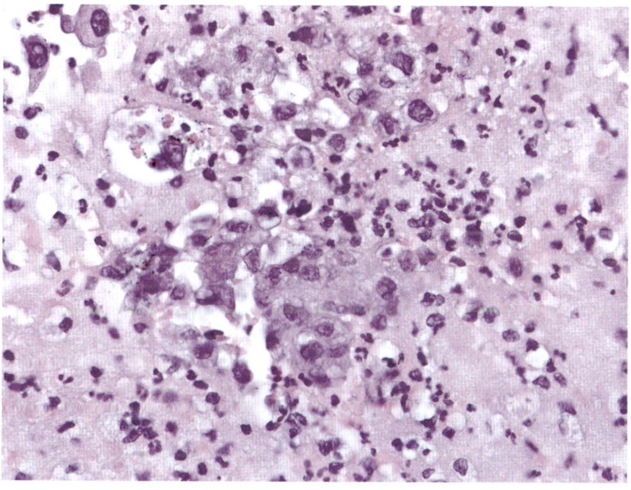

FIGURE 14.17 **Specimen mainly consisting of acute inflammation with scattered urothelial cells with vesicular nuclei and prominent nucleoli and rare atypical cells, favor reactive.** Follow-up was benign.

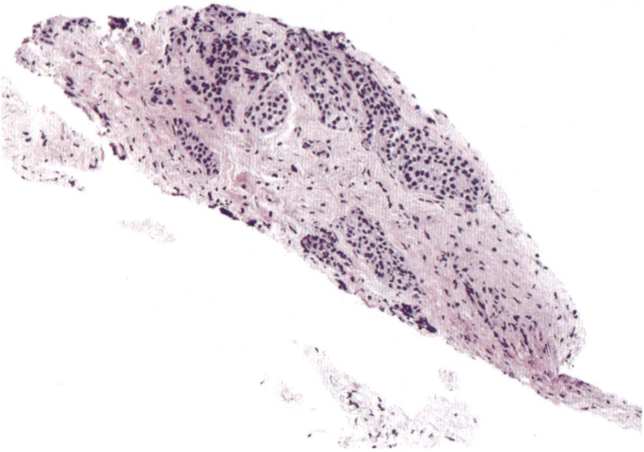

FIGURE 14.18 **Small specimen with a differential diagnosis of proliferation of von Brunn nests vs infiltrating urothelial carcinoma with nested features.** The patient had no evidence of disease at follow-up and subsequent biopsies.

Given this imperfect association between the presence of a clinical mass and the eventual diagnosis of a neoplasm, how can pathologists factor in this information in dealing with difficult ureter/pelvic biopsies? In a case where a low-grade papillary urothelial neoplasm is favored microscopically, knowledge that there is a presence of a mass can be helpful in ruling out an artifactual papillary formation. Conversely, in cases where there is some suggestion of papillary formation yet the cytology is totally benign and the urothelium is of normal thickness, the pathologist should

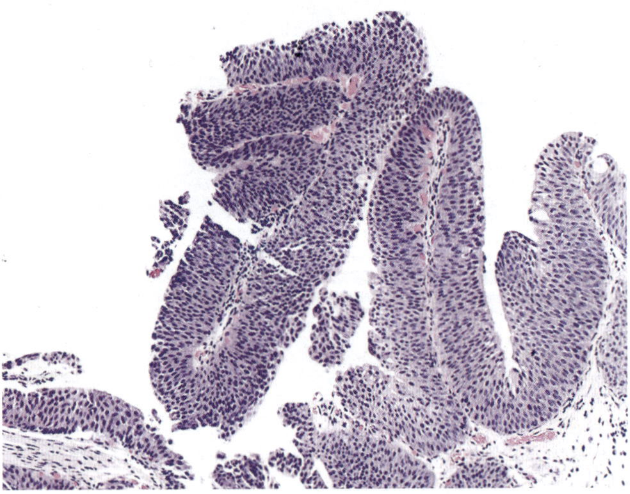

FIGURE 14.19 **Noninvasive low-grade urothelial carcinoma with unambiguous papillary formations.**

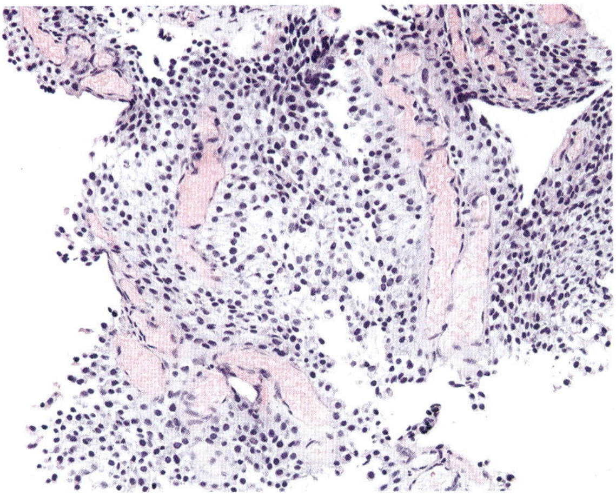

FIGURE 14.20 Low-grade papillary urothelial carcinoma from the ureter.

inquire if there is a mass present clinically and, if not, consider that the urothelial fragments may represent detached strips of benign or reactive urothelium mimicking a papillary neoplasm. In a case without a mass noted clinically, where histologic findings are not overtly neoplastic, it is reasonable to diagnose the lesion as atypical.

Caution must be exercised in the evaluation of limited specimens in the ureter and renal pelvis, especially in the absence of a gross lesion suspicious of a tumor, as overdiagnosis can result in radical nephroureterectomy. In a minority of cases, following the diagnosis of urothelial carcinoma on biopsy, there may be no residual carcinoma in the resection specimen. This may result from effective neoadjuvant chemotherapy or complete endoscopic treatment.[22] What needs to be avoided at all cost

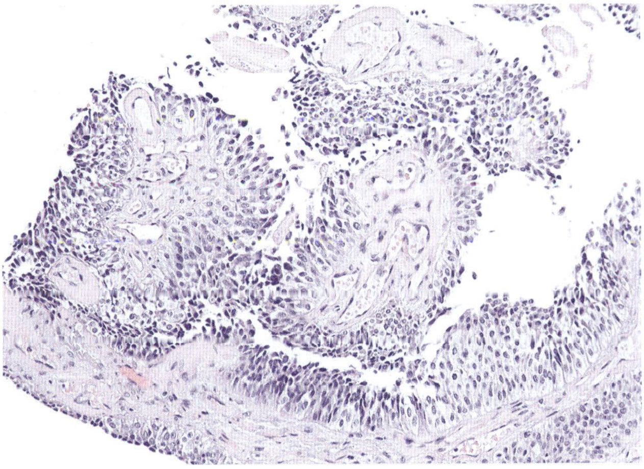

FIGURE 14.21 Low-grade papillary urothelial carcinoma from the renal pelvis.

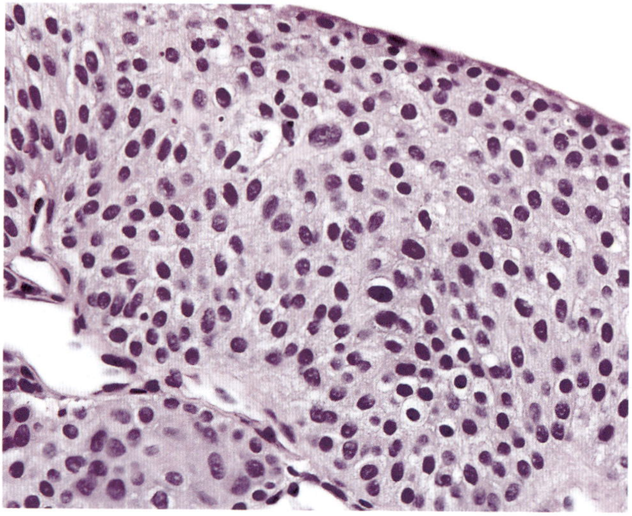

FIGURE 14.22 **Low-grade papillary urothelial carcinoma from the renal pelvis.**

is misinterpretation of the pathologic specimen resulting in a false-positive pT0.

The most important take home message for practicing pathologists is that because upper tract biopsies are technically difficult to obtain, they are often scant or small in size. Excessive blind manipulation while obtaining samples may result in artifactual stripping or balling up of reactive mucosa that may mimic neoplasm. Clinicopathologic correlation (mass lesion, previous bladder cancer, or history of stones and instrumentation) is imperative, as is correlation with urine or renal pelvic cytology samples. The clinical implications for both overdiagnosis and underdiagnosis (both of

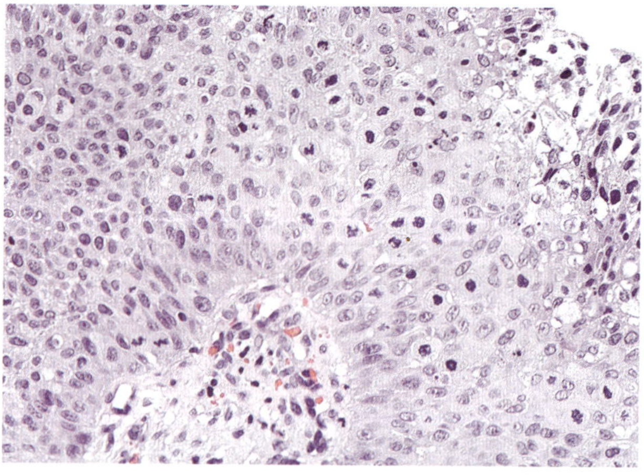

FIGURE 14.23 **High-grade papillary urothelial carcinoma from the renal pelvis.** Despite lack of prominent pleomorphism, there are many mitotic figures.

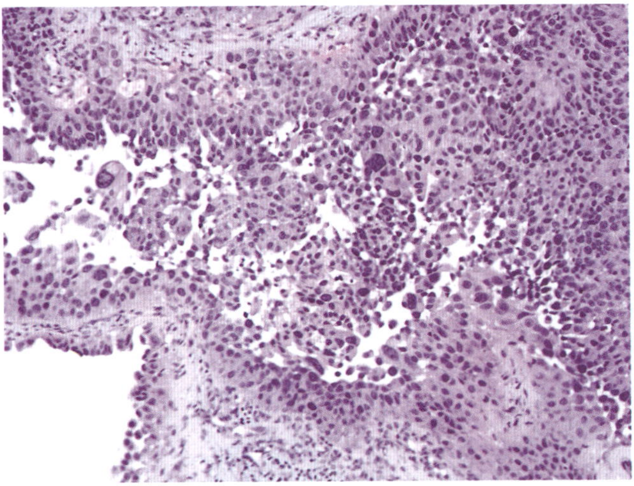

FIGURE 14.24 **Noninvasive high-grade urothelial papillary urothelial carcinoma.**

which can occur) are severe in upper tract biopsies; they remain diagnostically challenging and warrant excessive caution while being interpreted.

MOLECULAR CONSIDERATIONS

While the molecular features of upper and lower tract urothelial carcinoma overlap, upper tract tumors are more likely to exhibit *FGFR3* and *HRAS* but lower incidence of *p53*, *RB1*, and *ERBB2* genomic alterations.[23,24]

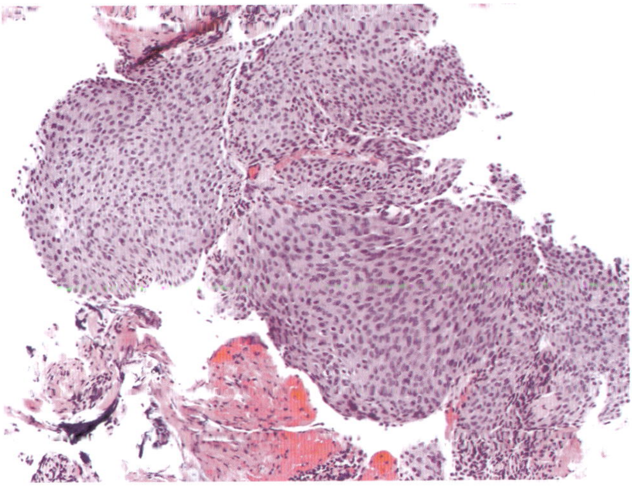

FIGURE 14.25 **Fragments of thickened urothelium without atypia or mitoses consistent with a low-grade papillary urothelial neoplasm where a grade could not be assigned.** Patient underwent nephroureterectomy to reveal a large PUNLMP with inverted growth pattern replacing the renal pelvis.

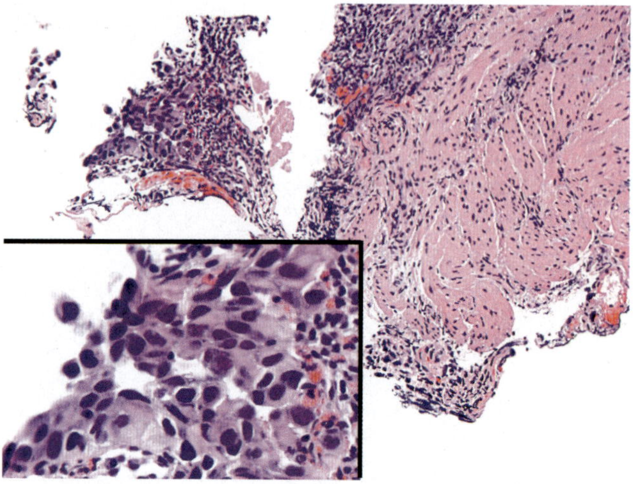

FIGURE 14.26 Although only a minute area of tumor is present, urothelial carcinoma *in situ* (CIS) is diagnostic with cells with high nuclear to cytoplasmic ratio, distorted architecture, nucleomegaly, and hyperchromasia (*inset*).

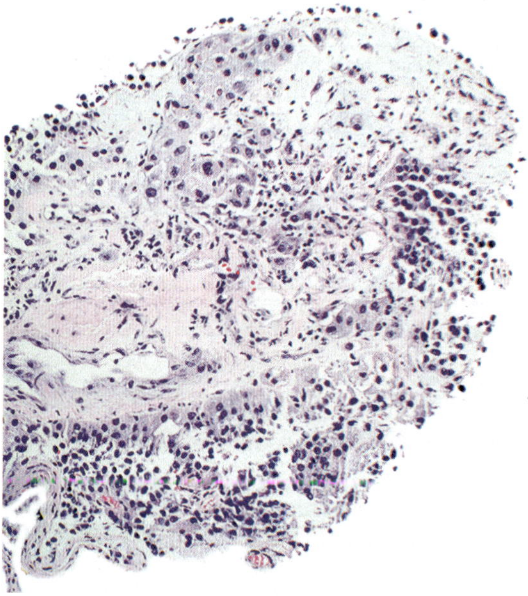

FIGURE 14.27 Invasive high-grade urothelial carcinoma on biopsy from the renal pelvis.

Molecular events in upper tract and bladder urothelial carcinomas can be shared or distinct,[23-27] although in most cases, the tumors are clonally related. There are two scenarios where pathologists are increasingly called upon for testing upper tract specimens for molecular-related events.

The first situation is in regards to defects in mismatch repair genes, either seen sporadically or associated with the Lynch syndrome.[28,29] The Lynch syndrome is caused by pathogenic germ-line variant in one of the mismatch repair (MMR) genes: *MHL1*, *MSH2*, *MSH6*, or *PMS2*. Following colorectal and endometrial cancer, upper tract urothelial carcinoma is the third most common cancer in this syndrome. Upper tract urothelial carcinoma develops in 2.2%-9.1% of Lynch syndrome individuals depending on the specific MMR variant and sex and may explain up to 21.3% of newly diagnosed upper tract urothelial carcinomas, often manifesting at a younger age than sporadic upper tract urothelial carcinomas. Rasmussen et al. reviewed patients in a systematic analysis of 12 studies of consecutively and predominately unselected cohort of upper tract urothelial carcinoma screened for MMR protein immunohistochemical loss.[30] From the pooled data, 140/1559 (9%) had tumors with loss, with 80.7% showing loss of MSH2, MSH6, or both. In 7 studies, genetic testing confirmed Lynch syndrome diagnosis for 20/970 (2.1%) patients. In 8 studies, 31 (2.6%) patients were given a clinical Lynch syndrome diagnosis. In total, 51/1087 (4.7%) patients with upper tract urothelial carcinomas were assumed or verified Lynch syndrome patients. It is recommend screening upper tract urothelial carcinoma using immunohistochemical staining for all four MMR proteins, although, as previously stated, MSH2 (particularly) and MSH6 are the most commonly altered proteins.[31]

Five programmed death-1 (PD-1)/programmed death-ligand 1 (PD-L1) inhibitors are currently approved for treatment of locally advanced or metastatic urothelial carcinoma of the bladder and the upper urinary tract. First-line treatment with atezolizumab and pembrolizumab in platinum-ineligible patients requires immunohistochemical PD-L1 positivity. PD-L1 assays in clinical trials include the 28-8 pharmDx (nivolumab), the 22C3 pharmDx (pembrolizumab), Ventana SP142 (atezolizumab), and the Ventana PD-L1 SP263 assays (durvalumab). PD-L1 testing is very complex due to intratumor heterogeneity, therapy-induced changes in expression, and differences in approved diagnostic PD-L1 antibody assays and the subsequent specific scoring algorithm, which is unique for each companion diagnostic assay. Since anti–PD-L1 immunohistochemistry is only indicated in patients with locally advanced or metastatic urothelial carcinoma, tissue sample should be selected with at least invasive urothelial carcinoma. When multiple tissue samples with invasive urothelial carcinoma are available, selection of the latest available tissue block with a sufficient amount of invasive UC (at least 100 tumor cells) and the lowest amount of cauterization artifact or necrotic areas is recommended. If available, biopsies of metastatic tumor is preferable, since there can be significant discrepancies of the PD-L1 status between primary and corresponding metastases. It is beyond this book to discuss different assays, scoring algorithms, cutoff systems, and reporting results, which are described in the review article by Eckstein et al. and in other sources.[32]

REFERENCES

1. Siegel RL, Miller KD, Fuchs HE, Jemal A. Cancer statistics, 2022. *CA Cancer J Clin.* 2022;72(1):7-33. doi:10.3322/caac.21708
2. Holmäng S, Johansson SL. Synchronous bilateral ureteral and renal pelvic carcinomas: incidence, etiology, treatment and outcome. *Cancer.* 2004;101(4):741-747. doi:10.1002/cncr.20395
3. Deuker M, Stolzenbach LF, Collà Ruvolo C, et al. Upper urinary tract tumors: variant histology versus urothelial carcinoma. *Clin Genitourin Cancer.* 2021;19(2):117-124.
4. Rolim I, Henriques V, Rolim N, et al. Clinicopathologic analysis of upper urinary tract carcinoma with variant histology. *Virchows Arch.* 2020;477(1):111-112.
5. Mori K, Janisch F, Parizi MK. Prognostic value of variant histology in upper tract urothelial carcinoma treated with nephroureterectomy: a systematic review and meta-analysis. *J Urol.* 2020;203(6):1075-1084.
6. Baydar D, Amin MB, Epstein JI. Osteoclast-rich undifferentiated carcinomas of the urinary tract. *Mod Pathol.* 2006;19(2):161-171.
7. Duplisea JJ, Petros FG, Li R, et al. Outcomes of nonmetastatic micropapillary variant upper tract urothelial carcinoma. *Urol Oncol.* 2019;37(6):354.e19-354.e26.
8. Lopez-Beltran A, Paner G, Blanca A, et al. Lymphoepithelioma-like carcinoma of the upper urinary tract. *Virchows Arch.* 2017;470(6):703-709.
9. Makise N, Morikawa T, Kawai T. Squamous differentiation and prognosis in upper urinary tract urothelial carcinoma. *Int J Clin Exp Pathol.* 2015;8(6):7203-7209.
10. Simon CT, Skala SL, Weizer AZ. Clinical utility and concordance of upper urinary tract cytology and biopsy in predicting clinicopathological features of upper urinary tract urothelial carcinoma. *Hum Pathol.* 2019;86:76-84.
11. Luo JD, Wang P, Chen J. Upper urinary tract inverted papillomas: Report of 10 cases. *Oncol Lett.* 2012;4(1):71-74.
12. Wobker SE, Zhong M, Epstein JI. Polypoid urothelial tumor with inverted growth pattern in the renal pelvis: morphologic and molecular characteristics of a unique diagnostic entity. *Hum Pathol.* 2017;59:26-33.
13. Vashistha V, Shabsigh A, Zynger DL. Utility and diagnostic accuracy of ureteroscopic biopsy in upper tract urothelial carcinoma. *Arch Pathol Lab Med.* 2013;137(3):400-407.
14. Subiela JD, Territo A, Mercadé A, et al. Diagnostic accuracy of ureteroscopic biopsy in predicting stage and grade at final pathology in upper tract urothelial carcinoma: systematic review and meta-analysis. *Eur J Surg Oncol.* 2020;46(11):1989-1997.
15. Margolin EJ, Matulay JT, Li G, et al. Discordance between ureteroscopic biopsy and final pathology for upper tract urothelial carcinoma. *J Urol.* 2018;199(6):1440-1445.
16. Tavora F, Fajardo DA, Lee TK, et al. Small endoscopic biopsies of the ureter and renal pelvis: pathologic pitfalls. *Am J Surg Pathol.* 2009;33(10):1540-1546.
17. Owens CL, Epstein JI. Significance of denuded urothelium in papillary urothelial lesions. *Am J Surg Pathol.* 2007;31(2):298-303.
18. El-Hakim A, Weiss GH, Lee BR, et al. Correlation of ureteroscopic appearance with histologic grade of upper tract transitional cell carcinoma. *Urology.* 2004;63(4):647-650.
19. Volmar KE, Chan TY, De Marzo AM, et al. Florid von Brunn nests mimicking urothelial carcinoma: a morphologic and immunohistochemical comparison to the nested variant of urothelial carcinoma. *Am J Surg Pathol.* 2003;27(9):1243-1252.

20. Fatima A, Russell DH, Epstein JI. Nested variant of urothelial carcinoma in the upper urinary tract: a series of 15 case (submitted for publication). *Am J Surg Pathol.* 2023;47:461-468.
21. Sheckley F, Nobert C, Stifelman M. Right renal pelvis renal cell carcinoma mimicking transitional cell carcinoma: case report. *J Endourol Case Rep.* 2020;6(4):536-539.
22. Rouprêt M, Xylinas E, Colin P, et al. Oncologic outcomes and survival in pT0 tumors after radical nephroureterectomy for upper tract urothelial carcinoma: results from of a large multicenter international collaborative study. *Eur Urol.* 2013;63(2):404-405.
23. Sfakianos JP, Cha EK, Iyer G, et al. Genomic characterization of upper tract urothelial carcinoma. *Eur Urol.* 2015;68:970-977.
24. Audenet F, Isharwal S, Cha EK, et al. Clonal relatedness and mutational differences between upper tract and bladder urothelial carcinoma. *Clin Cancer Res.* 2019;25:967-976.
25. Hassler MR, Bray F, Catto JWF, et al. Molecular characterization of upper tract urothelial carcinoma in the era of next-generation sequencing: a systematic review of the current literature. *Eur Urol.* 2020;78(2):209-220.
26. Moss TJ, Qi Y, Xi L, et al. Comprehensive genomic characterization of upper tract urothelial carcinoma. *Eur Urol.* 2017;72(4):641-649.
27. Necchi A, Madison R, Pal SK, et al. Comprehensive genomic profiling of upper-tract and bladder urothelial carcinoma. *Eur Urol Focus.* 2021;7(6):1339-1346.
28. Joost P, Therkildsen C, Dominguez-Valentin M, et al. Urinary tract cancer in Lynch syndrome; increased risk in carriers of MSH2 mutations. *Urology.* 2015;86(6):1212-1217.
29. Donahue TF, Bagrodia A, Audenet F, et al. Genomic characterization of upper-tract urothelial carcinoma in patients with Lynch Syndrome. *JCO Precis Oncol.* 2018;2018.
30. Rasmussen M, Madsen MG, Therkildsen C. Immunohistochemical screening of upper tract urothelial carcinomas for Lynch syndrome diagnostics: a systematic review. *Urology.* 2022;165:44-53.
31. Compérat E, Amin MB, Epstein JI, et al. The Genitourinary Pathology Society Update on classification of variant histologies, T1 substaging, molecular taxonomy, and immunotherapy and PD-L1 testing implications of urothelial cancers. *Adv Anat Pathol.* 2021;28:196-208.
32. Eckstein M, Cimadamore A, Hartmann A, et al. PD L1 assessment in urothelial carcinoma: a practical approach. *Ann Transl Med.* 2019;7(22):690.

15

URINARY TRACT CYTOPATHOLOGY

Christopher J. VandenBussche and Syed Z. Ali

While the microscopic examination of malignant cells in the urine began in the 19th century, the modern era of microscopic examination started with George Papanicolaou examining urinary sediment smears to diagnose urinary tract cancers in 1945; today, urinary tract specimens have become one of the most common cytopathology laboratory specimens after the PAP test.[1-3] The original purpose of urinary tract cytopathology, the detection of urothelial cancer, remains its mainstay.

The 2013 International Congress of Cytology in Paris, France established an international working group aimed at standardizing the terminology used in reporting urinary tract specimens and examining the practice patterns among different institutions. This effort arose due to the nonuniform practice of diagnosing and reporting of urinary tract cytopathology among cytopathologists, a lack of confidence among some pathologists when examining urinary tract specimens, and questions surrounding the clinical utility of urinary tract cytopathology. These factors both resulted in and were perpetuated by relatively high rates of "indeterminate" diagnoses at many institutions, sometimes approaching one-third of all urinary tract specimens.[4]

The result from the international working group was The Paris System for Reporting Urinary Cytology (TPS), which was finalized at the end of 2015 and endorsed by both the American Society of Cytopathology and International Academy of Cytology (Table 15.1). Another series of working groups updated the guidelines, which were released as a second edition in 2022. In short, TPS identifies the high positive predictive value (PPV) for high-grade urothelial carcinoma (HGUC) as the primary strength of urinary tract cytopathology. This strength is emphasized by the TPS, as it focuses almost exclusively on the use of urinary tract cytopathology to identify features of HGUC and stratify urinary tract specimens according to risk for HGUC and urothelial carcinoma *in situ* (CIS).

TABLE 15.1 Recommended Diagnostic Terminology in The Paris Classification (TPS)

Unsatisfactory/Nondiagnostic
Negative for high-grade urothelial carcinoma
Atypical urothelial cells
Suspicious for high-grade urothelial carcinoma
High-grade urothelial carcinoma
Other

BENEFITS AND DRAWBACKS OF URINARY TRACT CYTOPATHOLOGY

Voided urine specimens can be produced conveniently, cheaply, and noninvasively. Processing of these specimens is also relatively inexpensive and quick. Because specimens are concentrated during processing, relatively little time is required for their microscopic examination. Turnaround time can be same day if necessary. Because urine is produced from the kidneys in the upper urinary tract, a voided urine specimen represents a sampling of a patient's entire urinary tract. When samples are well preserved, the cytomorphologic features of HGUC are specific and a malignant diagnosis has a PPV that approaches 100%.[4-10]

The primary drawback to voided urine specimens is their relatively low sensitivity (50%-85%) for HGUC[11,12] and even much lower sensitivity for low-grade urothelial neoplasms (LGUNs) (10%-43.6%).[11,12] Diagnosis by urinary tract cytopathology requires neoplastic cells to be present in the urine specimen, but patients with dilute urine or a low tumor burden may have few to no malignant cells in a given sample. Therefore, the use of serial samples over time is recommended when a patient is being followed using voided urine specimens alone. Even large low-grade neoplasms shed tumor cells less frequently than high-grade lesions, and thus, urinary tract cytopathology has poor specificity and sensitivity for low-grade lesions. Because voided urine specimens represent the entire urinary tract, one cannot localize a lesion using voided urine specimens alone. Therefore, a malignant voided urine specimen needs to be correlated with cystoscopy, pyelogram, and/or radiographic results; in these instances, follow-up with location-specific urine specimens obtained through cystoscopy is often useful. Positive results may be especially difficult to clinically correlate in the case of flat (CIS) or small tumors, tumors in obscured locations, and tumors that mimic pathophysiologic and/or reactive processes such as stenosis or infection.[13,14] While this phenomenon of an "anticipatory positive" result may seem beneficial, early positive results can cause frustration for the urologist, who cannot treat a tumor until it is localized.

Urinary tract specimens obtained by instrumentation can help localize a neoplasm by washing (barbotage) or brushing a specific location of the urinary tract. These specimens can sometimes be taken directly from an abnormal area identified during cystoscopy and correlated with a concurrent tissue biopsy. Because the washing process disrupts urothelial cells, the cells obtained are generally better preserved and more numerous than those found in a voided urine specimen. Furthermore, instrumented specimens can improve the sensitivity for detecting HGUC in the upper tract when compared to voided urine specimens.[15] However, washing and brushing techniques also exert physical forces on the cells, which can result in cytomorphological artifacts. Additionally, normal urothelial lining can also be removed, resulting in very cellular specimens that, even if entirely benign, may give the impression of a neoplastic process. Compared to voided urine specimens, instrumented specimens are costlier to obtain, require a more invasive procedure, and are more inconvenient to the patient.

HIGH-GRADE UROTHELIAL CARCINOMA

A cytologic diagnosis of HGUC correlates with a histological diagnosis of either noninvasive high-grade papillary urothelial carcinoma or invasive HGUC. Because the primary goal of TPS is to identify HGUC, it is most important to be familiar with the cytomorphological features of HGUC (Figs. 15.1 and 15.2).[1,16,17] HGUC cells in the urine are pleomorphic and exist on a morphological spectrum, which at one end could be confused with benign, reactive urothelial cells.[18] Furthermore, most specimens contain degenerative changes that can alter the cytomorphologic critical features. Therefore, a urinary tract specimen may be very cellular and contain

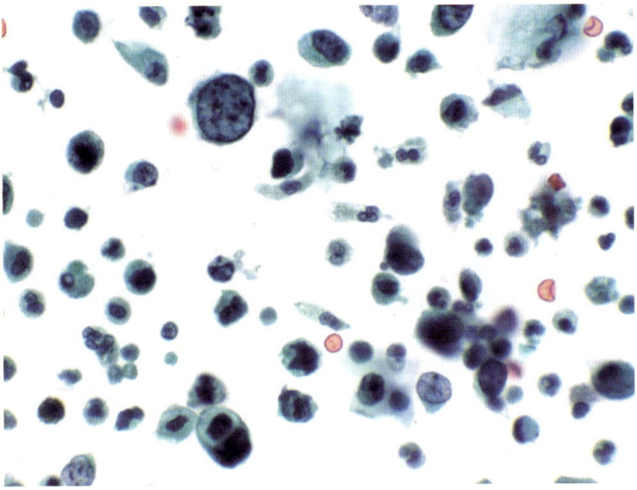

FIGURE 15.1 **High-grade urothelial carcinoma.** While high-grade urothelial carcinoma (HGUC) cells may be found abundantly in a urine specimen, only rare cells may demonstrate the required features: hyperchromasia; coarse, clumpy chromatin; irregular nuclear borders; and an N/C ratio that exceeds 0.7. Many cells in this field have degenerative changes and thus do not meet the N/C ratio requirement. A "cell-in-cell" morphology, as seen at the bottom, is commonly seen in HGUC.

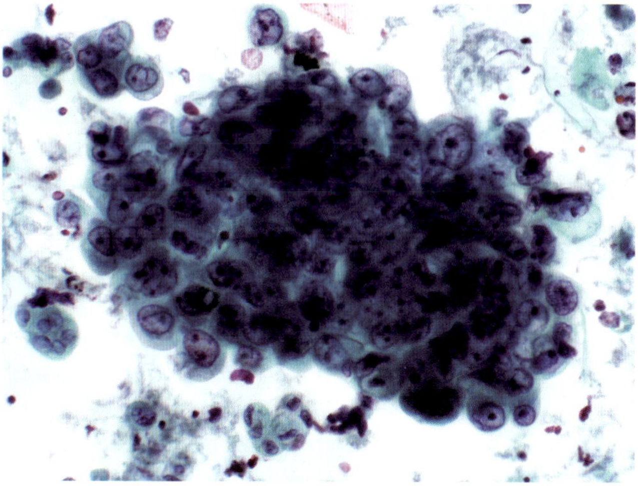

FIGURE 15.2 **Fragment of high-grade urothelial carcinoma.** While high-grade urothelial carcinoma usually presents with single cells in urinary tract specimens, occasionally overtly malignant tissue fragments can be found in instrumented or washing specimens. This fragment contains cells that meet the four criteria required for a diagnosis of high-grade urothelial carcinoma: coarse, clumpy chromatin; markedly irregular nuclear borders; elevated N/C ratios (above 0.7 in several cells); and severe hyperchromasia. Cells in tissue fragments may be difficult to assess, especially when determining the N/C ratio. If any doubt exists, do not make a definitive diagnosis of carcinoma in atypical tissue fragments alone and look carefully for individual malignant cells in the background.

abundant tumor cells, only a small fraction of which may contain all the diagnostic criteria for HGUC:

- High N/C ratio. Malignant cells should have an increased N/C ratio, of ~0.7 or greater, meaning that the nucleus occupies at least 70% of the cytoplasm. While HGUC cells tend to have larger nuclei than reactive than LGUN cells, the N/C ratio is a more specific feature because increase in cell size lags that of nuclear size increase.
- And *two* of the following:
  - Moderate to severe hyperchromasia. Practically, the amount of hyperchromasia should be sufficient to *clearly* distinguish the amount of chromasia from that of bystander benign urothelial cells.
  - Markedly irregular nuclear borders.
  - Coarse, clumpy chromatin.

The above cytomorphologic criteria must be present in at least 5-10 well-preserved urothelial cells to merit a diagnosis of HGUC. Because an HGUC diagnosis from upper tract specimens can contribute to the decision to perform a nephrectomy, it is recommended that an increased threshold be used to make a HGUC diagnosis in upper tract specimens.

While the quantity of malignant cells, presence of tumor diathesis, and level of atypia are all likely associated with a patient's tumor burden, there is no strong evidence to suggest that urinary tract cytopathology can reliably distinguish between invasive and noninvasive HGUC and no such commentary should be made.[5]

Carcinoma *In Situ*

Urinary tract cytopathology has tremendous utility in the diagnosis of CIS that can be difficult to identify and biopsy on cystoscopy. While some studies exist purporting to identify cytomorphological features distinguishing CIS from high-grade papillary urothelial carcinoma, the criteria used by TPS do not distinguish between HGUC and CIS.[19] Therefore, a diagnosis of HGUC on urinary tract cytology includes both high-grade papillary lesions and CIS.

"Hypochromatic" HGUC

Because HGUCs are pleomorphic, some HGUC cells may not possess the classic cytomorphologic features described above. In these instances, a strict interpretation using the TPS criteria would fail to detect some HGUC lesions. As an example, recent studies have reported the existence of paradoxically hypochromatic HGUC cells in some urinary tract specimens (Fig. 15.3). The chromatin in these cells is generally homogenous and lacks coarseness and granular clumps. Due to their bland chromatin, these cells may be overlooked,

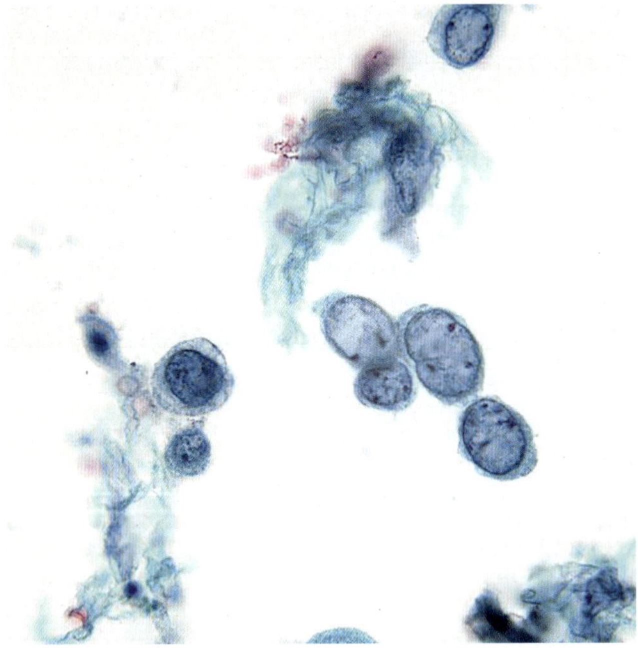

FIGURE 15.3 **Hypochromatic high-grade urothelial carcinoma cells.** A cluster of four HGUC cells (***center***) with hypochromatic nuclei can be seen adjacent to hyperchromatic HGUC cells. In addition to being hypochromatic, the cells lack the coarse clumps of chromatin often seen in HGUC cells. Recent studies have identified high-grade urothelial carcinoma cells that appear paradoxically hyperchromatic. Many of these cells still fulfill the TPS criteria for a malignant diagnosis, and oftentimes hyperchromatic forms are found in the same specimen.

especially in urinary tract washing specimens containing a background of benign urothelial cells. These cells usually maintain other atypical features such as anisonucleosis, high N/C ratio, irregular nuclear membranes, and increased nuclear and cellular size. While it was once speculated that these hypochromatic cells were associated with upper tract lesions, additional studies have shown they can be found in HGUC lesions arising in the lower tract as well.[20-22]

Histologic Variants of HGUC

Many histologic variants of HGUC are rare and do not have well-established features on urinary tract cytopathology, although some case reports exist purporting to associate certain features with particular variants.[23] Due to the lack of evidence regarding the cytologic correlations of these histologic variants, in most instances, it is not recommended to subclassify HGUC on urinary tract cytopathology alone. However, occasionally HGUC will be found with glandular, squamous, or small cell differentiation on urinary tract cytomorphology. Because these variants are the most commonly seen and possess distinct cytomorphological features, it is recommended that these be noted when seen. Given the difficulty of distinguishing these lesions from primary or secondary lesions when a HGUC component is not identified, it is only recommended to make this diagnosis when HGUC cells are present. For instance, in a urine specimen containing entirely carcinoma with squamous differentiation, it is impossible to distinguish a primary or secondary squamous cell carcinoma from a HGUC with squamous differentiation unless HGUC cells without squamous differentiation are also present (Fig. 15.4). Malignant or atypical specimens without a definite urothelial component

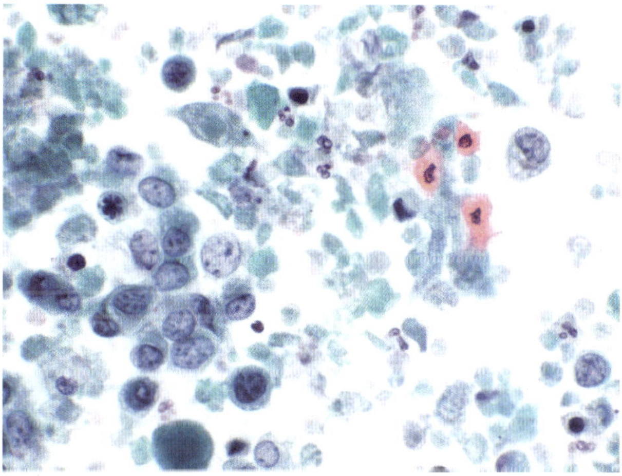

FIGURE 15.4 **High-grade urothelial carcinoma with squamous differentiation.** High-grade urothelial carcinoma may have focal areas of squamous differentiation. If high-grade urothelial carcinoma cells are present, a diagnosis of "high-grade urothelial carcinoma with squamous differentiation" can be made. Occasionally, only squamous carcinoma cells may be seen because the urothelial component is absent from the specimen—because of this, it is important not to assume such cells represent a primary squamous cell carcinoma of the bladder, which is much less common.

should be classified under the "Other" category using descriptors such as "carcinoma with squamous features" or "atypical squamous cells."

NEGATIVE FOR HIGH-GRADE UROTHELIAL CARCINOMA

The *Negative for High-Grade Urothelial Carcinoma (NHGUC)* category is used for specimens that lack HGUC cells and any atypical features concerning for HGUC. Specimens containing morphologic features suggestive of LGUNs are, therefore, classified in the *NHGUC* category.

Normal and Background Components

The typical components of a urinary tract specimen depend on the specimen type. Voided urine specimens often contain contaminating squamous cells and flora from outside the urinary tract. In some instances, squamous cells may greatly outnumber the urothelial cells. It is, therefore, critical to be familiar with urothelial cell morphology and examine these cells rather than becoming distracted by the contaminating squamous component. Washing and catheterized specimens should only contain urinary tract elements and the specimen should be interpreted in this context. Because instrumentation is disruptive to the urinary tract lining, these specimens typically contain a large number of urothelial tissue fragments while voided urine specimens rarely contain urothelial tissue fragments.

Normal urothelial cells are seen as parabasal-type cells and umbrella cells, and in tissue fragments that may contain a mixture of these two cell types. The parabasal-type cell is the most common type and is similar to parabasal cells seen in cervical PAP tests (Fig. 15.5). In a urine

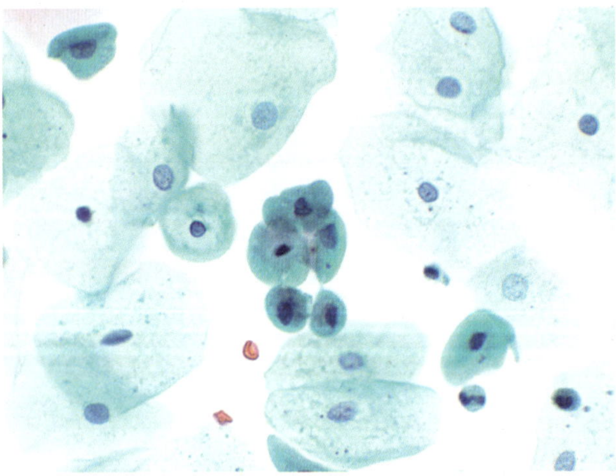

FIGURE 15.5 **Benign voided urine specimen.** This field demonstrates normal parabasal-like (or parabasal-type) urothelial cells surrounded by superficial squamous cells. The parabasal-like cells have similar cytomorphology as the parabasal cells seen in cervical Pap tests: dense cytoplasm, regular and round cytoplasmic borders, and granular chromatin. Superficial squamous cells are usually contaminants from outside the urinary tract and are commonly found in voided urine specimens.

specimen, the assumption is that parabasal-type cells are from the urinary tract because typically only superficial squamous cells contaminate urinary tract specimens. Parabasal-type cells have dense cytoplasm with regular cytoplasmic borders and contain a central small nucleus. They may loosely associate together and form cell clusters that mimic true tissue fragments.

Umbrella cells have abundant cytoplasm that may appear amphophilic. It is not unusual for umbrella cells to be binucleated and rarely umbrella cells may be packed with numerous nuclei. The size of umbrella cells may be distracting, but they typically do not contain features of HGUC. However, on occasion, specimens may contain enlarged malignant cells with abundant cytoplasm and multiple nuclei with hyperchromasia and irregular nuclear borders that resemble umbrella cells. Given their low N/C ratios, these malignant cells typically do not strictly meet the criteria of the *High-Grade Urothelial Carcinoma (HGUC)* category, though with careful examination more conventional-appearing malignant cells can be found in the specimen.[24]

Benign-appearing urothelial issue fragments are common in instrumented specimens and may occasionally be seen in voided urine specimens (Fig. 15.6). One major challenge in urinary tract cytology is the interpretation of tissue fragments, as the cellular overlap in fragments makes it difficult to evaluate important cytomorphological features such as hyperchromasia and N/C ratios. Furthermore, the intercellular junctions allow physical forces to be exerted across the cells, resulting in changes in cellular shapes. Therefore, the threshold for identifying atypia in urothelial tissue fragments should be higher than that for individual cells. This decision can be very subjective and is one reason why the evaluation of individual urothelial cells is a more critical task.

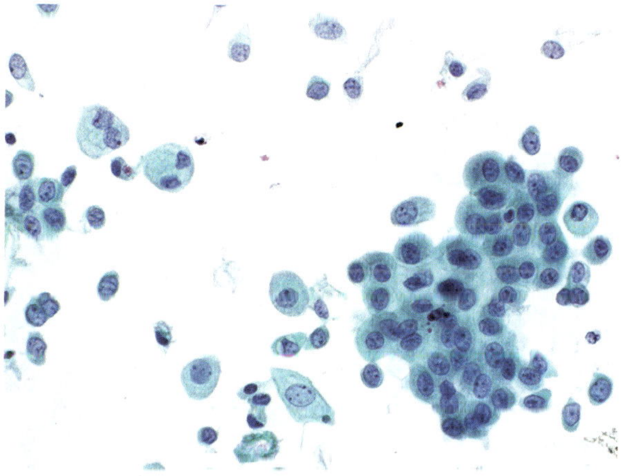

FIGURE 15.6 **Benign catheterized urine specimen demonstrating benign tissue fragments.** A catheterized urinary specimen is typically enriched for urothelial cells and lacks contaminant superficial squamous cells seen in a voided urine specimen. It is more common to see urothelial tissue fragments in instrumented urine specimens. Umbrella cells have more abundant cytoplasm and may be binucleated.

Renal tubular cells are occasionally shed and subsequently found in voided urine specimens. Although small, these cells typically appear hyperchromatic and have irregular nuclear borders. These features occasionally result in renal tubular cells being diagnosed as atypical urothelial cells (AUC). Renal tubular cells can usually be distinguished from urothelial cells by their very small size and high N/C ratios. While they may be found singly, renal tubular cells often form small clusters with hobnailed borders (Fig. 15.7). When seen together with casts, renal tubular cells may suggest that a patient with new-onset hematuria may have a non-neoplastic upper tract disease process.

Degenerative changes are common in voided urine specimens. The changes are tremendously variable and unpredictable. Some cells may have loss of cytoplasm, while other cells may have increased cytoplasm. Nuclear borders may become indistinct, or the nucleus may shrink and become pyknotic. The most well-described degenerative change is the presence of Melamed-Wolinska bodies, seen as dense and spherical cytoplasmic inclusions, which appear homogenously red or green on the Papanicolaou stain (Fig. 15.8).[25] Identifying the amount of degeneration present in a urinary tract specimen is important for two reasons. First, benign cells with degenerative changes may be flagged as atypical if they assume features that mimic HGUC. On the other hand, degenerated HGUC cells may lose diagnostic features. A urinary tract specimen may contain numerous HGUC cells, but extensive degeneration may mean rare to few HGUC cells meet the diagnostic criteria for the *HGUC* category. Degenerated HGUC cells often have pyknotic nuclei and expanded cytoplasm, resulting in N/C ratios below 0.7.[26,27]

Background components in a urinary tract specimen include bacteria, fungal elements, spermatozoa, proteinaceous debris, red blood cells,

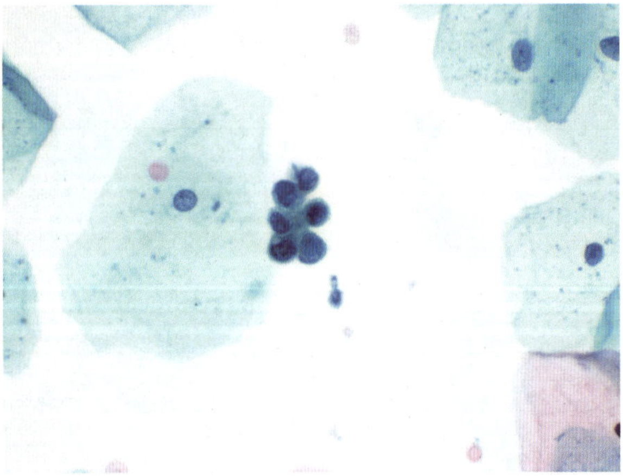

FIGURE 15.7 **Renal tubular cells.** Renal tubular cells are often very small and degenerated when found in urinary tract specimens. However, they are also hyperchromatic, which can cause distraction. Occasionally, these cells are misidentified as atypical urothelial cells. They may form clusters, which have a hobnailed appearance to their borders. When seen together with casts in a patient experiencing hematuria, a nonneoplastic renal process is favored.

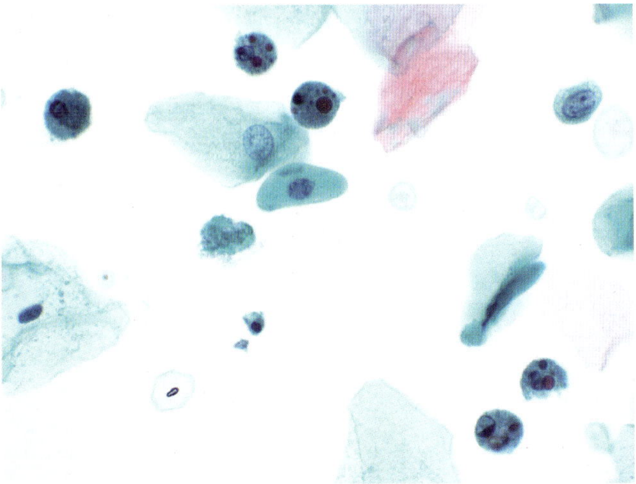

FIGURE 15.8 **Melamed-Wolinska bodies.** Melamed-Wolinska bodies are green and red dense, round inclusions found in the cytoplasm degenerated urothelial cells. They are found more commonly in voided urine specimens and simply serve as a marker specimen preservation.

casts, and crystals. While these factors are not necessarily normal and may represent a pathological process, they can distract from the primary goal of excluding HGUC and in most instances other laboratory tests are more appropriate for their clinical correlation. On occasion, macrophages may engulf spermatozoa, forming spermiophages, which can be distracting in urinary tract specimens[28] (Fig. 15.9).

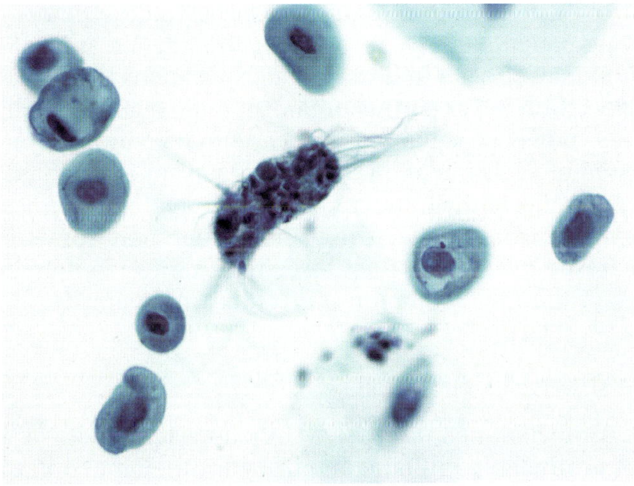

FIGURE 15.9 **Spermiophage.** A spermiophage is macrophage that has engulfed spermatozoa. The presence of spermiophages or spermatozoa in urinary tract specimens may be distracting but under most circumstances is not of clinical significance.

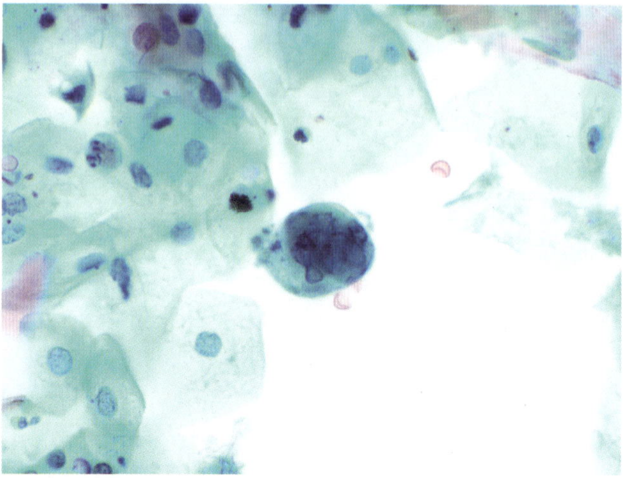

FIGURE 15.10 **Herpes simplex virus (HSV).** HSV can infect cells that originate from outside the urinary tract and be found as contaminants in urinary tract specimens. The morphology of multinucleated cells with molded nuclei containing glassy chromatin is typical of HSV seen in other cytology specimens. This clinically relevant finding should be reported.

Microbiological organisms may be contaminants from outside the urinary tract; a small number of organisms may grow into large colonies after specimen production and thus not correlate with a clinical infection. Occasionally, significant infections are present, which indicate a clinically relevant infection. The morphology of cytomegalovirus and herpes simplex virus infections is similar to that seen elsewhere, and these should be noted (Fig. 15.10). The most common parasites seen in urine specimens are contaminants from the gastrointestinal tract and include *Enterobius vermicularis.*[29] Among patients travelling or living in endemic areas, *Schistosoma haematobium* may be seen in urinary tract specimens (Fig. 15.11). There is a strong association between this organism and squamous cell carcinoma of the bladder; however, squamous cell carcinoma may arise in the bladder in the absence of such infection and the organism is rarely seen in laboratories outside the endemic areas. Vegetable material, typically present as a contaminant from outside the urinary tract, may sometimes be mistaken for parasite ova.[30] It is, therefore, important to be familiar with the morphology of the most common gastrointestinal parasites in the region of practice.

Low-Grade Urothelial Neoplasia

Low-grade urothelial neoplasia (LGUN) correlates with a histological diagnosis of urothelial papilloma, papillary urothelial neoplasm of uncertain malignant potential (PUNLMP), and low-grade urothelial carcinoma. Current literature and expert consensus do not support that such lesions can be diagnosed with enough accuracy that they deserve their own

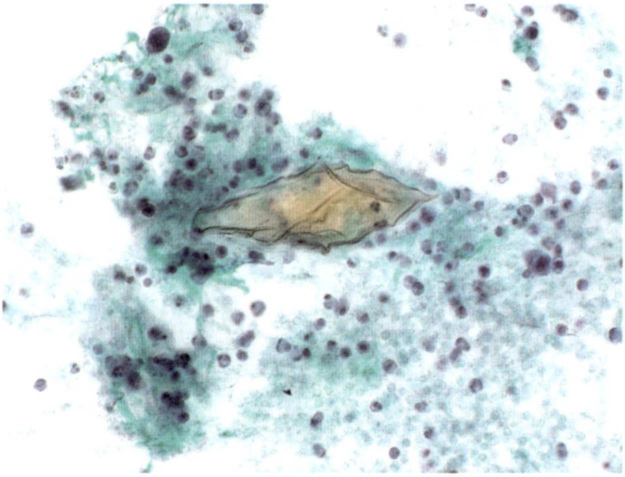

FIGURE 15.11 ***Schistosoma haematobium* ova.** *Schistosoma haematobium* ova may be found in patients from endemic areas (regions of the Middle East and Africa). The morphology can be similar to that of vegetable material or crystals, which are much more commonly found in urinary tract specimens. The most distinctive feature is the "terminal spine." *S haematobium* infection is a risk factor for primary squamous cell carcinoma of the bladder, but the parasite is often found in a background of inflammation and granular debris.

category or top-line diagnosis in urinary tract cytopathology. The second edition of TPS has removed LGUN as a distinct diagnostic category and recommends that such a diagnosis be made under the NHGUC category.[31] A note can be placed that states that features suggestive of LGUN are present. Cytomorphological features that have been reportedly associated with LGUN include three-dimensional cellular clusters, increased number of urothelial cells, cytoplasmic heterogeneity, and a slightly increased N/C ratio.[32-34] While some cytopathologists believe in some instances they can make an unequivocal diagnosis of LGUN, most evidence suggests that LGUN diagnoses in urinary tract cytopathology have poor PPV, sensitivity, and reproducibility.[5,17,32-40]

Although urinary tract cytology has poor accuracy for LGUN, it is acknowledged that LGUN can produce cytomorphological changes that can be identified in urinary tract specimens. These changes typically become more pronounced as the grade and size of the lesion increase–for instance, a large low-grade urothelial carcinoma is more likely to produce atypical findings than a small PUNLMP. Most often these changes are mild and cannot be distinguished from reactive changes, resulting in an atypical or indeterminate diagnosis. In some instances, true papillary fragments may be identified, which indicate the presence of a papillary neoplasm of indeterminate grade (Fig. 15.12). On occasion, the cytomorphological atypia may be present and result in a diagnosis of *Atypical Urothelial Cells* and rarely even *Suspicious for High-Grade Urothelial Carcinoma* (SHGUC) (see below).

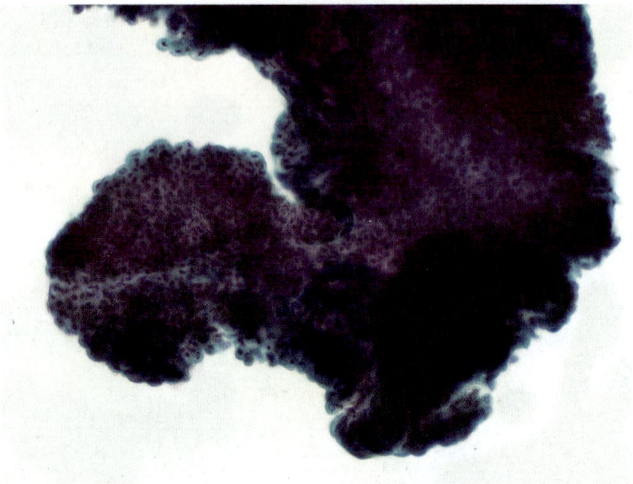

FIGURE 15.12 **True papillary fragments, indicative of a urothelial papillary neoplasm.** True papillary fragments contain vessels and are indicative of a neoplastic process, though these are only rarely found in urinary tract specimens. It is difficult to identify features of high-grade urothelial carcinoma (HGUC) in three-dimensional fragments, and thus, single cells in the background should be examined to help make this diagnosis. If features of HGUC are absent, grading papillary fragments by cytology alone is not recommended. In this particular instance, the patient had a papillary urothelial neoplasm of low malignant potential (PUNLMP) on follow-up biopsy.

Urothelial Tissue Fragments

The presence of urothelial tissue fragments in urinary tract specimens can often be explained by instrumentation; for instance, in a bladder washing specimen or in a patient with a urinary catheter. In other instances, pathophysiologic factors such as urolithiasis (either clinically detectable or inapparent) or infection may damage the tract and release urothelial tissue fragments into voided urine specimens. Other factors, such as recent exercise and prostatic massage, have been associated with urothelial tissue fragments in voided urine specimens. In most instances, the presence of urothelial tissue fragments cannot be identified.[41,42]

While in the past there has been some speculation that urothelial tissue fragments in voided urine specimens are associated with LGUN, a recent study has shown only an insignificant increased risk for a low-grade lesion when benign-appearing urothelial tissue fragments are present in voided urine specimens, and these findings are best diagnosed as *NHGUC* with a note describing their presence.[41] If the urothelial tissue fragments contain cells with atypical morphology (atypical urothelial tissue fragments) in a voided urine specimen, then the risk of HGUC becomes similar to the *Atypical Urothelial Cells* category (see below) and these specimens should be classified as such.[43] Interestingly, the study found no association between atypical urothelial tissue fragments and low-grade lesions, only HGUC.

The presence of urothelial fragments containing true papillae should be specifically noted, as they indicate the presence of a papillary lesion. Grading papillary lesions in the absence of diagnostic high-grade features is treacherous, as a papillary lesion with focal high-grade areas can potentially be misdiagnosed as a low-grade lesion. If no features of HGUC are identified, a diagnosis of *NHGUC* is most appropriate; otherwise, the specimen should be stratified into the appropriate category based on the atypical cytomorphological features present within the fragment or in individual cells.

BK (Polyoma) Virus Cytopathic Effect

TPS currently recommends that BK (polyoma) virus cytopathic effect be classified under the *NHGUC* category. BK virus remains dormant in most individuals and can occasionally be identified in cells shed into the urine from normal individuals. However, re-activation of BK virus occurs most commonly in immunocompromised patients, and in the past renal transplant patients have had their urine specimens monitored for the presence of BK cytopathic effect.[44]

The cytomorphological changes seen in BK cytopathic effect include an enlarged nucleus containing either homogenously "ground glass" chromatin or degenerated chromatin with a "spider web" type appearance (Fig. 15.13). Typically, the nucleus will have very smooth nuclear borders,

FIGURE 15.13 **BK (polyoma) virus cytopathic effect (CPE).** BK (polyoma) virus remains dormant in infected hosts, and urinary tract specimens may demonstrate BK cytopathic effect (CPE) even in asymptomatic, healthy patients. Typical cytomorphological features include a nucleus with smooth borders and chromatin with a "ground-glass appearance." Cells are often degenerated with little or absent cytoplasm; while the N/C ratio may be increased, BK CPE never results in the coarse, clumpy chromatin seen in high-grade urothelial carcinoma.

as opposed to the irregular borders typically seen in HGUC. The enlarged nucleus results in an increased N/C ratio, which may cause BK cytopathic effect to be mistaken for features of HGUC, thus the name *decoy cells* has been assigned to cells demonstrated BK cytopathic effect.[45] In addition to differences in chromatin quality and nuclear border regularity, decoy cells do not become as large as some HGUC and are rarely present in large numbers if the patient is immunocompetent.

Atypical Squamous Cells

In some patients, regions of the urothelial lining may be replaced by stratified squamous epithelium. This component may seem atypical compared to the typical superficial squamous cells in urine specimens. Under certain pathophysiological conditions, dysplastic cells may be present and represent a precursor to squamous cell carcinoma; in primary squamous cell carcinoma of the bladder or HGUC with squamous differentiation, rare atypical squamous cells may be seen if the lesion is not well represented in the specimen.

Dysplastic-appearing squamous cells or koilocytes may contaminate the urinary tract and represent infection with human papillomavirus (HPV). This is true regardless of whether the patient is male or female, and in many instances, it is not possible to determine an origin (urinary tract vs contaminant) based on urinary tract alone. Studies have shown that significant lesions can be identified on follow-up among women with such changes.[46,47] Therefore, changes should be noted as "atypical squamous cells of uncertain origin" with a note suggesting the possibility of an extraurinary tract origin.

Neobladder and Ileal Conduit Specimens

Following cystectomy, partial cystectomy, or cystoprostatectomy, a patient ideally will undergo reconstructive surgery to allow diversion of urinary flow. Most commonly, a segment of the small intestine can be used to create either a urinary neobladder, which preserves flow through the urethra, or an ileal conduit, which diverts flow through an abdominal stoma. Because these patients often have a history of infiltrating HGUC, they are at great risk for recurrence due to multifocal and/or residual disease. Specimens often contain a heavy background degenerating epithelial cells and debris and may only have few normal urothelial cells. It can be challenging to distinguish degenerating benign cells from degenerating carcinoma cells (Fig. 15.14A and B).

Given the high pretest probability of HGUC in these samples, extra time should be spent finding HGUC cells that may be obscured. Because these patients undergo frequent surveillance, indeterminate diagnoses are often not useful; furthermore, recurrence portends a poor prognosis as these patients have limited treatment options.[48]

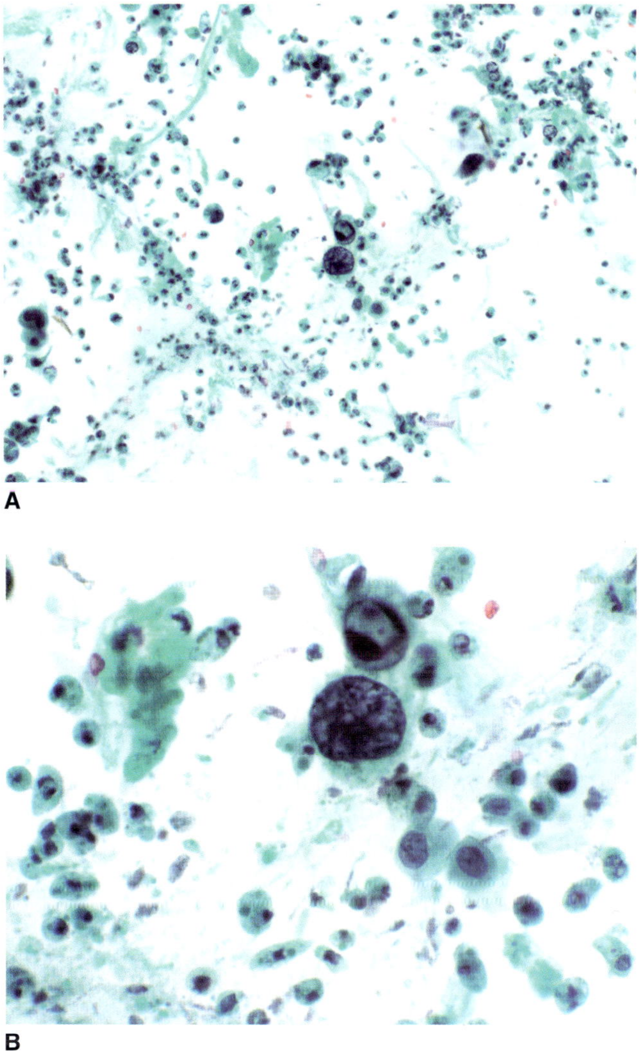

FIGURE 15.14 **Recurrent high-grade urothelial carcinoma in an ileal conduit specimen.** Specimens from patients with an ileal conduit or urinary neobladder usually contain a busy background with numerous degenerating and inflammatory cells. Urothelial cells may be rare and difficult to identify. Because these patients often have a history of infiltrating urothelial carcinoma, they have a high risk of recurrence, and the specimen should be examined carefully. Several hyperchromatic cells seen at low power **(A)** have features diagnostic for high-grade urothelial carcinoma when viewed at high power **(B)**.

Reactive Changes

The urothelial lining may be exposed to trauma (eg, urolithiasis or instrumentation) and infection, and reactive changes can sometimes mimic the atypia seen with urothelial neoplasia. Typically, cells will be enlarged with increased nuclear size; hyperchromasia and nuclear border irregularities may be present. In particular, "stone atypia" is used to describe changes secondary to urolithiasis: an increased amount of urothelial tissue fragments, nuclear enlargement, slightly increased N/C ratio, degenerative changes, and squamous metaplasia.[49,50] For this reason, following the criteria outlined by TPS is important to prevent an overdiagnosis of reactive changes. The presence of greatly elevated N/C ratios and/or coarse, clumpy chromatin is not typically due to benign reactive changes. Distinct nucleoli, a common finding in reactive glandular cells seen in other pathology specimens, are not a common feature of benign reactive urothelial cells.

Malakoplakia

The presence of histiocytes in a urinary tract specimen may be secondary to infection or treatment effect but careful consideration should include the possibility of malakoplakia. While traditional cytologic preparations make a definitive diagnosis difficult, special stains (eg, von Kossa) performed on residual material may confirm the presence of Michaelis-Gutmann bodies.[51]

Seminal Vesicle Cells

Seminal vesicle cells are rarely identified in urine specimens. Such cells are large with abundant cytoplasm and are primary distinguished by the presence of golden cytoplasmic pigment and associated spermatozoa.[52] These cells are typically just a distraction, though the abundant pigmented cytoplasm may result in them being mistaken for renal cell carcinoma (RCC), prostate adenocarcinoma, or melanoma.

Cystitis Glandularis

Cystitis glandularis occurs with glandular metaplasia of the urothelial lining, usually in response to chronic infections. Columnar cells are seen in the background, which may be mistaken for urothelial cells with cytoplasmic tails in washing specimens. Often patients have recurrent infections and thus inflammatory cells and/or bacteria may also be present. These findings are typically just distractors, though occasionally fragments of reactive glandular epithelium may appear more hyperchromatic and crowded, giving an atypical appearance compared to urothelial tissue fragments.[53]

Vesicoenteric Fistula

Patients with a history of abdominal or pelvic surgery, or with a history of Crohn disease, are at risk of developing microscopic vesicoenteric fistulas that result in recurrent urinary tract infections but may otherwise be subclinical. In these instances, findings in a urine specimen may be the first

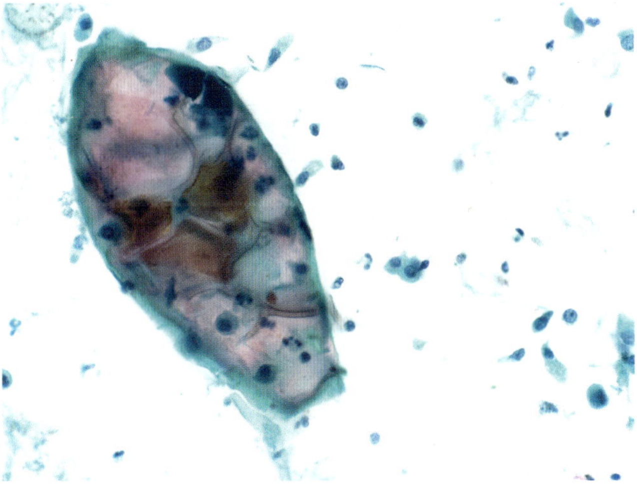

FIGURE 15.15 **Vegetable material.** Vegetable material is often a contaminant from outside the urinary tract in voided urine specimens. However, this patient had a history of Crohn disease, and the presence of inflammatory cells and glandular cells strongly suggested the possibility of a vesiculoenteric fistula. Such a diagnosis could be confirmed by a catheterized urine sample.

to suggest a fistula tract.[54] In addition to the discovery of certain infections or malignancy, this is an instance in which urinary tract findings are medically critical. The most striking finding is typically the presence of abundant foreign material, such as vegetable material or striated muscle (Fig. 15.15). The background typically contains columnar cells (representing gastrointestinal tract cells) as well as bacteria and inflammatory cells. Because the presence of vegetable material is the sole feature to distinguish this entity from cystitis glandularis with active infection, it is important to prove that the foreign material is not a contaminant. In patients with a history of surgery or Crohn disease, or with more obvious symptoms of a fistula (such as pneumaturia), the findings are strongly suggestive. A "clean catch" urine or catheterized urine should not be contaminated with vegetable material and confirms the diagnosis of a vesicoenteric fistula.

SUSPICIOUS FOR HIGH-GRADE UROTHELIAL CARCINOMA

The TPS category SHGUC should be utilized when the cytologic features seen in a specimen place the patient at high risk for having HGUC, but overall the specimen falls short of the criteria required for a HGUC diagnosis. This is usually due to an insufficient quantity of overtly malignant cells, though the *SHGUC* category can also be used when the amount of cytomorphologic atypia is concerning, but not diagnostic of, HGUC. Prior to TPS, the PPVs of the *SHGUC* and equivalent categories varies by institution and follow-up period but ranges from 37.8% to 79% given a 6-

month follow-up period.[7-9,55] When the follow-up period is extended, the PPV for this category approaches 95% in some institutions.[8] The largest of these studies demonstrated a similar PPV for patients with new symptoms as compared to those undergoing surveillance (79% vs 76%, respectively), though a second slightly smaller study demonstrated a higher PPV among the surveillance group than the nonsurveillance group (65.6% vs 56.2%). One issue with such analysis concerns the possibility that new (multifocal) lesions may arise during long follow-up periods, confounding interpretation of the results. Among laboratories implementing TPS, the risk of high-grade malignancy for the *SHGUC* category has ranged from 33.3% to 100%.[56] Given that the *SHGUC* category is not completely predictive of HGUC and the PPV rate varies greatly between institutions/pathologists, it is not recommended that significant treatment (eg, nephrectomy) be given based on a *SHGUC* diagnosis alone. However, given the historically overall poor PPV of indeterminate diagnoses in urinary tract cytopathology, a "suspicious" designation should convey to the clinical team that the patient is at high risk for HGUC. In some institutions, the *SHGUC* replaces indeterminate categories previously labelled with the phrase "cannot exclude HGUC." In such instances, it is important that clinicians be made aware that the *SHGUC* category is meant to convey the same risk.

TPS defines specific criteria to meet a diagnosis of *SHGUC* in order to preserve the predictive value of the category. These criteria are similar to those used for the *HGUC* category:

1. High N/C ratio. Atypical cells should have an N/C ratio of ~0.7 or greater.

   Additionally, two of the following three features must be present:

1. Markedly irregular nuclear borders
2. Coarse, clumpy chromatin
3. Moderate to severe hyperchromasia

According to TPS, the quantity of cells meeting these criteria will primarily determine whether the *HGUC* or *SHGUC* category should be used. TPS does not define an exact number of cells but recommends between 5 and 10 cells as a possible cutoff. The cutoff may vary between pathologists based on experience, though specificity for HGUC should remain high when using the *HGUC* category.

ATYPICAL UROTHELIAL CELLS

The atypical category has been criticized as being a "wastebasket" category in which many abnormal findings have been placed regardless of whether they are features concerning for HGUC.[57] While in part this has been due to the subjective nature and poor reproducibility of atypical diagnoses in cytopathology; in the past, specimens have been diagnosed as "atypical" over concern for the presence of *LGUN*. Now that TPS recommends the terminology *NHGUC*, pathologists can feel comfortable placing specimens in that category rather than labeling them "atypical," so long as features of HGUC are absent.

In order to preserve and improve the PPV of the *Atypical Urothelial Cells* category, the following feature is required to be present in the cells of question:

1. High N/C ratio. Atypical cells should have an N/C ratio of ~0.5 or greater.

   And one of the following:

1. Hyperchromasia. The hyperchromasia may not be as pronounced as in *HGUC* or *Suspicious for HGUC* but still distinct from what is seen in the surrounding benign urothelial cells.
2. Irregular cell borders.
3. Coarse, clumpy chromatin.

There is no required quantity of atypical cells to merit an *AUC* diagnosis; even a single atypical cell qualifies. However, studies have demonstrated that the number of atypical cells present correlates with risk for HGUC.[58] In many instances, atypical diagnoses result from scantly cellular specimens in which only rare cells are atypical; the presence of a single atypical cell in a specimen containing numerous benign urothelial cells is of questionable significance.

The *AUC* category should only be used to imply that the patient is at increased risk of HGUC. If atypical changes are believed to be secondary to infection, urolithiasis, specimen degeneration, BK cytopathic effect, benign-appearing tissue fragments, or other etiologies, then the specimen should not be classified as *AUC*. Historically, the PPV of atypical categories has ranged greatly (8.3%-37.5%) among institutions in published literature, and this was expected to greatly improve with the adoption of TPS.[4,10,39,49,55,59-63] Published studies from laboratories implementing TPS have shown the rate of high-grade malignancy of the AUC category to range from 12.3% to 60.9%.[56] Because some institutions are referral centers with an increased frequency of urothelial carcinoma, the *AUC* diagnosis rate likely correlates with the frequency of HGUC diagnoses.

OTHER DIAGNOSES

Primary Squamous Cell Carcinoma

Primary squamous cell carcinoma of the bladder is uncommon except in areas endemic for *S haematobium*, which generally includes regions of Africa and the Middle East. The parasite's preference for the vascular plexus surrounding the bladder results in inflammation and other factors that culminate in squamous cell carcinoma. In such instances, urothelial carcinoma is not a precursor lesion and is usually not present. *S haematobium* have a distinct morphology and are distinguished from other schistosome ova by the presence of a terminal spine, though other schistosome ova should not be present in urine specimens; if anything, vegetable material may be mistaken for *S haematobium* ova.[30,64] Even in primary squamous cell carcinomas secondary to *S haematobium*, the ova are not commonly seen.

Primary squamous cell carcinoma can also occur in the absence of *S haematobium* infection but is uncommon; in individuals from nonendemic region without the appropriate travel history, such an infection should not be suspected. Because the presence of squamous cell carcinoma in a specimen cannot entirely exclude an unsampled or absent urothelial carcinoma component, a direct diagnosis of squamous cell carcinoma is not possible with urinary tract cytology alone. It is recommended that such lesions be diagnosed as "carcinoma with squamous features." The cytologic features are as seen elsewhere for squamous cell carcinoma.

Primary Adenocarcinoma

Primary adenocarcinoma of the bladder is rare and typically has an intestinal differentiation.[65] The cytologic features are as seen elsewhere for adenocarcinoma. As previously mentioned, care must be taken to exclude a urothelial component, and thus, the presence of adenocarcinoma should be diagnosed as "carcinoma with glandular features" on urinary tract cytology alone. Clinical history may suggest involvement by a patient's known carcinoma, such as a colon primary.

Small Cell Carcinoma

Primary small cell carcinoma of the bladder is rare, and typically when small cell carcinoma is identified in urine specimens, the cells originate from the prostate. Small cell carcinoma can arise *de novo* in the prostate as a pure neoplasm or arise mixed with prostate adenocarcinoma. Approximately one-third of prostatic small cell carcinomas occur following chemoradiation of prostate cancer; therefore, the presence of small cell carcinoma may correlate with a history of prostate cancer. Very rarely does small cell carcinoma in the urine present as a metastasis from other sites, such as the lung. Cervical small cell carcinoma can also extend into the urinary tract. A patient's cancer history or newly diagnosed symptoms should suggest a secondary site, except in some cases of prostatic or urothelial small cell carcinoma.

Small cell carcinoma can be challenging to diagnose on urinary tract cytology because many of the classic features of small cell carcinoma are absent or reduced in liquid-based preparations.[66,67] In particular, necrotic cells and material may be washed away. Tumor cells tend to disassociate, which may reduce the amount of molding. The cells are better preserved due to reduced manipulation as compared to other preparations, and the Azzopardi phenomenon ("streaking artifact") may not be seen. The disassociated small cells may initially appear as lymphocytes and mimic lymphoma or inflammation, though lymphocytosis in urine specimens is rare.

The presence of only small cellular fragments limits the identification of geographic necrosis. Therefore, the proper identification of small cell carcinoma relies on the presence of numerous small cells with a neuroendocrine-type chromatin. On closer examination, the cells are larger than lymphocytes and lack the cytoplasmic rim usually seen in lymphocytes. A large number of the cells will be necrotic and appear as degenerated, small, disassociated blobs (Fig. 15.16).

If only small cell carcinoma is present, a diagnosis of small cell carcinoma can be rendered. However, careful examination for the presence of HGUC cells or prostatic adenocarcinoma cells should be undertaken, especially in patients without a known history of either malignancy. Unless poorly differentiated, a urothelial vs prostatic origin can usually be determined based on differences in cytomorphology alone. However, occasionally the accompanying malignant cells may be difficult to classify, in which case immunohistochemistry can be performed on any residual material. The presence of a urothelial component merits a diagnosis under the *HGUC* category rather than *Other* category–for example, "*HGUC with a small cell component*."

Prostate Carcinoma

Prostate carcinoma may involve the urinary tract by direct extension or metastasis. Prostate carcinoma cells have foamy cytoplasm, round nuclei

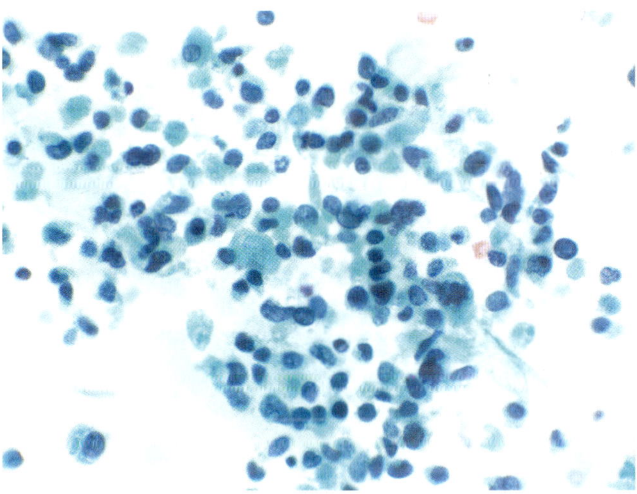

FIGURE 15.16 **Small cell carcinoma.** Small cell carcinoma in liquid-based preparations may be difficult to identify. The cells tend to disassociate, which may reduce the amount of nuclear molding that is otherwise seen in small cell carcinoma. Furthermore, necrosis may "wash away" in such preparations, and chromatin streaking artifact is not commonly seen. At first glance on low power, one may mistake the cells for lymphocytes. In the field shown, necrotic tumor cells intermingle with the carcinoma cells, providing a suggestion of geographic necrosis. Other important features include nuclei that are variably enlarged with nuclear border irregularities and speckled chromatin; these help distinguish the cells from lymphocytes.

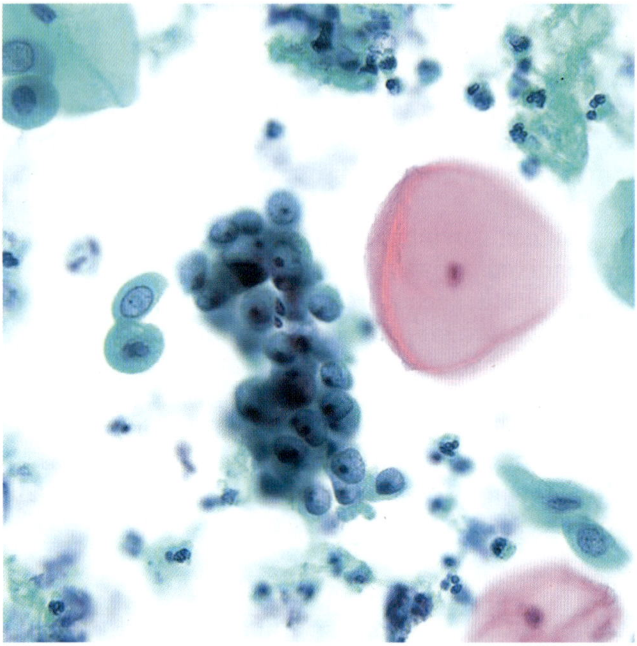

FIGURE 15.17 **Prostate carcinoma.** Prominent nucleoli are not commonly seen in high-grade urothelial carcinomas (HGUC) and suggest the possibility of prostate carcinoma involving the urinary tract. Typically, these cells have round and regular nuclear borders and maintain a greater amount of cytoplasm than HGUC cells. However, in some instances, it can be challenging to distinguish HGUC from prostate carcinoma cells using cytomorphology alone, and ancillary studies should be performed on residual material if possible.

with regular borders, and a prominent nucleolus (Fig. 15.17). Cells may exist singly or in fragments; if present, fragments may be sheetlike or have an underlying acinar pattern.[68] Single cells share cytomorphological overlap with RCC and melanoma, but occasionally, it may be difficult to distinguish prostate from urothelial carcinoma. Immunoperoxidase staining of residual material using prostate-specific markers (eg, PSA, NKX3.1, PSMA, or prostein) can allow for a definitive diagnosis if the patient does not have a known history of prostate carcinoma.

Renal Cell Carcinoma

Under most circumstances, nonurothelial tumors identified on imaging studies do not shed cells into the urinary tract. Imaging studies typically can distinguish between urothelial and nonurothelial tumors. On the rare occasion that nonurothelial renal neoplasms are found in urinary tract specimens, they are from renal cortical carcinomas, such as clear cell RCC. The cells usually maintain their classic cytologic appearance, possessing abundant granular cytoplasm, an eccentric nucleus, and a prominent nucleolus.[69] This cytomorphology may mimic that of melanoma and/or prostate cancer, thus in the absence of a RCC history or current renal tumor, care should be taken to suggest rather than definitively diagnosis RCC. If residual material remains, immunoperoxidase studies to identify a possible renal origin can be performed. Attempts to subclassify RCCs present in urinary tract cytology specimens are discouraged.

Lymphoma

Lymphoma of the urinary tract is rare and may involve the urinary tract primarily or secondarily; the most commonly seen lymphomas are MALT lymphoma and diffuse large B-cell lymphoma.[70] High-grade lymphomas can be identified by their malignant features, but ancillary studies may be required if the malignant cells do not have morphological features of a lymphoid origin.[71] Low-grade lymphomas may appear as lymphocytosis, which is uncommon in urinary tract specimens but may be secondary to infection or other benign processes.[72] Ancillary testing is required in such instances to prove whether a clonal population of lymphocytes exists.

Colonic Adenocarcinoma

Colonic adenocarcinoma typically involves the urinary tract through direct extension though metastasis is also possible. Colonic adenocarcinoma has a distinct morphology and produces malignant cells with hyperchromatic nuclei, glandular fragments with a "picket fence" appearance, and abundant necrosis and debris. Patients should have a history of colonic adenocarcinoma, or strong clinical suspicion of a gastrointestinal tract malignancy, by the time the urinary tract is involved. Special caution should be observed if this is not the case or the clinical history is unknown, because primary adenocarcinoma of the bladder typically has colonic differentiation and will appear similar.[65] Furthermore, high-grade dysplasia of glandular epithelium present in the bladder (eg, at sites of intestinal metaplasia or villous adenoma) may present with similar-appearing fragments.[73]

Anogenital Tract Lesions

In women, contamination from the gynecologic tract is common in voided urinary tract specimens. While the incidence of gynecologic tract squamous cell carcinoma has greatly decreased in the United States, gynecologic tract dysplasia secondary to HPV is not uncommon, and koilocytes (representing a low-grade squamous intraepithelial lesion [LSIL]) may be found in urinary tract specimens. High-grade squamous intraepithelial lesions (HSILs) are often more challenging to identify, especially if only present as rare cells. If koilocytic or dysplastic changes are seen, they should be noted in the report for the purpose of clinical correlation. Studies have shown that majority of women with these findings have nonurologic tract pathology on follow-up.

It is important to note that atypical squamous cells may also be contaminants from other regions of the anogenital tract where squamous dysplasia and carcinoma may arise from primary lesions of the bladder with squamous differentiation.[74] A catheterized urinary tract specimen containing such cells strongly suggests a urinary tract origin. In most laboratories, the same HPV testing methodology used for PAP tests has not been developed for use in urinary tract specimens, and in such cases, reflex HPV testing of the residual urine specimen is invalid and cannot provide a clinically reportable result. If a high-grade lesion is suspected, residual material can be tested using p16 immunoperoxidase staining or HPV *in situ* hybridization studies. In female patients without a recent PAP test, a follow-up PAP test may provide the quickest solution.

Nonprimary Squamous Cell Carcinoma

Squamous cell carcinoma typically invades from nearby anogenital region but may also be a contaminant from this region in voided urine specimens.[74] Because squamous cell carcinoma can also occur primary to the urinary tract, clinical correlation is often necessary to identify the primary site. Ancillary tests demonstrating the presence of HPV, or diffuse p16 immunoperoxidase staining in lesional cells, suggest an anogenital rather than urinary tract origin if not already clinically obvious.

Melanoma

Melanoma may involve the urinary tract as a metastatic disease and rarely as a primary tumor, but care must be taken to exclude the possibility that melanoma cells are not contaminants from outside the urinary tract.[75,76] Melanoma appears as it does in other cytologic specimens, typically as single cells with abundant cytoplasm, an eccentric nucleus, and a prominent nucleolus. This morphology overlaps with that of RCC and prostate carcinoma, which are always of concern in urinary tract specimens given their anatomic proximity. Pigment is not always produced, but its presence strongly suggests the possibility of melanoma. Benign seminal vesicle cells are occasionally seen in urinary tract specimens; these cells are pigmented and should not be overinterpreted as melanoma. If possible, immunoperoxidase staining can be performed on residual material to confirm the diagnosis.

SPECIMEN PROCUREMENT AND PREPARATION

Poor specimen preservation and/or preparation often limit the definitive interpretation of urinary tract cytology specimens. In addition to ensuring a good quality specimen preparation, the pathologist should help develop a system that allows the proper collection, storage, and transport of the specimen to the laboratory.

Urine is a toxic environment for cells, and degeneration is a common artifact in urinary tract specimens. Voided urine specimens always contain some amount of degeneration due to the time urothelial cells have spent in the bladder prior to the void. Thus, rapid transport to and processing by the cytopathology laboratory is critical to preserving the remaining cytomorphology. If urine specimens cannot be immediately processed, they should be immediately refrigerated and then processed the next morning. A concentration step must be performed before the cells can truly well preserved or fixed in additive solutions.

Overall, there is no recommended preparation method by TPS. Urine specimens may be prepared by a number of concentration techniques such as Cytospin, SurePath, or ThinPrep. Some laboratories use a filter paper preparation or conventional smears of urinary sediment. Specimens are then stained by either a Giemsa-based stain such as Diff-Quik or a Papanicolaou stain, with Papanicolaou staining being the most common. An H&E stain is sometimes used in laboratories that have low cytopathology volumes; in many instances, these H&E-stained preparations are of poor quality and limit the cytomorphological features that otherwise would provide a definitive diagnosis. It is recommended that residual specimens be stored until a final diagnosis is rendered; occasionally, residual specimens can be used for immunoperoxidase staining or other ancillary studies once the original slides have been reviewed.

ADEQUACY

Unlike several other cytopathology specimen types, urinary tract cytopathology has no well-defined criteria for adequacy and little scientific evidence exists to guide adequacy assignment. Some aspects of adequacy include specimen volume, the amount of urothelial cells present, obscuring features (inflammation and squamous cells), and the amount of specimen degeneration. Specimen type partially determines adequacy, since specimen volume applies to voided urine specimens and is irrelevant in washing specimens where a predefined volume is used. Conversely, it is not unusual for a large volume voided urine sample to have relatively few cells, whereas a sparsely cellular washing specimen may indicate an inadequately performed procedure.

Two studies of voided urine volumes indicated that specimens with <25-30 mL of urine volume were associated with an increased risk of a false-negative diagnosis.[77,78] This suggests that a minimum volume of voided urine should be submitted to the laboratory to properly exclude HGUC, though no consensus exists regarding the exact amount. A specimen containing few urothelial cells and low volume should be noted, and an early repeat sample has been shown to be beneficial in reducing the false positive rate.

The purpose of a washing specimen is to obtain an adequate sampling of urothelial cells. Therefore, a washing specimen with only few to rare urothelial cells should be noted and perhaps repeated. A study by Prather et al. found that a minimum of 2644 urothelial cells (20 per 10 hpf) statistically improves the PPV of a urinary tract washing specimen.[79] This study examined ThinPrep preparations; a second study from another laboratory using Cytospin preparations found that the false-negative rate was significantly increased when <10 urothelial cells per 10 hpf were present.[80]

The presence of extensive degeneration and/or obscuring factors should be noted, especially if the majority of urothelial cells are degenerated or obscured. The reason for degeneration should be identified and a fresh specimen should be obtained. The problem may be due to delay in transport to the laboratory or a delay in laboratory processing. The presence of numerous atypical degenerated cells may indicate an upper tract lesion in which the cells are too degenerated to make a definitive diagnosis. In such cases, cystoscopy to provide upper tract washing specimens may be indicated.

To eliminate obscuring squamous cells, the production of a "clean catch" specimen should be emphasized, although cystoscopy or catheterization may be indicated to prevent contamination from outside the urinary tract. This can be useful when the squamous cells contain some atypia and may represent a lesion from outside the urinary tract, such as squamous dysplasia in the gynecologic tract. If abundant bacteria and/or inflammation obscure cellular features, then the patient may need to submit an additional sample following treatment of a urinary tract infection. Because neoplasms may cause obstruction and/or necrosis, sometimes complete clearance may not be possible. Cystoscopy with sequential washing steps may be beneficial in such circumstances.

ANCILLARY TESTING

Several ancillary methods have been used either alone or in combination with urinary tract cytopathology to improve the sensitivity for detecting urothelial neoplasms. The most successful commercial method to date has been the use of fluorescence *in situ* hybridization (FISH) for chromosomal aberrations commonly found in urothelial carcinoma. The original test was developed by Abbott Laboratories and known as UroVysion. The examination of these ancillary testing techniques is outside the scope of this chapter, but UroVysion will be discussed as an example of how ancillary testing can enhance class urinary tract cytomorphology.

Ancillary tests can occur on whole urine, urine supernatants, or on the cells present in the urine specimen. If the urine specimen will also be used for cytologic analysis, then the specimen must at some point be split. Some tests detect the expression of abnormal proteins in urothelial neoplasms, which are found in tumor cells and/or in the urine specimen when the proteins are either excreted or leaked from degenerating tumor cells. These proteins can be detected in a laboratory using antibody-based techniques or developed into point-of-care testing (POCT) devices. Since

POCT may be conducted in an office or cystoscopy suite, the results of such tests may not be readily available to the pathologist for correlation with the cytology specimen. However, since these proteins are often dissociated from the tumor cells that produce them, such tests may have a positive result even if tumor cells are absent in the tested specimen.

Other methods may use genetic material and identify alterations, such as DNA mutations, commonly found in urothelial neoplasms. These assays typically require the presence of tumor cells, although investigation of "cell-free" genetic material is ongoing. Slide-based assays, such as UroVysion, require tumor cells to be present in a slide, which is then used for the assay. In the case of UroVysion, fluorescent probes have been designed to identify chromosomes 3, 7, and 17 as well as the locus 9p21 (Figs. 15.18 and 15.19). Other assays may use probes against specific genetic or protein targets and ultimately detected using a secondary probe associated with a fluorescent or chromogenic signal. One benefit of such assays is that the detected abnormality can be better associated with atypical cells, which allows for improved specificity.

Just as urinary tract cytopathology is associated with a "false false positive" or "anticipatory positive" phenomenon, the same phenomenon can be seen with ancillary tests.[81] This is due to the increased sensitivity of many of these tests over urinary tract cytopathology–a patient may have a positive test result before a positive urinary tract cytopathology result, and in turn a positive urinary tract cytopathology result prior to a positive cystoscopy and/or biopsy result. While frustrating, positive results can guide

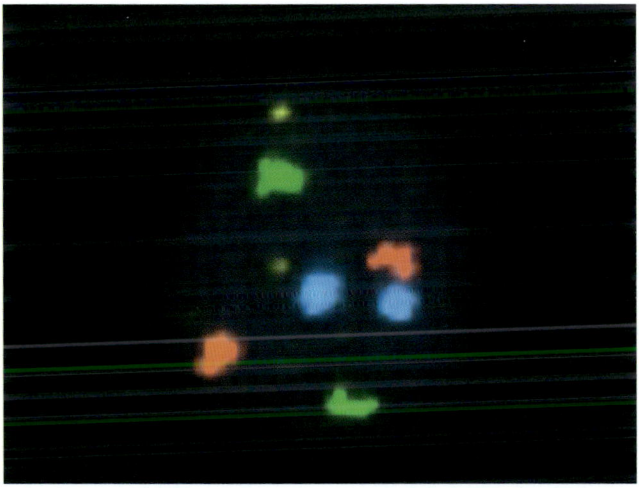

FIGURE 15.18 **UroVysion fluorescence *In situ* hybridization (FISH) assay, normal signal.** The UroVysion probe set looking for various colored fluorophores to specific DNA sequences matching the centromeres of chromosomes 3, 7, and 17. It also includes a locus-specific gold-colored fluoroprobe to 9p21 where several tumor suppressor genes, including p16, reside. In this instance, two signals for each probe are seen in a normal cell. (Image courtesy of Dr. Tehmina Z. Ali, Chesapeake Urology.)

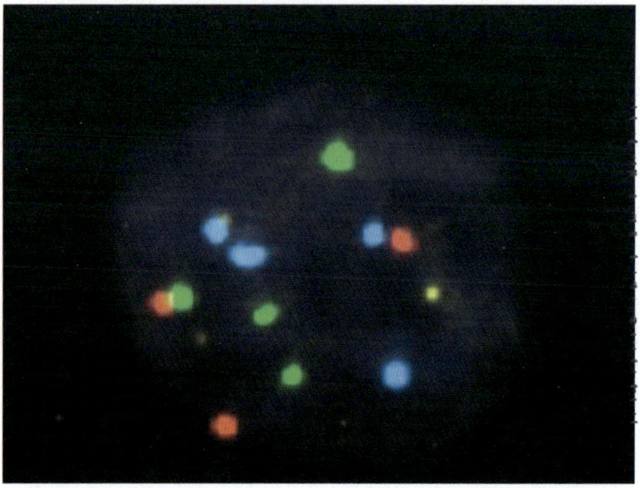

FIGURE 15.19 **UroVysion fluorescence *in situ* hybridization (FISH) assay, abnormal signal.** An abnormal UroVysion probe pattern, with more than two signals seen for the blue, green, and red probes. (Image courtesy of Dr. Tehmina Z. Ali, Chesapeake Urology.)

a more rigorous evaluation of the patient, leading to earlier detection of the lesion.[82]

UroVysion

UroVysion is an FDA-approved fluorescent *in situ* hybridization assay used for primary detection and surveillance of HGUC in urinary specimens (U-FISH). While U-FISH is currently the most commonly performed urinary tract ancillary test in the United States, it has not gained universal acceptance. U-FISH probes are specific to the 9p21 band and to the centromeres of chromosomes 3, 7, and 17 (Figs. 15.19 and 15.20). Proper interpretation requires the examination of multiple cells for patterns indicative for chromosomal aberrations. In general, the more subtle the genetic alterations (loss of signal to 9p21 or trisomy 7), the greater the number of cells required to view the FISH result as positive. Conversely, it takes fewer polysomic cells (defined as four or more cells with gains of two or more chromosomes) to establish a sample as positive and polysomic. The overall sensitivity and specificity has been reported to be 72% and 83%, respectively,[83] and the sensitivity ranges from 65% to 73% for pTa tumors and 95% to 100% for pT1-T4 urothelial carcinomas.[84,85] The phenomenon of anticipatory positive results is seen with U-FISH, with approximately two-thirds of surveillance patients testing positive U-FISH developing a recurrence in 29 months despite being negative by cytology and cystoscopy.[81]

In studies examining the usefulness of FISH performed on voided urine specimens for detecting upper tract urothelial carcinomas, the reported sensitivities ranged greatly from 35% to 87.5%. These data are inconclusive, but together with other studies suggest that upper tract malignancies might be better detected using FISH on upper tract washing specimens rather than voided urine specimens. Historically, results have been mixed regarding the use of U-FISH on equivocal cytology specimens, possibly due to inconsistent use of the atypical category prior to TPS. Studies of U-FISH among laboratories that have implemented TPS are limited. However, one recent study from a laboratory utilizing TPS found that 44% of AUC specimens were U-FISH positive and 89% of positive cases were associated with urothelial carcinoma on follow-up.[86] U-FISH may also be useful in patients receiving intravesical BCG treatment, with several studies demonstrating a higher risk of recurrence among patients with either cytologic HGUC diagnoses or positive U-FISH, compared to those with negative results.[87-89] Three months has been recommended as an interval for performing U-FISH after the initial transurethral resection of non–muscle-invasive bladder cancer.[89,90]

REFERENCES

1. Papanicolaou GN. Cytology of the urine sediment in neoplasms of the urinary tract. *J Urol*. 1947;57(2):375-379.
2. Papanicolaou GN, Marshall VF. Urine sediment smears as a diagnostic procedure in cancers of the urinary tract. *Science*. 1945;101(2629):519-520.
3. Pambuccian SE. The history of urinary cytology: the long and winding road to Paris 2.0. In: *The Paris System for Reporting Urinary Cytology*. Springer; 2022:267-315.
4. Rosenthal DL, Vandenbussche CJ, Burroughs FH, et al. The Johns Hopkins Hospital template for urologic cytology samples: part I-creating the template. *Cancer Cytopathol*. 2013;121(1):15-20.
5. Reid MD, Osunkoya AO, Siddiqui MT, et al. Accuracy of grading of urothelial carcinoma on urine cytology: an analysis of interobserver and intraobserver agreement. *Int J Clin Exp Pathol*. 2012;5(9):882-891.
6. Raab SS, Grzybicki DM, Vrbin CM, et al. Urine cytology discrepancies: frequency, causes, and outcomes. *Am J Clin Pathol*. 2007;127(6):946-953.
7. Sternberg I, Rona R, Olsfanger S, et al. The clinical significance of class III (suspicious) urine cytology. *Cytopathology*. 2011;22(5):329-333.
8. VandenBussche CJ, Sathiyamoorthy S, Owens CL, et al. The Johns Hopkins Hospital template for urologic cytology samples: parts II and III: improving the predictability of indeterminate results in urinary cytologic samples: an outcomes and cytomorphologic study. *Cancer Cytopathol*. 2013;121(1):21-28.
9. Ton Nu TN, Kassouf W, Ahmadi-Kaliji B, et al. The value of the "suspicious for urothelial carcinoma" cytology category: a correlative study of 4 years including 337 patients. *Cancer Cytopathol*. 2014;122(11):796-803.
10. Muus Ubago J, Mehta V, Wojcik EM, et al. Evaluation of atypical urine cytology progression to malignancy. *Cancer Cytopathol*. 2013;121(7):387-391.
11. Yafi FA, Brimo F, Auger M, et al. Is the performance of urinary cytology as high as reported historically? A contemporary analysis in the detection and surveillance of bladder cancer. *Urol Oncol*. 2014;32(1):27:e1-e6.
12. Li HX, Wang MR, Zhao H, et al. Comparison of fluorescence in situ hybridization, NMP22 bladderchek, and urinary liquid-based cytology in the detection of bladder urothelial carcinoma. *Diagn Cytopathol*. 2013;41(10):852-857.
13. Ramakumar S, Bhuiyan J, Besse JA, et al. Comparison of screening methods in the detection of bladder cancer. *J Urol*. 1999;161(2):388-394.

14. Karakiewicz PI, Benayoun S, Zippe C, et al. Institutional variability in the accuracy of urinary cytology for predicting recurrence of transitional cell carcinoma of the bladder. *BJU Int.* 2006;97(5):997-1001.
15. Messer J, Shariat SF, Brien JC, et al. Urinary cytology has a poor performance for predicting invasive or high-grade upper-tract urothelial carcinoma. *BJU Int.* 2011;108(5): 701-705.
16. Koss LG, Bartels PH, Sychra JJ, et al. Diagnostic cytologic sample profiles in patients with bladder cancer using TICAS system. *Acta Cytol.* 1978;22(5):392-397.
17. Layfield LJ, Elsheikh TM, Fili A, et al. Review of the state of the art and recommendations of the Papanicolaou Society of Cytopathology for urinary cytology procedures and reporting: the Papanicolaou Society of Cytopathology Practice Guidelines Task Force. *Diagn Cytopathol.* 2004;30(1):24-30.
18. Kern WH. The cytology of transitional cell carcinoma of the urinary bladder. *Acta Cytol.* 1975;19(5):420-428.
19. Koss LG, Deitch D, Ramanathan R, et al. Diagnostic value of cytology of voided urine. *Acta Cytol.* 1985;29(5):810-816.
20. Renshaw AA, Gould EW. High-grade urothelial carcinoma with hypochromatic chromatin in urine cytology. *J Am Soc Cytopathol.* 2021;10(1):25-28.
21. Xing J, Monaco SE, Pantanowitz L. Utility of the Paris system for reporting urinary cytology in upper urinary tract specimens. *J Am Soc Cytopathol.* 2018;7(6):311-317.
22. Stern ES, Siddiqui MT. Nuclear hypochromasia: shedding light on the "lightness" of high-grade urothelial carcinoma. *Diagn Cytopathol.* 2021;49(9):1032-1035.
23. Sakuma T, Furuta M, Mimura A, et al. Urine cytology of micropapillary carcinoma of the urinary bladder. *Diagn Cytopathol.* 2011;39(11):852-856.
24. Renshaw AA, Gould EW. High-grade urothelial carcinoma on urine cytology resembling umbrella cells. *Acta Cytol.* 2018;62(1):62-67.
25. Melamed MR, Wolinska WH. On the significance of intracytoplasmic inclusions in the urinary sediment. *Am J Pathol.* 1961;38:711-719.
26. Renshaw AA, Gould EW. High-grade urothelial carcinoma in urine cytology with jet black and smooth or glassy chromatin. *Cancer Cytopathol.* 2018;126(1):64-68.
27. Cowan ML, Rosenthal DL, VandenBussche CJ. Improved risk stratification for patients with high-grade urothelial carcinoma following application of the Paris System for reporting urinary cytology. *Cancer Cytopathol.* 2017;125(6):427-434.
28. Castelino-Prabhu S, Ali SZ. Spermiophages in a giant spermatocele. *Diagn Cytopathol.* 2010;38(11):816-817.
29. Avram E, Yakovlevitz M, Schachter A. Cytologic detection of *Enterobius vermicularis* and *Strongyloides stercoralis* in routine cervicovaginal smears and urocytograms. *Acta Cytol.* 1984;28(4):468-470.
30. Martinez-Giron R, Esteban-Sanchis JG, Doganci L. Parasite eggs in urine cytology: fact or artifact? *Diagn Cytopathol.* 2009;37(5):353-354.
31. VandenBussche CJ, Chandra A, Heymann JJ, et al. Chapter 3. Negative for high-grade urothelial carcinoma (NHGUC). In: Wojcik EM, Kurtycz DFI, Rosenthal DL, eds. *The Paris System for Reporting Urinary Cytology*. 2nd ed. Springer; 2022:21-62.
32. Murphy WM, Soloway MS, Jukkola AF, et al. Urinary cytology and bladder cancer. The cellular features of transitional cell neoplasms. *Cancer.* 1984;53(7):1555-1565.
33. Raab SS, Slagel DD, Jensen CS, et al. Low-grade transitional cell carcinoma of the urinary bladder: application of select cytologic criteria to improve diagnostic accuracy [corrected]. *Mod Pathol.* 1996;9(3):225-232.
34. Raab SS, Lenel JC, Cohen MB. Low grade transitional cell carcinoma of the bladder. Cytologic diagnosis by key features as identified by logistic regression analysis. *Cancer.* 1994;74(5):1621-1626.

35. Renshaw AA, Nappi D, Weinberg DS. Cytology of grade 1 papillary transitional cell carcinoma. A comparison of cytologic, architectural and morphometric criteria in cystoscopically obtained urine. *Acta Cytol.* 1996;40(4):676-682.

36. Renshaw AA. Compassionate conservatism in urinary cytology. *Diagn Cytopathol.* 2000;22(3):137-138.

37. Mai KT, Ball CG, Kos Z, et al. Three-dimensional cell groups with disordered nuclei and cellular discohesion (3DDD) are associated with high sensitivity and specificity for cystoscopic urine cytopathological diagnosis of low-grade urothelial neoplasia. *Diagn Cytopathol.* 2014;42(7):555-563.

38. Hughes JH, Raab SS, Cohen MB. The cytologic diagnosis of low-grade transitional cell carcinoma. *Am J Clin Pathol.* 2000;114(Suppl):S59-S67.

39. Brimo F, Vollmer RT, Case B, et al. Accuracy of urine cytology and the significance of an atypical category. *Am J Clin Pathol.* 2009;132(5):785-793.

40. Renshaw AA. Subclassifying atypical urinary cytology specimens. *Cancer.* 2000;90(4):222-229.

41. Onur I, Rosenthal DL, VandenBussche CJ. Benign-appearing urothelial tissue fragments in noninstrumented voided urine specimens are associated with low rates of urothelial neoplasia. *Cancer Cytopathol.* 2015;123(3):180-185.

42. Allison DB, Lisa Zhang M, Vohra P, VandenBussche CJ. The diagnostic dilemma of urothelial tissue fragments in urinary tract cytology specimens. *Diagnostics.* 2022;12(4):931.

43. Onur I, Rosenthal DL, VandenBussche CJ. Atypical urothelial tissue fragments in noninstrumented voided urine specimens are associated with low but significantly higher rates of urothelial neoplasia than benign-appearing urothelial tissue fragments. *Cancer Cytopathol.* 2015;123(3):186-192.

44. Drachenberg CB, Beskow CO, Cangro CB, et al. Human polyoma virus in renal allograft biopsies: morphological findings and correlation with urine cytology. *Hum Pathol.* 1999;30(8):970-977.

45. Koss LG. On decoy cells. *Acta Cytol.* 2005;49(3):233-234.

46. Owens CL, Ali SZ. Atypical squamous cells in exfoliative urinary cytology: clinicopathologic correlates. *Diagn Cytopathol.* 2005;33(6):394-398.

47. Hattori M, Nishimura Y, Toyonaga M, et al. Cytological significance of abnormal squamous cells in urinary cytology. *Diagn Cytopathol.* 2012;40(9):798-803.

48. Cimino-Mathews A, Ali SZ. The clinicopathologic correlates of cellular atypia in urinary cytology of ileal neobladders. *Acta Cytol.* 2011;55(5):449-454.

49. Deshpande V, McKee GT. Analysis of atypical urine cytology in a tertiary care center. *Cancer.* 2005;105(6):468-475.

50. Highman W, Wilson E. Urine cytology in patients with calculi. *J Clin Pathol.* 1982;35(3):350-356.

51. Melamed M. Urinary sediment cytology in a case of malakoplakia. *Am J Med.* 1962;33(2):471.

52. Sullivan PS, Chan JB, Levin MR, et al. Urine cytology and adjunct markers for detection and surveillance of bladder cancer. *Am J Transl Res.* 2010;2(4):412-440.

53. Pantanowitz L, Otis CN. Cystitis glandularis. *Diagn Cytopathol.* 2008;36(3):181-182.

54. Daniels IR, Bekdash B, Scott HJ, et al. Diagnostic lessons learnt from a series of enterovesical fistulae. *Colorectal Dis.* 2002;4(6):459-462.

55. Piaton E, Decaussin Petrucci M, Mege-Lechevallier F, et al. Diagnostic terminology for urinary cytology reports including the new subcategories 'atypical urothelial cells of undetermined significance' (AUC-US) and 'cannot exclude high grade' (AUC-H). *Cytopathology.* 2014;25(1):27-38.

56. Saieg M, Barkan GA, Brimo F, et al. Risk of high-grade malignancy (ROHM), Chapter 11. In: Wojcik EM, Kurtycz DFI, Rosenthal DL, eds. *The Paris System for Reporting Urinary Cytology.* 2nd ed. Springer; 2022:21-62.

57. Wojcik EM. What should not be reported as atypia in urine cytology. *J Am Soc Cytopathol.* 2015;4(1):30-36.
58. McCroskey Z, Bahar BH, Hu Z, et al. Subclassifying atypia in urine cytology: what are the helpful features? *J Am Soc Cytopathol.* 2015;4(4):183-189.
59. Barasch S, Choi M, Stewart J III, et al. Significance of atypical category in voided urine specimens prepared by liquid-based technology: experience of a single institution. *J Am Soc Cytopathol.* 2014;3(3):118-125.
60. Mokhtar GA, Al-Dousari M, Al-Ghamedi D. Diagnostic significance of atypical category in the voided urine samples: a retrospective study in a tertiary care center. *Urol Ann.* 2010;2(3):100-106.
61. Streeter EH, Turner GDH, McCormick R, et al. The significance of atypical urine cytology in the face of normal investigations–is extended investigation and follow-up required? *Br J Med Surg Urol.* 2008;1(3):131-135.
62. Kapur U, Venkataraman G, Wojcik EM. Diagnostic significance of 'atypia' in instrumented versus voided urine specimens. *Cancer.* 2008;114(4):270-274.
63. Bhatia A, Dey P, Kakkar N, et al. Malignant atypical cell in urine cytology: a diagnostic dilemma. *CytoJournal.* 2006;3:28.
64. Quiroga-Garza G, Nassar D, Khalbuss WE, et al. Vegetable cell contaminants in urinary bladder diversion cytology specimens. *Acta Cytol.* 2012;56(3):271-276.
65. Bardales RH, Pitman MB, Stanley MW, et al. Urine cytology of primary and secondary urinary bladder adenocarcinoma. *Cancer.* 1998;84(6):335-343.
66. Ali SZ, Reuter VE, Zakowski MF. Small cell neuroendocrine carcinoma of the urinary bladder. A clinicopathologic study with emphasis on cytologic features. *Cancer.* 1997;79(2):356-361.
67. Ainechi S, Pambuccian SE, Wojcik EM, et al. Cytomorphologic features and differential diagnosis of neoplasms with small cell features in liquid-based urinary tract cytologic specimens. *J Am Soc Cytopathol.* 2013;4(6):295-306.
68. Krishnan B, Truong LD. Prostatic adenocarcinoma diagnosed by urinary cytology. *Am J Clin Pathol.* 2000;113(1):29-34.
69. Piscioli F, Pusiol T, Scappini P, et al. Urine cytology in the detection of renal adenocarcinoma. *Cancer.* 1985;56(9):2251-2255.
70. Venyo AK-G. Lymphoma of the urinary bladder. *Adv Urol.* 2014;2014:327917.
71. Froehner M, Haase M, Hakenberg OW, et al. Urinary immunocytology for primary bladder B cell lymphoma. *Urology.* 2004;63(2):381-383.
72. Zaharopoulos P. Cytologic manifestations of cystitis follicularis in urine specimens. *Diagn Cytopathol.* 2002;27(4):205-209.
73. Chan L-P, Liu C-M, Ke T-Y. Villous adenoma found in voided urine cytology. *Urol Sci.* 2010;21(4):189-191.
74. Kawaguchi S, Shigehara K, Sasagawa T, et al. Liquid-based urine cytology as a tool for detection of human papillomavirus, *Mycoplasma spp.*, and *Ureaplasma spp.* in men. *J Clin Microbiol.* 2012;50(2):401-406.
75. Khalbuss WE, Hossain M, Elhosseiny A. Primary malignant melanoma of the urinary bladder diagnosed by urine cytology: a case report. *Acta Cytol.* 2001;45(4):631-635.
76. Piva AE, Koss LG. Cytologic diagnosis of metastatic malignant melanoma in urinary sediment. *Acta Cytol.* 1964;8(6):398-402.
77. VandenBussche CJ, Rosenthal DL, Olson MT. Adequacy in voided urine cytology specimens: the role of volume and a repeat void upon predictive values for high-grade urothelial carcinoma. *Cancer Cytopathol.* 2016;124(3):174-180.
78. Rezaee N, Tabatabai ZL, Olson MT. Adequacy of voided urine specimens prepared by ThinPrep and evaluated using The Paris System for Reporting Urinary Cytology. *J Am Soc Cytopathol.* 2017;6(4):155-161.

79. Prather J, Arville B, Chatt G, et al. Evidence-based adequacy criteria for urinary bladder barbotage cytology. *J Am Soc Cytopathol.* 2015;4(2):57-62.

80. Renshaw AA, Gould EW. Evidence-based adequacy criteria for instrumented urine cytology using cytospin preparations. *Diagn Cytopathol.* 2018;46(6):520-521.

81. Yoder BJ, Skacel M, Hedgepeth R, et al. Reflex UroVysion testing of bladder cancer surveillance patients with equivocal or negative urine cytology: a prospective study with focus on the natural history of anticipatory positive findings. *Am J Clin Pathol.* 2007;127(2):295-301.

82. van der Aa MN, Steyerberg EW, Bangma C, et al. Cystoscopy revisited as the gold standard for detecting bladder cancer recurrence: diagnostic review bias in the randomized, prospective CEFUB trial. *J Urol.* 2010;183(1):76-80.

83. Hajdinjak T. UroVysion FISH test for detecting urothelial cancers: meta-analysis of diagnostic accuracy and comparison with urinary cytology testing. *Urol Oncol.* 2008;26(6):646-651.

84. Halling KC, King W, Sokolova IA, et al. A comparison of BTA stat, hemoglobin dipstick, telomerase and Vysis UroVysion assays for the detection of urothelial carcinoma in urine. *J Urol.* 2002;167(5):2001-2006.

85. Bubendorf L, Grilli B, Sauter G, et al. Multiprobe FISH for enhanced detection of bladder cancer in voided urine specimens and bladder washings. *Am J Clin Pathol.* 2001;116(1):79-86.

86. Vlajnic T, Gut A, Savic S, et al. The Paris System for reporting urinary cytology in daily practice with emphasis on ancillary testing by multiprobe FISH. *J Clin Pathol.* 2020;73(2):90-95.

87. Savic S, Zlobec I, Thalmann GN, et al. The prognostic value of cytology and fluorescence in situ hybridization in the follow-up of nonmuscle-invasive bladder cancer after intravesical Bacillus Calmette-Guerin therapy. *Int J Cancer.* 2009;124(12):2899-2904.

88. Mengual L, Marín-Aguilera M, Ribal MJ, et al. Clinical utility of fluorescent in situ hybridization for the surveillance of bladder cancer patients treated with bacillus Calmette-Guerin therapy. *Eur Urol.* 2007;52(3):752-759.

89. Liem EIML, Oddens JR, Vernooij RWM, et al. The role of fluorescence in situ hybridization for predicting recurrence after adjuvant bacillus Calmette-Guerin in patients with intermediate and high risk nonmuscle invasive bladder cancer: a systematic review and meta-analysis of individual patient data. *J Urol.* 2020;203(2):283-291.

90. Bubendorf L, Caraway NP, Fischer AH, et al. Chapter 9. Ancillary studies in urinary cytology. In: Wojcik EM, Kurtycz DFI, Rosenthal DL, eds. *The Paris System for Reporting Urinary Cytology.* 2nd ed. Springer; 2022:21-62.

INDEX

Note: Page numbers followed by "*f*" denote figures; those followed by "*t*" denote tables.

D